COMMUNICATION DISORDERS
Remedial Principles and Practices

CONTRIBUTORS

Walter W. Amster, Veterans Administration Medical Center, Miami, and University of Miami School of Medicine

Gene J. Brutten, Southern Illinois University

Bertha Smith Clark, Bill Wilkerson Hearing and Speech Center, Tennessee State University, and Vanderbilt University

Louis M. Di Carlo, Veterans Administration Hospital, Syracuse

Stanley Dickson, State University College at Buffalo, New York

Marshall Duguay, State University College at Buffalo, New York

Joyce Fitch-West, Veterans Administration Medical Center, New York City; Hunter College of the City University of New York; and Teacher's College, Columbia University

M. N. Hegde, California State University, Fresno, California

Russell J. Love, Bill Wilkerson Hearing and Speech Center and Vanderbilt University

Edgar L. Lowell, John Tracy Clinic and University of Southern California

Freeman E. McConnell, Bill Wilkerson Hearing and Speech Center and Vanderbilt University School of Medicine

Doreen B. Pollack, Porter Memorial Hospital, Denver

James C. Shanks, Indiana University Medical Center

Ronald K. Sommers, Kent State University

Rolland J. Van Hattum, State University College at Buffalo, New York

COMMUNICATION DISORDERS

Remedial Principles and Practices

Second Edition

Stanley Dickson, General Editor
State University College at Buffalo, New York

Scott Foresman and Company   Glenview, Illinois
Dallas, Tex.   Oakland, N.J.   Palo Alto, Calif.
Tucker, Ga.   London, England

Acknowledgments
All credits appear on pages 508–509, which constitute a legal extension of the
copyright page.

Library of Congress Cataloging in Publication Data
Main entry under title:

Communication disorders.

  Bibliography
  Includes index.
  1. Communicative disorders.   I. Dickson, Stanley,
1927-   . [DNLM: 1. Communication. 2. Remedial
teaching. 3. Language disorders—Therapy. 4. Education,
Special. 5. Speech therapy.   WM 475 C7346]
RC423.C643 1984   616.85′5   83–20167
ISBN 0–673–15629–X

1 2 3 4 5 6 – MPC – 88 87 86 85 84 83

This book is dedicated to my wife, Marion, for her insights, under-standing, and assistance throughout my professional careeer. Her tolerance of my shortcomings was only exceeded by her attentiveness and love, without which none of this or any other professional accom-plishment could have been possible.

Preface

Communication Disorders: Remedial Principles and Practices, Second Edition, is intended for students in the field of Communication Disorders and for practicing clinicians. The text presents more than 120 diagnostic tests associated with the various types of communication disorders, and in addition, reviews a variety of remedial techniques, presenting the reader with an overview of the various remedial programs available for the major communication disorders. This presentation is placed within a historical framework to provide a sense of where the field has been, where it is now, and where it may be going in the future. Since no one is an expert in every area, leading experts in each area were asked to write the various chapters of this text; however, continuity has been maintained through the use of an overall editor. In addition, the text is abundantly illustrated—with case studies, charts, graphs, tables, photos, sample sessions, and case history forms. *The major feature of this text is its balanced coverage of the nature of each of the disabilities, the diagnostic-therapeutic continuum, and an overview of the major remedial practices available to work with each of the communication disorders presented.*

Chapter 1 reviews *diagnostic principles and practices* and includes a survey of more than sixty diagnostic tests available to the practicing clinician. In addition, the chapter places the evaluation process in perspective and cross-references subsequent chapters with appropriate commentary.

Chapter 2, by Love, Smith, and McConnell, focuses on *language disorders and remediation* and reviews a variety of available language tests, providing descriptions of and commentary on each test. The chapter categorizes the tests by how each assesses the various parameters of language behavior. In addition, an overview of the following remedial techniques is provided: the Johnson-Myklebust System, the McGinnis Association Method, Kirk and Kirk's Illinois Tests of Psycholinguistic Abilities Approach, the Bloom-Lahey Approach, Interactive Language Development Teaching, the Wiig-Semel Approach to language remediation, Goldman-Lynch's Auditory Program, and Adler's Approach to teaching culturally deprived children.

Chapter 3, on *articulation disorders*, not only reviews the current research on and orientation to the nature of articulation disorders, but also discusses the most up-to-date remedial techniques being used. Sommers describes and critiques each method, and he reviews both the early remedial techniques and some of the most current articulation remediation methods. Reviewed in chapter three are the remedial methods of Scripture; Stinchfield-Hawk and Young; Van Riper; Backus and Beasley; McDonald; Mysak; Winitz; Gerber; Holland and Mathews; Cooper; McReynolds; Costello and Bountress; Ingram; Weiner, Shriberg, and Kwiatkowski; Patrick and Wilcox; and Sommers.

Chapter 4, on *stuttering behavior*, describes current concepts on the nature of stuttering and applies sound learning theory to various aspects of stuttering behavior. Brutten and Hegde offer an informative perspective on the etiology and characteristics of stuttering behavior, and they comment extensively on the major approaches to stuttering remediation. They review practices advocated by such authorities as Johnson, Van Riper, Bloodstein, Wischner, Sheehan, Shames, and Brutten. This overview provides a perspective that cannot be obtained elsewhere.

Chapter 5, by Shanks and Duguay, covers *voice disorders* and has been recognized as an outstanding presentation on the remedial treatment of hypertonic and hypotonic voice disorders. As in the first edition, this chapter gives specific attention to the teaching of alaryngeal speech. In addition, the authors have revised the chapter in order to reflect current thinking and methodology, including discussion of the most recent surgical techniques.

Chapter 6, by Van Hattum, focuses on the *cleft palate* and concentrates on the remedial effort administered from the early speech and language developmental stage through the speech correction period. The text is complete, supplying information on the role of parents in the remedial program as well as the role of the clinical team. The author not only presents the major factors in the cleft palate habilitation program, but also describes clearly the major techniques used to remediate this communication difficulty.

The subject of chapter 7, by Di Carlo and Amster, is *cerebral palsy*. They achieve a balance between a description of the disorder in terms that are meaningful to the neophyte and a discussion of the necessary considerations for effective remediation of this complex problem. They identify the major elements that comprise the cerebral palsy disorder, and at the same time, devote considerable attention to the remediation, including a description of the necessary role of parents in the remedial effort. Reference to the methods of Bobath and Mysak are included.

The wealth of experience and vast knowledge of the literature that West brings to chapter 8, on *aphasia*, makes it essential reading for students of this disorder. She clearly describes the nature of aphasia and gives a thorough overview and review of the major remedial approaches, including the Stimulation Approach, the Programmed Instruction Approach, Melodic Intonation Therapy, Promoting Aphasics Communicative Affectiveness (PACE), Visual Communication Therapy (VIT), Visual Action Therapy (VAT), American-Indian Signing (Amer-Ind), Deblocking, the Preventative Method, and Helm's Elicited Language Program for Syntax Stimulation (HELPSS). Examples from her clinical experience with the Veterans Administration Aphasia Program further enrich the text.

Chapter 9, on *hearing rehabilitation*, offers the joint perspective of an authority on auditory remediation practices (Pollack) and an authority on education of the deaf (Lowell). Thus, this chapter provides students with an understanding of habilitation practices for the hearing impaired with major emphasis on audition and habilitation practices for the deaf with major emphasis on visual training and oralism. The chapter provides an overview of the nature of this disability and a discussion of remedial procedures that highlights the role of parents. Specific attention is given to language learning, the multisensory approach, speech remediation and the general language and speech pattern, and auditory remediation.

For help in reviewing the various chapters of this text, we are grateful to the following specialists: Martin R. Adams, University of Houston; Michael Casby, Michigan State University; Ronald Goldman, University of Alabama in Birmingham; John M. Hutchinson, Idaho State University; Jane E. Jarrow, Ohio State University; Patricia B. Kricos, University of Florida at Gainesville; Michael Rastatter, Bowling

Green State University; and Arthur H. Schwartz, University of Houston. We also wish to acknowledge the contribution of Michael Anderson, Lydia Webster, and Linda Bieze of Scott, Foresman for their valuable assistance with the manuscript.

In summary, the complete text strikes a sensitive balance between description of the nature of each of the communicative disorders presented, the diagnostic-therapeutic continuum, and an overview of a variety of remedial techniques designed to eliminate, circumvent, or minimize the communication difficulty. Throughout the text, use is made of past information and data that is still operative as well as current thinking and methodology. This combination provides a sound basis for additional study and review in the field of communication disorders without sacrificing attention to the remedial effort. Few other texts cover each of these areas as fully as this text does. In the final analysis it is the remedial aspect of our effort that is our *raison d'être*. Our clientele seek assistance from us to remediate their difficulty. To minimize attention to this area is less than appropriate. Similarly, to do justice to this area requires a broad overview of the *variety* of techniques and methods available. *Communication Disorders* attempts to provide that balance which is so difficult to obtain without doing injury to either the understanding of the nature of the disorder or its remediation. We have attempted to provide the reader with a background which is appropriate to make further study more meaningful and effective, thereby resulting in a more effective service to our clientele.

About the Authors

Walter W. Amster is Chief of the Audiology and Speech Pathology Service at the Veterans Administration Medical Center, Miami, Florida, and Adjunct Professor, Department of Otolaryngology, University of Miami School of Medicine. Dr. Amster completed his undergraduate studies at Indiana University, his M.A. at the State University of Iowa, and his Ph.D. at Syracuse University. He is a past president of the Florida Language, Speech, and Hearing Association and was previously affiliated with the United Cerebral Palsy Association of Miami. He is a Fellow of the American Speech-Language-Hearing Association and holds the Association's Certificates of Clinical Competence (CCC).[1]

Gene J. Brutten, Research Professor in the Department of Speech Pathology and Audiology at Southern Illinois University, is a Fellow in the American Speech-Language-Hearing Association and a holder of the CCC in Speech Pathology and Audiology. He obtained his B.A. degree from Kent State University, his M.A. from Brooklyn College, and his Ph.D. from the University of Illinois. He has gained wide recognition for his contributions to the behavioristic theory of stuttering and its remediation, and is the coauthor of a book on the two-factor theory of stuttering.

Bertha Smith Clark is associated with the Mama Lere (Parent-Child) Home of the Bill Wilkerson Hearing and Speech Center in Nashville, Tennessee, and is also Assistant Professor of Speech-Language Pathology and Aural Rehabilitation at Tennessee State University and Vanderbilt University. Specializing in work with children who manifest language disorders, Dr. Clark holds the CCC in Speech Pathology of the American Speech-Language-Hearing Association. She obtained her B.S. degree from Tennessee State University and her M.A. and Ph.D. from George Peabody College for Teachers of Vanderbilt University.

Louis M. Di Carlo, currently Chief of the Audiology and Speech Pathology Service at the Veterans Administration Hospital, Syracuse, New York, has been affiliated with the Department of Audiology and Speech Pathology at Ithaca College. He has received honors from the American Speech-Language-Hearing Association and is a Fellow, a life member, and a holder of the CCC in Speech Pathology and Audiology; in addition, he has been awarded honors from the New York State Speech and Hearing Association. Dr. Di Carlo did his undergraduate work at Union College and work leading to his doctorate at Columbia University. His many research publications attest to his interest in communication disorders related to dysfunctions of the central nervous system. The chapter on cerebral palsy in this book has grown partly out of his work at the Cerebral Palsy Center in Syracuse.

---

[1]See the Appendix for information concerning requirements for the Certificates of Clinical Competence.

Stanley Dickson, Professor of Communication Disorders at the State University College at Buffalo, New York, is a Fellow in the American Speech-Language-Hearing Association and holder of the CCC in Speech Pathology and Audiology. He received his bachelor's and master's degrees from Brooklyn College and his doctorate from the University of Buffalo. Dr. Dickson is a past president of the New York State Speech and Hearing Association. He has published articles on stuttering, language disorders, articulation disorders, hearing disorders, and attitudes toward the handicapped. Recently he has engaged in aerodynamic studies with cleft-palate children.

Marshall Duguay, Professor Communication Disorders at the State University College at Buffalo, received academic degrees leading to and including the Ph.D. from the State University of New York. He is a Fellow in the American Speech-Language-Hearing Association and a holder of the CCC in Speech Pathology. Professor Duguay is particularly active in the area of esophageal speech training and has achieved national recognition for his publications on voice disorders, his lectures throughout the country, and his videotapes on voice remediation.

Joyce Fitch-West, Ph.D., serves as Chief of Speech Pathology and Audiology at the Veterans Administration Medical Center in New York City. She also holds adjunct faculty appointments at Hunter College of the City University of New York, New York University, and Teacher's College, Columbia University. Dr. West's major research and clinical interests are in the field of adult aphasia, but she has had extensive experience working with the right brain-damaged patients as well. She was born and educated in the Midwest, receiving her B.S. degree from Central Michigan University, her M.A. degree from Ohio State University, and her Ph.D. from the University of Michigan. She is a fellow of the American Speech-Language-Hearing Association and holds the CCC in Speech. She has been active in numerous professional organizations.

M. N. Hegde is Professor of Communicative Disorders at California State University, Fresno, California. He is a member of the Association for Advancement of Behavior Therapy and the American Speech-Language-Hearing Association; he also holds the CCC in Speech Pathology. Editorial consultant to the *Journal of Speech and Hearing Disorders*, he is also the author of a textbook entitled *Behavior Therapy* and a frequent contributor to professional journals in the United States and abroad. He has published several papers on fluency and fluency disorders, language, language disorders, and clinical language training. Dr. Hegde obtained his B.A. and M.A. degrees from the University of Mysore, Mysore, India, and his Ph.D. from Southern Illinois University.

Russell J. Love is associated with the Bill Wilkerson Hearing and Speech Center, Nashville, Tennessee, as a consultant and research specialist. He is also Professor of Speech and Language Pathology at Vanderbilt University. Dr. Love received his Ph.D. from Northwestern University. He is a Fellow in the American Speech-Language-Hearing Association and holds the CCC in Speech Pathology. A number of publications attest to his interest in the remediation of language disorders in children.

Edgar L. Lowell has gained international recognition for his efforts in educating the deaf at the John Tracy Clinic, Los Angeles, which he serves as Administrator. In addition, he is Professor of Hearing Rehabilitation at the University of Southern California. Much of the writing for which he is known is associated with his work in educating the deaf and directing remedial activities for the hearing impaired. Dr. Lowell, a Fellow in the American Speech-Language-Hearing Association, was educated at Reed College (B.A.), Wesleyan University (M.A.), and Harvard University (Ph.D).

Freeman E. McConnell is Director Emeritus of the Bill Wilkerson Hearing and Speech Center, Nashville, Tennessee, and Professor Emeritus of Audiology, Division of Hearing and Speech Sciences at Vanderbilt University School of Medicine. The recipient of bachelor's and master's degrees from the University of Illinois, he obtained his Ph.D. from Northwestern University. Dr. McConnell has published widely in his discipline—currently focusing his research activities on language disorders. He has received honors from the American Speech-Language-Hearing Association and is a Fellow and holder of the CCC in Audiology.

Doreen B. Pollack is the Director of Speech and Hearing Services at Porter Memorial Hospital, Denver. Her identification with her area of competence began in England, where she received a diploma from London University and a licentiate from the College of Speech Therapists. The holder of the CCC in Speech Pathology and Audiology in the American Speech-Language-Hearing Association, Mrs. Pollack has written and lectured extensively on auditory techniques for the hearing impaired.

James C. Shanks, Professor and Clinical Director in Speech Pathology at the Indiana University Medical Center, is recognized as an authority on the subject of laryngeal dysfunction as a result of his research and clinical work in the remediation of voice disorders. Educated at Michigan State University (B.A.), the University of Denver (M.A.), and Northwestern University (Ph.D.), Dr. Shanks is a Fellow in the American Speech-Language-Hearing Association and holds the CCC in Speech Pathology.

Ronald K. Sommers has published extensively, particularly in the area of articulation disorders. Editorial consultant to the *Journal of Speech and Hearing Research*, Dr. Sommers is affiliated with Kent State University as Professor in the Division of Speech Pathology and Audiology. He received his B.S. at Kent State before going on to Northwestern for his M.A. and the University of Pittsburgh for his Ph.D. He is a Fellow in the American Speech-Language-Hearing Association and holder of the CCC in Speech Pathology and Audiology.

Rolland J. Van Hattum has served as President of the American Speech-Language-Hearing Association and Vice-President for Education and Scientific Affairs. He has also served on many committees and boards of directors of national and state organizations. His chief interests are cleft-palate speech remediations; speech, language, and hearing services in the schools; and communication problems of the mentally retarded. He has published extensively in a number of periodicals and has edited or authored three textbooks in his major areas of interest. He is Professor of the Communication Disorders Program at the State University College at Buffalo and a Fellow in the American Speech-Language-Hearing Association. He received his B.S. degree at Western Michigan University, his M.S. and Ph.D. at Pennsylvania State University, and holds the CCC in Speech Pathology and Audiology.

Overview

Contents

Chapter 2

LANGUAGE REMEDIATION IN CHILDREN 51

RUSSELL J. LOVE, BERTHA SMITH CLARK, AND
FREEMAN E. McCONNELL

Chapter 3

NATURE AND REMEDIATION OF FUNCTIONAL ARTICULATION AND PHONOLOGICAL DISORDERS   118

RONALD K. SOMMERS

Chapter 4

STUTTERING: A CLINICALLY RELATED OVERVIEW   178

GENE J. BRUTTEN AND M. N. HEGDE

Chapter 5

VOICE REMEDIATION AND THE TEACHING OF ALARYNGEAL SPEECH   240

JAMES C. SHANKS AND MARSHALL DUGUAY

Chapter 6

COMMUNICATION THERAPY FOR PROBLEMS
ASSOCIATED WITH CLEFT PALATE   288

ROLLAND J. VAN HATTUM

Chapter 8

APHASIA REHABILITATION   378

JOYCE FITCH-WEST

Chapter 9

REMEDIAL PRACTICES WITH THE
HEARING IMPAIRED   446

EDGAR L. LOWELL AND DOREEN B. POLLACK

FIGURES AND TABLES

1   Diagnostic Principles and Procedures

Stanley Dickson

In this chapter, we shall review the essential features of language, speech, and hearing disorders, and, by defining and explaining the discrete processes involved in identifying them and assessing their severity, set the stage for the succeeding chapters, whose authors may develop these topics further as a basis for presenting specific remedial principles and practices. The order in which we shall apply the principles of diagnosis to communication problems corresponds with the book's overall organization: language disorders first, followed by articulation disorders, stuttering, voice disorders, and hearing impairment.

Within this general framework, of course, given cases may reflect great variety and considerable overlap both in etiological patterns and in associated speech and language behaviors. This is particularly true of the multiple communication deficits associated with cleft palate, cerebral palsy, hearing impairment, and aphasia, to which separate chapters of this book are devoted. These types of disorders necessitate a combination of evaluative techniques. Cases representative of such broad problem areas figure in more than one discussion in this chapter. Frequent cross-referencing will thus be made to related discussions within and between chapters, a device employed whenever necesssary to link together supplementary discussions and to help the reader form a useful composite of the multifaceted phenomena called communication disorders.

Applied to speech and language behaviors, the diagnostic process may be used to determine whether or not the behaviors are abnormal, the ways in which they are abnormal, and whether the abnormalities are amenable to remediation. Emerick and Hatten (1974) state the purpose of diagnosis is to: (1) determine whether the speech pattern constitutes a handicap, (2) determine the etiology of the problem, and (3) provide therapy focus. Darley (1978) sees the diagnostic process as a five-step procedure: (1) the background—obtaining information about past development and status; (2) the appraisal—the communication problem and related aspects; (3) the diagnosis—the actual problem and causes from a study of information gathered; (4) the therapy plan; and (5) the prognosis. Van Hattum (1981) sees three stages in the diagnostic process: (1) screening, (2) differential diagnosis, and (3) remedial planning. We believe diagnosis encompasses all of these things and prefer to think of the process as a comprehensive procedure designed to determine whether an abnormal condition exists; if so, the nature of the condition and its cause; and, finally, what can be done about it to eliminate, circumvent, or minimize the consequences of the abnormal condition.

The terms *client* and *patient* may identify the person with the problem—the former term being preferred in most situations, unless the communication deficits are related to illness or physical handicap, making the term *patient* appropriate, as in a hospital setting. Somewhat interchangeable use also is made of the terms *clinician* and *diagnostician*, for one and the same person may perform functions denoted by either of these terms at different times. More frequent use is made of *clinician* because of its general applicability, while *diagnostician* refers more specifically to the individual in the performance of a given role. The final set of terms often used interchangeably concern the goal of therapy: *remediation*, *rehabilitation*, or *habilitation* may be used, depending on whether the effort is directed at improving, restoring, or developing adequate speech communication. Again, being the most general, *remediation* is the common choice.

PRINCIPLES OF DIAGNOSIS

Essentially, the diagnostic procedure involves assessing the symptoms of a communication disorder manifested by the client, relating these symptoms to causative factors whenever possible, exploring conditions that may maintain or aggravate the symptoms, and differentiating among disorders or syndromes of speech and language symptoms that may appear confusing upon cursory examination. Usually, in speech-language pathology and audiology, the diagnostic procedure precedes the initiation of the remedial program, for the quality of the latter hinges largely on the effort expended in the diagnosis. The manner in which the clinician proceeds will be indicative of the philosophy of diagnosis.

A Philosophy of Diagnosis

Clinicians have indicated three preferred ways of approaching the diagnostic-therapeutic continuum:

1. carrying on evaluation and remediation at the same time, viewing the program as one entailing ongoing diagnostic-therapeutic sessions;
2. completing the evaluation before initiating the remedial program; and
3. varying the diagnostic-therapeutic approach according to the type of communication problem presented, using the first for problems of differential diagnosis, for example, and the second for problems amenable to the sequential approach.

Procedure (2), completing the evaluation before initiating the remedial program, is probably used by most clinicians, for most cases, and it is our choice whenever applicable.

Rees (1978) and Emerick and Hatten (1974) differentiate between the medical model utilized in the diagnostic process and the educational model. The medical model is closely associated with discovering a category of pathology and the etiology. The second diagnostic procedure described above is usually applied when using this model. The educational model is primarily associated with identifying areas of communicative behavior that are defective and are descriptive in nature. This model is less concerned with etiology and pathology and has as a major focus remediation programs and their effects. Emerick and Hatten (1974) also describe the psychiatric model and the operant or behavioral model. These models stress adaptive behavior.

We are particularly impressed by the diagnostic philosophy, consistent with current scientific thinking and methodology, suggested by Schultz (1973). It is his view that the evaluation procedure is one in which hypotheses regarding the causes of the communication disorder are tested. Each observation by the clinician serves to alter the probability of each hypothesis until one alone stands out as the most probably correct. Therefore, the inductive-deductive procedure of stating a hypothesis, accumulating information from a variety of sources (tests, case studies, observation, other reports, etc.), evaluating this information, accepting or rejecting the hypothesis, and making appropriate recommendations, is an effective technique for assessing communication disorders, and it provides data directly relevant to the therapy program. Too often, failures in therapy occur because the diagnosis was incorrect or incomplete, and such defects of judgment can be obviated by collecting as much relevant information as possible. The more evidence there is for a diagnostic judgment, the greater the chance that judgment is correct and the greater the probability of a successful remedial effort.

In a somewhat similar vein, Ringel (1972) has suggested that the diagnostic procedure be approached much like a research project, as a questioning activity in which the clinician engages in all of the various analytical processes that help evaluate the disorder. Throughout the procedure the clinician should function as a listener and a collator of information who provides insights that other professionals are not likely to have. At times, the symptoms of communication difficulty are quite apparent and can be assessed with little effort, but some clients may have far more numerous or complex symptoms, with obscure and elusive causes. A differential diagnostic effort, which requires lengthy evaluation and study, is then necessary. However, the procedure should be only as extensive as necessary to obtain germane information.

Peterson and Marquardt (1981) emphasize the need to be descriptive. They point out that the diagnosis is a function of the descriptions collected, all of which may not have been quantifiable. As Rees (1978) has pointed out, there is no clear statement of unifying principles of diagnostic approaches in communication disorders. The personal preferences and predilections of the diagnostician, whether the model used be medical or educational, will determine the diagnostic protocol established. We have often observed that the planned remedial program is not a function of whether the approach is essentially medical or educational. It is rather dependent upon the experience and skill of the diagnostician. Suffice it to say our preference leans toward the medical model. It should be noted, however, that the remedial program does not invariably depend upon a specific, causal diagnosis. The full determination of the cause of a disorder may be impossible, and it clearly is not always essential. Often, diagnosis can be no more than a description of the symptoms presented by the client, but therapy does consist of treating symptoms, and the clinician must proceed with therapy techniques. An example can be found among some developmental language disorders. The causal factors may be unknown, but the clinician can treat these disorders successfully because people can and do modify their behavior.

Peterson and Marquardt (1981) characterize the diagnostic process as scientific when the process follows research organization by (1) defining the problem, (2) developing a hypothesis, (3) developing a procedure to test the hypothesis, (4) collecting the data, (5) analyzing the data, and (6) supporting or rejecting the hypothesis.

The Elements of Diagnosis

Diagnosis of a speech or communication disorder involves a number of fairly discrete procedures. The diagnostician must accumulate pertinent data, including information about prior assessments and attempts at remediation, in a case study; assess the symptom complex through testing and observation; relate the speech and language differences to etiological factors in order to achieve the best possible explanation for the atypical behavior when possible, and make a statement concerning the prognosis for improvement; and, finally, outline techniques and treatments to be included in a remedial program, where one is indicated.

The Case Study. The case study, a major part of the diagnostic procedure, is a questioning process aimed at getting information about the disorder from the client or a responsible person who is able to answer for him or her. Areas of inquiry include the client's birth, growth, development, and educational history; medical, psychological, and social history; and speech, language, and hearing ability. The resulting data should provide the clinician with a description of the symptoms, should suggest possible causes of the symptoms as well as factors that may have a bearing on them, and should assist in estimating what the client's communication abilities are likely to be with or without therapy. Before beginning the interview, the clinician should always advise the client (or the person who is to supply the case history information) that the information disclosed will be held confidential.

Darley (1978) includes a basic case history outline specifying (1) the complaint, (2) individual or agency referral source, (3) history of the speech problem, (4) developmental history, (5) medical history, (6) school history, (7) social history, (8) family history, and (9) comments on the interview that are deemed important.

A case history form (see figure 1-1) is a useful tool for assembling the data in an orderly and complete way. Such a form should have spaces for all of the important information to be obtained, with specific attention focused upon how the client perceives the problem and what he or she thinks should be done about it. While extremely useful as a guide to exploration, the form should not be rigidly adhered to. The clinician should try to conduct a spontaneous and insightful interview, and should adapt the questions to the client's educational, social, and communicational levels. If the nature of the communication difficulty is known, e.g., articulatory, phonatory, stuttering, etc., a case study form specifically designed to explore the specific impairment may be useful.

When completed, the case history may indicate that certain areas deserve additional investigation by other specialists. For example, often a client will report behaviors that suggest central nervous system impairment. If the client is a child, the clinician may then ask the parent to have this possibility checked with a neurologist or the family physician. If mental deficiency is suspected, reports from a psychologist may be desirable. Such reports may, in fact, already be available, but frequently the speech clinician may be the first professional person to see the child. In any event the

Figure 1–1. Example of a Case History Form. The general information section in this form can be used with the specific case history forms that follow.

Examiner _____

Supervisor _____

Name _____ Date _____

Address _____ Phone _____

      (Street)   (City)   (Zone)

Date of Birth _____ Age _____ Sex _____

Parent or Guardian _____ Occupation _____

School _____ Grade _____ Principal's Name _____

Referred by _____ Referred to _____

Family Doctor _____ Siblings _____

Diagnosis _____ Prognosis _____

Parents' concept of speech problem: _____

_____

I. HEALTH HISTORY

A. BIRTH HISTORY   COMMENTS
Term baby _____

Delivery _____

Difficulties at birth _____

    "   shortly after _____

Mother's age at birth _____

Mother's health (pregnancy) _____

Rh factors _____

Cyanosis _____

Jaundice _____

B. DEVELOPMENTAL HISTORY   COMMENTS
Sat up _____

Crawled _____

Walked _____

Talked _____

Toilet trained _____

Sucking _____

Swallowing _____

Chewing _____

C. ILLNESSES   COMMENTS (Fever, etc.)
Measles _____

Mumps _____

Scarlet fever _____

Chicken pox _____

Whooping cough _____

Convulsion _____   DOCTOR:

D. OPERATIONS   COMMENTS
Cleft palate _____

T and A _____

Other _____

E. HEALTH AT PRESENT TIME   COMMENTS
Handicaps (dental, visual, hearing, etc.)

II. SOCIAL HISTORY

A. ENVIRONMENTAL ADJUSTMENT
1. Parents' attitude (to speech, behavior) _____
2. Family relationship _____
3. Discipline of child:
   who _____
   how _____
   most effective _____
4. Tensions in the home _____
5. Behavior problems:

Tantrums _____	Enuresis _____
Nervousness _____	Sleeplessness _____
Shyness _____	Nightmares _____
Rejection _____	Strange persistent fears _____
Aggression _____	Thumb sucking _____
Extreme jealousy _____	Talking in sleep _____
Extreme possessiveness (people, objects) _____	Crying in sleep _____

6. Child reflects:
   Stable adjustment _____
   Insecurity _____
   Excessive tension _____
   Overprotection _____
   General maladjustment _____
   Examiner's impression:
   _____
   _____

COMMENTS

B. SCHOOL ADJUSTMENT AND ACHIEVEMENT

III. PSYCHOMETRIC EVALUATION   COMMENTS

Impression of IQ _____
Tests administered

_____
M.A. _____
C.A. _____
IQ _____

IV. SPEECH HISTORY   COMMENTS
A. PRESENT PROBLEM
Regressing _____
Improving _____
Parents' impression of speech problem
1. Severe _____
2. Moderate _____
How do you help him? _____
_____

B. SPEECH DEVELOPMENT
1. Onset of speech (date and words) _____
   (phrases) _____
2. Factors affecting speech: (bilingualism) _____
   (others) _____
3. Vocabulary (how many words) _____
4. Comprehension _____

5. Speech & hearing problems in family _____

6. Handedness: (client) _____ (siblings) _____

C. SPEECH EXAMINATION (Artic., Voice, Rhythm, Rate)

1. Phonetic analysis: (Artic. Test attached) _____

_____

_____

2. Hearing tests: _____

_____

3. Physical exam:
    Teeth _____
    Palate _____
    Lips _____
    Tongue _____
    Tonsils _____
    Nose _____
    Pharynx _____
    Velum _____

4. Other tests administered: (Voice, Rhythm, Phonetic Discrimination, Auditory Memory)

_____

5. If delayed development:
    What attempt to communicate?
    Jargon _____
    Gestures _____
    Babbling _____
    Eye contact _____

Impression of present speech _____

_____

_____

V. SUMMARY

    DIAGNOSIS

    PROGNOSIS

    COMMENTS

VI. RECOMMENDATIONS

VII. PROCEDURES INITIATED (Dates)

clinician should be prepared to recommend what seems to be the appropriate course of action.

Emerick and Hatten (1974) discuss eleven errors that beginning interviewers may make that should be avoided. Among those are: asking questions that may be answered simply by a yes or no response; talking too much; asking questions that do not permit freedom of response; making negativistic or moralistic responses; asking questions that do not permit the interviewee to express feelings and attitudes; making aimless or insignificant responses that tend to wander into areas of little or no significance; and trusting to memory instead of recording all pertinent responses. Emerick and Hatten (1974) also review a number of things the interviewer can do to improve interviewing skills (pp. 40–41). Hutchinson et al. (1979) admonish the interviewer to control reactions to all types of behaviors and attitudes. An accepting interviewer who possesses good listening skills, instills confidence, and develops good rapport will often obtain the most significant information. A perceptive, attentive, and skilled interviewer will obtain all important information.

Assessment of the Symptoms. The symptom complex revealed in the case study should be assessed wherever possible by objective and semiobjective tests, observation of behavior during assigned tasks, and spontaneous communication. The clinician should also assess whatever information from other sources might help explain the symptoms and, in particular, should not ignore previous diagnoses and attempts at treatment, for they may reveal related problems which may need to be considered for a more effective program.

Objective and Semiobjective Instruments. The term *objective instrument* refers to a test requiring specific responses to presented tasks whose validity and reliability have been demonstrated and for which there are established norms. Three questions can be asked in an effort to determine whether a test meets the necessary criteria:

1. To what extent does the test measure what it purports to measure? Does it do the job it is intended to do? If so, the test has validity.
2. Is the test consistent in measuring whatever it measures? Then it has reliability.
3. Can the test's results be evaluated in relation to the test performance of a specific appropriate comparison group? Then it meets the need for a standardization of norms.

As an example, when giving a child an auditory discrimination test the clinician wants to be sure that the procedures actually do test the child's auditory discrimination ability, so that the test is *valid*. The test is therefore planned to give the child an opportunity to discriminate all of the standard English sounds in their various positions in words. If the child were given the test on two different days, or by two different people, the same results should be obtained; the test should be *reliable*. The test is *standardized* by giving it to many children in the same age group so that any one score can be compared to an average, or norm, to reveal the degree to which the obtained score deviates from the norm.

Emerick and Hatten (1974) list a number of factors to consider when selecting a test. In addition to the factors mentioned above, they include specific characteristics of the tests that make for ease of administration, scoring, and interpretation. Hutchinson, Hanson, and Mecham (1979) suggest a positive correlation between objectivity, sensitivity, reliability, and validity of a test and its use and the need for precision and accountability. The greater the need for precision and accountability, the greater the need for objectivity, sensitivity, reliability, and validity. There are many tests which, while unable to be statistically evaluated, do produce valuable and clinically appropriate measurements. Some of these tests have demonstrated reliability but must rely for their effectiveness on the education and training of the speech clinician using them. An example may be found in the technique of reviewing X-ray films to evaluate the anatomical and functional competence of cleft-palate children. The value of judgments concerning the objective features of such films hinges upon the ability of the clinician to interpret what is seen.

Many tests are available for assessing speech, language, and related behaviors for which we have little or no information regarding their validity, reliability, or standardization data. Frequently, students or new clinicians will assume, in the absence of such information, that the test is not valid or is unreliable. Actually, if no such information is available, then the test may or may not be valid or reliable. Students frequently assume that if validity and reliability data is available, then the test is valid and reliable. Again the assumption may or may not be accurate. A review of how validity, reliability, and standardization data was obtained is appropriate. It may well be that the manner in which such data was gathered leaves much to be desired. Sample size may be small; statistical techniques used may be less than satisfactory; and other limitations may be apparent when the data is examined. Darley (1974) and Buros (Mental Measurement Yearbook) review many tests, and their ideas may be helpful to the beginning student in that regard.

Observation and Selected Tasks. When there is no standardized test to assess an apparently objective and atypical parameter of behavior, the speech clinician can use any of several techniques for eliciting responses related to the behavior in question. To assess language comprehension, for instance, the clinician may direct the client to perform specific tasks such as "turn off the light" or "open the curtains." Failure to respond to directions may suggest an impairment of language comprehension or memory.

It is important to note that the tasks that will provide material for informal observation should be chosen carefully. They should not be taken haphazardly from standard batteries of tests, such as the Stanford-Binet or the Illinois Test of Psycholinguistic Abilities, in which each item is meant to contribute to an evaluation of the subject's global performance. Taken out of context, the results of any one or several such tasks may be extremely misleading.

More often than not, the speech clinician's appraisal of speech and language disorders consists of empirical observation of self-evident conditions. As Van Riper has remarked, such a problem as stuttering, nasality, or lisping is a problem because it "calls attention to itself, interferes with communication, or causes its possessor to be maladjusted" (1972, p. 29). An experienced, astute observer can often identify aberrant behaviors, overlooked by the young clinician, which may be of significant importance in planning the remedial program.

Hypothesis and Prognosis. From an examination of the data gathered in the case history, and from objective tests and informal observations, the clinician may tentatively or conclusively identify the speech disorder and its causes by eliminating unsupported hypotheses, as Shultz (1973) has suggested. At this time, too, the clinician should make some statement of the prognosis for improvement, based both upon the data accumulated during the diagnostic interview and upon the impressions obtained. While it may be difficult to predict the results of treating some cases, optimism is justified with many. The clinician should not, however, engage in therapy knowing that it will be ineffective, unless the treatment is experimental and clearly defined as such.

The prognosis should be reached by applying specific criteria to the data collected in the diagnostic procedure. Its accuracy will depend upon the experience of the examiner, the age of the client, and the cause of the disorder, but because it will involve learning, or the deliberate modification of behavior, it will also depend upon the client's intelligence and motivations.

The prognosis should be phrased in terms of the probability that the client will respond favorably to the suggested remedial program. Such statements as "The prognosis for language recovery is favorable" (or "guarded" or "poor") are often used. The failure of a client to respond to the remedial treatment despite a favorable prognosis should suggest that the diagnosis was not correct, that the diagnostic data upon which the prognosis was based were not complete, or that the remedial techniques applied to the case were not well chosen.

Recommendations for a Remedial Program. A properly designed remedial program, based on careful study of the client's symptoms and their causes, should eliminate, circumvent, alleviate, or minimize the effects of the disorder on the client. It should address itself to those factors whose adverse effects on the client's communication skills were disclosed during the diagnostic procedure, and it should take advantage of any specific learning procedures that may have been suggested by positive responses to any of the diagnostic tests. These targets and suggestions should be carefully recorded by the diagnostician, usually in a part of the diagnostic report titled "Recommendations." Such data can be especially valuable to another clinician who may have responsibility for the remedial program.

A recommendation frequently noted in diagnostic reports is that the problem be given further study by a person in a related specialty, such as a psychiatrist, maxillofacial surgeon, or neurologist. When such consultation services are obtained, the diagnostician should be sure to add the information so provided, together with interpretations and recommendations, to the existing battery of diagnostic data. Such information may be very relevant to the remedial program. But the diagnostician should not, even when they are obviously indicated, make medical decisions on recommendations; these are best left to the physician and parents.

Other recommendations noted in the diagnostic report usually pertain specifically to the remedial program, and should, together with the specific diagnosis, serve as a guide for the development of treatment procedures. West (chap. 8) and Van Hattum (chap. 6) discuss descriptive therapy based upon an evaluation of the symptom complex. What the clinician does in remediation is directly related to the data obtained and conclusions reached after the diagnostic review.

The clinician in charge of the remedial program will usually have the responsibility of evaluating the client's progress, but occasionally the diagnostician will see the client again to assess the client's gains. If the gains are less than expected, the clinician should look for the factors impeding the program, perform further diagnostic procedures, or suggest that the remedial techniques be modified. Diagnostic judgments and planned remedial programs should never be so dogmatic that new information cannot be considered. They should always be aimed at making the client's communicative abilities more acceptable, both personally and to other people.

Case Examples. Before we begin to discuss the diagnostic approaches appropriate to the various communication disorders discussed in this book, it may be useful to present two cases exemplifying different types of speech and language difficulties. The descriptions, evaluations, and recommendations associated with these cases will illustrate the kinds of difficulties confronting a client and a clinician. Problems in each require differential diagnosis; one case involves diagnostic appraisal of a child with delayed language, and the other, an ongoing diagnostic-therapeutic process for a child with an articulation problem.

Case 1

Albert, age four to six, was seen for a speech and hearing evaluation at the Speech and Hearing Clinic upon referral by the nurse at the County Public Health Clinic.

According to his mother, Albert's gestational and neonatal history had been clinically uneventful. He had walked without support at nine and one-half months, used his first meaningful words at fifteen months, and was toilet-trained by twenty-three months. He had had none of the childhood diseases and no operations. His only illness had been a streptococcus throat infection at six months, with a very high fever and, according to his mother, two or three febrile convulsions. His mother described his present health as good and said the home situation was reasonably free of tension. Both parents generally disciplined their children by "taking away . . . treats." Albert occasionally had temper tantrums and had shown that he could be affected by his own "word magic," that is, when he made up stories about ghosts, he would sometimes have subsequent nightmares. This evidence of hypersensitivity was strengthened by reported nervousness, possessiveness, and jealousy. These traits appeared to be brought out by criticism of Albert's speech by peers and adults.

In contrast to the mother's judgment of Albert's state of adjustment, the clinician found him to be a very cooperative child who adjusted readily to a new situation.

An evaluation of Albert's fine and gross motor adaptive function (using the Oseretsky Tests of Motor Proficiency) showed that he performed at a level about one year below that expected for his age. He could complete the simple motor tasks used for the evaluation successfully, but not the more complex ones. His failure to complete some of the tasks geared to four-year-old abilities suggested some delay in motor development.

Hearing sensitivity, evaluated by pure-tone air-conduction threshold testing, was judged to fall within normal limits. The Illinois Test of Psycholinguistic Abilities indicated that on another aspect of auditory function—auditory-vocal sequential ability—he was essentially normal, but that language ability was about one year below the norm for his age—test items for receptive and expressive language development (encoding and decoding) showed him functioning at approximately a three-and-one-half-year-old's level. In summary, the ITPA revealed that Albert was somewhat below average in visual motor tasks and verbal expression although his auditory reception and association responses were essentially normal; he did not use plurals, the future tense, or pronouns correctly; he did not give his last name; he could not complete most "opposite analogies"; and he showed generally poor expressive language usage.

On the Peabody Picture Vocabulary Test, used to evaluate vocabulary recognition ability, Albert earned a language age of three to five, which was consistent with the degree of language lag indicated by the ITPA results and suggested that Albert might accurately be viewed as a slow learner.

Albert's connected speech was not very intelligible; he was judged to be understandable on only about 25 percent of his spontaneous utterances. When the Hejna Test was used to assess his word articulation ability, he was found to articulate the /h/ sound consistently well, but to make substitution or omission errors on all other consonants tested. Errors occurred in as many as two positions within words on the consonants /p/, /b/, /m/, and /w/—that is, in four out of the five consonants normally mastered by the age of three and one-half. Omission errors were almost always associated in the sounds in the final position; and for the most part /h/ and /b/ were the sounds used in errors of substitution. Two-element blends, such as /gl/, tended to be articulated as one, such as /g/. In general, Albert's articulatory repertoire was very limited; he had not yet achieved a three-year-old's level of development, though he did appear to be stimulable for improvement on /p/, /b/, and /k/.

An evaluation of the appearance and function of the peripheral oral structures showed that Albert's dental occlusion and bite were normal, the hard palate was normal in height and width, and the soft palate moved well on phonation; there was no indication of sucking, swallowing, or chewing difficulty, and spontaneous smiling was noted; yet he had poor control of his lip and tongue movements, being unable to imitate elevation of the tongue to the hard palate and movement of the tongue from one corner of the lips to the other. These manifestations of dysfunction, together with his inability to pucker his lips on command, suggested an oral dyspraxia.

The Stanford-Binet Test, form L-M, was administered by a psychologist at the Child Study Center. The results revealed an intelligence quotient of 87, placing him in the dull normal range, but it was felt that his poor verbal facility may have penalized him on the verbal items of the scale, and therefore the score may have been an underestimate of his intellectual potential.

At its conclusion, the diagnostic appraisal had led to a delineation of the nature of Albert's speech and language difficulty and an awareness of possible etiological factors. The consistent lag of about a year in Albert's language and nonlanguage functions warranted the impression of delayed speech. His poor oral motor control and inability to initiate certain movements of the articulators suggested the presence of an oral dyspraxia. The "febrile convulsions," or seizures, mentioned by his mother were possibly related to some central nervous system dysfunction.

In view of the stimulability observed, however, the prognosis seemed good for improvement. Accordingly, it was recommended that Albert be given speech therapy for two half-hour sessions a week. The immediate goals would center around improvement in intelligibility. In addition, the consonants would be systematically taught in their developmental sequence. It was also suggested that a neurological evaluation of the child through a referral by the family physician would be advisable, and that within the next year there might be a need to consider educational planning.

Discussion of the Diagnostic Procedure. Our case study of Albert revealed little of clinical significance—other than his early febrile convulsions and his hypersensitive behavior. The test results showed a delay of about a year in language behavior and a year and a half in articulation growth. His average performance on some scales of the language test but poor performance on other scales suggested that his articulation problems might be interfering with his performance of tasks requiring expressive language use.

Albert's poor performance on tasks involving the function of the articulatory musculature, together with the results of the Hejna Test, suggested that his communication difficulty was an oral apraxia (articulation errors due to central nervous system impairment). There was no oral paralysis or oral reflexive difficulty, but an impaired capacity to control the oral musculature and the sequencing of muscle movements for the production of phonemes. There was thus a strong possibility that brain damage was a causative factor of Albert's overall communication problem.

Subsequent remedial efforts were designed to reduce and circumvent the effects of the oral apraxia and promote Albert's personal growth and development, and they seemed to result in his relatively prompt acquisition of intelligible speech. After a year of speech and language remediation, his communication had improved greatly. He was readily intelligible, and his score on the Peabody Picture Vocabulary Test was within average limits. A number of articulation errors still remained, but were expected to respond to future remedial efforts.

Case 2

Matthew, a male of average appearance, was first seen at the speech clinic when he was three years and three months old. He had been referred by a local Hearing and Speech Center for diagnostic speech and language therapy.

During the first interview at the college clinic, no formal testing was done. Matthew was observed in a play situation with his sister and during the interview with his parents, and he appeared to be a healthy, normal, active three-year-old with incomprehensible speech. His language abilities appeared more than adequate; he was interested, alert, talkative, and played very well. His behavior was purposeful, his attention span good.

All of the consonant sounds appeared severely distorted. There was considerable hypernasality, and the grimaces that ordinarily accompany difficulty in building up oral pressure were beginning to appear. Matthew also appeared to have a prognathic mandible.

A résumé of the report sent from the Hearing and Speech Center revealed no abnormalities in the areas of birth history, family problems, genetic development, medical history, and social behavior. Matthew was the fifth of six children and he lived on a farm, although his father was employed in industry. His mother was a competent and gracious person, very eager to do her best for all her children.

In the area of speech and orofacial activities, the mother reported that Matthew's speech originally consisted of grunting and nasal sounds and that he had had difficulty in suckling after birth and in chewing and swallowing food later, suggesting some abnormality of the velopharyngeal mechanism. His use of language developed rapidly in his third year, but although his speech remained quite incomprehensible to outsiders, the family itself had no difficulty in understanding him.

Hearing acuity was reported as normal and appeared to be so during the first interview. The reports of articulation testing revealed poor speech intelligibility, with most consonant and vowel sounds distorted, and gross and imprecise articulatory movements. Matthew was able to produce /b/, /k/, /g/, and /w/ in isolation, but was unable even to approximate any of the other sounds. There was also a pervasive use of glottal stops and a consistently hypernasal voice quality.

Although Matthew refused to cooperate in test situations for any length of time, informal observations indicated that his language, perceptual, visual, and motor functioning and motor behavior were normal. He was reluctant to leave his parents, as are many three-year-olds.

At the end of the first session, it was suggested to the parents that therapy might be delayed in order to allow Matthew to mature, though he would be kept on an active evaluation status. The family, particularly the mother, found this suggestion helpful, for the family was large and it would have been difficult for the mother to bring the child to the clinic regularly at this time.

Because the observations of hypernasality and difficulties in suckling, chewing, and swallowing were felt to be significant, and because Matthew's frenulum had had to be clipped a few days after birth, the final suggestion was made that his velopharyngeal competence would have to be assessed by a competent orofacial surgeon at some later date.

One year after Matthew was seen at the college clinic, he was recalled for a reevaluation. At this time his articulation was still severely distorted and there was severe hypernasality. Unable to achieve oral pressure on the consonant sounds, Matthew was substituting marked distortions, glottal stops, and nasally emitted fricatives and sibilants. There had been considerable growth in language, however, and Matthew talked away at great length, experiencing no difficulty communicating with his mother and sister. He still clung to his mother and acted quite spoiled when an attempt was made to assess his speech formally, but it was possible, using his older sister as a model, to examine his production of some sounds such as the /g/ and /s/ in isolation. These were very clear and it appeared that there was good velopharyngeal function in these instances.

The mother still complained of Matthew's disturbed chewing behavior, saying, "He doesn't chew; he mushes his food." Again, the question of orofacial neurological dysfunction arose related to the velopharyngeal dysfunction and the difficulty in suckling at birth. The tendency toward a prognathic mandible was more marked than it had been previously.

At this time an evaluation was made of the orofacial structures. Chewing was disturbed, as was velopharyngeal competency during speech. Although the velum appeared long, flexible, and mobile, the child's nasality and his inability to build up intraoral pressure suggested either a functional or an organic difficulty.

The mother was advised to attempt to place Matthew in a kindergarten. He appeared eager and ready for the additional stimulation, and it seemed time that he learned to relate to a larger group than the family on the farm. Since Matthew's father was on strike and the family was experiencing some anxiety at home, no other recommendations were made.

A month later Matthew was brought back to the clinic for a reevaluation. The mother was delighted with Matthew's response to kindergarten, although the well-meaning teacher had at first tried to correct Matthew's speech. When the mother suggested that since the clinic was watching Matthew's speech very closely, the teacher should refrain from teaching him to say his sounds, the teacher agreed and had been very cooperative.

An additional problem at kindergarten was a social one. Matthew was experiencing difficulty in making himself understood and also in his relationships with his peers. Also, the new language he acquired in connection with his new experiences made it difficult for his family to understand him. The tension at home caused by worry over the father's job had cleared up, only to be replaced by tension related to Matthew's disordered speech. Consequently, definite action was recommended, namely, that Matthew be taken to the family physician to be referred to an orofacial surgeon for an assessment, not only of the velopharyngeal mechanism, but also of the oral physiology as it related to sucking, chewing, and swallowing. Matthew's mother readily agreed and, at the end of the interview, expressed concern about Matthew's intelligence and hearing. She was again counseled that both appeared to be within average limits. She promised to call back as soon as the appointments were made, and a few days later she reported that Matthew had an appointment to see the orofacial surgeon at the university clinic.

Discussion of the Diagnostic Procedure. Most of the information we obtained about Matthew had to be gained through casual, informal, but sophisticated observations of his behavior. Such a situation is not unusual, for the clinician must often "play it by ear" and be able to fit the pieces of diagnostic information together through careful observation and interpretation. In the case of Matthew, the parent was very cooperative though the child was not. The boy's willingness to enter into a situation already shared by his sister and the ease with which he could enter into a play situation with another child, however, made the evaluation easier. At the same time, we remembered that Matthew was only one part of a family and that other people had to be considered in our recommendations.

Support for the family was an important aspect of our overall approach. While we did not minimize Matthew's problems, we did not maximize them either. We reassured the parents and allayed their fears.

When the time came to find a kindergarten for Matthew, we made recommendations as to why Matthew should be accepted in the situation, and, on the basis of our recommendations, the school did place him.

In the referral to the family physician, the mother was again given support. We clearly stipulated what we wished from the family physician, and this worked out to everybody's satisfaction. Finally, we assured the mother that after Matthew was seen by the oral surgeon, we would confer with her about his findings.

This case points up the need to see the whole child. To be flexible, approachable, and pragmatic in the use of methods—but more than that, to understand, to be humane—is an integral part of the diagnostic-remedial process.

APPLICATION OF DIAGNOSTIC PROCEDURES

The later chapters of this book will go into some detail concerning the diagnosis of particular communication disorders, but a few words should be said first about how the case history, objective and semiobjective instruments, and observations and selected tasks may be advantageously used in the initial diagnosis of the various kinds of problems. The brief discussions below represent attempts to generalize from the specific disorders to the larger problem of *diagnosis* which all speech clinicians, whatever their specialty or orientation, must share. Combined with the fuller treatment of individual topics in subsequent chapters, these discussions should provide the reader with a more comprehensive and subtle understanding of the principles and practices of diagnosing communication disorders.

We shall take up language disorders first, because of their basic nature and broad range, as well as their close relationship with all of the other communication problems. We shall then consider articulation disorders, perhaps the most pervasive of all communication problems, and stuttering, followed by the phonatory disorders, and hearing impairment. Each of these topics, however, does not correspond to a single one of the later chapters in this book, for material relevant to each of them may be found in more than one chapter.

Diagnostic Procedures for Language Disorders

Language behavior is a "structured system of arbitrary vocal sounds and sequences of sounds that is used in interpersonal communication and which rather exhaustively catalogues the things, events, and processes of human communication" (Carroll, 1961). This definition, while providing a key to normal language function, gives no clue to the nature of language disorders. For that, it is necessary to consider Bangs' (1968) definition of language disordered children as those who do not follow an orderly pattern or sequence in learning the language code, as well as the division of language-disordered clients into three groups, as suggested by West and Ansberry (1968). The three groups are:

1. Those children, like Albert in the first of the case studies above, who do not seem to be developing language normally. Love, Clark, and McConnell, in chapter 2 of this book, have subdivided this group further into the hearing impaired, neurologically impaired, environmentally deprived, and those with idiopathic etiology.
2. Those mature adults who have developed language, have functioned successfully, and have, through some traumatic insult, suffered a disturbance of the language function. The disorder may be related to central nervous system dysfunction or dysphasia.
3. Those aged individuals in whom the anatomical structures subserving the language function are degenerating and for whom the abilities to learn, remember, and speak are rapidly disappearing. The anatomical bases of their problems may be the same as for the other two groups.

Darley (1978) differentiates between the developmentally delayed language disorders and the acquired language dysfunctions. He states that mental retardation is the most common of the delayed language disorders, which include those who have a significant hearing loss, autistic children, and children who have language delay in the absence of an organic or emotional disorder "disproportionate to their other cognitive abilities" (p. 481). Among those with acquired language dysfunction, Darley includes aphasia, those with "confused language," dementia, akinetic mutism, and emotional disturbance.

Language disorders may take the form of difficulty with receptive language—the ability to understand what is heard or read—or with expressive language—the ability to communicate orally or graphically (in writing)—or with both. In addition, language disorders may be classified in relation to the three areas of language development, namely, into phonemic, syntactic, and semantic disorders. As Bangs (1968) has remarked, language disorders in children are concerned with "a child's inability to comprehend the meaning of single words and connected discourse, and/or his faulty application of semantics and the syntactic and morphologic rules in his oral output" (p. 13). That the adult may have very similar problems is indicated by West in chapter 8 of this book.

Because remedial efforts require a thorough linguistic evaluation of language ability and disability, diagnostic procedures for persons with language disorders should include a general evaluation of their receptive and expressive language abilities and a specific assessment of the semantic, syntactic, and phonemic parameters of their language behavior. Love, Clark, and McConnell, in chapter 2, point out the need for a differential diagnosis for non-language children. Four possible major causes to be considered are: (1) hearing impairment, (2) neurological impairment, (3) developmental delay and/or mental retardation, and (4) emotional disturbance. They identify typical behaviors of children with these disorders.

The Case Study. All obtainable data that is pertinent to a given case should be gathered and correlated with the symptoms presented by the client. For the child, Bangs (1968) has suggested the inclusion of data on birth and medical history; motor development; language and speech history; and interpersonal, family, and school relationships. For the aphasic adult, the data should cover not only the medical history, but also information about the early language, educational, and family background, and the family's present attitudes toward the disability. The clinician should also explore such factors as the patient's threshold of fatigue, sense of direction, sensory difficulties, personality characteristics, and recreational habits.

Obviously, the more complete and specific the information that can be gathered about a client with a language disorder, the better the remedial program will be. When the interview data have all been correlated with the information obtained from objective and semiobjective tests and other observations, the case study will be useful in diagnostic assessment and remedial planning. It may also prove useful to other professionals who may be working with the client.

Objective and Semiobjective Instruments. In chapter 2 of this book, Love, Clark, and McConnell list many tests suitable for assessing receptive and expressive language and related abilities in children, including the Houston Test for Language Development (Crabtree, 1963), the Illinois Test of Psycholinguistic Abilities (Kirk, McCarthy, and Kirk, 1968), the Peabody Picture Vocabulary Test (Dunn, 1980), the Utah Test of Language Development (Mecham, Jex, and Jones, 1967), the Verbal Language Development Scale (Mecham, 1959), the Wechsler Intelligence Scale for Children (Wechsler, 1949), the Wechsler Preschool and Primary Scale for Children (Wechsler, 1967), the Northwestern Syntax Screening Test (Lee, 1969), and the Michigan Picture Language Inventory (Lerea, 1958). More recent tests such as the Clinical Evaluation of Language Functions (Semel and Wig, 1980), the Token Test for Children (DiSimoni, 1979), the Environmental Language Inventory (MacDonald, 1978), and others have been added to the clinical armamentarium of professional workers with the language impaired. (See tables 2–6, 2–7, and 2–8 for more reference information and descriptions.)

Of the above-mentioned tests, Van Hattum in chapter 6 of this book recommends the Verbal Language Development Scale, the Northwestern Syntax Screening Test (applicable to three- through eight-year-olds), and the Michigan Picture Language Inventory (1962) for assessing the language abilities of cleft-palate children.

One of our preferences among available tests for evaluating psycholinguistic abilities of children below the age of ten is the ITPA as it has been revised (Kirk, McCarthy, and Kirk, 1968). Now having a more diagnostic character than it did originally, this test delineates (through twelve subtests, two of which are intended only for children thought to have spelling and reading difficulties) specific abilities and disabilities in ten discrete areas of language. (A description of the ITPA may be found in chapter 2.) Such an analysis of the child's language disorder allows us to plan a remedial program addressed specifically to the areas of weakness. Dickson (1967) found that clinical judgment of language delay correlates highly with low scores on the ITPA with children in the primary grades.

Another test that is exceedingly useful as a clinical tool is the Peabody Picture Vocabulary Test (Dunn, 1980). Designed to provide an estimate of the two-and-one-half- to eighteen-year-old clients' verbal intelligence and recognition vocabularies, it is effective with persons of average IQ, and, because it requires no reading skill, it can be used with children who have reading disabilities. Further, because responses do not have to be verbal, it is an appropriate test for the expressive aphasic, the stutterer, the autistic, and the cerebral-palsied patient. It may be given to any speaker of American English—after all, it was only standardized for that vocabulary—and it permits the clinician to extract estimates of intelligence from the derived scores. When a more precise measurement of IQ is needed, the client should be referred to a qualified psychologist for a complete psychometric evaluation.

The speech clinician is frequently confronted with children who have apparently developed no language system. They have not, as has the aphasic, lost a language capability, but seem never to have acquired it, usually because of mental retardation, hearing impairment, neurological impairment, or an emotional disorder such as childhood schizophrenia or autism. In order to make a differential diagnosis, the clinician must rely on those assessments available for each etiological factor and consider carefully the differences in responses typical of each group, as described by Love, Clark, and McConnell in chapter 2 of this book.

There is also a group of children whose language abilities are similar in nature and range to those of the neurologically impaired, although they do not show the gross neurological signs which suggest central nervous system impairment and there is nothing of clinical significance in their birth and medical histories. Despite this, they perform linguistically—and behaviorally, in some ways—as if they do have a central nervous system impairment. Such children are often described as suffering from "minimal brain dysfunction," a disorder which has also been called "brain damage syndrome" (Hardy, 1965), or "Strauss syndrome" (Stevens and Birch, 1967). Labels applied to such children include "non-motor brain-damaged" and "psychoneurological learning disordered," but regardless of what one chooses to call these children, the presence of a language impairment requires that they be evaluated in much the same way as other language-disordered clients.

For those who have language losses after some cerebral trauma or cerebral vascular accident, the Minnesota Test for Differential Diagnosis of Aphasia (Schuell, 1965) identifies patterns of impairment that correlate significantly and meaningfully with neurological findings. A short form of the test (Schuell, 1967) is reported to have predictive validity and high reliability, although it has not been standardized. West (chap. 8) reviews the Schuell Test and others that may be used to assess the language behavior of the aphasic. In addition she includes a description of some of the more current and widely used tests with aphasics such as the Boston Diagnostic Aphasia Examination (BDAE), the Porch Index of Communicative Ability (PICA), the Communicative Abilities in Daily Living (CADL), the Functional Communication Profile (FCP), the Token Test, and others. Other instruments available are the Examining for Aphasia test (Eisenson, 1954), and the Halstead-Wepman Aphasia Screening Test (Halstead and Wepman, 1949).

Informal Observation and Selected Tasks. Informal, subjective impressions can often add to the information obtained from the standardized tests. Indeed, in some types of problems they may provide the only means of assessing a client's capabilities. If a child, for example, will not pay attention to a standardized testing procedure, a more informal presentation of tasks and observation of behavior will be required. Bangs (1968) has described some tasks and features of behavior useful for this purpose:

1. recognition of objects and pictures;
2. naming objects and pictures;
3. responding to action agents;
4. defining words and describing pictures;
5. categorizing (pictorial identification, association, and analyses);
6. dealing with numbers;
7. understanding spatial concepts;
8. following serial directions;
9. using jargon, echolalia, or gestures;
10. remembering words, sentences, visual objects (pictures);
11. demonstrating a perceptual-motor pattern;
12. showing visual perception; and
13. indicating handedness preference

Obtaining a language sample is a widely used technique to assess the language behavior of children. Byrne (1978) describes four purposes for obtaining a language sample. They are (1) to describe the language use of an individual, (2) to compare the linguistic performance with that of a peer group, (3) to assist in planning a remedial program, and (4) to evaluate progress in therapy. Lynch (1978) suggests that the sample be obtained in a carefully controlled setting such as a "play" room. The manner in which the sample is to be analyzed is of importance. Frequently used techniques were the ones suggested by Lee (1974), Muma (1973), Bloom and Lahey (1978), and Crystal, Fletcher, and Garman (1976). Observation of such features of spontaneous speaking activity as grammatical usage, mean length of response (MLR), mean length of utterance (MLU), number of one-word responses, and amount of social speech, may also prove useful in identifying and assessing language disorders. Figure 1–2 is an example of a language case summary form that may be used in planning for therapy.

Figure 1–2. Pre-therapy Case Summary (Language)
State University College at Buffalo
Speech-Language-Hearing Clinic
Dr. Nancy J. Lund

Previous Evaluations & Therapy (dates, agency, and summary of report)

Past Language Test Results (date, test, scores and interpretation)

Related Test Results (intelligence, motor, reading, etc.)

Phonological Analysis
Name of Articulation Test _____Date _____
From Language Sample Date _____
Substitution Analysis (indicate substitution or omission for target sound)

  Stops

  Fricatives

  Affricates

  Nasals

  Glides

Feature pattern summary:

Assimilation/coalescence errors:

Syllable structure patterns (cv, cvc, cvcv, etc.)

Language Sample Analysis—Date of Sample _____
(Note if imitated)   MLU _____
Morphological Analysis:
Indicate forms present and correct, or show which are omitted (X) or not sampled (NS)

Noun Forms
 plural irregular
 plural regular
 possessive (*'s*)
 articles (*a, the*)

Verb Forms
 Lexical forms:
  third person singular
  past regular
  past irregular
 Auxiliary forms:
  progressive: *am*   + *-ing*
                  are
                  is
                  was
                  were
 perfective (have + past participle)
 modals
 do- forms

Copula forms: *am*   *was*
               are   *were*
               is

Adjective/Adverb Forms
Comparative
Superlative

Syntactic Analysis:
 Clause Structure
 Give examples of each clause-type noted:
  Subject-verb
  Subject-verb-object
  Subject-copula-complement
  Subject-verb-object-dative

 Compound clause
 Relative clause
 Subordinate clause

Pragmatic Analysis from Language Sample
 Intentions Expressed (indicate what child said or did)
 requesting help
 requesting object
 requesting action
 rejecting action
 directing attention
 others:

Topic Selection
 physically present objects/events as topics
 non-present topic referents
 inappropriate topic shifts
 greater number of turns on one topic

Listener Perspective Taking
 orienting terms
 relative pronouns/descriptive adjectives
 deictic terms

Ability to Initiate/Engage in Speech Event (indicate event)
 initiates activity/dialogue
 responds to other's initiation
 takes turns
 responds only to routines
 inappropriate responding

Phrase Structure
 Give examples of most complex noun phrases noted:

Prepositions
 Spatial:
 Temporal:
 Other:
 Errors:

Negative Forms:

Question Forms:
 yes/no
 intonation

inverted auxiliary
do- form
tag
wh- question forms used
with auxiliary
without auxiliary

Pronoun Forms

	Subject	Object	Possessive
first			
second			
third			
other:			

Parental Perception of Communication Ability

Factors That Might Act As Deterrents to Therapy

Factors That Might Facilitate Therapy

For the diagnosis of aphasia, there are so many objective and semiobjective tests available that most speech clinicians do not rely as heavily upon informal observation as they do for other language disorders. But even here, some clinicians may prefer to gain their impressions of areas of disability and intact function in the aphasic individual informally. Head (1963) has suggested that the patient be asked to name or describe the use of common objects and that familiar sounds be used to assess the possibility of auditory agnosia. Tasks to be carried out on command, which may be helpful in evaluating the existence of apraxia, have been suggested by Longerich and Bordeaux (1959); these involve the patient's ability to protrude his tongue, to use his hands in buttoning his shirt, and to carry out activities composed of several different tasks. West, in chapter 8, describes some of the communication problems experienced by the apraxic. In chapter 7, Di Carlo and Amster discuss the evaluation of language disorders in cerebral-palsied children.

As they gain experience with individuals with language disorders, most clinicians will develop their own preferred tasks and find features of behavior and speech which are, to them, most informative. It should be borne in mind, however, that the use of such informal techniques becomes meaningful only when combined, as a complement and supplement, with all of the data amassed from the case study and the objective testing.

Diagnostic Procedures for Articulation Disorders

Of all types of communication disorders, articulation problems occur most frequently. They are seen in as many as 80 percent of the school-age children who find occasion to visit a speech-language clinician; and three quarters of the speech-language clinicians functioning today in schools, clinics, and hospitals are doing so because of the prevalence of articulatory defects in the population. It is therefore essential that the clinician know how to assess and treat these problems well.

Articulation problems occur when speech is characterized by substitutions, omissions, or distortions of speech sounds. They are classified as organic when they are caused by abnormalities of the organs or systems of speech and as functional when they are judged to represent abnormal behavior patterns related to faulty learning and faulty use of the organs. The usefulness of this classification has its limits, however; the reader is referred to the discussion of the organic-functional dichotomy in chapter 3.

Organic causes of articulation disorders, described in professional literature, include:

1. central nervous system pathologies, resulting in dysarthria and dyspraxia;
2. structural anomalies of the organs of articulation, such as cleft palate and related maxillofacial disorders, and malocclusion and related dental abnormalities;
3. emotional disorders based upon psychopathology, such as schizophrenia and autism;
4. reduced hearing levels due to a pathology of the end organ of hearing, such as sensory neural loss resulting from rubella or viral diseases.

Darley (1978) describes the disorders of articulation based upon sensory deficits, physiological limitations, learning factors, and a combination of these factors. The sensory deficits include hearing loss and oral anesthesia; physiological limitations include palatopharyngeal incompetence, neuromotor impairments (dysarthria, apraxia), dental deviations, and lingual defects. Learning factors include mental retardation, language disability, and functional articulatory defects. Since the cause of Matthew's problem (pp. 13–15) was suspected to be of the second type, the assessment called for examination of his velopharyngeal mechanism and overall oral physiology. It was also possible that Matthew's problem was functional in nature.

Functional articulation disorders, as impairments in the specific function of the articulatory structures, are of unknown origin (Darley, 1978); that is, an organic cause is not clearly evident. In the review of the research in chapter 3, inadequate development of articulatory skills is linked to such factors as auditory (including pitch) discrimination, motor skills, oral sensation, mental age, intelligence, and socioeconomic status, within an overall context of faulty learning. In addition, basic importance is attached to such speech factors as stimulability and consistency of correct sound production in a variety of acoustic contexts and situations, each of which may be viewed in the light of linguistic theory as related to the laws of sound acquisition (Winitz, 1969). Menyuk (1968), for example, has suggested that sound productions of children with articulation problems may be described by applying the distinctive feature theory of sound production (discussed by Jakobson, Fant, and Halle, 1952). More on this subject will be found in chapter 3, where Sommers discusses distinctive feature theory, especially in relation to his wedge approach for planning articulation therapy.

Sommers describes a variety of remedial techniques that are used to correct articulation problems. While their treatment of the subject focuses on functional articulation disorders, the techniques they describe may have some application to organic problems as well. The latter, however, may require additional remedial techniques, such as those suggested by Van Hattum (chapter 6) for helping the cleft-palate child improve intraoral pressure for better articulation; by Di Carlo and Amster (chapter 7) for coordinating the breathing, phonation, and articulation of the cerebral-palsied child; and by Lowell and Pollack (chapter 9) for enhancing the development of articulation in the hearing-impaired child. The creative clinician will use whatever techniques seem appropriate, and will borrow from all legitimate sources to enhance the effectiveness and the communication skills of the client.

The Case Study. The client will frequently have been referred to the speech clinician by another professional, and much of the necessary case history information will be contained in the referral report. The clinician should study this material thoroughly before seeing the client and try to avoid needless repetition of questions during the diagnostic interview, although the clinician should be guided primarily by experience and training in collecting case history data.

The material to be covered in the case study will vary according to the etiology of the disorder, but certain basic data (as indicated in figure 1–1) must be obtained. That is, the clinician needs information concerning

1. physiological factors which appear significant;
2. psychodynamic factors, such as sibling rivalry, family tensions, and bizarre home or school situations; and
3. environmental influences, such as foreign language background, atypical speech models, and deprivation.

The clinician should use this information to start remedial therapy as soon as possible, for not only will an immediate sense of progress have a very positive effect on the client, and the parents, too, if they are involved, but it will facilitate the collection of further data.

Objective and Semiobjective Instruments. Many of the tests for assessing articulation ability use pictures intended to elicit as responses the various sounds of speech both in isolation and at the beginning, middle, and end of words. The client may also be asked to read, if able, certain sentences or paragraphs aloud. Such tests must be formulated with an eye to the consistency of the examiner's judgment and of the client's responses, as well as to the extent of agreement among examiners. The reliability of the tests demands a consensus as to the normality of the sounds whose production is being evaluated, and it is attained by training the examiners to know the normal and to recognize the abnormal. The consistency of the client's responses is an important factor in testing, for on it depend suggestions for therapy. For example, a five-year-old who sometimes uses the sounds of speech appropriate to that age, but often does not, may not need treatment, but an eight-year-old who consistently lateralizes the sibilants and who cannot produce a correct sound in isolation should be given therapy.

There are essentially three types of articulation tests. One, used particularly for rapid screening of large numbers of children, consists of presenting material for oral reading, suitable to the grade level of the child and supplemented by a few questions to elicit germane responses. The paragraph, "My Grandfather" (Van Riper, 1972), which contains all of the American English consonant and vowel sounds, is frequently used. Other sample passages are suggested by West and Ansberry in *The Rehabilitation of Speech* (1968). The clinician should not, however, depend solely on oral reading tests, for frequently children who are nonreaders are being tested. If the child cannot read, the difficulty should be noted quickly and a nonreading articulation test substituted. Hutchinson et al. (1979) describes a number of screening tests available for detecting children who may have articulation difficulty (pp. 159–160). Van Riper and Ericksen (1973) developed a screening test in an attempt to predict who will spontaneously outgrow articulation errors by third grade without formal articulation therapy. This test is primarily based upon the child's degree of stimulability as a predictor for articulatory maturation. Emerick and Hattan (1974), extolling the predictive value of this instrument, argue for sound clinical judgment rather than just test scores. We would also suggest that children with articulatory defects based upon organic factors or adverse environmental circumstances may not spontaneously outgrow articulation errors. There is no substitute for a thorough clinical analysis and subsequent diagnostic judgment based upon all the information accumulated.

The second type of test which the clinician should have in the diagnostic repertoire is the horizontal test for assessing the articulation of single sounds. An example is the Goldman-Fristoe (1969) articulation test designed to assess consonant sounds on a chronological development scale. The levels of the scale are the ages at which children may be expected to have mastered the sounds and twelve blends for /s/, /l/, and /r/. The results are recorded on a scoring sheet, supplied with the test, which also gives instructions on the order of presentation of the pictures and provides the age at which the child should have stabilized production of each phoneme. When the testing has been completed, the examiner should have some idea of just where the child is in relation to the normal range of development of articulatory abilities. The results can then serve as a guide to whether the child needs therapy and, if so, which sounds should be emphasized first. We have found the test useful in counseling parents, since it provides some indication of where their child stands with respect to the maturation level of peers—and therefore why their fears may sometimes be unjustified—and why the child may not be in need of therapy.

Other types of horizontal tests available for use that are popular with many clinicians include the Templin-Darley Tests of Articulation (Templin and Darley, 1968), the Fisher-Logemann Test of Articulation Competence, (Fisher and Logemann, 1970), the Hejna Developmental Articulation Test (Hejna, 1955), and the Photo Articulation Test (PAT) (Pendergast et al., 1969). Clinicians often find the stimulus material attractive to children and conducive to obtaining appropriate responses. An examination and review of these tests may help the clinician in selecting one more appropriate for the child being tested. Love, Clark, and McConnell, in chapter 2, briefly describe a number of these tests.

The third type of test, designed to assess sounds in context, is the deep test, such as that developed by McDonald (1964) to evaluate speech sounds as the results of syllabic movement patterns. It requires that the examiner learn beforehand which sounds are most frequently misarticulated by the child and then select pairs of pictures which, when named as connected syllables, will evoke those sounds. At the beginning of the test, the examiner demonstrates to the child how to name the pairs of pictures, connecting them as "tub-vase, tub-sheep, teach-sheep." When the child has practiced naming the pictures long enough to know how to respond, the examiner turns to the picture that ends with the sound to be deep tested, such as /s/. By linking pairs of pictures, the examiner may then assess the child's ability to produce the /s/ sound in many fundamental phonetic contexts. If, during the test, the examiner can identify contexts in which the sound is correctly articulated, this forms a basis for starting to correct the sound immediately.

If given routinely, deep tests can be extremely useful for research purposes and the accumulation of data, but there are a number of other tests frequently used in diagnosing articulation defects. Van Hattum (chapter 6), for example, suggests observation of children's speech during play and also the use of the Bzoch Phonetic Analysis (Philips and Bzoch, 1969), wherein the examiner asks the subject to repeat a test word three times. He suggests the use of rating scales for judging the severity of errors, the rate of articulation, and intelligibility, and places importance on stimulability, the ability of a subject to repeat a sound correctly when asked.

Another test Van Hattum describes is the Iowa Pressure Articulation Test (Morris, Sprietersbach, and Darley, 1961), which is used with cleft-palate subjects to infer the extent of oral pressure and velopharyngeal function during the articulatory process. These test results require recording not only the errors made but the type of error, substitution, distortion, or omission. Once recorded, an analysis of test results is appropriate. Darley (1978) suggests the following type of analysis: "1) comparison with norms, 2) types of errors, 3) consistency of errors, 4) response to stimulation, 5) comparison with contextual speech, 6) search for patterns of errors, and 7) rating of intelligibility," (pp. 237–245). In addition, Michel (1978) suggests charting articulative errors based upon their place, manner, and voicing characteristics. Weiner and Bernthal (1978) suggest the application of distinctive features to misarticulations for a thorough understanding of error patterns.

Informal Observation and Selected Tasks. The first indication of a need for testing a person's articulation is often the informal observation, by parents, teachers, friends, or students, of such aberrations of speech as the distorted /r/, the lateral /s/, or the omitted /l/. Indeed, such informal observations often lead a client to the speech clinician, who will initially confirm or dismiss the existence of a problem by similar attention to the client's speech. The speech clinician will not, however, stop there, but will often examine the client's oral structures in an attempt to determine their adequacy for articulation or test a child's general motor coordination by having the child skip, hop, jump, or tie shoelaces. The clinician may also try to make some estimate of the client's laterality preference by asking the client to throw or kick a ball.

Hutchinson et al. (1979) review diagnostic instruments that can be used to assess concomitants of articulation difficulties and relate them to possible etiologies. They provide a review of personality tests, including personality inventories and projective tests, measures of social maturity, intelligence tests, aptitude tests, perceptual-motor tests, achievement tests, school readiness tests, reading tests, and neurological tests (pp. 70–105). To keep up with the instruments being published requires a periodic review of *Asha*, which describes tests and tells where they may be obtained. Some of these tests may also be reviewed in Buros' *Mental Measurements Yearbook*.

Specific disability groups, however, require a more careful appraisal of articulation, for to treat them effectively the clinician must know precisely what the communication difficulty is. To do this, the clinician must evaluate, both individually and as a total communicative system, such essential parameters of speech and language behavior as the structural and functional integrity of the oral musculature and linguistic mechanisms, respiratory function, phonatory ability, resonance and articulation, language itself, and audition. Suitable techniques include the use of kymographic tracings to assess respiratory function; spectrographic recordings to visualize the utterances of cerebral-palsied children; stroboscopic evaluations of laryngeal function; cineradiography or cephalometrics to examine oral activity during speech; and some of the specific techniques recommended by each of the authors in their respective chapters in this book.

The parameters more directly related to articulation, such as language, may be somewhat more difficult to evaluate because they are not easily identifiable. McDonald and Chance (1964) have suggested specific language tasks, but the recently revised and standardized Illinois Test of Psycholinguistic Abilities (Kirk, McCarthy, and Kirk, 1968) may be more suitable. Gaining a complete understanding of a cerebral-palsied child's status may require the assessment of mental function by the use of standardized intelligence tests, or sections from several such tests. Some authorities, however, feel that standardized testing procedures are inappropriate for this task (McDonald and Chance, 1964). For that reason, some psychologists have developed original tests or have used single items from several existing tests (Haeussermann, 1958).

The disabling consequences of such disorders as cerebral palsy often force the diagnostician to rely on observation of specific performances when evaluating a child's developmental status and its relationship to articulation ability. Else Haeussermann (1952), for instance, selected tasks from a variety of sources to evaluate the developmental level of the multiple-handicapped child by revealing the child's ability to perform the task and to circumvent some of the obstacles, such as lack of dexterity, presented by the disability.

For cleft-palate children, articulation may be evaluated by the various techniques discussed by Van Hattum in chapter 6 for assessing velopharyngeal competence as it relates to valving proficiency, nasal air escape, and nasality. These techniques include observation of the specific nature of the articulation difficulty; the use of an oral manometer to measure oral pressure; direct observation of the velopharyngeal and laryngeal areas during phonation with fiber optic study; and the study of still and moving X-ray films of the speech apparatus as a whole. Further research with these techniques may be expected to clarify many aspects of articulatory problems that are enigmatic.

An examination of the peripheral oral mechanism is essential to a careful diagnosis of any articulation disorder (Darley, 1964; Counihan, 1960), for, as Westlake and Rutherford (1966) have suggested, facial structures, postures, and movements may have serious acoustic and cosmetic effects on speech production. While informal observation and such selected tasks as tongue manipulation may help clarify the structure and function of the oral musculature, the correct interpretation of results requires long experience and familiarity; moreover, such observation must be supplemented by other procedures. The case study must also be made, and auditory, perceptual-motor, intellectual, and language function, as well as articulation itself, must be assessed. Figure 1–3 and figure 1–4 are examples of forms that may be used to assess various parameters of articulatory impairments.

Diagnostic Procedures for Stuttering

Stuttering has been defined as a disturbance in the rhythm or fluency of speech manifested in repeated and prolonged sounds, words, or phrases; or pauses, blockings, or other hesitancies; but a characterization of the disorder as including an "anticipatory, apprehensive, hypertonic avoidance reaction" differentiates it best

Figure 1–3. Pre-therapy Case Summary (Articulation)
State University College at Buffalo
Speech-Language-Hearing Clinic
Dr. Donald Hess

Examination Findings

Articulation Test Results

Test(s) Employed _____Date _____

Phonetic Errors (specify)

Patterns of Misarticulation Represented by These Errors

	Prosodic
Voicing	Factors
Place of Articulation	Phonologic
	Factors
Manner of Articulation	

Stimulability Test Results

Sounds		Stimulable in		
	Isolation	Nonsense Syllables	Words	Sentences

Are errors consistent in all "positions" and phonetic contexts? Explain

Are errors in connected speech consistent with errors in words? Explain

Are there "key words" that are correctly articulated? (specify these and underline sound)

Intelligibility in connected speech (state as percentage)
 Careful, slow, guarded speech
 Fast, unguarded speech
 With topic known to examiner
 With topic unknown to examiner
What other factors seem to affect intelligibility?

Hearing (date)

Oral Examination (date)

Oral Motor Coordination and Function (dates) (including diadochokinetic rates, etc.)

Auditory Perceptual Function (dates)
Auditory Discrimination

Auditory Memory Span

Other Auditory Factors (synthesis, closure, vocal phonics)

Visual Motor Function

Language Measures (e.g., PPVT, ITPA, etc.)

Voice (pitch, loudness, quality)

Previous Therapy
When?

By Whom?

Attitude of Case Toward Problem (and therapy)

Prognosis
General

Factors that might facilitate therapy

Factors that might act as deterrents to therapy

Special considerations re: therapy planning based on special diagnostic findings

from normal nonfluencies, according to Johnson et al. (1967). Some clinicians attribute its etiology to learned behavior patterns resulting from instrumental conditioning (Shames and Sherrick, 1963), while others impute it to a combination of classical and instrumental conditioning (Brutten and Shoemaker, 1967). The specific etiology is elusive, but it seems clear that faulty learning is an important factor, particularly if one accepts Van Riper's (1971) definition of stuttering as including the speaker's reactions to his own halting speech.

The weight of the evidence suggests that the speech clinician should concentrate on those learned behaviors associated with stuttering. Since stuttering appears to include

Figure 1–4. Pre-therapy Case Summary (Oral Examination)
State University College at Buffalo
Speech-Language-Hearing Clinic

ORAL EXAMINATION

I. Examination of lips and peripheral structures

    A. Lips
        Ability to round _____
        Ability to retract _____
        Ability to vary degree of roundness _____
        Appearance (if abnormal, describe)
    B. Facial structures (if abnormal, describe)

II. Examination of jaw (mandible)

    A. Appearance:
        Normal _____ Prognathic _____ Retrognathic _____
    B. Function: (if abnormal, describe)

III. Examination of the teeth

    A. Class of occlusion _____ Subdivision _____
    B. Type of bite:
        Normal _____ Open _____ Closed _____ Overbite _____ Crossbite _____
        Edge-to-edge _____ Overjet _____
    C. Individual teeth variations: (if abnormal, describe)

IV. Examination of the tongue

    A. Appearance (if abnormal, describe)
    B. Function
        1. Ability to groove _____
        2. Ability to elevate to rugae _____
        3. Ability to touch corners of lips _____
        4. Ability to encircle lips of open mouth _____
        5. Ability to protrude _____
        6. Ability to elevate dorsum of tongue to velum _____

V. Examination of the hard palate

    A. Vaulting
        1. Normal _____ 2. Abnormalities? Describe _____
        _____
        3. Height _____ 4. Width _____
    B. Deformities (if present, describe)

VI. Examination of the soft palate

    A. Appearance
        1. Faucial pillars (if abnormal, describe; also note size and condition of tonsils)

        2. Function during phonation

VII. Pharynx (if abnormal, describe)

behavior that the stutterer has learned as a consequence of a variety of experiences tending to reinforce the stuttering behavior, we are interested in how the laws of learning apply to a given situation. Thus, we are primarily interested in the experiences that have some direct influence on an individual's learning to stutter, that person's attitudes about stuttering, what the person does when anticipating stuttering, the actual stuttering moment, and, finally, the individual's reaction to the stuttering. The diagnostic interview should be structured to obtain as much information as possible about these things.

Because stuttering generally is not considered a medical problem, the speech clinician is often the first professional to see the individual who stutters. The young stutterer is referred most frequently by teachers or by concerned parents. The older stutterer may be referred similarly or may personally recognize the problem and seek help. If the stutterer has been to other speech clinics, reports may be available and should be obtained and studied.

The Case Study. The case study should be devoted to obtaining specific information about the onset and early development of stuttering, as well as the client's reactions to these dysfluencies and perception of the reactions of others to them. In the course of it, the clinician should discuss with the client the social aspects of the problem and their relation to educational and vocational plans. The clinician should try to gain some understanding of the depth of emotional involvement the stutterer and family and friends have in the problem. The clinician should determine what specific sounds, words, or situations provoke stuttering, and should note any reports of periods of fluency for longer than usual periods of time.

In addition to the standard inquiries we have suggested in The General Case Study Review, Williams (1978) listed additional considerations for the stutterer as follows:

1. Onset and development of the stuttering problem;
2. Variability of the disfluency;
3. Attitudes and beliefs about stuttering of the parents, teachers, and the stutterer;
4. The stutterer's experience with the problem educationally, socially, and vocationally;
5. The stutterer's view of the future, goals, and estimates of the realization of those goals.

The clinician should also carefully note any discrepancies between parental reports and the client's perceptions of any of these questions. Darley and Spriestersbach (1978) have identified three factors of major importance in examining the stuttering problem. They are:

"(1) The attitudes and reactions of listeners to the speaker and his speech,
 (2) the attitudes and reactions of the speaker to those of his listeners and to himself and his own speech, and
 (3) the speech behavior of the speaker," (p. 284).

The last of these is essential to a determination of the goal of the remedial program, while the first two may help the clinician see ways to approach the task of remediation.

Objective and Semiobjective Instruments. A diagnosis of stuttering must emerge from an analysis of the many behaviors that constitute the client's global reaction to his or her inability to speak smoothly or freely. The stuttering behavior itself is self-evident, but careful assessment involves the tasks of estimating its severity and the nature and location of the disturbance in the flow of speech. For that assessment the clinician can use one or a few of the many tests, scales of severity, and indices that have been devised by speech pathologists. These include tests for determining the frequency and duration of blocks, degree of tension, complexity of secondary symptoms, attitudes toward stuttering, feared words and situations, and physiological fear responses.

Rating scales are probably the most frequently used means of describing and evaluating stuttering behavior. Besides being helpful in planning therapy, the rating scales have a value when used periodically to determine the changes in stuttering behavior brought about by remedial efforts. The speech clinician should become thoroughly familiar with several of these checklists and rating scales, such as the Iowa Scale for Rating Severity of Stuttering (Sherman, 1952), which determines the degree of severity through the use of predetermined criteria.

The forms found useful by Darley and Spriestersbach (1978) include (1) a checklist of stuttering behavior; (2) a scale for rating the severity of stuttering; and (3) stutterer's self-ratings of reactions to speech situations. Johnson (1968) also recommended the use of the Iowa Scale of Attitude Toward Stuttering. Brutten and Shoemaker recommend the use of the "Speech Situations Checklist" to identify situations evoking negative emotion associated with fluency failure (1974a). They also recommend the use of their Behavior Checklist (1974b) and the Southern Illinois Modification of the Geer Fear Survey Schedule (Brutten and Shoemaker, 1974c). Two other instruments available for clinical use are the Riley Stuttering Severity Instrument (Riley, 1972) and Woolf's Perceptions of Stuttering Inventory (PSI), (Woolf, 1967). Cooper's (1976) Chronicity Prediction Checklist may help to predict recovery from stuttering or may be a useful predictor of success with treatment. Hood (1978) describes a number of instruments available for the assessment of stuttering (pp. 556–59). A review of this listing should provide the clinician with an awareness of the major methods available to assess a variety of factors related to stuttering behavior.

Measurements of the adaptation and consistency shown by stutterers have been standard procedures ever since Johnson and Knott (1937) demonstrated that the frequency of stuttering is reduced with each consecutive reading of a selected passage (adaptation) and that the stutterer tends to stutter on the same words in each successive reading (consistency). The interpretation of these phenomena has been varied, but some clinicians believe that adaptation is prognostic for eventual improvement (Johnson, Darley, and Spriestersbach, 1963). Williams (1978) questions the value of such measures as part of a routine clinical evaluation, and so do we.

Because speech clinicians are frequently concerned about the personal adjustment of stutterers, they may wish to see results of such personality assessment tests as the Taylor Manifest Anxiety Scale (Taylor, 1953) and the Minnesota Multiphasic Personality Inventory (Welsh and Dahlstrom, 1956). These tests can be properly administered and interpreted only by clinical psychologists, so the clinician should not hesitate to refer a client to a psychologist or psychiatrist for consultation whenever it might yield useful information for planning the therapy program.

Chapter 4 includes Brutten and Hegde's review for developing a profile of a stutterer, which can serve as a guide to the clinician in organizing the symptom picture and in making a prognosis. These authors are also concerned about the stutterer's escape and avoidance, and they recommend identifying stimulus situations that elicit anxiety and listing the theme areas (such as using the telephone) around which remediation efforts can be planned. The Southern Illinois Checklists and Scales mentioned above (Brutten and Shoemaker, 1974) may help to accomplish that objective.

Informal Observation and Selected Tasks. Because of the nature of stuttering, most of the information necessary to a diagnosis must be obtained in the interview, for it is only during speech that the secondary symptoms and the character of the stuttering block reveal themselves and can be evaluated. During the initial interview, the speech clinician can form some impression of the client's reading and speaking rate and of his or her affective reactions during spontaneous speech. Some clinicians may also ask the stutterer to write an autobiography that includes family background, with the idea that it will reveal attitudes and behavioral tendencies relevant to the remedial program. It has been our experience, however, that the initial interview does not reveal very much. Getting to know the stutterer takes several sessions, during which time the stutterer also gains self-knowledge, a development which we feel is an important aspect of the therapeutic process.

In addition to the interview situation where stuttering behavior can be observed, Hutchinson et al. (1979) suggest a comprehensive analysis of the five processes of speech: respiration, phonation, resonation, articulation, and cerebration. They state that "malfunction of any of the parts of the system affects the efficiency of the integrated whole" (p. 265). Although we agree that such an assessment should be made, comprehensive and thorough review need to be undertaken only when one or more than one of these processes are noted to be defective.

The relative emphasis placed on various parts of the diagnostic protocol will probably depend upon the stuttering concepts emphasized by the diagnostician. Brutten and Hegde (chap. 4) would place great emphasis on the stimulus events and situations associated with stuttering behavior, while a more psychoanalytically oriented clinician might rely heavily on the stutterer's verbalized and implied attitudes and expressions as noted during the diagnostic interview. We would urge each clinician to use experience to develop a diagnostic protocol consistent with the kind of remedial practices discussed in chapter 4. Figure 1–5 is an example of a case history form that may be used with stutterers.

Diagnostic Procedures for Phonatory Disorders

In describing voice, "appropriateness" is the term ordinarily applied to normal function, while similarly subjective terms are used in labeling abnormalities— "breathiness," "hoarseness," "harshness," "nasality," "denasality," and the like. Judgments based on the perception of such vocal characteristics as pitch, quality, and loudness have a certain validity, even without the benefit of scientific measurement, and indeed they bring many clients to the attention of the speech clinician. While the latter's impressions of a client's voice are expressed in similarly subjective terms, diagnostic experience sharpens the ability to use them accurately. That is, the clinician will recognize differences between voice defects per se and differences, as in

Figure 1–5. Pre-therapy Case Summary (Stuttering)
State University College at Buffalo
Speech-Language-Hearing Clinic
Dr. Donald Hess

A. *History of Stuttering*

When was the stuttering first noticed? _____

Who noticed it? _____ What did they do or say? _____

Can you associate it with any physical injury, emotional crisis, or geographical move? _____

Have you ever discussed your speech with anyone? _____

Who? _____ What did they tell you? _____

Have you had any previous therapy? _____ When? _____

Where? _____ What kind? _____

By whom? _____

Has anyone become impatient with your speech or filled in a word for you as you were about to stutter? _____

Did you ever think people felt sorry for you because of your speech? _____

Have you ever failed to give an answer that you knew because you were afraid to speak? _____

Have any of your past teachers made a point of not calling on you because of your speech problem? _____

How did you feel about that? _____

Have you ever substituted a word for another in order to avoid stuttering? _____

Have you ever chosen not to participate in verbal activities? _____

Have you ever avoided asking for or giving information? _____

Have you ever felt you could not do something (job, etc.) because of your speech? _____

Did you ever have another person speak for you in a difficult situation (restaurant, etc.)? _____

B. *Problems with Stuttering at the Present*

Is your speech behavior fairly consistent in all situations? _____

How do your friends react to your speech? _____

Do you avoid talking to people in authority? _____

Do you ever use gestures as a substitute for speaking? _____

Are some sounds, words, or situations harder than others for you? _____

_____ Which ones? _____

Do you use your stuttering as a reason to avoid a speaking activity? _____

Do you have general body tension during speech attempts? _____

Do you ever practice what you are going to say long before you speak? _____

Do you know when you are going to stutter before you actually do? _____

Do you coordinate or time your speech with a rhythmic movement (foot tapping, etc.)? _____

Do you avoid talking to others of your own age group? _____

Do you feel that your speech has limited you socially? _____

Do you become more inhibited in front of large groups? _____

Do you use any tricks to disguise your stuttering (circumlocution, telegraphic speech)? _____

Do you have any words, sounds, or actions that help you start a sentence?

_____ Which ones? _____

How do you release yourself from a stuttering block? _____

Are there any situations you fear the most (telephone, etc.)? _____

Which ones? _____

C. *Examinations*

1. *Stuttering Severity Instrument*

   score:

   degree of severity:

2. *Predictive stuttering ability*
   # predicted stuttered words:
   # actual stuttered words:
   results of comparison:
3. *Rereading same paragraph for comparison (adaptation, consistency)*
   results of comparison:
4. *Taping conversational speech*
5. "Arthur, the Young Rat"—test for adaptation effect
   adaptation %
   consistency %

D. *Examination Results and Observations—Overt and Covert Behaviors*
   postponements:
   circumlocutions:
   interruptors:
   release mechanisms:
   air stream:
   sequence of secondaries during blocks:
   pitch or volume changes:
   duration of blocks:
   Physical Concomitants
   facial grimaces
   lip contortions
   head movements
   dilating nostrils
   gestures
   eye contact
   body movements
   other

E. *Clinicians' Impressions of Client's Self-Concept*
   self-hostility
   defensive
   frustrated
   overly concerned of other person's impression
   embarrassed
   motivated to correct
   reaction to hearing self on tape

F. *Future Therapy Prognosis*

G. *Diagnosis*

H. *Recommendations*

quality or inflection, associated with the speaker's milieu. Because voice is associated with personality and culture, the clinician will realize that the "abnormality" may exist in the ear of the listener; that is, "strange" voices may be appropriate, and hence normal, in their owners' proper contexts.

Although the symptoms of a voice disorder can be accurately described by the trained speech pathologist, we must bear in mind the unequivocal observation of West and Ansberry (1968) that

> so many abnormalities of voice are symptoms of underlying pathologies that the cooperation of the speech clinician and physician is extremely important . . . . He [the speech clinician] should refer all patients for a final determination of procedures—therapy or no therapy (p. 366).

Fox (1978) lists five possible causes of vocal dysfunction. They are (1) vocal misuse or abuse, (2) structural abnormalities, (3) neurological abnormalities, (4) endocrine or other systemic disorders, and (5) psychological or environmental stress. Aronson (1978) suggests classifying voice disorders into two main groups: organic voice disorders and psychogenic voice disorders. It is necessary, therefore, to differentiate between those vocal problems that are due to an organic pathology and those that are essentially functional in nature. Fox (1978) points out that it requires the expertise of a number of specialties to effectively determine the "etiology, type, and the treatment of the vocal dysfunction" (p. 504). Therefore, the diagnostic interview should always include a laryngeal examination by a qualified physician, as Shanks and Duguay indicate in chapter 5, and as Boone (1977) indicates elsewhere.

The diagnostic procedures may be concerned with (1) an organic voice disorder, caused by defective structures of speech or (2) a functional one, caused by malfunction of normal structures. Those of the first type may accompany cerebral palsy, or occur as a result of laryngeal pathology. Loss of the larynx through surgical intervention for some purpose unrelated to speech is usually included in this classification. The functional disorders, which are equated with abuse or misuse of the phonatory structures with regard to pitch, loudness, and time of utterance, can lead to organic changes of the kind described by Shanks and Duguay in the first section of chapter 5. Misuse or abuse of the vocal cords and faulty training or maladaptive adjustment to the environment typically account for functional disorders.

Not only must the laryngologist have the primary responsibility for determining whether the function of the vocal apparatus is pathological, he or she also should determine the proper treatment approach. Under no circumstances should vocal therapy be initiated without the recommendations of the laryngologist, for it could have serious consequences if the condition behind the phonatory disability were a carcinoma or laryngeal papilloma.

Shanks and Duguay in chapter 5 suggest that phonatory disorders are best measured and understood by means of several analytical procedures. The first of these is a thorough analysis of the physiological characteristics and of phonation, including studies of air flow and air pressure; observation of the vocal folds and their physical characteristics; and neuromuscular analysis of laryngeal muscle function. In addition, they recommend psychological and auditory analyses of phonation, including the subjective impressions of pitch, loudness, and quality; the objective measurement of frequency, intensity, and duration of vocal behavior; and a final clinical analysis to suggest that maintaining the appropriate tension in laryngeal muscles during the respiratory-phonatory effort is the essence of normal phonation. They admit, however, that it is not always a simple matter to teach a client to correct an abnormal tension. The ability of the muscles to function properly can be affected by anything that changes the mass, size, or approximation characteristics of the vocal folds, including vocal nodules, polyps, ulcers, carcinomas, granulomas, laryngitis, and pubertal changes (Boone, 1977).

The Case Study. The factors pertinent to the diagnosis of many voice disorders may have been determined before the client is seen by the speech clinician, for often the suspected etiology and apparent pathology have been defined and, in some cases, surgery has already been carried out. When this is so, the speech clinician must still collect important information related to the medical factors, such as the type of problem, date of onset, and variability; and the date of any surgery, its extent, and postoperative complications. The clinician should also be concerned with the client's general physical condition, auditory behavior, emotional status, and such social factors as educational and vocational background. Boone (1977) has described the kinds of information that should be collected, and Morris and Spriestersbach (1978, pp. 218–220) have furnished an example of a form that can be used in recording the data. They include such items as onset and duration of the problem, incidents of vocal misuse, family history of voice and speech problems, medical problems including respiratory difficulties, and personal and social adjustment. Fox (1978) lists the broad categories of congenital or acquired structural differences, environmental or psychic stress, and hyper- or hypofunction of the phonatory mechanism as the differential diagnostic etiological factors. She notes that changes in vocal function may be a danger signal of significant importance thereby requiring a thorough case history to assess the "inter-relationships of vocal function and medical, physical, social, and psychological data" (p. 505). Figure 1–6 is a pre-therapy form used to summarize the pertinent findings of the diagnostic procedures.

Shames, Font, and Matthews (1963) have devised a questionnaire for extracting similar data from patients who will have to learn alaryngeal speech. Such data are necessary because, as Diedrich and Youngstrom (1966) have shown, the likelihood of success in these cases depends upon physical and psychological factors. From a negative standpoint, the most important psychological factors cited by Snidecor (1969) are depression and the fear of recurrence of cancer, and support for his view has been provided by Bisi and Conley (1965), Damste, Van den Berg, and Moolenaar-Bijl (1956), Stoll (1958), and others.

Objective and Semiobjective Instruments. The close relationship between the respiratory and phonatory functions suggests the importance of making some assessment of the patient's respiratory capability. Several methods are available: fluoroscopy and cinefluorography may be used to view the activity of the respiratory mechanism as a whole; X-ray techniques may be used to examine the movement of the diaphragm and thoracic cavity; kymographic and electromyographic recordings may be made to evaluate the thoracic and abdominal respiratory movements and the use of the muscles in breathing and during speech; and wet or dry spirometric readings may be used to determine lung capacity measurements, such as the vital and tidal capacities. Emerick and Hatten (1974) review six areas of concern requiring diagnostic assessment. They are air volume, respiratory type, respiratory rate and ratio, durational aspects, associated tension, and associated sounds (pp. 274–276). In addition, it is suggested that each of the vocal characteristics of pitch, loudness, and quality be evaluated.

The value of air flow studies for assessing aerodynamic competence has been stressed by Shanks and Duguay in chapter 5, although most authorities agree that no one type of breathing pattern produces a "best" voice quality. Moreover, there are no appropriate norms against which observations of breath control may be evaluated. The clinician can, however, infer such aerodynamic factors as nasal leakage and velopharyngeal sphincteric action from measurements of intraoral air pressure, obtained with the oral manometer or the spirometer, and of air flow, obtained with the pneumotachograph or a thermistor placed within the oral cavity.

The physical characteristics of the vocal cords may be observed with various

Figure 1–6. Pre-therapy Case Summary (Voice)
State University College at Buffalo
Speech-Language-Hearing Clinic
Dr. Marshall Duguay

Nature of Onset _____

Duration of Problem _____

Previous Therapy _____

Voice Quality _____

Relevant Medical History _____

Hearing Evaluation _____

PHONATION

	YES	NO
A. History of laryngeal pathology (growths, inflammations, chronic pain or tickling)	___	___
Complaint of "tired throat"	___	___
Evidence of "pinched throat" during phonation	___	___
Can you palpate the thyroid notch?	___	___
What is the effect of depression of thyroid notch on the voice?	___	___
What is the effect of tilting head to either side on the voice?	___	___
What is the effect of tilting head up or down on the voice?	___	___
Muscular contractions exhibited during phonation which are similar to those exhibited during swallowing	___	___

If the answer to any of the items above is yes, give the relevant details.

Does the speaker exhibit any of the following during phonation?
hard glottal attach_____ two-toned voice _____ infrequent pitch _____
breaks _____ frequent pitch breaks _____ phonation interspersed with
whispering _____ tremulous voice _____

Give the relevant details concerning any of the items that have been checked above:

Has speaker done any formal singing: Yes_____ No_____
If yes, what vocal part has he or she sung? (tenor, soprano, etc.)
Can the speaker sing up and down the musical scale? Yes_____ No_____
Can the speaker match a musical pitch? Yes_____ No_____
Can the speaker imitate inflectional patterns? Yes_____ No_____

ASSOCIATED VARIABLES

1. *Pitch:*
   Total range (number of tones including falsetto)

   Habitual pitch level (range)

   Natural pitch level (range)

   Number of tones habitual pitch level is above lowest tone

Inflection

Rate

2. *Pitch and Loudness:*
Quality changed under any of the following conditions:

If "yes"
describe the change

Sustained Vowels:
lower than habitual pitch level: Yes _____ No _____   _____
higher than habitual pitch level: Yes _____ No _____   _____
softer than habitual loudness level: Yes _____ No _____   _____
louder than habitual loudness level: Yes _____ No _____   _____
Oral Reading
softer than habitual loudness level: Yes _____ No _____   _____
louder than habitual loudness level: Yes _____ No _____   _____
Degree of "Harshness"
Does the degree of harshness of the vowels appear to be modified by certain adjacent consonants?
Yes _____ No _____
If yes, specify _____

3. *Non-Speech Activities:*
Does the patient's voice quality change when he or she:
Sighs
Coughs
Clears throat
Laughs
Grunts
Hums
Vocalizes a yawn
Describe the change:
Description of how voice is used in daily activities:

B. *Respiratory Mechanism:*
Breath supply and control appear to be adequate: Yes _____ No _____
*Is there any air "wastage"? Yes _____ No _____
Does he or she appear to be speaking on "residual air"? Yes _____ No _____
Any apparent muscular tensions of the chest and neck which appear to be related to faulty breath
supply and control? Yes _____ No _____
Describe and discuss any such deviations:
Vital Capacity _____

C. *Articulatory Mechanism:*
Activity of lips and jaws (extent of mouth opening) while speaking:
        immobile and clenched _____ slight movement _____ average movement _____
        above average movement _____
Quality when nostrils occluded during sustained phonation of vowels:
        changed _____ unchanged _____
Pressure ratio: nostrils open _____ nostrils occluded _____ ratio _____
Discuss the significance of any deviations noted above:

D. *Resonators:*
Size of velopharyngeal space: depth: shallow _____ normal _____ deep _____
                              width: narrow _____ normal _____ wide _____
Tonsils: none _____ small _____ moderately large _____ very large _____
Nasal obstructions: right nostril: none _____ some _____ complete _____
                    left nostril: none _____ some _____ complete _____
Discuss the significance of any deviations noted above:

        Palatal Sufficiency _____
        Palatal Mobility _____

E. *Posture:*
    Overall posture of the body generally adequate: Yes _____ No _____
    Head held in reasonably upright position during speaking: Yes _____ No _____
    Is the position of the larynx in the neck symmetrical: Yes _____ No _____
    If the answer to any of the items above is no, describe the deviation and discuss any possible relationships it may have to the voice problem.

F. *Miscellaneous—Physical:*
    Any evidence of post-nasal drip
    Allergies
    Smoking
    Mouth Breathing
    Other
    *Clinician may also wish to refer to Beckett's procedure for determining spirometric quotient, *JSHD*, February, 1971

PERSONAL AND SOCIAL ADJUSTMENT

What is the degree of obvious concern that the speaker has about his or her voice problem? None _____ Some _____ Marked _____

Does the language which the speaker uses tend to be well qualified, normally cautious, specific, or does it tend to be rigidly either-or-ish, absolute, inappropriate to the situation, etc.?

Does the speaker's interpretation of objective events tend to be competent, impersonal, factual, or does it tend to be exaggerated, self-defensive, vague, etc.?

Does the speaker tend to have a relaxed appearance, a smooth, rhythmical gait, firm handshake, direct gaze, or does he or she tend to appear physically tense, move jerkily, remain quietly at ease only with difficulty, refuse to look directly at the examiner, etc?

Does the speaker tend to appear hostile (curt, cryptic, indifferent), extremely dependent, generally insecure, or does he or she tend to appear cooperative, pleasant, helpful, interested, etc?

In talking about the voice problem itself is the speaker reticent, apologetic, embarrassed, depressed, and self-defensive, or does he or she discuss it freely in a forthright manner, with an interested, objective, problem-solving attitude?

Specify and discuss any other aspects of the speaker's behavior which appear to be indices of adjustment.

Do the speaker's maladjustments, if any, appear to be related largely to specific problems and situations or do they appear to be characteristic of his or her behavior generally? List any situations to which the speaker appears to adjust poorly.

How would you rate the speaker's overall adjustments?
    above average _____ average _____ below average _____

Ask the following questions; give ample time for response and then summarize response.
1. What do you think about your voice?

2. What do others think about your voice?

3. What kind of voices do you like? Dislike? Why?

4. What impression does your voice really make?

5. Should a man's voice be masculine?

6. Should a woman's voice be feminine?

7. What should a good voice be?

8. What kind of voice do you want?

9. How important is it to you to improve your voice?

radiographic and stroboscopic instruments. More recently, the oral panendoscope and fiber optic instruments have permitted indirect laryngoscopy and have gained wide usage, though some clinicians still prefer to use mirrors to view the vocal cords and adjacent structures.

Spectrographic recordings may be made to evaluate the fundamental frequency and some of the harmonics of the sound produced; and the level of achievement of the esophageal speaker may be determined by tests such as those of Berlin and Zobell (1963), Snidecor and Curry (1960), and Wepman, MacGahn, and Neilson (1953). They have all developed sets of norms or scales that can be used, but aside from these there are few objective scales for evaluating the status of the laryngectomee, or for predicting success in learning alaryngeal speech. Perhaps the developing interest in this area of remediation and the increase in the number of laryngectomees will provoke the invention of additional measures for making sound diagnostic judgments.

Informal Observation and Selected Tasks. During the diagnostic interview, the clinician should carefully observe and evaluate the pitch, quality, and intensity of the client's voice, as well as related problems with register and articulation. This is also the time to note the type of breathing pattern used (thoracic, clavicular, or abdominal) and the sites of muscular tension (neck, face, body, etc.). The clinician can assess the client's habitual pitch level by using a pitch pipe or piano or can use more accurate methods such as the PAD pitch meter (PAD Laboratories, 1962). To estimate optimum (most effective) pitch, Peterson and Marquardt (1981) describe eight different techniques used by clinicians including the Fairbanks (1960) twenty-five percent method. The thirty-three and one-third percent method described by Hahn, Lomas, and Vandraegan (1957) may also be used. The former places the optimum pitch at a point twenty-five percent up from the lowest pitch in the range and the latter places it thirty-three and one-third percent up from the lowest pitch in the total range, excluding falsetto. Two alternative methods have been described by Boone (1977). Peterson and Marquardt (1981) also mention less elaborate procedures described by Murphy (1964) and Boone (1977). They include such sound-producing behaviors as "grunting," "coughing," sighing," "yawning," and saying "ah" or "uh-huh."

Informal observations and judgments of the client's performance of selected tasks may yield useful insights for formulating and initiating a remedial progam. They may help to identify factors responsible for an imbalance in laryngeal muscle activity which need correction, or—in the case of laryngectomees—they may indicate how well a patient can produce alaryngeal sound so that the clinician can proceed from there in tailoring speech instruction to individual capabilities.

Diagnostic Procedures for Hearing Impairment

A person with severe hearing loss associated with damage to the auditory nerve may have difficulties with articulation, language, and phonation. The greater the degree of hearing impairment, the more likely it is that each of the other parameters of communication behavior will become impaired. For example, a deaf child can acquire neither language nor speech without some remedial effort, while a child whose hearing loss is only partial may—if the loss is of certain kinds—experience only articulation difficulties. For the adult who suffers a complete hearing loss remedial effort must be initiated to prevent deterioration of speech. The consequences of hearing loss may extend beyond the immediate area of communication difficulties. As Myklebust (1964) has observed, visuomotor, intellectual, and learning impairments may accompany the hearing loss, and the diagnostic procedure should attempt to assess these parameters of behavior as well.

It is not practical to attempt in this book a review of all of the contributions of audiologists to the remediation of hearing impairments. Perhaps it is enough to say that the audiological practitioner is often the one who, in conjunction with the otologist, has the major responsibility for evaluating auditory behavior in a way that will enable the remediation specialist and others to understand a given case and the consequences of auditory impairment for communication. The audiologist uses a battery of diagnostic tests as the basis for making specific remedial recommendations; for example, the data gathered may suggest the need for special educational placement, use of amplification, lipreading instruction, auditory training, language training, or speech training. If any of these recommendations are to be made with confidence, a thorough evaluation of the patient is essential.

The discussion of the deaf and hard of hearing by Lowell and Pollack in chapter 9 stresses key factors in remediation: the patient's age at onset of the hearing loss, the etiological factors, the type and configuration of the loss, and the presence or absence of other handicaps—all will have a definite bearing on the patient's development of communication skills and response to remedial efforts. In that chapter, which focuses on auditory remediation and remedial practices for the deaf, the authors distinguish between the deaf and the hard of hearing. They present remediation programs suitable for children who are completely deaf and must be taught to "hear" primarily with their other senses, and for those who have some usable hearing and must be taught by emphasizing the development of auditory skills.

The Case Study. The case study interview should include, besides the routine medical history questions, specific questions and tests pertaining to auditory behavior. If the patient is a child, the responses to such acoustic stimuli as the ringing of a bell or the sound of a car horn are of diagnostic interest.

Special attention should be paid to any illnesses, such as rubella and chronic otitis media, that are often related etiologically to reduced hearing; and in addition, note should be made of any familial history of deafness. This attention to a child's developmental history is essential because failure to respond to language and delay in speaking may be associated not only with severe hearing loss, but also with such other disorders as mental retardation, autism, and central nervous system impairment.

Murphy and Shallop (1978) suggest that a developmental assessment be made prior to testing and should include a study of the child's motor abilities and general alertness. They state that much of the child's behavior can be observed while taking the case history. They recommend that the person taking the case history should be the professional who also administers the test and interprets results. They also suggest a team evaluation of a child suspected of having a severe hearing loss, using psychological, educational, social, medical, speech-language, and audiological evaluations, as appropriate.

A careful case history will help the diagnostician differentiate among possible etiologies, for, as Myklebust (1954) has pointed out, such factors as the patient's age at the onset of the hearing impairment are "influential in determining the symptomatology and [serve] as a background against which the diagnostic possibilities can be evaluated" (p. 35). Myklebust has stressed the need to investigate the types of response shown by the patient because of their etiological implications. Thus, if a child's parents report that there are evidences of inconsistencies of response—responding at times to faint sounds, but at other times, not to even very loud ones—there may be a central auditory disorder such as receptive aphasia.

Objective and Semiobjective Instruments. Many of the instruments used for assessing auditory integrity have been shown to have satisfactory validity, reliability, and standardization norms. The standard battery of such tests includes the pure tone audiometric test and speech audiometric tests.

Various workers have adapted some of these tests for young children. For example, Dix and Hallpike (1947) have reported on the "peepshow" procedure, which is an adaptation of the pure tone test, and other adaptations of speech audiometry for children have been made by Keaster (1947); Siegenthaler, Pearson, and Lezak (1954); and Sortini and Flake (1953). Electrophysiological techniques such as the EDR (electrodermal response) and the EEG have been used with children, and Frisina has discussed their reliability and validity in Jerger's *Modern Developments in Audiology* (1963). Jerger (1978) aptly identified the major developments within recent times that have influenced the assessment of hearing function, especially in children. Impedance assessment and evoked response audiometry have added immeasurably to the evaluation of hearing disorders. Brain stem evoked responses (BSER) and sensitivity predictions from acoustic reflex measurements (SPAR) have enabled audiologists to add to their diagnostic battery in an effort to estimate hearing sensitivity loss independent of behavioral audiometric procedures for difficult-to-test patients. Murphy and Shallop (1978) review other procedures designed to estimate hearing levels for children who present problems in testing. Included in this battery are the sound localization tests, visual reinforcement audiometry (VRA), tangible reinforcer operant conditioning audiometry (TROCA), and play audiometry. We would be remiss if we would not refer to the third major development Jerger (1978) referred to as part of the diagnostic battery and that is the addition of speech tests as part of the "site of lesion" testing. Included among the more recent speech tests are the synthetic sentence identification test (SSI—Jerger, Speaks, and Trammell, 1968), the staggered spondaic word test (SSW—Katz, 1968), and the performance versus intensity for PB (phonetically balanced) words (PI-PB—Jerger, 1973). Jerger (1973) identified a diagnostic test battery in order to differentiate various sites of hearing pathology. In addition to the tests mentioned above, he included Bekesy audiometry, short increment sensitivity index

(SISI), alternate binaural loudness balance test (ABLB), and tests for tone decay. Electronystagmography and filtered speech tests may also be used as part of the audiological diagnostic battery, when appropriate.

A word should also be said for the neonatal hearing evaluation techniques being used in many nurseries throughout the country by audiologists. Altman et al. (1975) developed the "Accelerometer Recording System" (ARS) to detect the responses of infants to auditory stimulation at 90dB SPL at the ear of the infant, for a signal 500 msec. duration. Simmons and Russ (1974) developed the "crib-o-gram," a technique designed to detect changes in motor activity of infants after auditory stimulation. Downs and Steritt (1967) developed a technique for neonatal hearing screening which is very popular. They used a 3 kHz tone of 90dB SPL with a 100 dB SPL used if no responses are elicited. The clarity of the infant's response is graded on a five-point scale, and children suspected of having a hearing loss are scheduled for further evaluation (auditory brain stem response, ABR).

Anderson and Davis (1978) note that there are no language tests specifically designed to evaluate the language ability of hearing-impaired children. They point out some necessary safeguards that should be taken if available standardized tests are used. Among them are avoiding visual cues and structuring and controlling the testing environment.

Factors which may affect a child's auditory behavior—such as social maturity and mental and motor capacity—are most often evaluated by using one or more of the standard psychological tests for which their authors have attempted to demonstrate validity, reliability, and standardization norms. The safeguards mentioned by Anderson and Davis (1978) should be taken for these tests as well.

Informal Observation and Selected Tasks. While objective tests may provide a wealth of quantitative data concerning a child's auditory behavior and the mental, social, emotional, and linguistic capacities related to it, a full and insightful understanding of the hearing-impaired child requires observation of spontaneous behavior.

Myklebust (1954) has suggested evaluation of auditory behavior during spontaneous play and has described a few techniques for assessing auditory behavior informally:

1. Sound Instrument and Toy Test;
2. Imitation of Vocalization Test;
3. Voice Test;
4. Verbal Comprehension Test;
5. Sound-Field tests; and
6. Tests of Auditory Perception (Music and Voice).

The Myklebust text is also a source for a group of selected tasks, drawn from several standardized mental tests, which can be used to assess the intellectual growth of young children with auditory disorders; it lists specific behaviors that are indicative of emotional adjustment and that may be observed as a child engages in spontaneous play with people, with toys, and alone. Northern and Downs (1978) suggest the use of a screening checklist developed by the Committee on Children with Handicaps, American Academy of Pediatrics (p. 125). The checklist is for infants from one month to five years to assess major developmental patterns. They offer a number of procedures for observing responses to auditory stimuli introduced into the young child's environment. Murphy and Shallop (1978) describe the maturation of infants in four stages. These stages provide a basis for further observation of children's responses to sound sources and hearing acuity.

The use of standardized tests, the case study, and a careful analysis of the child's spontaneous behavior and responses to a variety of tasks related to auditory behavior should afford the diagnostician the best possible means of making an accurate estimate of the auditory integrity of the child. This estimate, in turn, should permit planning of the most effective remedial program.

SUMMARY

We have applied the term "diagnosis" essentially to a questioning procedure in which the clinician, acting as a listener and a collator of information, engages in a sequence of processes. That is, the clinician collects pertinent information in the case study, assesses the symptom complex through testing and observation, relates the speech and language differences to etiological factors for purposes of discovering causes and making a prognosis for improvement, and, finally, outlines remedial techniques and treatments.

The initial general discussion was followed by two case studies that illustrated problems in differential diagnosis. One case in particular, that of three-year-old Matthew, showed how the diagnostic-remedial process can take cognizance of and serve the needs of the whole person in relation to the milieu. The evaluation, for instance, took into account the child's readiness for therapy and the family situation as well; specific recommendations relating to educational and social activities and medical examinations were delayed to give the child a chance to mature; and assurance and support were given to the parents throughout the entire period.

In the second section of this chapter we applied the principles of diagnosis to the five problem areas of language and articulation disorders, stuttering, voice disorders, and hearing impairments. For each of them we discussed the kinds of information essential to the case study, the kinds of objective and semiobjective tests that are particularly appropriate, and the kinds of informal observations and selected tasks that are useful in certain circumstances. In so doing, we referred the reader to later chapters where fuller treatment of techniques may be found.

A number of times, we have indicated a preference for tests which we have found to be especially useful. While this implies that a clinician may rely more heavily on some testing procedures than on others, it does not deny the obligation to know as much as possible about all current testing procedures. Only by continually reviewing the literature and becoming familiar with the characteristics and purposes of the various diagnostic tools available can we make the best choice among them for application to a given set of circumstances.

BIBLIOGRAPHY

Altman, M., Shenhav, R., and Schaudinschky, L., Semi-objective method for auditory mass screening of neonates, *Acta Otolaryngologica*, **79,** 46–50 (1975).
Anderson, C. V., and Davis, J. M., The appraisal of auditory functioning. In F. L. Darley and D. C.

Spriestersbach (Eds.), *Diagnostic Methods in Speech Pathology*. (2nd ed.) New York: Harper and Row (1978).

Aronson, A. E., Differential diagnosis of organic and psychogenic voice disorders. In F. L. Darley and D. C. Spriestersbach (Eds.), *Diagnostic Methods in Speech Pathology*. (2nd ed.) New York: Harper and Row (1978).

Bangs, T. E., *Language and Learning Disorders of the Pre-Academic Child*. New York: Appleton-Century-Crofts, Inc. (1968).

Berlin, C., and Zobell, D. H., Clinical measurement during the acquisition of esophaegeal speech. II. An unexpected dividend. *J. Speech Hearing Dis.*, **28,** 389–392 (1963).

Bisi, R. H., and Conley, J. J., Psychological factors influencing vocal rehabilitation of the post-laryngectomized patient. *A.M.A. Ann. Otol. Rhinol. Laryngol.*, **67,** 1073–1078 (1965).

Bloom, L., and Lahey, M., *Language Development and Language Disorders*. New York: John Wiley (1978).

Boone, D. R., *The Voice and Voice Therapy*. (2nd ed.) Englewood Cliffs, N.J.: Prentice-Hall, Inc. (1977).

Brutten, E. J., and Shoemaker, D. J., *The Modification of Stuttering*. Englewood Cliffs, N.J.: Prentice-Hall, Inc. (1967).

Brutten, G., and Shoemaker, D., *Speech Situation Checklist*. Carbondale, Ill.: Southern Illinois University (1974a).

Brutten, G., and Shoemaker, D., *Behavior Checklist*. Carbondale, Ill.: Southern Illinois University (1974b).

Brutten, G., and Shoemaker D., *The Southern Illinois Modification of the Geer Fear Survey Schedule*. Carbondale, Ill.: Southern Illinois University (1974c).

Buros, O. K., *Mental Measurements Yearbook*. Highland Park, N.J.: Gryphon Press (1975).

Byrne, M., Appraisal of child language acquisition. In F. L. Darley and D. C. Spriestersbach (Eds.), *Diagnostic Methods in Speech Pathology*. (2nd ed.) New York: Harper and Row (1978).

Carroll, J. B., Language acquisition, bilingualism, and language change. In S. Saporta (Ed.), *Psycholinguistics: A Book of Readings*. New York: Holt, Rinehart & Winston, Inc. (1961).

Cooper, E. B., The development of a stuttering chronicity prediction checklist: A preliminary report. *Jr. Speech and Hearing Dis.*, **38,** 215–223 (1973).

Counihan, D. L., Articulation skills of adolescents and adults with cleft palate. *J. Speech Hearing Dis.*, **25,** 181–187 (1960).

Crabtree, M., *The Houston Test for Language Development*. Houston: Houston Test Company (1963).

Crystal, D., Fletcher, P., and Garman, M., *The Grammatical Analysis of Language Disability: A Procedure for Assessment and Remediation*. New York: Elsevier Publishing Co., Inc. (1976).

Damsté, P. H., Van den Berg, J. W., and Moolenaar-Bijl, A., Why are some patients unable to learn esophageal speech? *Ann. Otolaryngol. Rhinol. Laryngol.*, **65,** 998 (1956).

Darley, F. L., *Diagnosis and Appraisal of Communication*. Englewood Cliffs, N.J.: Prentice-Hall Inc. (1964).

Darley, F. L., Appraisal of articulation. In F. L. Darley and D. C. Spriestersbach (Eds.), *Diagnostic Methods in Speech Pathology*. (2nd ed.) New York: Harper and Row, (1978).

Darley, F. L., Differential diagnosis of language disorders. In F. L. Darley and D. C. Spriestersbach, *Diagnostic Methods in Speech Pathology*. (2nd ed.) New York: Harper and Row, (1978).

De Renzi, E., and Vignolo, L. A., The Token Test: A sensitive test to detect receptive disturbances in aphasics. *Brain*, **85,** 665–678 (1962).

Dickson, S., Clinical judgment of language delay and I.T.P.A. measurements. *Journal of Communication Disorders*, **6,** 35–40 (1967).

Diedrich, W. M., and Youngstrom, K. C., *Alaryngeal Speech*. Springfield, Ill.: Charles C. Thomas (1966).

DiSimoni, F., *The Token Test for Children*. Bingham, Mass.: Teaching Resources (1979).

Dix, M., and Hallpike, C., The peep show: A new technique for pure tone audiometry in young children. *Brit. Med. J.*, **2,** 719 (1947).

Downs, M. P., and Steritt, G. M., A guide to newborn and infant screening programs. *Arch. of Otolaryngology*, **85,** 15–22 (1967).

Dunn, L., *Peabody Picture Vocabulary Test, Revised*. Minneapolis: American Guidance Service, Inc. (1980).

Eisenson, J., *Examining for Aphasia*. (Rev. ed.) New York: The Psychological Corporation (1954).

Emerick, L. L., and Hatten, J. T., *Diagnosis and Evaluation in Speech Pathology*. Englewood Cliffs, New Jersey: Prentice-Hall, Inc. (1974).

Fairbanks, G., *Voice and Articulation Drillbook*. (2nd ed.) New York: Harper & Row (1960).

Fisher, H., and Logemann, J., *The Fisher-Logemann Test of Articulation Competence*. Boston: Houghton Mifflin Company (1970).

Fox, D. R., Evaluation of voice problems. In S. Singh and J. Lynch (Eds.), *Diagnostic Procedures in Hearing, Speech, and Language*. Baltimore: Univ. Park Press (1978).

Frisina, A., Measurement of hearing in children. In J. Jerger (Ed.), *Modern Developments in Audiology*. New York: Academic Press (1963).

Goldman, R., and Fristoe, M., *Goldman-Fristoe Test of Articulation*. Circle Pines, Minn.: American Guidance Service, Inc. (1969).

Goldman, R., Fristoe, M., and Woodcock, R., *Goldman-Fristoe-Woodcock Test of Auditory Discrimination*. Circle Pines, Minn.: American Guidance Service, Inc. (1970).

Haeussermann, E., *Evaluating the Developmental Level of Pre-School Children Handicapped by Cerebral Palsy*. New York: United Cerebral Palsy Association (1952).

Haeussermann, E., *Developmental Potential of Pre-School Children*. New York: Grune & Stratton, Inc. (1958).

Hahn, E., Lomas, D. E., Hargis, D., and Vandraegen, D., *Basic Voice Training for Speech*. New York: McGraw-Hill (1957).

Halstead, W. C., and Wepman, J. M., *Manual for the Halstead-Wepman Screening Test for Aphasia*. Chicago: University of Chicago Clinics (1949).

Hardy, W. G., On language disorders in young children: A reorganization of thinking. *J. Speech Hearing Dis.*, **30**, 3–16 (1965).

Head, H., *Aphasia and Kindred Disorders of Speech*. New York: Hafner Publishing Co., Inc. (1963).

Hejna, R., *Developmental Articulation Test*. Storrs: University of Connecticut (1955).

Hood, S. B., The assessment of fluency disorders. In S. Singh and J. Lynch (Eds.), *Diagnostic Procedures in Hearing, Speech, and Language*. Baltimore: Univ. Park Press (1978).

Hutchinson, B. B., Hanson, M. L., and Mecham, M. J., *Diagnostic Handbook of Speech Pathology*. Baltimore: The Williams and Wilkins Co. (1979).

Jakobson, R., Fant, C., and Halle, M., *Preliminaries to Speech Analysis: The Distinctive Features and Their Correlates*. (2nd ed.) Cambridge, Mass.: The M.I.T. Press (1952).

Jerger, J., Diagnostic audiometry. In J. Jerger (Ed.), *Modern Developments in Audiology*. (2nd ed.) New York: Academic Press (1973).

Jerger, J., Introduction. In S. Singh and J. Lynch (Eds.), *Diagnostic Procedures in Hearing, Speech, and Language*. Baltimore: Univ. Park Press (1978).

Jerger, J., Speaks, C., and Trammell, J. L., A new approach to speech audiometry. *Jr. Speech and Hearing Dis.*, **33**, 318–28 (1968).

Johnson, W., Brown, S. F., Curtis, J. F., Edney, C. W., and Keaster, J., *Speech Handicapped School Children*. (3rd ed.) New York: Harper and Row (1967).

Johnson, W., Darley, F. L., and Spriestersbach, D. C., *Diagnostic Methods in Speech Pathology*. New York: Harper & Row (1963).

Johnson, W., and Knott, J. R., The distribution of moments of stuttering in successive readings of the same material. *J. Speech Dis.*, **2**, 17–19 (1937).

Katz, J., The SSW Test: An interim report. *Jr. Speech and Hearing Disorders*, **33**, 132–146 (1968).

Keaster, J. A., A quantitative method of testing the hearing of young children. *J. Speech Dis.*, **12**, 159–160 (1947).

Kirk, S., McCarthy, J., and Kirk, W., *The Illinois Test of Psycholinguistic Abilities*. (Rev. ed.) Urbana: University of Illinois Press (1968).

Lee, L., *The Northwestern Syntax Screening Test*. Evanston, Ill.: Northwestern University Press (1969).

Lee, L. L., *Developmental Sentence Analysis*. Evanston, Ill.: Northwestern University Press (1974).

Lerea, L., *The Michigan Picture Language Inventory*. Ann Arbor: University of Michigan Press (1958).

Longerich, M., and Bordeaux, J., *Aphasia Therapeutics*. New York: Macmillan (1959).

Lynch, J., Evaluation of linguistic disorders in children. In S. Singh and J. Lynch (Eds.), *Diagnostic Procedures in Hearing, Speech, and Language*. Baltimore: University Park Press (1978).

MacDonald, J., *Environmental Language Inventory*. Columbus: Charles E. Merrill Pub. Co. (1978).

McDonald, E., *A Deep Test of Articulation*. Pittsburgh: Stanwix House, Inc. (1964).

McDonald, F., and Chance, B., *Cerebral Palsy*. Englewood Cliffs, N.J.: Prentice-Hall, Inc. (1964).

Mecham, M., *The Verbal Language Development Scale*. Minneapolis: American Guidance Service, Inc. (1959).

Mecham, M., Jex, J., and Jones, J., *The Utah Test of Language Development*. (Rev. ed.) Salt Lake City: Communication Research Associates (1967).

Menyuk, P., The role of distinctive features in children's acquisition of phonology. *J. Speech Hearing Res.*, **11**, 138–146 (1968).

Michel, L. I., Evaluation of articulatory disorders: Traditional approach. In S. Singh and J. Lynch (Eds.), *Diagnostic Procedures in Hearing, Speech, and Language*. Baltimore: University Park Press (1978).

Morris, H. L., and Spriestersbach, D. C., Appraisal of respiration and phonation. In F. L. Darley and

D. C. Spriestersbach, (Eds.) *Diagnostic Methods in Speech Pathology.* (2nd ed.) New York: Harper and Row (1978).

Morris, H. L., Spriestersbach, D. C., and Darley, F. L., An articulation test for assessing competency of velopharyngeal closure. *J. Speech Hearing Dis.*, **4,** 48–55 (1961).

Muma, J. R., Language assessment: The co-occurring and restricted structure procedure. *Acta Symbolica,* **4,** 12–29 (1973).

Murphy, A., *Functional Voice Disorders.* Englewood Cliffs, New Jersey: Prentice-Hall, Inc., (1964).

Murphy, K. P., and Shallop, J. K., Identification of hearing loss in young children: Prenatal to age six. In S. Singh and J. Lynch (Eds.), *Diagnostic Procedures in Hearing, Speech, and Language.* Baltimore: Univ. Park Press (1978).

Myklebust, H., *Auditory Disorders in Children.* New York: Grune & Stratton, Inc. (1954).

Myklebust, H., *The Psychology of Deafness.* New York: Grune & Stratton, Inc. (1964).

Northern, J. L., and Downs, M. P., *Hearing in Children.* (2nd ed.) Baltimore: Williams and Wilkins Co. (1978).

PAD Pitchmeter. Cleveland, Ohio: PAD Laboratories (1962).

Pendergast, K., Dickey, S. E., Selmar, J. W., and Soder, A. L., *Photo Articulation Test.* Danville, Illinois: Interstate Printers and Publishers (1969).

Peterson, H. A., and Marquardt, T. P., *Appraisal and Diagnosis of Speech and Language Disorders.* Englewood Cliffs, New Jersey: Prentice-Hall, Inc. (1981).

Philips, B. J., and Bzoch, K., Reliability of judgments of articulation of cleft palate speakers. *Cleft Palate J.,* **6,** 24–34 (1969).

Porch, B., *Porch Index of Communicative Ability.* Palo Alto, Calif.: Consulting Psychologists (1967).

Rees, N. S., Art and science of diagnosis in hearing, language, and speech. In S. Singh and J. Lynch (Eds.), *Diagnostic Procedures in Hearing, Speech, and Language.* Baltimore: University Park Press (1978).

Riley, G. D., A stuttering severity instrument for children and adults. *Jr. of Speech and Hearing Dis.*, **37,** 314–322 (1972).

Rinegel, R. L., The clinician and the researcher: An artificial dichotomy. *Asha,* **14,** 351–353 (1972).

Schuell, H., *The Minnesota Test for Differential Diagnosis of Aphasia.* (Rev. ed.) Minneapolis: University of Minnesota Press (1965).

Schuell, H., A re-evaluation of the short examination of aphasia. *J. Speech Hearing Dis.*, **31,** 137–147 (1967).

Schultz, M. C., The bases of speech pathology and audiology: Evaluation as the resolution of uncertainty. *J. Speech Hearing Dis.,* **38,** 147–155 (1973).

Semel, M., and Wiig, E., *Clinical Evaluation of Language Functions.* Columbus: Charles E. Merrill Publishing Co. (1980).

Shames, G., Font, J., and Matthews, J., Factors related to the speech proficiency of the laryngectomized. *J. Speech Hearing Dis.*, **28,** 273–287 (1963).

Shames, G., and Sherrick, G. E., Discussion of non-fluency and stuttering as operant behavior. *J. Speech Hearing Dis.*, **28,** 3–18 (1963).

Sherman, D., *Iowa Scale for Rating Severity of Stuttering.* Danville, Ill.: Interstate Printers and Publishers (1952).

Siegenthaler, B., Pearson, J., and Lezak, R., A speech reception threshold test for children. *J. Speech Hearing Dis.*, **17,** 360–366 (1954).

Simmons, F. B., and Reuss, F. N., Automated newborn hearing screening, the crib-o-gram. *Arch. of Otolaryngology,* **100,** 1–7 (1974).

Snidecor, J. C. (Ed.), *Speech Rehabilitation of the Laryngectomized.* (2nd ed.) Springfield, Ill.: Charles C. Thomas (1969).

Snidecor, J. C., and Curry, R., How effectively can a laryngectomee expect to speak. *Laryngoscope,* **70,** 62–67 (1960).

Sortini, A., and Flake, C. G., Speech audiometry testing for preschool children. *Laryngoscope,* **63,** 991–997 (1953).

Stevens, G. D., and Birch, J. W., A proposal for clarification of the terminology used to describe brain injured children. In E. C. Frierson and W. B. Barbe (Eds.), *Educating Children with Learning Disabilities: Selected Readings.* New York: Appleton-Century-Crofts, Inc. (1967).

Stoll, B., Psychological factors determining the success or failure of the rehabilitation program. *Ann. Otolaryngol. Rhinol. Laryngol.,* **67,** 550–557 (1958).

Taylor, J. A., A personality scale of manifest anxiety. *J. Abnorm. Soc. Psychol.,* **48,** 285–290 (1953).

Templin, M., *Templin Sound Discrimination Tests.* Minneapolis: University of Minnesota Press (1943).

Templin, M., and Darley, F., *Templin Darley Tests of Articulation*. Iowa City: Bureau of Educational Research and Service, The University of Iowa (1968).

Van Hattum, R. J., Diagnosis of communication disorders. *Seminars in Speech, Language, and Hearing*. New York: Thieme-Stratton Inc., VI, No. 1, Feb. (1981).

Van Riper, C., *The Nature of Stuttering*. Englewood Cliffs, N.J.: Prentice-Hall, Inc. (1971).

Van Riper, C., *Speech Correction: Principles and Methods*. (5th ed.) Englewood Cliffs, N.J.: Prentice-Hall, Inc. (1972).

Van Riper, C., and Erickson, R., *Predictive Screening Test of Articulation*. Kalamazoo, Michigan: Western Michigan University, Continuing Education Office (1973).

Wechsler, D., *The Wechsler Intelligence Scale for Children, Revised*. New York: The Psychological Corporation (1967).

Wechsler, D., *Wechsler Preschool and Primary Scale of Intelligence*. New York: The Psychological Corporation (1967).

Weiner, F. F., and Bernthal, J., Articulation feature assessment. In S. Singh and J. Lynch (Eds.), *Diagnostic Procedures in Hearing, Speech, and Language*. Baltimore: Univ. Park Press, (1978).

Welsh, G. S., and Dahlstrom, W. G., *Basic Readings on the Minnesota Multiphasic Personality Inventory in Psychology and Medicine*. Minneapolis: University of Minnesota Press (1956).

Wepman, J. M., MacGahn, J. A., and Neilson, J. R., Objective measurement of progressive esophageal speech. *J. Speech Hearing Dis.*, **18**, 247–251 (1953).

West, R., and Ansberry, M., *Rehabilitation of Speech*. (4th ed.) New York: Harper and Row (1968).

Westlake, H., and Rutherford, D., *Cleft Palate*. Englewood Cliffs, N.J.: Prentice-Hall, Inc. (1966).

Williams, D. E., The problem of stuttering. In F. L. Darley and D. C. Spriestersbach (Eds.), *Diagnostic Methods in Speech Pathology*. (2nd ed.) New York: Harper and Row (1978).

Winitz, H., *Articulatory Acquisition and Behavior*. New York: Appleton-Century-Crofts, Inc. (1969).

Woolf, G., The assessment of stuttering as struggle, avoidance, and expectancy. *British Jr. Disorders of Communication*, **2**, 158–171 (1967).

2 Language Remediation in Children

Russell J. Love
Bertha Smith Clark
Freeman E. McConnell

Disorders of communication cannot be considered separately from disorders of language, since communication and language are highly interdependent functions. Although communication may be defined simply as an interaction that occurs between living organisms, the more common connotation (and the one underlying this discussion) is that communication occurs through some form of *verbal interaction* between two or more people. Thus, verbal communication employs heard, spoken, read, or written language, which is comprised of words having a symbolic meaning to the human primate who hears them. Because it is a purely human method of communicating ideas, feelings, and desires by means of a system of voluntarily produced symbols, it transcends the animal limitation of communication to the here and now.

Language as a form of human behavior has a specific biological foundation. It is present in all cultures of the world; it is age-correlated in all cultures; and it has only one acquisition strategy, which is the same for all babies everywhere in the world (Lenneberg, 1969). It also may be impaired specifically by brain lesions which may leave other mental and motor skills relatively unaffected. It is developmental, like physical growth, in that it correlates better with motor development than with chronological age. Hence, language may be said to be inherent in the child's maturation, and the appropriate environment triggers and enhances a process which has been anticipated in millions of years of evolutionary development.

THE NORMAL DEVELOPMENT OF LANGUAGE

Principles of language remediation, with which we shall deal later, can be better applied to children with disordered, delayed, or different language if normal language development is first explained.

50

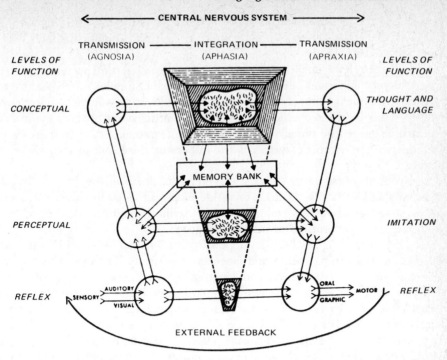

CENTRAL NERVOUS SYSTEM

TRANSMISSION ——— INTEGRATION ——— TRANSMISSION
(AGNOSIA)   (APHASIA)   (APRAXIA)

LEVELS OF   LEVELS OF
FUNCTION   FUNCTION

CONCEPTUAL   THOUGHT AND
                                             LANGUAGE

MEMORY BANK

PERCEPTUAL   IMITATION

REFLEX   SENSORY AUDITORY   ORAL MOTOR   REFLEX
                   VISUAL   GRAPHIC

EXTERNAL FEEDBACK

Figure 2–1. A Receptive-Expressive Language Model

Receptive-Expressive Language Models

Figure 2–1 presents a language model originally devised by Wepman, Jones, Bock, and VanPelt (1960), in which the central nervous system (CNS) incorporates at least a three-part system of language components: (1) an *input* system specific to the sense modalities (vision and audition in particular); (2) an *output* system, also specific to the motor modalities of oral (or spoken) language and graphics (or written language); and (3) an integrating and mediating system between the input and output systems, which may be referred to as the *symbolic* system and in any degree could adversely affect communicative language functioning.

As Wepman et al. explain their model, the ear and the eye are the two sensory receptors (lower left in Figure 2–1), forming the periphery of the input transmission system. Moving up, the diagram depicts several levels of CNS functions.

The lowest level is primarily *reflexive*, such as the startle reflex shown by infants a few weeks old when loud sounds are presented near the ear. Although such a stimulus may pass through the CNS in order to mediate the motor-action corollary of the response, there is no recall nor use made of memory, and no apparent trace within the system.

When an input stimulus reaches the next higher level of transmission, the *echoing* level, the organism transmits percepts that leave their trace on the memory bank but have no meaning to the individual. An example is the echoic language of infants, which merely parrots the input stimulus. The central process provides the necessary transmission from the decoding (receptive handling) to the encoding (expressive processing) of the message in terms of previously learned patterns. The higher-order process of conceptualization is not required in repeating auditory stimuli nor in copying printed stimuli.

At the highest level in the transmission system is *conceptual* functioning, which leads to the very important integrative process where the stimulus is freed of its input modality. The mediation which now occurs results in a conscious selection of language symbols (the semantic process) and the articulation of those symbols in connected language (the syntactic process). This integration of the two transmission modalities via the symbolic system is the important third link in communicative language.

There will, of course, be a close relation and feedback among the three levels, both horizontally and vertically. Damage or maldevelopment along the input side would limit the stimuli reaching the cerebral cortex; such limiting in turn would be reflected in the integrative and output functions of language.

A second model (figure 2–2) developed by Nation and Aram (1977) provides needed detail concerning speech and language processing. The model shows three major components: (1) a speech and language environmental component, which identifies the various levels of processing in both speech and language input; (2) an internal speech and language processing component, which illustrates how receptive auditory functions relate to expressive speech production functions at various levels of processing; and (3) a speech and language product component which indicates levels of critical processing in speech and language output. The terminology of this model matches current linguistic analysis and psychological processing theory and adds newer detail about probable processing mechanisms for speech and language not found in the Wepman model. The terms used in this chapter are generally those used in the Nation and Aram model.

The Developmental Sequence

Although the study of communicative disorders has given considerably more attention to the expressive than the receptive aspects of language, it is clear that language comprehension must precede production in the earliest stages of language development. The implications of this observation for therapy will be dealt with later in this chapter. For the present, we are concerned principally with the developmental sequence.

Receptive Language Development. Audition plays a pervasive role in receiving and sending information from the very beginning of life. The newborn child enters the world with a hearing mechanism capable of responding immediately to sound stimuli. Eisenberg and Friedlander (1970) have shown that the infant, from the first day of life, can actively regulate auditory stimulus events; thus, the individual is not simply a passive recipient of external forces. On the contrary, the child's attempts at preverbal language in these first weeks and months of life outwardly manifest the need to become a communicating member of the family unit. Parents who recognize this need and provide positive reinforcement of these preverbal attempts enhance their child's verbal language development.

In the first weeks of life the infant will respond reflexively to a variety of sounds, particularly those that are sudden and loud. Selective listening begins soon, however, along with the ability to differentiate between moods and emotional values in the

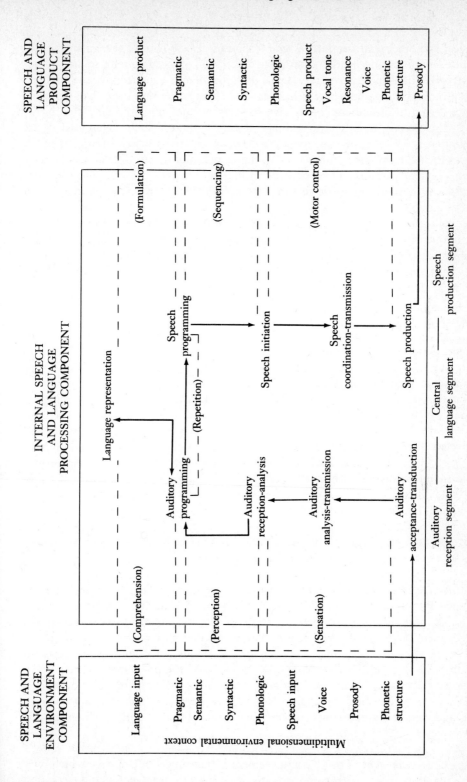

Figure 2-2. Speech and language processing model

voices of those around the child. When the infant coos and smiles in response to a person talking in a soothing voice next to the ear, he or she is reflecting a state of physical and emotional comfort. These responses also show that the infant has developed an auditory perception, that is, an association of meaning with sound source. These perceptions increase rapidly, expanding the infant's knowledge of the environment through the distance sense of hearing while yet restricted to the crib or playpen. Data reported by Eisenberg (1976) have shown that human infants can, from birth, respond selectively to different auditory signals, although such differential signal recognition is less refined than the acoustic discriminations which become possible later in their development. Infants as young as one month can discriminate among certain phonetic parameters of speech, according to Eimas (1975), who suggested they possess a system of "linguistic feature detectors" that are progressively adapted to speech sounds.

By the age of six months, children have learned to move their eyes to locate sound and, frequently, to vocalize in response to the intonations of others' voices. Their first vocalizations consist primarily of vowel sounds, sometimes combined with more easily made consonant sounds, such as /m/ and /b/. In the second six months, speech sounds gradually begin to acquire meaning associated with past experiences. The year-old child is able to respond globally to simple instructions, such as "Show me your nose," or "Go get your teddy bear," even though the ability to produce such a complexity of syntax or even to recognize the verbal components individually is not present. Between eighteen months to two years of age, most children enjoy listening to nursery rhymes because of their rhythmic patterns, even though little or none of the verbal meaning is comprehended. These prosodic features of language are important at this stage, and children around eighteen months imitate them in their own jargon, which is a personal version of the connected speech of adults. Not until children are about three years old can they be expected to follow simple stories and connected discourse through the auditory modality alone. By age four, they have progressed in their handling of receptive stimuli so that they can participate in a conversation with competence, although their attention span is still somewhat limited. The relative importance of audition and the learning of language and speech is highlighted by Pollock in chapter 9.

Expressive Language Development. Spoken language has four main elements—phonemic, syntactic, semantic, and pragmatic.

Phonemic Development. Speech is comprised of a vast array of sounds, which may be arranged into a small set of distinctive speech-sound categories. A phoneme is a minimum meaningful unit of speech in terms of acoustic parameters or speech-sound category that can be produced by the human vocal apparatus. Infants as young as one to four months can discriminate between speech sounds, although it is not expected that they have yet ascribed any linguistic meanings to the phonemes (Eimas, 1975). Vocalization produced in the early months of life consists of a repertoire of the various phonemic units that make up spoken language; however, a child normally does not learn to articulate all these units correctly in connected speech until reaching approximately seven years in age.

Syntactic Development. The syntactic element is that aspect of language which must be mastered in order to arrange words into a meaningful utterance. Thus, in syntax one deals with the grammar of a language, which is the set of rules relating sounds of language to meaning. Syntax allows for an infinite variation within a system that uses a finite number of sounds and words, and it serves as a tool to translate inner thought into the acoustical phenomenon which is spoken communication.

Semantic Development. The semantic element of language is concerned with meaning, or what a given word symbolizes. The word *bird* stands for a certain two-legged creature, although acoustic features of the word have no direct connection with the creature itself. *Bird* is simply an arbitrarily agreed-upon symbol which triggers an image in the English-speaker's mind. In contrast to phonemic and syntactic development, semantic development is never complete because vocabulary growth takes place all through life.

Pragmatic Development. Pragmatic development refers to the use of language and encompasses two aspects. One is concerned with the functions or goals of language, and is dependent on the child's desire and intent to communicate with the environment. Another aspect of pragmatics deals with the influence of both linguistic and non-linguistic contexts of language usage in determining communication goals.

Periods of Language Growth. In the discussion of receptive language, we began to trace the sequence of stages in which children learn to speak. They begin the process by mentally storing the many auditory images heard in the environment; thereupon, they soon learn to associate those images that are most frequently repeated in relation to their physical and psychological needs with their appropriate meanings. In the first year, the infant's responses in the form of cooing, vocal play, and babbling lay the foundation for the first words, which are spoken in imitation of those most often heard. By one year of age, most children will produce spontaneously from one to three single words.

During the second year of life the child uses vocal expression abundantly, and often in meaningless utterances, yet the vocalization is rich in inflection and emotional content, marking the onset of connected spoken language. Single words spoken increase from twenty to twenty-five by eighteen months, to more than two hundred by the age of two years (Lillywhite and Bradley, 1969). By age three, the child can narrate simple experiences, and shows interest in the environment by using endless queries like "What's that?" and "What's this?"

In the period between two and one-half and four and one-half years, the average child has progressed from the ability to produce a few short telegraphic sentences to fully developed comprehension and production of language and all of its basic syntactical elements. For example, comprehension of relationships is mastered in the knowledge that a ball is *on* the table instead of *under* the table. The child says, "Three big yellow oranges," instead of "yellow three big oranges" because an intuitive grasp of the appropriate word order in language has been acquired through the auditory modality. Once this level of competence is reached, children merely increase vocabulary, lengthen sentence span, and refine and polish their use of language. The production of more difficult phonemes and phoneme combinations is mastered up to about the age of seven years; but normally the basic foundations of spoken language are well laid by the age of four and one-half (table 2–1).

In recent years increased attention has been focused on the close relationship between the child's cognition (or mental abilities) and language use (Lund and Duchan,

Table 2-1. Looking at Language Learning

AGE RANGE	CHILD'S LINGUISTIC BEHAVIORS	MODE OF COMMUNICATION	ACQUISITION OF SPEECH SOUNDS	INTELLIGIBILITY OF SPEECH	MOTOR BEHAVIORS	SELF-HELP BEHAVIORS
0–6 MONTHS	Responds to the sound of mother's voice; Cry changes with emotional or bodily state; Turns eyes and head toward source of a sound; Infant is aware of his own sounds; Makes soft vowel sounds: "uh" and "ah"	Smiles Babbles Cries	Rate of development varies among children, but the sequence of development follows the same general pattern for all children.		Holds head up; sits with support, rolls over; Plays with hands and fingers; Holds rattle; Puts objects to mouth; Reaches for familiar objects and persons	Actively sucks; Opens mouth for bottle or food; Drinks from cup when held to lips
7–10 MONTHS	Turns head and shoulder toward soft, familiar sounds; Imitates intonational patterns of familiar phrases using some vowel and consonant combinations; Practices different intonational and inflectional patterns; Understands simple phrases such as "bye, bye," "no-no," "hot," own name; Directs vocalization and gestures toward people and objects	Smiles Cries Grunts Squeals Vocalizes "m-m-m" when crying Buzzes lips	In general, the sequence of acquisition of speech sounds is governed by the following principles: 1 motorically simple to motorically complex; e.g., (m) as in "mama" to (kw) as in "queen" 2 acoustically simple to acoustically complex; e.g., (p) as in "pie" to (thr) as in "throw" 3 visible to less visible; e.g., (b) as in boy to (r) as in red	The intelligibility of the child's speech will be affected by his mastery of speech sounds and other features of his speech such as stress patterns, fluency, and rate. It is expected that the overall average intelligibility of the child's speech will be . . .	Crawls; Transfers objects from hand to hand; Shakes or waves rattle; Stands with support; Puts feet to mouth; Grasps with thumb opposition but has poor pincer grasp	Holds bottle Feeds self crackers
11–16 MONTHS	Says first words; Uses several words consistently; Points or looks to familiar objects or persons when asked to; Imitates and jabbers in response to human voice; Frowns when scolded; Imitates sounds he hears; Vocalizes using inflected jargon and some words; Expresses wants and needs by body responses and vocalizations	Extensive babbling Single words			Stands alone; Walks alone; Helps turn pages in a book; Imitates scribble vigorously; Rides mobility toy; Begins to walk up stairs with help	Eats with fingers Removes socks
18 MONTHS	Begins to identify body parts; e.g., able to point to nose and eyes; Uses several meaningful words which may not be articulated correctly (e.g., "ba-ba" for bottle, "tu-tee" for cookie, or "ga-gee" for doggie); May use one word to represent several things (e.g., "wa-wa" may mean "I want water" or "Look at the water" or "I spilled the water")	Points Uses word combinations such as "big doggie"		20–25%	Runs stiffly; Seats self in small chair; Climbs onto objects from standing position; Pushes, pulls, or carries objects while walking; Throws a ball; Builds a tower of 3 blocks	Drinks unassisted from a cup; Eats with a spoon; Cooperates in dressing; Picks up toys
2 YEARS	Follows simple commands without visual clues; Enjoys books; likes being read to if book is familiar; Points out familiar pictures in books or magazines; Develops a sense of "mine" and "me"; Uses a variety of common words consistently heard in the environment (approximately 10–20 words); Refers to self by name; Puts familiar words together to make simple sentences like "daddy bye-bye" or "milk all gone"; Talks mainly about self; Imitates animal or object sounds	Words Phrases Simple 2-word sentences (noun-verb combinations)	Correctly articulated sounds are incorporated into the child's speech in a generally predictable sequence. Before the fourth birthday, it is expected that the child will have mastered the following groups of sounds:		Runs well; Walks up and down stairs, holding on and not alternating feet; Imitates vertical stroke; Turns pages one-at-a-time; Kicks ball; Stands on one foot with help; Squats and rises without using hands	Removes coat or dress; Can unzip zippers; Verbalizes toilet needs; Unwraps candy

			Sounds	%	Gross Motor	Self-Help
2½ YEARS	Likes listening to music or mother's singing Sings short rhymes or songs Imitates 3–4 word sentences Reacts to sound by telling what is heard or running to look at source of sound Expresses refusal by saying "no"	Word vocabulary grows Uses more simple sentences	(b), (p), (d), (t), (g), (k), (f) (m), (n), (ng) (w), (h), (y)	60–65%	Jumps with both feet Throws large ball 4–5 feet Holds crayon with fingers when drawing Copies vertical line	Dries hands Eats with fork Picks up toys and puts them away Begins buttoning
3 YEARS	Understands and uses simple verbs, pronouns, prepositions, adjectives, and adverbs such as "me," "in," "big," "go," "more" Uses plurals Understands contrasts such as yes/no, come/go, run/stop Uses complete sentences frequently Answers simple questions appropriately Uses "I" and "me"	Phrases 3–4 word sentences		75–90%	Rides a tricycle Walks up and down stairs, alternating feet, holding onto rail or wall Begins to use scissors Walks on tiptoes Strings large beads Establishes hand preference	Undresses self Puts on coat or dress Washes hands Feed self with little spilling Becomes toilet trained
4 YEARS	Gives full name when asked Asks questions, especially "what" and "where" Gives accurate, connected account of some recent experience Carries out a sequence of two simple commands Names common colors	Uses more complex sentences Uses slang expressions	Sounds usually mastered after the fourth birthday include: (s), (z), (sh), (zh), (v), (th), (ch), (j)	90%	Skips on one foot Climbs very well Jumps onto or over objects Throws a ball overhand Catches ball in arms Walks up stairs, alternating feet, without support	Laces shoes Brushes own teeth Washes and dries face
5 YEARS	Uses speech that is intelligible although some sounds may be substituted or distorted Carries on meaningful conversation with adult or child if vocabulary is familiar Uses pronouns correctly Asks meaning of unfamiliar words Uses language that matches the dialect of peers and adults in the family and neighborhood	Uses fully developed complex sentences Uses 7–8 word sentences Uses many new words from his expanding vocabulary			Plays running games Can imitate some letters correctly Folds paper diagonally Can skip on alternate feet Walks down stairs, alternating feet, without support	Dresses without assistance, except tying Washes self without wetting clothes Cuts with knife

Developed by Janet E. Coscarelli,
Patricia F. Casey, and
Kathryn B. Horton

© 1977 K. B. Horton & J. E. Coscarelli

WHO HELPED US

1. Boone, Daniel, Infant speech and language development. *Volta Review*, 1965, 67, 414–419.
2. Cattell, Psyche, *The Management of Intelligence in Infants and Young Children*. New York: Psychological Corporation, 1940.
3. Gesell, A. L., et al, *The First Five Years of Life*. New York: Harper and Row, 1940.
4. Gesell, A. and Katherine S. Amatruda, *Developmental Diagnosis: Normal and Abnormal Child Development*. New York: Paul Hoeber, Inc., 1960.
5. Wood, Barbara S. *Children and Communication: Verbal and Nonverbal Language Development*. Englewood Cliffs, N.J. Prentice Hall, Inc., 1976.

1983). However, in some populations, such as hearing impaired and autistic children, cognitive levels may be more advanced than language levels (Piaget and Inhelder, 1969; Wetherby and Gaines, 1982).

Much of the current interest in the influence of mental development on language development has been sparked by the Swiss cognitive psychologist, Jean Piaget. Thus, in many clinics, cognitive assessments are a part of the diagnostic and/or management programs, especially for nonverbal children. Piaget (Piaget and Inhelder, 1969) described four hierarchially arranged but qualitatively different stages of cognitive development. These stages are the sensorimotor period (zero to eighteen months), the preoperational period (two to seven years), the concrete operations period (seven to eleven years) and the formal operations period (eleven years to adult). Since this chapter is concerned primarily with the infant and young child, the first two periods of Piaget's cognitive theory will be reviewed briefly. Other excellent references give comprehensive coverage of Piaget's theory (Beard, 1969; Flavell, 1977; Ginsburg and Opper, 1969; Gruber and Vonéche, 1977; Piaget and Inhelder, 1969). During the sensorimotor period, the infant develops knowledge of the world through mastery of various behaviors or schemes. These schemes involve the child's coordination of the senses (seeing, hearing, tasting, touching) and the child's motor (movement) abilities. Early in the child's development (zero to three months), the child masters oral or sucking schemes. As the infant's capabilities enlarge, the infant is able to coordinate two or more schemes such as looking and grasping. Progressively, the child develops the ability to respond to and act on different objects to accomplish a goal. Toward the end of this period, the infant can mentally retain symbols and can perform tasks such as searching for an object which has been hidden under one of three different screens. This ability to internalize symbols marks the infant's highest achievement during the sensorimotor period and is believed to be the basis for language.

During the ten-to-eighteen-month period, when the infant begins to say the first true words, labels for events or people are tied closely to the child's sensory experiences. Such words as *mama, car, daddy, bottle, good*, are common examples of first words.

At the eighteen-to-twenty-four-month period, the child begins to combine two-word utterances such as *ball gone, daddy gone*. This marks the beginning of Piaget's second cognitive period, the preoperational period. At this time, the child is able to discover new ways of solving problems through physical acts as well as through mentally internalized combinations of schemes. A refinement of language and sensorimotor schemes continues as the child at this age learns to count, classify, and seriate objects. The preoperational child can also tell the position of objects in space and is developing a refined sense of time and causality concepts.

LANGUAGE DISORDERS, LANGUAGE DELAY, AND LANGUAGE DIFFERENCES

Definitions

The term *language disorders* represents both deviations from an orderly pattern in the learning of the language code and delayed language represented by an orderly pattern of learning that is inappropriate to chronological age. Since both language deviancy and language delay are language disorders and major causes of learning disabilities, they require specific remedial efforts.

A given language disorder can include one or more of several types of deficits. A semantic disorder, for example, can include reduced vocabulary usage and/or reduced vocabulary comprehension. Disorders of syntax and morphology (the smallest meaningful unit contained within a language) include disorders of comprehension and of the use of connected discourse. A phonologic disorder involves the deviant production of speech sounds, which may be the result of central or peripheral disorder or deficit.

Depending on the severity of the impairment, language disorders may be restricted in nature or may encompass the entire range of verbal functioning. Several of the former type appear to be related to auditory processing deficits, such as those involving poor auditory discrimination, auditory sequencing, and auditory memory (Zigmond, 1968; Wiig and Semel, 1976). Some children, for example, may confuse fine, but not gross, differences in sounds; that is, they may be able to distinguish between a knock on the door and a telephone ringing, but not between the telephone and the doorbell ringing. Others may be unable to handle the sequencing of auditory events, which may result in their inability to learn the days of the week or the months of the year, and may show in pronunciations such as *aminal* for *animal*, or *bakstet* for *basket*, or in confusion of compound words, such as *sitterbaby* and *wipeshield winders*. Still other children may exhibit defects of auditory memory; they may have no difficulty in comprehending single words, but their ability to recall verbal information may be too limited to follow a series of commands, such as "Take the paste to the cabinet; wash the paste brushes; and then return to your seat until the bell rings for dismissal."

Classification and Characteristics

Language learning difficulties may be broadly classified as being associated with hearing impairment, neurologic impairment, environmental deprivation, or idiopathic etiology.

Problems of the Hearing Impaired. Sensory deprivation of hearing from the prelingual years is a major barrier to language learning. The child who hears the spoken word partially or not at all is unable to progress in the normal sequence of language mastery. This includes the development of capacity to comprehend verbal messages, to produce intelligible speech conveying one's thoughts and feelings to others, and to read and write. Since chapter 9 is devoted exclusively to the deaf and hard of hearing, the reader is referred to those authors for more detailed treatment of language disorders related to hearing impairment.

Problems of the Developmentally Language Impaired. In this category we are concerned with the failure of some children to develop adequate language because of obvious or presumed central nervous system dysfunction. (Adults who sustain a reduction in or loss of language functioning because of acquired neurological disease or trauma are described by West in chapter 8.) Recent evidence from the Collaborative Perinatal Project of the National Institute of Neurological and Communicative Disorders and Stroke, titled *Early Correlates of Speech, Language and Hearing* (Lassman et al., 1980), indicates that reduced language performance in a sample of 27,558 children was frequently associated with such perinatal factors as prematurity, breech delivery, use of forceps, low birth weight, and reduced Apgar scores (a rating scale that assesses neonatal well-being, including heart rate, breathing effort, muscle tone, reflex irritability, and skin color). These same factors are also often related to neurological abnormalities other than language impairment. Earlier Perinatal Project data of the National Institute of Neurological Diseases and Stroke indicated that from 12 to 15 percent of children show neurological abnormalities by one year of age (Subcommittee on Human Communication and Its Disorders, 1969). It may be expected that a considerable number from this group will be affected by central language problems, such as dyslexia (difficulty in reading) and other significant auditory and visual perception problems creating language disabilities, in addition to the childhood aphasias. In the study cited, the Subcommittee on Human Communication and Its Disorders has estimated that at least 1.5 million children in this country suffer from central communicative disorders affecting the linguistic processes. DiCarlo and Amster, in chapter 7, review the etiological bases and subsequent language and speech impairments associated specifically with cerebral palsy.

Central language disorders can involve any portion or combination of portions of the central nervous system and at any level, as depicted by the language model presented earlier in figure 2–1. Disorders of auditory receptive language may range from complete inability to respond to verbal stimuli, in which case the child may function as deaf, to specific disabilities related to recognition of the sound elements in spoken language (auditory discrimination), retention of these units of information in the memory bank (auditory memory), integration of the symbolic relationships of these units as language concepts, and the comprehension of language symbols through the previous stages of auditory perceptual function (Sabatino, 1969).

Auditory Comprehension Deficits. A primary characteristic of children with auditory comprehension deficits is an inability to understand the spoken word, although the degree of involvement may vary from quite mild to severe. For example, a child at the extreme end of the severity continuum might not even be able to recognize or respond to name words. Others may function adequately as long as the verbal message is concrete but have no capacity to handle language abstractions pertaining to quality, reason, and feelings. Similarly, they may not be able to understand the variations in tense accomplished by morphologic endings, and thus are restricted to the use of the present tense. Other children may be able to repeat what others say to them, but not to answer appropriately by initiating their own linguistic responses. These children may learn to read orally quite acceptably, since they simply change the visual symbols on the printed page to auditory symbols. Questioning them about the content, however, reveals they have no understanding of the message. Such readers are merely word callers: the central mediating process (see figure 2–1) is apparently bypassed in the transduction of the input stimuli to the output modality.

The degree of language involvement sometimes is demonstrated primarily by a difficulty in reading (dyslexia) and difficulty in writing (dysgraphia). The written excerpt below illustrates a language disability confined primarily to the school learning skills of reading and writing.

Wins (once) when a boy *cane hone fone school* (came home from school) he *what* (wanted) something to eat so he *clopd* (climbed) on a *shlf* (shelf) and got the *cookees* (cookies) *a* (and) he *siarted* (started) to eat *then* (them) when his dog *cane* (came) in and *what sone* (wanted some) so he gave *hin sone* (him some). Then he *pt* (put) the *cookie baak an* (cookies back and) then his mother *what sone* (wanted some) and *fond* (found) out *ther ws* (there was) no cookies and *shee called* (she called) the boy and *spcot hin* (spanked him) and the dog ran off and *boe cry* (both cried) and *nother* (mother) made *sone* (some) more.

The writer of the story was a ten-year-old boy with neurological language impairment. His comprehension and use of oral language was considered adequate, although he had been slow in learning to talk and his parents had considered his locomotor development clumsy. The written sample demonstrates that he was able to construct a sequence of ideas, even though he "strung" these ideas together in two long sentences with an excessive number of conjunctions. His major difficulty was in word-sound association as reflected in poor performance on tasks of speech-sound discrimination and auditory blending. This boy's ability to handle the syntax of written language contrasts with that of deaf children who, because of their limited auditory experience, tend to confuse word order in a way that markedly alters the thought content.

Oral Expressive Language Deficits. There are many children with obvious neurological impairment or suspected impairment who have little or no problem in understanding the spoken word, but are unable to express themselves with any degree of oral competence. A common difficulty is misarticulation of speech sounds. Traditionally, disorders of speech articulation involving the phonologic level of the language system have been separated from disorders involving the syntactic, semantic, and pragmatic levels of the system, but it is now recognized that phonologic rules and performance are part of the total language system. The majority of phonologic disorders in children usually have been considered functional rather than neurogenic in origin, and the misarticulation problems of the many children assisted in public schools have been viewed primarily as functional disorders. Some disorders of articulation, however, involving the processes of speech programming, speech initiation, and speech coordination-transmission (see fig. 2–2), clearly have a neurological basis and are one aspect of a central language disorder. These disorders are characterized by problems in motor programming, sequencing, control, and transmission in the nervous system. They are known as motor speech disorders and include dysarthria and speech apraxia. Both these disorders may occur in children as well as in adults. Developmental or childhood dysarthria is an articulation and/or voice problem that results from paralysis, weakness, or incoordination of the muscles resulting from a lesion in the nervous system, generally in subcortical structures. It is most common in children who have generalized neuromotor disorders such as cerebral palsy or muscular dystrophy, but on rare occasions a child may have isolated paralysis of the speech muscles which will produce a speech disorder characterized primarily by defective phonology. Physicians call this significant but uncommon motor speech disorder congenital suprabulbar paresis (Worster-Drought, 1974); it is labeled a developmental or childhood dysarthria by speech-language pathologists (LaPointe, 1975).

Developmental speech apraxia is a motor programming problem in which the child shows difficulty in performing the motor actions for speech, even though the muscles are free from paralysis. Voluntary initiation of the movements of speech are very difficult for the child. Articulation errors are often highly inconsistent and frequent omissions and distortions of sounds are heard. The articulation problem is typically severe and often resistant to therapeutic intervention (Macaluso-Haynes, 1978). In the past, developmental speech apraxia was often confused with severe articulation problems of a functional nature (Yoss and Darley, 1974).

Dysfunction at levels in the central nervous system higher than the motor level may include a variety of oral expressive disorders of phonology, syntax, and semantics in the central language system proper. The most commonly used label for this disorder in the past was childhood aphasia. One objection to this term is that the clinical picture of language disability in the child often fails to fit the clinical descriptions of the classic aphasias of adulthood. In fact, a language disorder in a child usually presents a totally different clinical picture. A second objection is that the concept of aphasia usually implies a clear-cut etiology of neurologic origin and demonstrable signs of a neurologic lesion. However, in children the language symptoms are usually associated with developmental abnormality of the nervous system rather than obvious focal cerebral damage. Evidence of neurologic injury is often absent on neurologic examination and in the case history of a child with such a language disorder. Many writers, therefore, have abandoned the term childhood aphasia when describing these children with language delay or disorder and have substituted the term developmental language disability, childhood language disability, or childhood language disorder (Bloom and Lahey, 1978; Weiner, 1980).

Recent studies have attempted to delineate empirically the types of expressive oral language disturbance characteristic of developmental language disability. It is clear, however, that children with this problem do not come from a homogeneous population, nor do they present a common and consistent picture of expressive language difficulties. For example, Wolfus, Moscovitch, and Kinsbourne (1980) studied nineteen children with normal intelligence and language impairment. They classified the children into two distinct groups based on the results of a series of language tests. The first group of children, called the expressive disability group, was characterized by deficits in the production of syntax and phonology. A second group, called the expressive-receptive disability group, was more impaired on measures of phonologic discrimination, memory for digits, and semantic ability, together with global deficits in syntax. Aram and Nation (1975) studied forty-seven children, using a series of tests to assess comprehension, formulation, and repetition at phonologic, syntactic, and semantic levels. They identified six patterns of language deficits:

1. a repetition strength pattern in which children were able to repeat syntactic and phonologic test materials at high levels, but performed at lower levels on other tests;
2. a non-specific formulation-repetition deficit pattern in which there was low performance on phonologic and syntactic formulation and repetition tasks compared to other language tasks;
3. a generalized low performance pattern in which children were globally depressed in all comprehension formulation and repetition tasks;
4. a phonologic comprehension-formulation-repetition deficit pattern in which children scored high on all tasks except the phonologic test as well as on a test of syntactic formulation and on a test of syntactic repetition;
5. a comprehension deficit pattern in which higher scores occurred on formulation and repetition tasks than on comprehension tasks; and
6. a formulation-repetition deficit pattern in which comprehension task scores were higher than formulation and repetition task scores.

Psycholinguistic research involving children with developmental language disabilities has also been directed at determining whether such children display a deviant or a delayed pattern of linguistic development. This considerable body of research has been recently reviewed by Menyuk (1978), Leonard (1979), and Weiner (1980), who conclude that, by and large, the speech of language-impaired children resembles that of normal children at an earlier level of linguistic rule development in phonology, syntax, semantics, and pragmatics. However, studies (Menyuk, 1969; Menyuk and Looney, 1972; and Johnston, 1980) indicate these children sometimes make use of deviant rather than immature linguistic forms. This finding has practical implications for language remediation. If a language-impaired child shows grossly deviant linguistic rules and language forms, or presents a different pattern of usage from that of the normal child, immediate and intensive intervention is imperative. If, however, accurate predictions can be made of the future course of language development in a language-delayed child, as opposed to a language-deviant child, this child will require neither intensive nor extensive therapeutic management.

Several theories have been set forth to explain the basis for language impairment in children. Tallal and Piercy (1978) have presented evidence to suggest that auditory processing may be slower in dysphasic children than in normal children. Others (Menyuk, 1969; Menyuk and Looney, 1972) have implicated short-term memory deficits in language-impaired children. Still other investigators (Morehead and Ingram, 1973; Rees, 1973; Morehead and Morehead, 1974; Cromer, 1978; and Leonard, 1979) have argued that cognitive deficits in one form or another play a role in language disability. This view is supported by the fact that many of these children show delays in representational play and imagery as well as in oral expressive language.

Any single theory of the cause of the language deficit is probably open to some criticism on the grounds of oversimplification, since it is more likely that a number of factors affecting various levels of functioning will interact differently from child to child to produce the varied array of patterns of language disability observed in children in clinics and schools. At this time a complex theory of language deficit is more appealing than any single cause theory.

Language and Cultural Influences. Traditionally, the speech-language pathologist is trained to evaluate and remediate all deviations from normal patterns in the reception and production of language and speech, including those related to cultural heritage. Frequently, these deviations have been referred to as deficiencies when they varied from the supposed norms of white middle-class speech. The rapidly increasing multicultural composition of the United States population has forced a reexamination of the manner in which persons who differ from the middle-income members of the primary culture are viewed. Thus, children who are not members of the predominant culture group and whose social and ethnic background differ from that of the speech-language pathologist's background present a unique challenge. The speech-language pathologist is faced with determining if a true disorder exists or whether this behavior is typical of the behaviors of the child's cultural group. This challenge is underscored if the speech-language pathologist has had little or no formal training in separating cultural language-speech differences from those which result from other causes (Bountress, 1980).

In this chapter, the term *culturally different child* will be used to represent all those whose language and speaking skills are different from those of the primary cultural group. Included are such diverse groups as Native Americans, Afro-Americans (blacks), Appalachian whites, Hispanic-Americans, and Asian-Americans (Banks, 1977; Cole, 1980). While it is recognized that all cultural groups are of equal importance, the current discussion will highlight the language and speech of non-standard black speakers and of Spanish-speaking children, since these populations comprise the two largest minority groups in the United States.

Two premises are of significance when studying language and speech differences. First, they should be studied and analyzed with reference to the particular norms of the cultural group to which the speaker belongs. Taylor (1971a) and Bauman (1971) emphasized the need for viewing language as a part of the cultural context in which it develops, or from an ethnographic orientation. This basic orientation is vitally important in obtaining an accurate assessment of the child's current level of function-ing, in both the comprehension and production of language. Second, all languages (whether they represent the communication of the middle class population or that of the culturally different child) are organized in a systematic way which conveys information through use of a predetermined or rule-governed structure (Bauman, 1971; Taylor, 1971a; Naremore, 1980). Thus, the language and speech of the cultur-ally different child represent a highly developed and systematic form of communica-tion.

Nonstandard Black Language and Speech. The largest number of minority children in the United States are urban blacks (Taylor, 1980). However, it is projected that by 1990, Hispanic-Americans will become the largest single urban minority (U.S. Census, 1982). The language and speech of black Americans have been referred to as Black English (Williams and Wolfram, 1974), Black-English vernacular (Labov, 1972), Black dialect, Negro nonstandard dialect (Naremore, 1980), and American Negro dialect (Stewart, 1970). Two theories regarding black language dominate the literature. These are the "deficit" and "difference" theories; each has been used to explain the nonstandard patterns that are used, in varying degrees, by a substantial number of black persons. Not all black persons speak nonstandard dialect, nor do all persons who speak nonstandard Black English conform to a pattern of using all of the characteristics of the dialect. The extent of use is subject to wide variation among speakers.

The deficit theory appears to be a result of the overgeneralization which charac-terized the War on Poverty era in the 1960s. Williams (1970) notes that "cultural deprivation," a term used to define children who came from economically im-poverished backgrounds, was extended to mean language deprivation. Persons who espouse the deficit theory state that such a child's language is an inferiorly developed system which, though similar to the developmental patterns of white middle-class Americans, occurs at a slower rate of development (Bereiter and Engelmann, 1966). They suggest that urban black children use a vocabulary that is more limited than that of middle-class children and that overall linguistic performance levels are somewhat lower than those of middle-class white children (Osser, Wang, and Zaid, 1969).

It is true, of course, that language reception, production, and use are influenced by socioeconomic variables (Poag, 1968; Schachter, 1979; LaBenz and LaBenz, 1980). Poag (1968) compared the grammar performance (syntax and morphology) of four groups of preschool children on both a racial and a socioeconomic basis. A total of 127 children were studied, divided approximately evenly into black middle-class, white middle-class, black lower-class, and white lower-class populations. An adaptation of

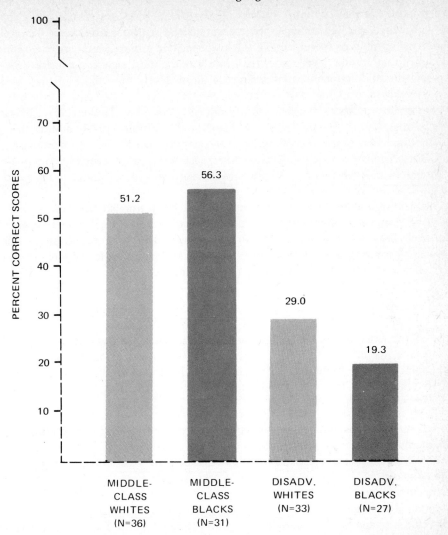

Figure 2–3. Comparison of Mean Scores on Grammar Performance Test for Two Socioeconomic Groups Divided into Racial Subgroups. The testing procedure followed that of Berko (1961), but it included the use of specially selected stimulus pictures.

the test of morphology and syntax by Berko (1961) was administered to each subject. The results, shown in figure 2–3, clearly demonstrated that the grammar performance levels were significantly higher in the middle-class groups. Their mean scores were at least twice as high as those of the two lower-income groups. Thus, differences were related to socioeconomic rather than cultural factors. In a related study, Schachter (1979) studied the linguistic input (spontaneous and responsive talk) of three groups of mothers to their toddlers. Two higher-income groups—one black group of ten mothers and one white group of ten mothers—were compared with one group of ten lower-income black mothers. Schachter found that while the black higher-income group's total amount of talk exceeded the white higher-income group's performance, there was no statistically significant difference between these two groups. However, the verbal total talk performance for each of these two groups was approximately double the number of speech acts of the lower-income group of mothers. Schachter concluded that income level rather than race was the most significant factor differentiating the middle-income mothers' verbal input levels from those of the lower-income mothers.

The "difference" theory has been most eloquently voiced by Taylor (1971a, 1971b, 1980), Adler (1971), Baratz (1970), Williams and Wolfram (1974), and Williams (1970). Proponents of this theory state that the language used by speakers of nonstandard Black English is a richly developed language which is governed by an equally sophisticated and systematic set of phonologic, morphologic, semantic, and syntactic rules.

The most frequently observed characteristics of Black English are summarized in table 2–2. Sample productions in Black English and standard English are presented with each brief description. In the first example, illustrating reduction of final consonant clusters characteristic of Black English, the sample word or production is "tes;" in standard English the counterpart production is "test."

Language and Speech of Hispanics. The speech of Spanish-speaking children has also received much attention in recent years. Naremore (1980) uses the term *Latino* to describe residents within the continental United States who are of any Spanish background, including Cubans, Mexicans, Puerto Ricans, and others. These same individuals are more frequently spoken of as the Hispanic population. Attention has centered on some of the issues similar to those for the black urban child. These are

1. Does the child possess a true disorder of communication or is the communication adequate?
2. Does the speech-language pathologist possess adequate skills to make an appropriate diagnosis?
3. Are culture-sensitive assessment instruments available to enable a diagnosis representing a true measure of the child's language functioning?
4. Is referral to another person or agency with expertise in meeting the needs of this cultural group indicated to best serve the child's needs?
5. Is the use of standard English an important goal to the parents and the child?

The Spanish-speaking child, just as the speaker of Black English, may have phonologic, semantic, and syntactic differences as compared to the speaker of standard English. Thus, the speech-language pathologist must be thoroughly familiar with the Hispanic child's language and speech forms in order to make accurate diagnoses and plan appropriate management strategies. An overview of some of the phonologic and syntactic-semantic contrasts between Hispanic-English and standard English is presented in table 2–3. Reference to table 2–2 shows that several similarities exist between Black English and Hispanic-English, such as the use of the d/th phoneme, the absence of the plural marker, and the absence of the third person tense marker.

Table 2–2. Some Differences Between Nonstandard Black English (B.E.) and Standard English (S.E.)

Phonologic Aspects	Black English	Standard English
1. Reduction of final consonant clusters	tes, was, des, lef, min, col, miss, desses, ghosses, rub	test, wasp, desk, left, mind, cold, missed, desks, ghosts, rubbed
2. Disappearance of /r/ after /p/, /b/, /k/, /th/, and /g/	bovva, potec	brother, protect
3. Substitution of phonemes		
a. skr/str	skreet	street
b. v/th	bruvah, ravah, baving	brother, rather, bathing
c. d/th (initial position)	de, dey	the, they
d. t/th	sout	south
e. f/th	baftub, aufur, nofin, Ruf, toof	bathtub, author, nothing, Ruth, tooth
f. b/v	balentine, sebm, haeb	valentine, seven, have
4. Dropping of /r/ and /l/		
a. If these precede a consonant	hep, taught, cat, toe	help, torte, carrot, told
b. After initial consonant	th'ow, th'ough	throw, through
c. At end of words	show, doe, foe	sure, door, four
d. *they-their, you-your* May sound alike	It is they book. It is you book.	It is their book. It is your book.
e. Between vowels /r/ or /l/ may be absent	ca'ol, sto'y	carol, story
5. Devoicing of /b/, /d/, and /g/ may make some words sound more similar. Not all words sound alike due to the length of the vowel, for example *u* in *bud* is longer than *u* in *butt*	rib, stupit	rip, stupid
6. Deletion of /d/	ba' man, goo' soldier	bad man, good soldier
7. Nasalization changes occur		
a. Nasalized vowel may be used at end of word instead of nasalized consonant	ma', ru', bu'	man, run, bun
b. /i/ and /e/ do not contrast in nasalized ending words	pin, tin	pen, pin ten, tin

Semantic-Syntactic Aspects	Black English	Standard English
1. Reduction of *-ed* suffixes which indicate past tense, past participial forms, and derived adjectives, due to the consonant reduction rule. Sample Word: finished, cashed, forged, cracked, named	finish, cash, forge, crack, name	finisht, casht, forgd, crackt, namd
2. *Been* as a means of distant time designation	I *been* had it there for about six years.	I *have* had it there for about six years.
3. Absence of present tense marker for third person singular	She *walk.* The lady *walk.*	She *walks.* The lady *walks.*
4. Absence of *has* and *does* third person forms	She *have* a bike. She always *do* silly things.	She *has* a bike. She always *does* silly things.

Semantic-Syntactic Aspects	Black English	Standard English
5. Hypercorrections: Marking of first and second person singular, third person plural forms	I *walks*. You *walks*. The children *walks*.	I *walk*. You *walk*. The children *walk*.
6. *Gonna* as an indicator of future tense (*is, are* often omitted when *gonna* used)	He *gonna* go. You *gonna get* in trouble.	He *will be going*. You *will get* into trouble.
7. Reduction of *gonna* to *nga, mana, mon, ma*.	I 'ngna go. I 'mana go. I 'mon go. I 'ma go.	No corollary structure.
8. Dropping of /l/ may cause confusion of future forms such as *will*	Tomorrow *I bring* the thing.	Tomorrow *I will bring* the thing.
9. *Be* as a main verb.	I *be here* in the evening. Sometime *he be* busy.	*I'm* usually here in the evening. Sometimes *he is* very busy.
10. *Be* as a non-specific tense used to define "an object or event distributed intermittently in time"	I *be* good.	(Meaning) I'm good sometimes.

11. Absence of copula *is-are*
a. Is
b. Are
  1. Used less often than *is*
  2. Changes to *ah*, or *uh* when pronounced
	He *a* man. He *bad*. She *running* to school.	He *is a* man. He's *bad*. She *is running* to school.

12. Negation a. *Ain't* used by some black speakers to mean *didn't* b. Preposed negative auxiliary c. Negative auxiliary used d. Negative concord across clause boundaries	She *ain't* go home. *Couldn't nobody* do it. *Nobody didn't* do it. *Ain't no cat can't get into no coop*.	She *didn't* go home. *Nobody could* do it. *Nobody did* it. *No cat can get into any coop*.
13. Possessive a. Common noun possessive case indicated by word order b. Personal names, *'s* used with the first name in double noun forms	The *boy hat*. *John's Dawson* car	The *boy's hat*. *John Dawson's* car
14. Plural a. Absence of *-s* or *-es* b. Regular plurals and irregular nouns, *-s* suffix used by some speakers with irregular nouns	He took five *book*. *two foots, two deers*	He took five *books*. *two feet, two deer*
15. Pronominal apposition (pronoun used in addition to the noun subject within a sentence)	*My sister, she bigger* than you.	*My sister is bigger* than you.
16. Relative clauses—relative pronoun deletion	*That's the dog bit me.*	*That's the dog that bit me.*
17. Questions a. Indirect question form used for direct question	*I want to know where did she go?*	*Where did she go?*

Semantic-Syntactic Aspects	Black English	Standard English
18. Uninverted forms	*What that is?*	*What is that?*
19. Existential *it* used instead of *there*.	It's a store on the corner.	There's a store on the corner.

20. Pronouns
  a. Nominative/objective neutralization forms used as objective may be used as subject
  b. Non-possessive case for possessives
	Him ain't playing.
	
	She want *she* mother.
		He's not playing.
		
		She wants *her* mother.

21. *Done* as an indicator of completed action	I *done* tried.	I *have* tried.

Table 2–3. Some differences between Hispanic English and standard English

Phonologic Aspects	Hispanic English	Standard English

1. Plosives
  a. Initial position plosives always voiced
  b. Final position plosives always voiceless
	got
	cop, bic
		cot
		cob, big

2. Fricatives and affricates
  a. /th/ nonexistent in Hispanic; /d/ often substituted for voiced /th/; /s/ often substituted for voiceless /th/
  b. No distinction made between /b/ and /v/
  c. The /s/ and /ch/ sounds are present but the cognates /zh/ and /j/ are not, /s/ often substituted for /z/
  d. Nonexistence of "h" fricative, but similar Hispanic fricative used
	de, sum
	
	bote
	sip
	
	-orse or Hispanic velar fricative may be substituted for /h/
		the, thumb
		
		vote
		zip
		
		horse

3. Liquids: /r/ and /l/. Pronounced differently in Hispanic-English than in standard English.
  a. *R* is "rolled" in a standard Hispanic production. Thus, the Hispanic /r/ may be substituted for the English /r/.
  b. /l/ sound is pronounced like /y/ (as in llama) in Hispanic. Therefore, Hispanic /l/ may be substituted for the English /l/.		

4. Vowels
  a. The /i/ sound, as in *did* or *bit*, is nonexistent in Hispanic. Thus, /ee/ may be substituted for /i/.
  b. The /ae/ sound, as in *bag*, is nonexistent. Thus, the vowel sound /e/ as in *bet* may be substituted.
  c. The /u/ sound, as in *bun* and *done*, is nonexistent. Thus, a sound that rhymes with the Spanish word, Juan, may be substituted.
	b$\overline{ee}$g
	
	beg
	
	buan
		big
		
		bag
		
		bun

Semantic-Syntactic Aspects	Hispanic English	Standard English
1. Endings of words		
a. Comparatives	That one is *more big*. That girl is *most pretty* of the girls.	That one is *bigger*. That girl is *prettiest*.
b. Singular verbs: third person	She *walk* very fast.	She *walks* very fast.
c. Plurals	The *cat* are gone.	The *cats* are gone.
d. Past tense	We *play* there last week.	We *played* there last week.
e. Possessive	This is the dress *of my sister*.	This is *my sister's* dress.
2. Order of words		
a. Questions	*Pablo can go?*	*Can Pablo go?*
b. Pronouns as subjects	Pablo is my brother. *Is big*.	Pablo is my brother. *He is big*.
c. Not sentences	Maria *no is* here.	Maria *is not* here.
d. Adjective position	The *water blue* is nice.	The *blue water* is nice.
3. Function words		
a. *Do* omitted from questions	— you like it?	Do you like it?
b. *Don't* commands	*No do* that.	*Don't* do that.
c. *Be* verbs	He *have* hunger.	He *is* hungry.
d. Prepositions	It is *in* the chair.	It is *on* the chair.
e. Articles	*Is Mexican child.* *Is teacher.*	*Maria is a Mexican child.* Mrs. Gomez *is the teacher.*

EVALUATION PRINCIPLES AND PROCEDURES

Differential Assessment of the Auditory Capacity of Nonlanguage Children

If a child has developed no intelligible spoken language, four major causes must be considered: (1) hearing impairment; (2) neurological impairment; (3) developmental delay and/or mental retardation; and (4) emotional disturbance. Both auditory intake and oral speech output processes must be evaluated, even though the use of formal standardized measures is often not feasible. Instead, the examiner must rely heavily on careful observation of behavior and on clinical judgment.

To rule out deafness, a major cause of failure to develop language, the child's auditory capacity should be considered first. The examiner must ask:

1. Does this child use hearing or vision as the primary sense modality?
2. If the child does not use hearing as the primary modality, is it used secondarily or not at all?
3. Does the child use sound inconsistently?

Response of the Child with Severe to Profound Hearing Impairment.
The deaf child is likely to be more consistent in a test situation than children with other disorders. Deaf children respond readily to sounds at intensity levels above their threshold. A startle response, induced by a rapid rise in loudness (recruitment), may suggest sensorineural hearing impairment. Parents may report that their child

does notice loud environmental sounds, such as a low-flying airplane or a car horn. Loud speech at a distance of one foot behind the ear will frequently make the deaf child respond with eye movement, momentary cessation of activity, or turning toward the source. In presenting such stimuli, the examiner must not allow breath movement or other tactile clues to reach the child. In all such tests, it is important to set the stage so that the child's attention is only mildly diverted to a play activity in which an examiner seated opposite is engaged. If the child participates to any active degree, the opportunity to elicit attention to sound is greatly lessened.

Response of the Neurologically Impaired Child. The child with neurological impairment will frequently ignore all sounds except those with which meaning has been previously associated. These children are apt to demonstrate a very labile attention span. For example, they may respond once or twice to sounds produced by noisemakers, but will ignore such stimuli shortly thereafter, once conditioning to the sound has occurred. As in the case of emotionally disturbed children, questioning the parents may reveal that neurologically impaired children will also respond to specific stimuli associated with a meaningful experience; but for the most part, speech falls on "deaf" ears. Observation of play behavior is always valuable for assessing any types of vocalizations that may be produced. Left undisturbed in a play environment and presented with a toy car or animal, these children will frequently vocalize readily in imitation of the sound associated with the toy object. Often their inflection pattern and voice quality will illustrate that they have used auditory feedback principles to monitor their own voices.

Response of the Developmentally Delayed Child. The developmentally delayed or severely retarded child will likely respond quite erratically to sound stimuli. These children usually require intensities greater than actual threshold before indicating a response. Pure tone signals have limited value, unless combined with more meaningful stimuli and use of play-conditioning techniques. Animal and bird sounds filtered to narrow octave bands have been found valuable in testing the retarded child. Children at the lowest levels of mentality (below about 40 IQ level) often will pay no attention to sound stimuli of any kind, but this behavior results from lack of attention and interest rather than inability to hear. In such cases, if the examiner will faintly rattle a spoon against a plate or produce some other common sound associated with physical comfort, they will turn instantly toward the source. Children of higher mentality levels (ranging from 40 up to about 60 IQ) will often respond to speech sounds, but not to pure tones.

Response of the Emotionally Disturbed Child. The child with severe emotional disturbance may ignore nearly all sounds, even those ranging in intensity up to pain threshold level. To rule out deafness, it is necessary to explore carefully with the parents the child's auditory behavior in the home. Given the information on specific kinds of sounds to which a child has been attentive in the past, the examiner may be able to elicit responses to those stimuli at very low intensities, even though the child may ignore all other sensory stimuli. Conversation generally will fail to stimulate such a child, but stressful situations (for example, separation from the parents) may motivate the child to produce intelligible speech, such as "No, No," or "Daddy! Daddy!" thus indicating that the auditory intake has not been impaired.

In summary, one of the more difficult and challenging tasks in assessing children who have failed to develop spoken language is to differentiate between cases caused by hearing impairment as compared with those with other causes. The examiner must also determine the relative significance of hearing impairment when it is superimposed on other handicaps. Only increasing experience and ability to use clinical skills of observation can bring about competence in this area. The large number of children who fail to develop spoken language requires continued attention and effort on the part of audiologists and speech-language pathologists to develop proficiency in determining the cause of the condition, for certainly that must be defined in planning a remedial program for a particular child. There is good evidence to suggest that these conditions exist in combination in many children, and in all degrees, just as does hearing impairment itself. Imagine, for example, the complexity of accurate diagnosis in the case of a child with damaged cortical functioning, high-frequency-hearing loss, and mild developmental delay. Depending on severity of the handicap, progress in speech, language, and communication may be anticipated in varying amounts. As we emphasize in a later section, intensive training of such children in the early preschool years holds the most promise for maximum development.

Assessment of Deviant Receptive-Expressive Language

In dealing with deviations in receptive-expressive language, the assessment procedure involves the classification of the language problem, the diagnosis of specific abilities and disabilities, and an analysis of the child's linguistic system.

Assessment Techniques and Goals.
Classification procedures usually include obtaining the child's history, making clinical observations, administering tests, and sampling spontaneous language behavior. These procedures help point to an appropriate general category for the child's language problem. Tests which yield global scores are particularly useful at this point. For instance, the information derived from the performance and verbal subtest scores from such instruments as the Wechsler Intelligence Scale for Children—Revised (Wechsler, 1974) and the Wechsler Preschool and Primary Scales of Intelligence (Wechsler, 1967) or other tests utilizing performance and language subscales are initially useful in determining whether the child, in fact, has a language problem. Other language scales, such as the Illinois Test of Psycholinguistic Abilities (Kirk, McCarthy, and Kirk, 1968) will yield a global score—a psycholinguistic language quotient—which can be compared to normative data and used for initial identification and classification purposes.

Differential diagnosis of specific abilities, on the other hand, aims at detecting strengths and weaknesses in the various processes of language functioning which might explain the specific nature of the language impairment or delay. This type of information is particularly helpful in planning remedial programs that involve specific channels of language input and output.

Sampling of spontaneous behavior in natural situations rather than highly structured test situations is another assessment technique that is now widely used by speech-language pathologists. Analysis of a language sample allows the examiner to establish the linguistic rules the language-impaired child is currently using. By comparing these rules to the linguistic rule system of a normal child of the same age, the rules and linguistic structures needing therapeutic attention can be determined.

A comprehensive assessment of a language disorder should also include information about its possible etiology, and its past, present, and future status. Typically, information concerning the past status of the problem includes a determination of the nature of the disorder at onset as well as a history of early development of speech and language. This information is routinely gained from a complete case history. An excellent discussion of the case history and an example of a practical case history form appropriate for children may be found in Nation and Aram (1977).

The present status of the language behavior may be clarified through parental report, observation of behavior, and administration of formal and informal tests and scales. Often the parents' discription of a problem provides the language diagnostician with useful information on the type of disorder manifested and its degree of severity. Because parents frequently are discerning observers, they can provide working hypotheses which may be further verified or rejected by the examiner's own observation and testing. Although parents occasionally will be inaccurate, biased, or confused in describing their child's language behavior, the fact that they are ongoing observers of this behavior each day gives them certain advantages over a clinician who has only a limited time to observe the child.

Although, as earlier noted, language assessment should imply etiologic diagnosis, in many cases the direct cause of the impairment remains obscure. For instance, the impairment in a deaf child may be clearly related to rubella, meningitis, kernicterus, or any of several other causes, but an etiologic determination may be less obvious in certain types of intellectual retardation, psychosis, or neurologic disease. Neurologic dysfunction has often been suspected as a cause of language impairment in children, and structural damage and abnormal brain function have been documented in several cases (Dreifuss, 1975; Cohen, Caparulo, and Shaywitz, 1976; and Ferry, Culbertson, Fitzgibbons, and Netsky, 1979). However, in a number of children, even when neurologic dysfunction is suspected, a clear-cut history of cerebral insult or disorder and gross signs of abnormal neurologic functioning have not been found. In such cases, some examiners have assumed the cause to be minimal brain dysfunction (MBD) and have considered the problem to be one form of "psychoneurological learning disability" (Johnson and Myklebust, 1967). However, Weiner (1980) casts doubt on the idea that minimal cerebral dysfunction, as it is currently defined, can be considered the predominant etiology in child language impairment. Many clinicians, while admitting the possibility of cerebral dysfunction as one etiology, believe that such a diagnosis is premature. They would prefer simply to treat the pattern of disability—explaining the problem in terms of psychologic or linguistic deficit instead of neurologic deficit. However, in view of the known relation between brain and language disorders as particularly demonstrated in the area of adult aphasia, caution is warranted in discounting underlying neurogenic dysfunction as a pivotal issue in child language impairment. The interdisciplinary study of language problems by speech-language pathologists, linguists, and neuroscientists must not be impeded by our current inability to assess fully the critical neurologic parameters in the etiology of the majority of child language disorders. Likewise, at the service level, the need for interdisciplinary effort is also vital. The passage of the Education for All Handicapped Children Act of 1975 (PL 94–142) demands an integrated approach to the diagnosis and management of the language-impaired child in the classroom. This approach involves not only speech-language pathologists, but classroom teachers, special education specialists, psychologists, social workers, medical personnel, and parents.

The Developmental Approach. Most often, the language-impaired child acts much as a younger normal child would. Consequently, the developmental approach to assessment of language disorders in children provides a frame of reference that is most useful in acquiring clinical information. Within definable limits of error that result from individual variation in growth and development, the examiner may assign to all, or any part of, a receptive or expressive behavior a "language age" which indicates when this behavior is present in the normal child. Not only can the level of verbal behavior be characterized, but comparisons can be made with certain aspects of nonverbal behavior which reveal whether the child manifests specific language problems or whether the language delay is only one feature of a generalized depression of performance.

Generalized depression of all performance is typical of the developmentally delayed or mentally retarded child, for example. It is also common for these children to score somewhat higher on performance items than on verbal items on standardized tests. It has been demonstrated that the acquisition of the speech and language milestones for the developmentally delayed child will occur in an orderly sequence, but that completion of this sequence will take longer than for the normal child (Lenneberg, 1967). For the developmentally delayed child, single words usually emerge between the ages of one and six, with the average age being three years; sentences are formed between the ages of two and eight years, with average onset at four years, depending on the severity of retardation (Morley, 1965).

The developmental approach to language disorders is logically tied in with the concept of critical periods for the acquisition of language. Lenneberg (1967) has presented evidence to suggest that the emergence of language is a correlate of cerebral maturation. When brain growth slows, a sharp decline occurs in the facility to acquire language. This decline begins between the ages of ten and twelve years. Furthermore, in the normal child, the thirty-six-month period between the ages of two and five appears to be extremely propitious for language development (Krashen, 1975). Basic mastery of grammar, in terms of understanding rules and acquiring strategies for comprehending and generating sentences, is achieved by the fourth birthday. Obviously, then, early identification, diagnosis, and therapeutic intervention can capitalize on the biological timetable that sets the pace for language acquisition.

Several general developmental scales and intelligence tests with language subsections (summarized in table 2–4) are available for assessment of language behavior and other behavior extending from earliest infancy to later maturity. Developmental language scales which emphasize preverbal as well as verbal stages of development are of special merit because preverbal vocalizations, with some noticeable exceptions, generally appear to be prerequisites for normal oral language development. In many neurologically impaired children, an abnormal cry, plus the lack of preverbal babbling, provide the first clue that special intervention will be required to foster adequate use of language.

It should be mentioned that detailed testing of developmental language skills may not be necessary to reveal significant deviations in language. Rather, as has been persuasively argued by Lenneberg (1969), the major developmental milestones of receptive and expressive symbolic behavior clearly show the child's capacity and potential for language development. Such easily obtainable data as the age at onset of the first word (nine to twelve months), emergence of two-word phrases (eighteen to twenty-four months), ability to follow directions (thirty to thirty-six months), and

Table 2–4. Selected General Developmental and Intellectual Scales with Language Subscales

Author(s)	Reference Source	Brief Description
Anderson, R., Miles, M., and Matheny, P.	*Communication Evaluation Chart.* Cambridge, Mass.: Educators Publishing Service (1963).	Both language and performance items selected from various preschool intelligence tests and developmental scales are included. Suitable for children between three months and five years old.
Doll, E.	*Vineland Social Maturity Scale.* Circle Pines, MN: American Guidance Service (1965).	Measures social competence from birth to twenty-five years. Communication items are included.
Doll, E.	*Preschool Attainment Record, Experimental Edition.* Circle Pines, MN: American Guidance Service (1966).	Eight checklist subscales for determining level of preschool behavior from birth to seven years. One subscale deals with communication.
Frankenburg W. and Dodds, J.	*Denver Developmental Screening Test.* Denver: Ladoca Project and Publishing Foundation (1975).	Detects delay in development in ages zero to six years. Assesses social, fine motor, gross motor, and language skills. Subscale age levels can be obtained.
Goodenough, F., Maurer, K., and Van Wagenen, M.	*Minnesota Preschool Scale.* Circle Pines, MN: American Guidance Service (1949).	Well-known standard preschool intelligence test which allows establishment of verbal and nonverbal percentile scores and IQ. Estimates IQ as early as eighteen months.
Kaufman, A.S. and Kaufman, N. L.	*Kaufman Assessment Battery for Children (K-ABC).* Circle Pines, MN: American Guidance Service, (1982).	Provides an individual assessment of intelligence and achievement for normal and exceptional children within 2-1/2 to 12-1/2 years.
Knoblock, H. and Pasamanick, B. (eds.)	*Gesell and Armatruda's Developmental Diagnosis* (3rd ed.). New York: Harper and Row (1974).	Classic pediatric scales and test items for assessing stages and sequences of developmental behavior from four months to three years. Language development is one of the five areas assessed.
McCarthy, D.	*McCarthy Scales of Children's Abilities.* New York: Psychological Corporation (1972).	Widely used intellectual and motor scales for children 2-1/2 to 8-1/2 years. Yields overall IQ and scores in six areas, one of which is verbal ability.
Wechsler, D.	*Wechsler Preschool and Primary Scale of Intelligence* (WPPSI). New York: Psychological Corporation (1967).	Well-known intelligence test for children ages 4 to 6-1/2 years. Can obtain Verbal and Performance IQs and Full Scale IQ.
Wechsler, D.	*Wechsler Intelligence Scale for Children—Revised (WISC-R).* New York: Psychological Corporation (1974).	This test is for ages six to sixteen years. Similar IQs as above can be obtained.

spontaneous construction of syntactically complex sentences with fair intelligibility (thirty-six to forty-eight months) may be better indices of capacity to develop language than information from more precise, standardized tests which assess vocabulary, syntactical complexity of sentences, and proficiency of articulation. In fact, these latter measures may simply reflect the varying linguistic environments of the child and the specific deficiencies of these environments.

Other simple and useful measures are mean length of response (Johnson, Darley, and Spriestersbach, 1963) and mean length of utterance (Brown, 1973). Mean length of response is tallied in number of words per utterance, and mean length of utterance is based on the number of morphemes per utterance. Utterances are elicited by pictures and toys, and although the reliability of these measures varies with the number of utterances judged, the stimulus material, and the individual child, these simple average measures serve as an impressive estimator of language maturity. Roughly, the average two-year-old uses two-word responses; the three-year-old, five-word responses, and the eight-year-old, eight-word responses (Brown, Darley, and Gomez, 1967). Thus, despite varied environmental influences, consistency of developmental patterns is pivotal in language development and becomes an important concept for assessment.

Comprehensive Language Tests. The recent burgeoning literature on language development and its disorders, in addition to a notable increase of language-impaired children in the caseloads of speech-language pathologists, has prompted the construction of several tests designed to assess various aspects of language behavior separated from other developmental behaviors. Several of these tests—notably the Illinois Test of Psycholinguistic Abilities (Kirk, McCarthy, and Kirk, 1968); the Porch Index of Communicative Ability in Children (Porch, 1975); the Preschool Language Scale (Zimmerman, Steiner, and Evatt, 1979); the Receptive-Expressive Emergent Language Scale (Bzoch and League, 1971); the Sequenced Inventory of Communication Development (Hedrick, Prather, and Tobin, 1975); the Houston Test of Language Development (Crabtree, 1963); and the Utah Test of Language Development Scale (Mecham, 1978)—all incorporate a developmental framework in which normative data are used to establish language performance expectations at each age level. These tests and scales attempt to provide comprehensive measures of language function, usually assessing aspects of both comprehension and expression. The Illinois Test of Psycholinguistic Abilities, for instance, has ten subtests plus two supplementary tests, which purport to measure reception, association, and expression on "representational" and "automatic levels." Other subtests involve sequential memory and closure. The Preschool Language Scale, a widely used comprehensive developmental scale, provides separate language ages for auditory comprehension and for verbal ability, as well as a single language age from a combination of subtests. Each of the three language ages may be converted to a quotient. Test results on the Preschool Language Scale are based on direct observation of performance rather than reports from informants. The Sequenced Inventory of Communication Development uses both receptive and expressive responses and a combination of informant reports and observation of the child's actual performance. Receptively, the scale proceeds developmentally from sound localization responses to comprehending linguistic contrasts and speech sound discriminations. Expressively, the items move from prelingual behavior to picture naming and responses to questions. In addition to highly specific expressive subtest items, there is opportunity to take a language sample, and scoring procedures are provided for a full range of syntactic constructions in this sample. A separate articulation test is provided, but its score is not included in the derived expressive communication age. The test broadly samples language and is clearly a comprehensive test rather than a prescriptive test, such as the ITPA, which profiles specific abilities and disabilities.

Two older tests, the Houston Test for Language Development and the Utah Test of Language Development, also are broad in assessment. The Houston Test measures general areas of reception, conceptualization, and expression, including such items as melody, accent, gesture, articulation, vocabulary, grammatical usage, and drawing. The Utah Test assesses comprehension and expression in such areas as recognition vocabulary, expressive naming vocabulary, sentence length, digit memory, color naming, copying geometric designs, and reading. Although these tests lack some of the linguistic sophistication of the more modern comprehensive tests, they served in their time to alert the speech-language pathologist to the need for broad-based assessment instruments for the diagnosis of language impairment in children.

The Porch Index for Communicative Ability in Children (PICAC) was constructed in a format similar to the Porch Index of Communicative Ability (Porch, 1969; 1971), a highly successful test for assessment of aphasia in adults. The PICAC is available in only an experimental edition. The basic and advanced batteries of the PICAC contain a total of thirty-five subtests evaluating the verbal, gestural, reading, reading auditory, visual, and graphic modalities. A complex, multidimensional scoring system, similar to that of the PICA, is employed for judging the child's responses. Although the PICAC retains many of the strengths that made its adult companion, the PICA, appealing to clinicians, its present incompleteness makes it a less popular comprehensive language test for children.

Two widely known comprehensive tests, the Verbal Language Development Scale and the Receptive-Expressive Emergent Language Scale (REEL), are based primarily on parent or informant interview. The Verbal Language Development Scale extends the communication items on the Vineland Social Maturity Scale (Doll, 1965) and tests items in listening, speaking, reading, and writing from birth to fifteen years. A language age equivalent score is derived from the total score. The REEL Scale, on the other hand, yields three scores, a receptive language age, an expressive language age, and a combined age. A total language quotient also may be derived. The age range is zero to thirty-six months.

A major criticism of some of these tests, particularly the older ones, is that, although broad in scope, they sometimes miss certain aspects of language functioning that appear important to the understanding of language disorders. The linguistic analysis of oral language derived from Chomsky (1957; 1965; 1972; 1975; 1976) and other linguists has stressed the role of syntax as well as semantics and pragmatics in understanding how sentences are comprehended and produced. This linguistic approach has seemed more relevant to the problem of understanding language disorders than assumptions in developmental and psychological processing theory that underlie many of the older comprehensive tests. Nevertheless, selected subtests from the older comprehensive tests are often very useful in assessing certain aspects of language behavior, even though the examiner may prefer a major test battery with more emphasis on current linguistic concepts. More recent comprehensive tests, such as the Clinical Evaluation of Language Functions (Semel and Wiig, 1980), have a strong

Table 2–5. Comprehensive Tests of Language

Author(s)	Reference Source	Brief Description
Bzoch, K. and League, R.	*Receptive-Expressive Emergent Language Scale.* Gainesville, FL: Tree of Life Press (1971).	Developmental language scale for ages zero to thirty-six months.
Crabtree, M.	*The Houston Test for Language Development.* Houston: Houston Test Company (1963).	Receptive and expressive test items for ages eighteen months to six years cover a broad range of speech and language skills.
Hammill, D. D., Brown, V. L., Larsen, S. C., and Wiederholt, J. L.	*Test of Adolescent Language (TOAL).* East Aurora, NY: Slosson Educational Publications (1982).	A test covering ten areas of language function designed for children six to twelve years. Is one of a series of language measures that includes the Test of Early Language Development (TELD) for children at least three years of age.
Hedrick, D., Prather, E., and Tobin, A.	*Sequenced Inventory of Communication Development.* Seattle: University of Washington Press (1975).	An inclusive language test of both receptive and expressive behavior for ages four months to four years.
Horstmier, D. and MacDonald, J.	*Environmental Pre-Language Battery.* Columbus: Charles E. Merrill (1978).	For children who are nonverbal or at a single word level.
Kirk, S., McCarthy, J., and Kirk, W.	*The Illinois Test of Psycholinguistic Abilities* (Rev. ed.). Urbana: University of Illinois Press (1968).	A widely used test containing ten subtests (two supplementary ones) for ages two to ten. Provides for individualized remedial programs.
MacDonald, J.	*Environmental Language Inventory.* Columbus: Charles E. Merrill (1978).	Tests grammatical-semantic rules in imitation, conversation, and free play of young children.

linguistic base. This test includes a complete diagnostic battery, as well as two screening tests which assess syntax, semantics, phonology, and memory in thirteen subtests. Six of these tests are in areas of language processing, five in language production, and two tests assess receptive and expressive phonology. Table 2–5 lists and briefly describes these tests, as well as others that may be considered comprehensive language tests.

Language Screening Tests. Relatively short tests designed to distinguish the language-impaired child from the normal child and identify broad areas of disorders are always welcomed by speech-language pathologists who must evaluate a number of children rapidly. Such language screening tests are available to the clinician. These tests do not aspire to the completeness of the more comprehensive tests; they serve only to aid the clinician in recognizing the child who needs in-depth diagnostic assessment and, possibly, therapeutic management later.

A popular and well-known screening test is the Northwestern Syntax Screening Test (NSST) (Lee, 1971). It provides both receptive and expressive subtests to assess the level of the child's syntactic development between three and eight years of age.

Author(s)	Reference Source	Brief Description
Mecham, M., Jex, J., and Jones, J.	*Utah Test of Language Development.* Salt Lake City: Communication Research Associates (1978).	Arranges items compiled from other tests by child's age, from one to fifteen years, to provide a functional language age.
Mecham, M.	*Verbal Language Development Scale.* Circle Pines, MN: American Guidance Service (1971).	Extends the communication items from the *Vineland Social Maturity Scale* in an informant interview scale for ages ranging from zero to fifteen years.
Moog, J. and Geers, A.	*Scales of Early Communication Skills for Hearing Impaired Children.* St. Louis: Central Institute for the Deaf (1975).	Receptive and expressive skills are assessed in imitation and comprehension, as well as spontaneous production, in ages three through eight years.
Porch, B.	*Porch Index of Communicative Ability for Children.* Palo Alto: Consulting Psychologists Press (1975).	Twenty-two subtests assess the verbal, gestural, reading, auditory, visual, and graphic modalities. For preschoolers and children ages six to twelve. Incomplete research edition.
Wiig, E. and Semel, E.	*Clinical Evaluation of Language Functions: Diagnostic Battery.* Columbus: Charles E. Merrill (1980).	Contains thirteen subtests assessing language processing, language production, and receptive and expressive phonological factors.
Wolski, W. and Lerea, L.	*Michigan Picture Language Inventory.* Ann Arbor: University of Michigan (1962).	Assesses receptive and expressive vocabulary and nine aspects of language structure for ages ranging from four to six years.
Zimmerman, I., Steiner, V., and Pond, R.	*Preschool Language Scale, Revised edition.* Columbus: Charles E. Merrill (1979).	For children eighteen months to seven years, this scale assesses both comprehension and use, yielding quotients.

Twenty items each in the receptive and expressive subtests assess the same linguistic structures. Normative data are provided. This test has received considerable attention in the research literature; those interested in a summary of comments on its merits and deficits are referred to Darley (1979, pp. 39–42). The Oral Language Sentence Imitation Screening Test (Zachman, Huisingh, Jorgenson, and Barrett, 1977) also screens syntactic development using the popular psycholinguistic research techniques of sentence imitation. Sixty test sentences are employed. Unlike the Northwestern Syntax Screening Test, the test has no normative data available to determine the adequacy of response, and the examiner must rely on personal clinical judgment.

The Bankson Language Screening Test (Bankson, 1977) and the Screening Tests of the Clinical Evaluation of Language Functions (CELF) (Semel and Wiig, 1980) are instruments that also reflect current linguistic concepts, but they do not limit themselves to syntactic development alone. The Bankson Test utilizes seventeen subtests to assess basic vocabulary and semantic knowledge; early syntactic and morphologic features; and auditory and visual tasks involving matching, association, discrimination, memory, and sequencing. The CELF screening tests assess language processing and production with such tasks as phrase and sentence imitation, phrase completion, serial recall, antonyms, phoneme recall production, and abstraction and formulation of attributes.

Several screening batteries are aimed at assessing speech and language development only in the preschool or early elementary grade child. Often, articulation tests plus selected sensitive language items are included; examples are the Picture and Language Screening Test (Rodgers, 1976), the Riley Articulation and Language Test (Riley, 1971), the Compton Speech and Language Evaluation (Compton, 1978), the Vane Evaluation of Language Scale (Vane, 1975) and the Merrill Language Screening Test (Mumm, Secord, and Dykstra, 1979). Finally, the reader should note that screening tests for Spanish-English speakers are now present on the commercial test market. Descriptions and sources of language screening tests are found in table 2–6.

Tests for Assessing Specific Aspects of Language. The speech-language pathologist will find it convenient and useful to assess language behavior in a systematic fashion, organizing the evaluation to sample receptive and expressive aspects of the semantic, syntactic, and phonologic levels of language functioning. Useful tests are not equally available at every level of this organizational scheme, however. Note that tests to assess pragmatic functions cannot be represented in such an organizational scheme because commercial tests at this level are not widely available as yet. To assist the reader, a listing of a representative selection of receptive and expressive language tests is offered in tables 2–7 and 2–8, respectively.

Receptive Semantic Level. Since the process of recognizing words and associating them with objects, actions, and relationships appears to be one of the earliest language functions acquired by the young child, growth of vocabulary has been a long-time index of language development (McCarthy, 1954). There have been methodological problems in estimating total vocabulary, and because of them, current tests have emphasized the measurement of lexicon development as an age-graded function. Receptive vocabulary tests are frequently used because of their ease of administration and their appropriateness for children whose speech is not intelligible. Those such as the Peabody Picture Vocabulary Test (Dunn, 1965), the Peabody Picture Vocabulary Test, Revised (Dunn, 1980), and the Ammons Full-Range Vocabulary Test (Ammons and Ammons, 1948) are suitable for preschoolers and school-age children, and the latter two applicable for adults as well. Although originally designed to assess verbal intelligence, these tests are more appropriate for assessing the current level of word recognition in the language-impaired child, and should not be used as definitive estimators of intellectual functioning. Bangs (1975) has developed a receptive vocabulary test called the Vocabulary Comprehension Scale, which tests the ability to comprehend semantic concepts expressed in pronouns and words of position, size, quantity, and quality.

Tests of vocabulary definition are also measures of word recognition, but in addition they allow for a judgment of the maturity level of the concept underlying word comprehension. Vocabulary definition subtests from standard intelligence tests, such as the Wechsler Intelligence Scale for Children and the Stanford-Binet, may be used to assess ability to define words. Love (1964) has proposed a method for assessing the quality of vocabulary definitions of certain words from the Peabody Picture Vocabulary Test. A disadvantage of vocabulary definition tests for language-impaired children is that they require a verbal response.

Table 2-6. Screening Tests of Language

Author(s)	Reference Source	Brief Description
Bankson, N.	*Bankson Language Screening Test.* Baltimore: University Park Press (1977).	Linguistically based test with norms for five-, six-, and seven-year-olds.
Carrow-Woolfolk, E.	*Screening Test for Auditory Comprehension of Language, English/Spanish.* Boston: Teaching Resources Corporation (1974).	Screens syntax comprehension in ages three to six. Uses twenty items.
Compton, A.	*Compton Speech and Language Screening Evaluation.* San Francisco: Carousel House (1978).	Brief test uses objects to elicit several language functions for children ages three to six.
Dailey, J.	*Language Facility Test.* Alexandria, VA: Allington Corporation (1977).	Quick test for ages two to fifteen. Story telling is judged on a zero-to-nine scoring system.
James, P.	*James Language Dominance Test.* Austin: Learning Concepts (1974).	For grades K–1; test yields a measure of language dominance or bilingualism in both reception and expression in Spanish and English.
Lee, L.	*Northwestern Syntax Screening Test.* Evanston:Northwestern University Press (1971).	Evaluates comprehension and expression of morphologic and syntactic structures by children from three to eight years.
Mumm, M., Secord, W., and Dykstra, K.	*Merrill Language Screening Test.* Columbus: Charles E. Merrill (1979).	Five-minute screening test in which the child retells story and answers questions about it; sentence repetition is employed.
Riley, G.	*Riley Articulation and Language Test.* Los Angeles: Western Psychological Services (1971).	Articulation and language proficiency is scored from a short language sample. Norms for Headstart and K through 2.
Rodgers, W.	*Picture Articulation and Language Screening Test.* Salt Lake City: Word Making Productions (1976).	Assesses verbal description of actions, naming, and articulation. Ages three to five years.
Toronto, A., Leverman, D., Hanna, C., Rosenzweig, P., and Maldonado, A.	*Del Rio Language Screening Test, English/Spanish.* Austin: National Education Laboratory Publishers (1975).	Screens five language functions in ages four to six years. For children of southwestern United States.
Vane, J.	*Vane Evaluation of Language Scale.* Brandon, VT: Clinical Psychology Publishing Company, Inc. (1975).	Assesses receptive and expressive language, memory, and handedness in ages 2-1/2 to six years.
Wiig, E. and Semel, E.	*Clinical Evaluation of Language Functions: Screening Tests.* Columbus: Charles E. Merrill (1980).	Assesses forty-eight items in grades K through 5, and fifty-two items in grades 5 through 12. Current linguistics concepts tested.
Zachman, L., Huisingh, R., Jorgenson, C., and Barrett, M.	*The Oral Language Sentence Imitation Screening Test.* Moline, IL: Linguistic Systems (1976).	Screens syntactic performance using sentence imitation techniques.

Table 2–7. Selected Tests for Assessment of Receptive Language Behavior: Semantic, Syntactic, and Phonologic

Author(s)	Reference Source	Brief Description
I. Semantic Level		
Ammons, R. and Ammons, H.	*Full-Range Vocabulary Test.* Missoula, MT: Psychological Test Specialists (1959).	Provides norms for recognition vocabulary, for clients ranging from two years old to the superior adult level.
Bangs, T.	*Vocabulary Comprehension Scale.* Boston: Teaching Resources Corporation (1975).	Assesses pronouns, and words of position, size, quantity, and quality.
Dunn, L.	*Peabody Picture Vocabulary Test; Revised.* Circle Pines, MN: American Guidance Service (1980).	Revision is restandardized with new stimulus pictures and extended norms.
Dunn, L.	*Peabody Picture Vocabulary Test.* Circle Pines, MN: American Guidance Service (1965).	Provides age equivalents, quotients, and percentile for recognition vocabulary, ranging from eighteen months to eighteen years.
Toronto, A.	*Toronto Tests of Receptive Vocabulary: English/Spanish.* Austin: Academic Tests (1977).	Picture vocabulary test for children between four and ten years.
II. Syntactic Level		
Carrow-Woolfolk, E.	*Test for Auditory Comprehension of Language, Spanish/English.* Boston: Teaching Resources (1974).	Tests five aspects of comprehension of syntax. Normed for children ages three to six years.
DiSimoni, F.	*Token Test for Children.* Hingham, MA: Teaching Resources (1979).	Identifies receptive language function in children four to twelve years. Tests lexicon and syntax.
Foster, R., Giddan, J., and Stark, J.	*Assessment of Children's Language Comprehension.* Palo Alto: Consulting Psychologists Press (1969, 1973).	Assess child's ability to understand varied word classes in different length and complexity combinations.
Zachman, L., Huisingh, R., Jorgenson, L., and Barrett, M.	*The Oral Language Sentence Imitation Diagnostic Test.* Moline, IL: Lingui-Systems (1977).	Tests of syntactic performance using sentence imitation techniques.
III. Phonologic Level		
Aten, J.	*Denver Auditory Phoneme Sequencing Test.* Houston: College Press (1979).	Assess single phoneme discrimination and sequenced phoneme abilities in children.
Flowers, A.	*Flowers Auditory Test of Selective Attention, Experimental Edition.* Dearborn, MI: Perceptual Learning Systems (1975).	Audiotape directs child to point to pictures under a series of directions requiring close attention.
Flowers, A. and Costello, M.	*Flowers-Costello Test of Central Auditory Abilities.* Dearborn, MI: Perceptual Learning Systems (1970).	Tests response to low-pass filtered speech and response to competing messages.

Author(s)	Reference Source	Brief Description
Fudula, J., Kunze, L., and Ross, J.	*Auditory Pointing Test.* San Rafael, CA: Academic Therapy Publications (1974).	Measures short-term word memory span and sequencing abilities in children from five to twelve years.
Goldman, R., Fristoe, M., and Woodcock, R.	*Goldman-Fristoe-Woodcock Auditory Selective Attention Test:* Circle Pines, MN: American Guidance Service (1976).	Listening task in competing noise of varying types and intensity. Age range is three to eighty years.
Goldman, R., Fristoe, M., and Woodcock, R.	*Goldman-Fristoe-Woodcock Auditory Memory Tests.* Circle Pines, MN: American Guidance Service (1974).	Prerecorded tests of recognition memory, memory for content, and memory for sequence. Norms for three to eighty-five years.
Goldman, R., Fristoe, M., and Woodcock, R.	*Goldman-Fristoe-Woodcock Sound-Symbol Tests.* Circle Pines, MN: American Guidance Service (1974).	Seven subtests of auditory ability presented on audiotape. Norms are for three through eighty years with emphasis on ages three through twelve years.
Goldman, R., Fristoe, M., and Woodcock, R.	*Goldman-Fristoe-Woodcock Test of Auditory Discrimination.* Circle Pines, MN: American Guidance Service (1970).	Prerecorded test of discrimination, controlling for vocabulary, designed for persons three years, eight months to adulthood. Also assesses discrimination in noise.
Irwin, O.	*A Test of Sound Discrimination.* In *Communication Variables of Cerebral Palsied and Mentally Retarded Children.* Springfield, IL: Charles C. Thomas (1972).	Discrimination tests used in research with cerebral palsied and retarded children for ages six to sixteen.
Kimmell, G. and Wahl, J.	*Screening Test for Auditory Perception.* San Rafael, CA: Academic Therapy Publications (1959).	Five tests of aural perception designed as a screening test. Still in experimental edition.
Lindamood, C. and Lindamood, P.	*Lindamood Auditory Conceptualization Test.* Boston: Teaching Resources (1971).	Tests ability to recognize differences in speech sounds as well as number and order of sound sequences in sound patterns.
Mecham, M., Jex, J., and Jones, J.	*Test of Listening Accuracy in Children.* Salt Lake City, UT: Communication Research Associates (1968, 1973).	Words for auditory discrimination are presented in noise by audiotape. Norms by grade level.
Pather, E., Miner, A., Addicott, M., and Sunderland, L.	*Washington Speech Sound Discrimination Test.* Danville, IL: Interstate Printers and Publishers (1971).	A sound discrimination test utilizing five words to avoid confounding by vocabulary knowledge.
Provonost, W.	*Boston University Speech Sound Discrimination Test.* Cedar Falls, IA: Go-mo Products (1953, 1974).	Has a long and short form, using same-different responses.
Reagan, C. and Cunningham, S.	*Differentiation of Auditory Perceptual Skills—Experimental Edition.* Tucson, AZ: Communication Skills Builder (1975).	Screening test for ages five to eight years, measuring auditory cadence, auditory distinction, auditory imagery, syllable completion, and auditory reasoning.

Author(s)	Reference Source	Brief Description
Templin, M.	*Sound Discrimination Test.* In *Certain Language Skills in Children.* Minneapolis: University of Minnesota (1957).	Presents fifty auditory discrimination items standardized for children three to five years.
Wepman, J.	*Auditory Discrimination Test.* Chicago: Language Research Associates (1973).	Requires the child to give a same-different response to forty pairs of words; for ages five to eight years.
Wepman, J. and Morency, A.	*Auditory Memory Span Test.* Chicago: Language Research Associates (1973).	Tests ability to recall single-syllable words in series of two to six words; for children five to eight years old.
Wepman, J. and Morency, A.	*The Auditory Sequential Memory Test.* Chicago: Language Research Associates (1974).	Digit sequences are presented to test sequential memory. Designed for children five to eight years of age.

The Auditory Reception subtest of the ITPA is also an age-graded test of the ability to understand the meaning of words placed in short interrogative sentences. Attempts were made to reduce syntax that might give clues to meaning in the sentence form. In this subtest, for example, the subject is asked to respond with a "yes" or "no" to such questions as "Do dials yawn?" and "Do logs burn?" The number of correct answers is totaled and converted to an age equivalent.

Semantic measures like these tend to yield only limited, superficial measures of the development of a child's lexicon and little information about the categorization of the semantic aspects of his or her grammar. It may well be that the language-impaired child is employing different semantic rules and features than those used by the normal child.

Receptive Syntactic Level. Psycholinguistic research has emphasized the central role of syntactic rules—probably innate—that are necessary for comprehending and generating language. Establishing how the child comprehends and employs syntax is therefore critical for the diagnosis of a language disorder. Johnson and Myklebust (1967) reported that disorders of syntax make up a major group of psychoneurological learning disorders in children; more recent researchers in language impairment have studied the use of syntax in developmental language disorders to a greater extent than any other aspect of language functioning (Leonard, 1979).

Several major tests at this level have developed that may be applied clinically. The Michigan Picture Language Inventory, developed by Lerea (1958a; 1958b) and modified by Wolski (Wolski and Lerea, 1962) contained a receptive vocabulary test and comprehension of certain language structures, including pronouns, possessives, comparative forms, adjectives, demonstratives, articles, adverbs, and three verb tenses. The Northwestern Syntax Screening Test (Lee, 1971), first developed in 1969, also distinguished clearly between receptive and expressive aspects of grammar. Several of the more recent screening tests and comprehensive tests discussed above also have independent receptive language sections which may be used to assess receptive syntax.

A well-known test of receptive syntax is the Assessment of Children's Language Comprehension developed by Foster, Giddan, and Stark (1969). Carrow-Woolfolk (1974c; 1974d) has published two tests, one a diagnostic battery and the other a

Table 2–8. Selected Tests for Assessment of Expressive Language Behavior: Semantic, Syntactic, and Phonologic

Author(s)	Reference Source	Brief Description
I. Semantic Level		
Bankson, N.	Bankson Language Screening Test. Baltimore: University Park Press (1977).	Many items in this test measure basic expressive vocabulary and semantics.
Hedrick, D., Pather, E., and Tobin A.	Sequenced Inventory of Communication Development. Seattle: University of Washington (1975).	Expressive tests require picture naming and describing of function. Ages four months to four years.
Kirk, S., McCarthy, J., and Kirk, W.	Vocal Expression Subtest, The Illinois Test of Psycholinguistic Abilities (Rev. ed.). Urbana: The University of Illinois Press (1968).	Measures the quantity of expressive verbal concepts for describing four objects.
Kirk, S., McCarthy, J., and Kirk, W.	Auditory-Vocal Association Subtest, The Illinois Test of Psycholinguistic Abilities (Rev. ed.). Urbana: The University of Illinois Press (1968).	Gives an expressive measure of word association ability.
Love, R.	Oral language behavior of older cerebral palsied children. J. Speech Hearing Res. 7, 349–362 (1964).	Describes procedures for using the first fifty-five words of the PPVT as an expressive naming test. Also describes a definitions test using thirty-nine words from the same source.
MacDonald, J.	Environmental Language Inventory. Columbus: Charles E. Merrill (1978).	This comprehensive test for expressively delayed children focuses on assessing semantic-grammatical rules.
Semel, E. and Wiig, E.	Clinical Evaluation of Language Functions: Diagnostic Battery. Columbus: Charles E. Merrill (1980).	Subtests include expressive naming.
Terman, L. and Merrill, M.	Vocabulary Test. Stanford-Binet Intelligence Scale (Form L–M). Boston: Houghton Mifflin Company (1960).	May be used to assess vocabulary definition.
Wechsler, D.	Vocabulary Subtest, The Wechsler Intelligence Scale for Children. New York: The Psychological Corporation (1949).	Vocabulary definitions on vocabulary subtest may be scored on a three-point scale.
Wolski, W. and Lerea, L.	Michigan Picture Language Inventory. Ann Arbor: The University of Michigan (1962).	Test battery includes picture naming items for ages four to six years.
II. Syntactic Level		
Bloom, L. and Lahey, M.	Language Development and Language Disorders. New York: John Wiley (1978).	Provides discussion of procedures for analyzing a language sample.
Carrow-Woolfolk, E.	Carrow Elicited Language Inventory. Austin: Teaching Resources (1974).	Diagnostic test of productive grammar. Identifies errors in specific grammatical structure. Uses imitation.

Author(s)	Reference Source	Brief Description
Lee, L.	*Developmental Sentence Analysis.* Evanston, IL: Northwestern University Press (1974).	Allows scoring of language sample for developmental level. Includes Development Sentence Types and Developmental Scoring techniques.
Tyack, D. and Gottsleben, R.	*Language Sampling, Analysis and Training.* Palo Alto: Consulting Psychologist's Press (1974).	A method for analyzing a 100-sentence sample of spontaneous speech.

III. *Phonologic Level*

Blakeley, R.	*Screening Test for Developmental Apraxia of Speech.* Tigard, OR: C. C. Publications, Inc. (1980).	Ten-minute screening test for children four to twelve.
Carrow-Woolfolk, E.	*Austin Spanish Articulation Test.* Boston: Teaching Resources (1974).	Single-word articulation test designed for use with Spanish-speaking children. No provisions for variations of Spanish dialect.
Compton, A. and Hutton, J.	*Compton-Hutton Phonological Assessment.* San Francisco: Carousel House (1978).	Close transcriptions of articulation error patterns may be compared to a list of sound errors. Designed for ages three to ten years.
Fisher, H. and Logemann, J.	*The Fisher-Logemann Test of Articulation Competence.* Boston: Houghton-Mifflin (1971).	Records production of phonemes allophonically and analyzes them in terms of manner and place of production. Emphasizes analysis of geographic and socioeconomic class dialects.
Goldman, R. and Fristoe, M.	*Goldman-Fristoe Test of Articulation.* Circle Pines, MN: American Guidance (1969).	Tests phoneme proficiency in words and sentences and in conditions of maximum oral-visual stimulation.
McDonald, E.	*Deep Tests of Articulation.* Pittsburgh: Stanwix House, Inc. (1964, 1968).	Assesses phonemes in contexts where the test phoneme is one of an abutting pair.
McReynolds, L. and Engmann, D.	*Distinctive Feature Analysis of Misarticulations.* Baltimore: University Park Press (1975).	Application of Chomsky-Halle distinctive feature theory to sound errors.
Shirberg, L. and Kwiatkowski, J.	*Natural Process Analysis* (NPA): *A Procedure for Phonological Analysis of Continuous Speech Samples.* New York: John Wiley (1980).	Methods of articulation analysis that allow feature analysis, developmental analysis, and grammatical morpheme analysis in speech samples.
Templin, M. and Darley, F.	*The Templin-Darley Tests of Articulation.* Iowa City: Bureau of Educational Research and Service, The University of Iowa (1969).	Characterized by age-graded norms for articulation proficiency; provides data for ages three through eight years.
Toronto, A.	*Southwestern Spanish Articulation Test.* Austin: Academic Tests (1977).	A single-word articulation test for the Spanish-speaking child.
Weiner, F.	*Phonological Process Analysis.* Baltimore: University Park Press (1978).	Twenty phonological processes are tested in response to sentence completion and recall to 136 pictures.

screening test of auditory comprehension. The diagnostic battery is called the Test for Auditory Comprehension of Language, English/Spanish and the screening test is called the Screening Test for Auditory Comprehension of Language, English/Spanish.

The Token Test for Children (DiSimoni, 1979), based on a well-known adult test for studying comprehension in adult aphasia, assesses receptive language in the areas of lexicon and syntax. It was designed to identify higher-level receptive dysfunction in children four to twelve years of age.

Receptive Phonologic Level. Throughout the history of speech-language pathology, there always has been a vital and continuing interest in the various parameters of the perception of speech sounds. The ability to recognize and interpret phonemes has been studied primarily from the standpoint of discriminating phonemes, but in recent years particular attention has been paid to auditory memory for phonemes and auditory sequencing of phonemes, as well as the more generalized function of auditory attention. The most popular techniques for assessing the accuracy of the individual's reception of phonemes have been phonetically balanced word lists (O'Neill and Oyer, 1966) and tests of auditory sound discrimination. Two widely used tests have been those devised by Wepman (1958) and Goldman, Fristoe, and Woodcock (1970). Despite the widespread use of auditory discrimination tests, it is still not clear, however, just what effect a disability in auditory discrimination may have on other aspects of language functioning (Bloom and Lahey, 1978). Likewise, the effect of problems in auditory sequencing, auditory memory, and auditory attention on language are also equivocal at this time. There are some clinical indications that in some children poor auditory discrimination is related causally to inadequate phoneme production. On the other hand, evidence exists that poor auditory discrimination in most instances does not necessarily retard syntactic and semantic development (Bloom and Lahey, 1978). At present, the best data available on auditory discrimination skills are restricted to normative information. Valuable as these data are, they provide little or no knowledge about the actual process involved in recognition and interpretation of phonemes nor information on the relation of speech discrimination to production. This, of course, also holds true for the other auditory processes of auditory memory, sequencing, and attention that are subsumed under speech perception. Thus, clinicians must be very careful in test selection; if we do not yet truly understand the underlying processes of speech perception, it is unlikely that a given clinical test can accurately measure the parameters of that process. Some assistance in test selection is available in evaluative reviews of tests used in speech-language pathology, such as those found in Darley (1979). Instead, the clinician can use an alternative approach in lieu of assessing receptive auditory perceptual processes in relation to speech production. The analysis of a spontaneous expressive speech sample can indicate the child's errors in speech and language production, and a custom-designed program can then be developed to remediate them. In this way, any tenuous assumptions about supposed auditory processing deficits as causes of errors in speech and language performance are circumvented.

Expressive Semantic Level. Even an untrained observer is aware that the ability to recall words and demonstrate knowledge of lexical and semantic concepts is a good measure of linguistic maturity. Many of the comprehensive and screening tests discussed above include some form of expressive naming tests or vocabulary definition tests for gaining information about the child's semantic concepts. For example, in the Utah Test of Language Development, items are included on assessing extent of expressive vocabulary and type and number of verbal concepts; on this test "Naming Common Pictures" and "Naming Colors" occurs at two-to-three-year, three-to-four-year, and four-to-five-year levels. Picture naming is also present in more recently developed tests such as the Bankson Language Screening Test, the Preschool Language Scale, the Sequenced Inventory of Communication Development, and the Clinical Evaluation of Language Functions.

A recent test, the Environmental Language Inventory (MacDonald, 1978), is of interest at the semantic level because it provides a means for analyzing the semantic-grammatical rules found in the utterances of children. Semantic word classes in utterances are examined after objects and food are used as stimuli to elicit language to study early semantic rules. Language is also assessed in free play in this inventory to assess the semantic system.

Facility at associating verbal concepts can be tested with the Auditory Vocal Association subtest of the ITPA. This subtest contains forty-two orally presented analogies such as, "I cut with a saw; I pound with a ———." The child must respond orally, and the score can be converted to an age equivalent to determine specific disabilities in verbal association.

Another test of semantic functioning that goes beyond word recall and simple verbal association is one requiring children to express their own verbal concepts about common objects. Designed for this purpose is the Verbal Expression subtest of the ITPA, which requires the child to produce a series of discrete, relevant, and factual verbal concepts about five items: a nail, a ball, a block, an envelope, and a button. Shown each of these items, for example, the child is asked, "Tell me all about this." The amount and quality of the verbalizations are evaluated and converted to an age equivalent.

The importance of assessing the child's lexicon and semantic concepts is highlighted by many writers. Bloom and Lahey (1978) described problems in word recall in children and called them "content and form interaction" disorders. Earlier, Johnson and Myklebust (1967) described one of the three groups of children with impairments of expressive language whom they studied as having a "deficit primarily in reauditorization and word selection." They wrote:

> These children understand and recognize words but they cannot remember (or retrieve) them for spontaneous usage. . . . In some instances it appears that the words of greatest consequence to meaning are the hardest to remember. For example, they recall ejaculations (okay or all right) but cannot remember the words for transmitting an idea. (pp. 114–115)

The preschool child who demonstrates this type of semantic disability, traditionally called "dysnomia," will resort to gesture and pantomime, while older children will use nonspecific circumlocutions such as "junk," "stuff," and "whatchamacallit" as substitutes for specific nouns that cannot be recalled. Other common errors occur in the production of words closely associated in memory with the one required. For instance, a dog may be misnamed a cat, or a fountain pen may be called a writer.

Expressive Syntactic Level. The contention of contemporary linguists and psycholinguists that an analysis of the grammatical rule systems governing the language performance of the developing child will ultimately explain the mechanisms of language acquisition has had a profound effect on test construction and assessment techniques in the area of child language impairment. Probably more tests and scales have been developed to evaluate expressive syntactic functioning than any other aspect of language. Some language tests deal almost exclusively with the assessment of expressive syntactical development and use techniques for analyzing a spontaneous language sample.

Lee (1974) has provided a method for analyzing the syntactic development of young children with two techniques, Developmental Sentence Types (DST) and Developmental Sentence Scoring (DSS), which may be applied to a spontaneous language sample. Together, they are called Developmental Sentence Analysis (DSA). They are described more fully in the section of this chapter titled Language Sampling. Similar techniques for syntactic analysis of a language sample have been described by Tyack and Gottsleben (1974) and Bloom and Lahey (1978). These language sampling analysis techniques which emphasize expressive syntax seem to be powerful approaches for the language pathologist, not only because they separate the normal child from the language-impaired child, but because they isolate the specific deficit areas in a child's language system that provide the basis for a language intervention program. Further, it is clear from research using language sampling techniques for studying syntactic rules that syntactical disorders are pivotal in the description of the majority, if not all, of the children classified as language-impaired. Tools which can measure change over time such as those developed by Lee, Tyack, and Gottsleben, and Bloom and Lahey are important advancements in the study of language disorders.

A standardized test for the study of expressive or productive syntax that has been widely used for assessing syntactic defects and delays is the Carrow Elicited Language Inventory (CELI) (Carrow-Woolfolk, 1974b). This diagnostic test used one phrase and fifty-one sentences in sentence imitation. A series of grammatical categories is elicited with emphasis on verb forms. As a test of expressive syntax, the CELI provides an inventory of several grammatical forms in a briefer time than is required to administer and score a language sample. A more recent test battery, similar in design, is the Oral Language Sentence Imitation Diagnostic Inventory and the Oral Language Sentence Imitation Screening Test (Zachman, Huisingh, Jorgeson, and Barrett, 1977). It provides imitative testing of twenty-four morphological and syntactic features highlighted in generative linguistic theory. This test battery also purports to provide information about syntactic behavior more rapidly than traditional language sampling.

Expressive Phonologic Level. Expressive phoneme proficiency typically is measured with an articulation test designed to assess the child's mastery of sound production—the standards for comparison being the productions expected for chronological age or adult proficiency (Fisher and Logemann, 1971; Goldman and Fristoe, 1969; and Templin and Darley, 1969). While such tests catalog errors, they do not emphasize the underlying phonologic processes that are disturbed in the phonologically defective child, nor do they indicate what mechanisms operate to bring about normal development of articulation. More recent clinical test materials based on linguistic theory, however, provide the clinician with some insights into phonologic processes that may be operative in children with such disorders. For example, McReynolds and Engmann (1975) have described a procedure for analyzing articulation errors using a distinctive feature analysis based on the work of Chomsky and Halle (1968). Phonologic rules are tested also in the Compton-Hutton Phonological Assessment (Compton and Hutton, 1978) and Weiner's Phonological Process Analysis (Weiner, 1978). Shriberg and Kwiatkowski (1980) have described procedures to study phonologic disorders in continuous speech samples rather than in single words. Data concerning feature analysis, developmental analysis, and grammatical morpheme analysis can be gathered from speech samples. A special group of tests (Carrow-Woolfolk, 1974a; Toronto, 1977) assess Spanish-English phonology.

If neurologic deficits are accepted as part of the clinical picture in language-impaired children, the concepts of developmental dysarthria and developmental apraxia of speech are important to consider in the spectrum of phonologic disorders of speech in the language-impaired child. Groups of children with expressive disorders have been identified as primarily apraxics by several writers (Brown, Darley, and Gomez, 1967; Johnson and Myklebust, 1967; Yoss and Darley, 1974; and Macaluso-Haynes, 1978). These children cannot recall the motor pattern for speech sounds and sound sequences, yet they are free of obvious paralysis, motor weakness, and incoordination in the muscles of articulation. Blakeley (1980) has developed a screening test of developmental apraxia of speech with norms for children from ages four to twelve years which may be helpful in identifying these children.

Developmental dysarthria, on the other hand, is a specific motor impairment affecting the muscles and motor control of the muscles of articulation; it generally involves paralysis, weakness, and incoordination in both speech and non-speech activities such as chewing and swallowing. Higher central control centers for motor programming and sequencing are not involved. Formal test procedures for the acoustic-perceptual analysis of the childhood dysarthrias are not available as they are for the adult dysarthrias; neither are there well-documented patterns of speech and voice characteristics of such children, as for adults (Darley, Aronson, and Brown, 1975). If, however, the developmental dysarthric symptoms are mild and primarily affect the articulation of phonemes, a standard oral peripheral examination will usually be sufficient to indicate to the examiner the basis of the dysarthria and will suggest how the motor involvement of the speech muscles is interfering with the normal production of phonemes. For a discussion of severe dysarthria in children, see chapter 7.

Language Sampling. Many child language specialists believe that after a language disorder has been identified by one of the formal standardized tests described above, more complete observation of a child's actual language performance should be conducted in a natural, everyday setting by procuring what is known as a language sample. A language sample is a body of language that provides a representative sample of oral language behavior that allows the language pathologist to generate hypotheses about the developmental maturity of the linguistic rules in a child's language system. It is typical to elicit a language sample in a natural setting such as the home, classroom, or clinic. The situation is generally low-keyed and relaxed to avoid a testing atmosphere and to prevent attempts to elicit specific words or linguistic structures. Stimuli for language sampling have usually included describing pictures, talking about toys, or responding to probes offered by an interviewer. Because young children sometimes find it difficult to describe a picture, their connected speech may be more spontaneous when a few simple objects and activities are used to elicit speech.

Some objections have been raised about the efficacy of obtaining a language sample and using the resulting linguistic analysis to formulate an intervention plan for individual case management as contrasted to using the results of standardized tests to formulate an intervention plan. Some have argued that acquiring and analyzing a language sample is extremely time consuming and is better suited for research than for clinical purposes. This criticism may be countered with the argument that a well-analyzed language sample probably provides the most accurate and complete picture of the child's language system available. The significant information about pho-nologic, syntactic, semantic, and pragmatic language functioning derived from a good language sample provides a highly informative and knowledgeable approach to ther-apy intervention. Since most standardized language tests stress only identification of deficit areas, they do not give as comprehensive a view of a child's language behavior as does a language sample.

A second objection to language sampling is that a given sample may not be completely representative of the child's language system at the time of sampling. It is well documented that such samples are subject to environmental influences (Long-hurst and Schrandt, 1973), but it can be argued that a language sample taken in a natural setting may be more, or at least as, representative of typical language perform-ance as that elicited in an artificial test situation which is highly structured.

There is some debate about what sampling conditions are required to yield a representative and useful corpus of language. Most authors (Lee, 1974; Tyack and Gottsleben, 1974) have recommended fifty to one hundred utterances and Bloom and Lahey (1978) have suggested a minimum of a half hour of direct observation of both language and nonlanguage behavior. Ideal sampling will include sampling over a period of days and use of a videotape recorder to document behavior. Audiotaping with hand notes may also be used. It is conventional to establish a developmental language age for the child or children sampled in terms of the mean length of utterance (MLU). Brown (1973) has established a widely used set of guidelines for determining this measure. Also, a system for recording and transcribing observations has been proposed by Bloom and Lahey (1978, pp. 600–609).

Several systems have been developed for analyzing language responses. Lee (1974), in a widely known system called Developmental Sentence Analysis (DSA), estab-lishes normative data which will allow identification of a language disorder from a sample and provides a developmental sequence of eight grammatical forms that are used in sentences containing a subject and a predicate. The grammatical forms include indefinite pronouns, personal pronouns, main verb elaborations including gerunds and infinitives, negative forms, conjunctions, interrogative reversals, and *wh*-question forms. The developmental sequence is divided into eight levels and yields a sequence both within each of and among all of the eight grammatical features. Goals can be determined for each of these eight grammatical features in sentences that contain both a subject and a predicate. Several features are omitted from the DSS analysis, and it is implied that forms such as articles, plurals, and possessives develop early and are first-level goals. A companion analysis called Developmental Sentence Types (DST) is used for earlier stages of language development. This analysis is divided into three levels: single words, two-word combinations, and constructions or utterances of more than two words that do not include a subject and a verb. Within these levels are two subcategories for elaborations or modifications such as plurals, possessives, or questions. Utterances are placed in one of five categories, according to sentence type.

Tyack and Gottsleben (1974) include a syntactic structure analysis of a child's utterance and an adult gloss of the utterance. A word-morpheme index can be computed to place the child at a developmental level and a score sheet allows analysis according to linguistic features and basic construction types. Hutchinson, Hanson, and Mecham (1979, pp. 202–205) have provided information which allows analysis of basic syntax from a language sample; Crystal, Fletcher, and Garman (1976) also have provided methods to analyze language form in a developmental sequence. Muma (1973) and Bloom and Lahey (1978) have described other procedures for analyzing a language sample which focus on concurring/restrictive structures and content of verb categories respectively.

In summary, use of language sample analysis has allowed the language pathologist to describe developmental deficits in language systems and to plan therapy programs for remediation that rely on determining the rule system of language rather than determining remediation on assumptions about performance according to etiologic category such as deafness, emotional disturbance, aphasia, mental retardation, or neurologic impairment. It also has allowed the language clinician to go beyond the sometimes limited data available for planning remediation from test scores, language ages, and percentiles derived from formal tests.

Informal Nonstandard Approaches to Language Assessment. Despite the recent increase in the number of standardized tests for assessing language performance in children and the wide use of language sampling techniques, several child language specialists (Aram and Nation, 1977; Bloom and Lahey, 1978; and Leonard, Prutting, Perozzi, and Berkley, 1978) have called for the use of nonstandardized clinically constructed measures as a necessary supplement to the use of standardized language tests and language sampling techniques. The purpose of developing nonstandard measures is to acquire sufficient knowledge about the child's language system to devise effective management strategies not revealed by other techniques. Language tasks may be derived from the extensive research literature on child language acquisition or devised by the creative clinician. These tasks will highlight some feature of the language system that has not been tapped in standardized language tests or a syntactic analysis of the language. As an example of a nonstandard measure, Leonard et al. (1978) offer an illustration of a nonstandardized testing item which will allow an examiner to assess, for example, a child's pragmatic ability to describe an object using information available to the listener rather than basing the description on information available only to the child. A spontaneously evoked task may be employed: being shown a geometric shape, a child may be asked to give instructions in sufficient detail to permit a listener behind a visual barrier to draw an identical shape. The examiner transcribes the child's utterances, noting whether they contain information useful to the listener—like the sentence, "Draw a line along the top of the paper." An utterance like, "Draw a line like this," spoken as the child points to a line on the shape outside the listener's view, will indicate the child's inability to convey information with appropriate communicative intent. An alert clinician may use this information to devise therapy tasks which will facilitate the child's pragmatic use of language.

PRINCIPLES AND METHODS OF LANGUAGE REMEDIATION

Any type of treatment or educational approach for the language-impaired child should begin with a consideration of remediation principles. Those set forth below have grown out of the discussion in the preceding sections, and they lead to a discussion of programs for children with specific impairments.

In recent years, child language therapists have been greatly influenced by the psychologist Jean Piaget and by others from his school of thought (e.g., Flavell, 1977) who have emphasized cognitive aspects of language. Also, the work of Dore (1975) and Halliday (1975) has largely determined that the functions or pragmatics of language are essential aspects of the intervention process. The work of Lee, Koenigsknecht, and Mulhern (1975) has influenced speech-language pathologists in the form or grammatical aspects of language. Bloom and Lahey (1978) have also addressed issues of semantic content, form, and use of language. Thus, the theoretical and practical bases for many current language intervention programs have come from these researchers. It is expected that future programs will incorporate cognitive and pragmatic theory into the language intervention process.

Remedial Principles

Sensitivity to Individual Needs. To be effective, any program in language development must be relevant to the current social, economic, and cultural patterns of the persons it serves (Bountress, 1980; Abernathy, 1970). Inherent in this statement is the principle that any program designed for the language-different or language-impaired child must be sensitive to a child's linguistic needs and interests and to the cultural milieu in which the individual will ultimately be communicating. This concept is particularly critical when designing programs for the child with language differences. Consistent with this tenet is an emphasis on using appropriate diagnostic and teaching materials standardized for a child's cultural situation, as well as on employing teaching personnel who are familiar with and concerned about the needs and characteristics of the specific group. Taylor (1971a) has suggested that we should view language as a culturally transmitted developmental process rather than as a criterion for evaluating different ethnic classes.

Early Intervention and Parental Involvement. A second basic principle of language is that intervention programs must occur early to maximize and enrich language development for the linguistically impaired child. The research of McNeill (1970) and Lenneberg (1967) suggests that there are critical periods for the acquisition of language, the most important of which fall within the early preschool years. Parental involvement in the understanding and facilitation of language development for handicapped children is essential, inasmuch as they normally play the most important role in stimulating language development in those first critical years. Parents need specific training in overall child development, including the nature of language development and methods of stimulating and reinforcing language regardless of the cause of their child's language deficiency. Studies reviewed by Bron-fenbrenner (1974) showed that a child's affective and cognitive development is enhanced when the parents are actively involved in the intervention program. Bron-fenbrenner indicates that the parent's involvement in intervention helps to insure long-term benefits of the program even after the intervention ends. Finally, Sameroff and Chandler (1975) completed an extensive review of the literature on high-risk factors and later developmental problems. They concluded that the mother's educational level (and her presumed intervention with the child) was the best single predictor of the child's future success in language. Thus, all intervention programs, consistent with Public Law 94–142, must involve the parents throughout the management process.

Naturalness of Communication. Because communication is a two-way, mutually influenced act, the intervention program must provide natural opportunities for the child to master language. Practice should be given in the dual roles of speaker and listener in contexts which are natural and meaningful to the child. Toward this end, an experiential, action-oriented approach should be used. Since language is both a cognitive and affective act, the intervention must consist of a great deal of positive interaction between the speech-language pathologist and the child.

Training in Cognitive and Communicative Functions. The language intervention program should provide training in the cognitive and communicative functions of communication. Muma (1978) stated that

> [b]oth cognitive and communicative functions are more important than form because verbal behavior is used in the service of cognitive and communicative functions. Early language learning exhibits a priority for cognitive development and for communicative functions (semantic and relational). After the basic syntactic mechanisms are learned, there is an emphasis on learning to become adept in the use of these mechanisms and on learning to use listener feedback in realizing effective communication. Intervention programs that reflect verbal functions are consistently more effective than those aimed at learning form, such as sentence making, vocabulary building, etc. (p. 298)

Ongoing Diagnostic Approach in Teaching. The remediation of language deficits involves an ongoing diagnostic approach in teaching. It is widely recognized that the effects of language deficiency in a child are generally long-lasting and may cross several modalities of language input (Wiig and Semel, 1980; Wiener, 1971). It is only through recognition of the various levels of modality deficit and intensive stimulation in these or in more intact areas of language input that successful remediation and reversal of such deficits will occur. Moreover, the speech-language pathologist must be able to change teaching methods in accordance with the changing needs of the child. Myers and Hammill (1969) have defined diagnostic teaching as an extension and continuation of the diagnostic process in which the teacher, through careful observation and reporting, is aided in arriving at a behavioral description of the child's specific disability. To be an adaptive and dynamic process sensitive to the changing patterns of the child, the training program must provide these components:

1. a pleasant and stimulating atmosphere in which learning can occur:
2. an individually determined curriculum which emphasizes the child's strengths and weaknesses;

3. the development and use of valid assessment instruments for ongoing diagnosis; and

4. the coordination and involvement of a multiprofessional team of specialists in special education, speech pathology, audiology, social service, medicine, and related health disciplines to provide for the total welfare of the communicatively handicapped child.

A Review of Current Teaching Methods

The remainder of this section is devoted to a review of current teaching methods for the language-impaired or language-different child. We make no attempt to endorse or propose any single teaching approach for any specific language disorder; rather, our purpose is to treat briefly some of the approaches which may be used, separately or in combination, to meet the needs of the child with a particular language problem. Selected references on methods and materials for language remediation appear in table 2–9.

Educating the Hearing Impaired. Remedial treatment of the deaf and the partially hearing is discussed in chapter 9; consequently, the language remediation of hearing-impaired children will be omitted here. Suffice it to say that hearing-impaired children, whether their deficit is mild to moderate in degree or severe to profound, require highly specialized methods of language development and remediation. As with other types of language retardation, the earlier intervention is begun, the more effective it will be. Educators of the deaf and the partially hearing vary in their approaches. Some espouse early exploitation of residual hearing from infancy and thus emphasize auditory learning through the natural language approach, while others believe that all such children must depend primarily on visual and tactile approaches for language learning.

Educating the Developmentally Language Impaired. A number of language remediation programs have been developed for children who demonstrate developmental learning problems. Space limitations preclude an adequate treatment of all of these programs, but it is important to recognize, first of all, that language deficits will usually require a long-term educational approach. That fact has required speech-language pathologists to carefully consider the relation between a communication disorder and educational programming, for if a communication disorder derives from a basic language deficit, it follows that the child's learning capacity will be affected, resulting in an educational as well as a communication problem.

Establishing Auditory Learning. When a primary learning disability involving language development can be identified early in life (at preschool age or sooner), the parents are in the best position to help the child overcome the language handicap. Since many such problems arise from a primary disability in the perceptual-sequential-associative levels of the auditory system, the early emphasis should be on the comprehension of language input. Teachers and speech-language pathologists can best help the child by helping the parents, at this early period, in obtaining a more insightful analysis of their own auditory environment so that they may better orient their child to listening skills. The following practices are appropriate in establishing auditory learning, whether a child suffers from sensory hearing impairment or from

Table 2–9. Selected Reference Sources on Methods and Materials for Language Remediation

Author(s)	Reference Source	Brief Description
Ausberger, C.	*Syntax One.* Tucson, Ariz.: Communication Skill Builders (1976).	A step-by-step program for the child whose syntactic skills are one to five years behind other language-related skills. Uses visual motor cues to facilitate learning.
———	*Syntax Two.* Tucson, Ariz.: Communication Skill Builders (1980).	Uses a wide number of materials, including a manual, syntax wheels, pictures, games, and sample lesson on cassette. Aimed at the language delayed, the bilingual, the developmentally delayed, and those with reading disorders.
Bricker, D., Dennison, L. and Bricker, W.	*A Language Intervention Program for Developmentally Young Children.* MCCD Monograph Series, No. 1, Mailman Center for Child Development, Miami: University of Miami (1976).	This program emphasizes a cognitive, action sequence, and semantic orientation toward language learning.
Blockcolsky, V., Frazer, J., Kurn, B., and Metz, E.	*Peel and Put Speech and Language Programs.* Tucson, Ariz.: Communication Skill Builders (1968–77).	A series of five hundred pressure-sensitive, full-color pictures. Designed to facilitate vocabulary, listening, speaking, concept formation, and overall language developments. Aimed at language delayed, bilingual, and developmentally delayed.
Bush, C. S.	*Language Remediation and Expansion: 100 Skill-Building Reference Lists.* Tucson, Ariz.: Communication Skill Builders (1979).	Consists of one hundred lists for promoting communication and experientially based language training. Provides lists in the areas of phonology, morphology and syntax, semantics and comprehension, cognition, and nonverbal communication. May be used with language delayed, culturally different, articulatorily impaired, voice and fluency cases.
Coughran, L. and Liles, B. A.	*Developmental Syntax Program* (Rev. ed.). Hingham MA: Teaching Resources Corporation (1980).	A sequentially based syntax development program for eleven most often observed errors. Uses ear training, production, and generalization to elicit and stabilize syntactic constructions.
Developmental Language and Speech Center Staff, Grand Rapids, Michigan	*Teach Your Child to Talk: A Parent Handbook.* New York: (EBCO/Standard Publishing Company) (Copyright claimed until 1975).	Offers guidance for parents concerning their child's speech and language development.
	Peabody Language Development Kits (Revised). Circle Pines, MN: American Guidance Service, Inc. (1981).	Four newly revised items designed to stimulate overall language and cognitive development.

Author(s)	*Reference Source*	*Brief Description*
Dunn, L. M., Horton, K. B., and Smith, J. O.	Level P—Revised (for average four- and five-year-olds)	Uses a carefully researched manual of lessons and activities which are conducted through use of pictures, puppets, audiotapes, and other novel materials. May be used with normally functioning or language-impaired children.
Dunn, L. M., Smith, J. O., Dunn, L. M., and Smith, D. D.	Level 1—Revised (for average six-year-olds and advanced five-year-olds)

Level 2—Revised (for average seven-year-olds and advanced six-year-olds)

Level 3—Revised (for average eight-year-olds and advanced seven-year-olds) | |
Fitzgerald, E.	*Straight Language for the Deaf*: A System of Instruction for Deaf Children. Washington, DC: The Volta Bureau (1949).	A method of structuring language for the deaf which has also been found useful in dealing with other language handicaps. The system is essentially a key consisting of headings, such as *who*, *what (verb)*, *where*, and *when*, which help the child organize language concepts. For preschool to intermediate levels.
Fokes, J.	*Fokes Sentence Builder*. Hingham, MA: Teaching Resources (1976).	A device for developing comprehension, verbal expression, and construction of sentences through a structured approach to grammar. Training provided in *who*, *what*, *is doing*, *which* and *where*. An expansion of the categories *whose*, *how*, and *when* is also available separately. Aimed at language delayed children.
Goldman, R. and Lynch, M.	*Goldman-Lynch Sounds and Symbols Development Kit*. Circle Pines, MN: American Guidance Service, Inc. (1971).	A phonically oriented program with one symbol for each sound. Uses a manual of lessons and stories, pictures, symbol cards, and puppets for teaching speech production. For preschool to primary levels.
Hermann, G. G., Ogana, D. F., and Olsen, P. H.	*What to Do About Bill?* Tucson, Ariz.: Communication Skill Builders (1976).	A handbook for remediation of language problems in secondary students.
Johnson, D. and Myklebust, H.	*Learning Disabilities—Educational Principles and Practices*. New York: Grune & Stratton, Inc. (1967), chapters 4–6.	Detailed description of procedures used for teaching children with auditory, reading, and writing language disorders.
Johnson, O. and Smith, R. H.	*Developmental Language Stories, Parts 1 and 2*. Hingham, MA: Teaching Resources (1980).	Fourteen different language structures are taught in thirty-one stories which are based on Lee's DSS Chart. May be used with mildly or severely language-impaired children and as a means of auditory comprehension training for normal children.

Author(s)	*Reference Source*	*Brief Description*
Leff, S. L. and Leff, R. B.	*Talking Pictures*. Milwaukee, WI: Crestwood Company (1980).	A set of 110 functional pictures which represent the necessities of everyday living. Five different languages are used: English, Spanish, German, French, and Italian. Designed for those with limited verbal communication abilities.
Lindamood, C. and Lindamood, P.	*Auditory Discrimination in Depth* (A.D.D.). Boston, MA: Teaching Resources Corporation (1969).	Developmental program in auditory perception which provides "in-depth" experiences in auditory discrimination through training at three levels. Emphasizes the visual, auditory, and kinesthetic modalities as the phonological structure of language is taught. For preschool to adult levels.
McLean, J. E. and Snyder-McLean, L. K.	*Transactional Approach to Early Language Training*. Columbus, Ohio: Charles E. Merrill (1978).	This strongly research-based model of language training emphasizes the cognitive, linguistic, and social functions in the communication training of severely language-delayed children. It also provides an excellent overview of current research and its relationship to the three areas of the transactional model.
McGivern, A. B., Rieff, M. L., and Vender, B. F.	*Language Stories: Teaching Language to Developmentally Disabled Children*. New York: The John Day Company (1978).	This method is an adaptation of Interactive Language Development Teaching for use with developmentally delayed children. Contains two sets of stories. Set I is for ages five to ten; Set II is for ages ten to fifteen.
Mowery, C. W. and Replogle, A.	*Developmental Language Lessons, Level 1 and Level 2*. Hingham, MA: Teaching Resources (1980).	This program of 710 lessons stresses the eight grammatical categories in Lee's DSS procedure. Instead of stories, verbal-action oriented sequences are used to teach grammar. May be used with language-delayed, developmentally delayed, and hearing-impaired persons.
Muma, J. R.	*Language Handbook: Concepts, Assessment, Intervention*. Englewood Cliffs, NJ: Prentice-Hall (1978).	Provides a "principle-oriented" model of assessment and intervention; includes cognitive, language, and communicative processes and systems; integrates research from other disciplines and individualizes language assessment and training. Designed especially for beginning clinicians.
Woodcock, R. and Clark, C.	*The Peabody Rebus Reading Program*. Circle Pines, MN: American Guidance Service, Inc. (1967).	Picture word approach to teaching reading. Uses individual workbooks and readers to introduce and develop an understanding of the semantic and syntactic systems of language. For preschool to primary levels. May be used with the child with limited language abilities.

difficulty in transmission and integration of auditory stimuli in the central nervous system auditory pathways:

1. selecting appropriate sounds to which to call their child's attention;
2. responding visibly and appropriately to these sounds, thereby stimulating the child's response;
3. consistently associating all sounds with their sources;
4. gaining an appreciation of the need for repetition of the sounds selected, and for consistency in responding to their child's reactions to these sounds in a manner to provide positive reinforcement; and
5. understanding the need for, and the techniques through which, listening to and responding to sound can be made fun for the child.

Developing Linguistic Competence. When the child has begun to recognize that verbal auditory stimuli have a communicative (language) intent, the succeeding stages of parental guidance must be directed toward the nature of the linguistic competence of the child. The following practices will be important:

1. consistently using short, simple, appropriate sentences and phrases;
2. talking about the here and now (the immediate environment which is relevant to the young child);
3. using consistent, meaningful, and somewhat exaggerated patterns of inflection and intonation to give the child stimulating language filled with variety and interest;
4. talking close to the child if any sensory deficit of hearing is suspected, and, if the child has been fitted with a hearing aid, talking directly into the microphone of the instrument;
5. capitalizing on all talking times as well as creating opportunities for talking during everyday activities;
6. expanding the child's speech utterances through consistent feedback in order to stimulate syntactic and morphological growth; and
7. talking at the child's ear and eye level.

The Johnson-Myklebust System. Johnson and Myklebust (1967) view the neurologically impaired child as one whose perceptual and integrative organization differs from that of the normal child and who, therefore, learns differently. Materials presented through auditory, visual, and tactile channels must be modified appropriately to compensate for the child's deviances. Although other workers, such as Strauss and Lehtinen (1947), Cruickshank (1961), and Wiig and Semel (1976, 1980) have emphasized the crucial role of perceptual deficits in training the language-impaired, Johnson and Myklebust hold that not all (perhaps not even the majority of) language-impaired children have perceptual disturbances. Hence, not all of these children require specific structuring of the environment or of incoming stimuli.

To deal effectively with the child, the teacher must isolate the psychological level of disability-perception, imagery, symbolization, or conceptualization. In addition, the teacher must identify the type of involvement—nonverbal-nonsocial, social-nonverbal, or verbal. This analysis emphasizes meaning versus nonmeaning and verbal versus nonverbal factors in learning.

A basic principle of the Johnson-Myklebust system is that input takes precedence over output in teaching; that is, the child must learn to comprehend before learning to speak, read, or write. Consideration of disorders of input versus those of output is therefore important. On a perceptual level, input disorders are known as agnosias; output disturbances on a motor level are known as dyspraxias. Input disorders, particularly at the level of the auditory language system, are very critical. The clinician, while teaching to the auditory modality to develop language, must be aware of the reciprocal relations between visual, auditory, and graphic modalities in verbal as well as in nonverbal learning.

Teaching to deficit areas is considered a limited concept by Johnson and Myklebust because it fails to consider interneurosensory learning, and the conversion of learning to other sensory modalities must be achieved. Likewise, teaching to a single integrity area, such as vision or audition, may heighten learning in that modality at the expense of others, and total integration of information is not achieved. They contend that the child with a psychoneurological learning disorder presents multiple readiness levels, and that these levels must be met in the teaching play by multisensory stimulation techniques that avoid training only the deficits or only the integrities. Overstimulation, or overloading, also must be avoided, since it precludes recognition of neurological and psychological tolerance levels resulting from cerebral dysfunction.

Johnson and Myklebust emphasize techniques for remediation of both receptive and expressive auditory language disorders. Receptively, training begins on a non-speech level. First, the child must learn to understand the meaning of environmental sounds and the prosodic features of speech. Early in the training, the child is made aware of the presence and absence of sound, after which the individual is given noise-producing toys to explore. Next, the child is required to localize sound by indicating whether the stimulus is from the left or the right and by following a sound source about the room. Noisemakers are matched to the sounds they make. Training in auditory memory tasks follows. In selected cases, amplification of sound may be used. Special emphasis is placed on recognizing and comprehending the inflection and rhythmic patterns of speech. On a verbal and auditory-verbal comprehension level, problems should be dealt with early, emphasizing meaningful units of speech, such as nouns. Extraneous language is reduced and carrier phrases are shortened to stress the meaning of critical words. Spoken language is carefully timed with experience to ensure exact associations, and the same words and concepts are repeatedly used to reverse memory problems. Vocabulary is carefully selected so as to stress common concrete words; isolated sound and syllable drills are avoided because they are not meaningful. After simple nouns are taught, verbs, prepositions, adjectives, adverbs, and pronouns are added.

The disorders of auditory expressive language recognized by Johnson and Myklebust are (1) dysnomia based on reauditorization and word selection problems, (2) apraxia based on sensorimotor deficits, and (3) formulation and syntactic problems. For reauditorization and word selection problems, sentence completion techniques, word association drills, and rapid-naming techniques are some of the therapeutic methods employed. For the apraxic child, a motor plan for control of the oral musculature is stressed by emphasizing awareness of sounds and movement patterns for sounds. After awareness of sounds is achieved, the sounds are placed in meaningful symbolic units. To establish motor plans for speech, visual cues, verbal instructions, and motokinesthetic approaches are used. Syntactic or formulation problems are approached by teaching structured rules through use of noun-verb sequences in the child's immediate experience. More complex syntactic sequences are added and are reinforced with selected use of pictures, scrambled sentences, and story completion techniques.

McGinnis Association Method. The Association Method of McGinnis (McGinnis, 1963), so called because of the close association between three processes of learning (attention, retention, and recall) employs an analytic and phonologically oriented approach in the development of language competence, proceeding from the recognition and production of individual phonemes to combinations of two sounds, then to words, and finally to sentences. The five basic principles embodied in this approach are that

1. words are taught by a phonetic or elemental approach;
2. each sound is learned through emphasis on precise articulation production;
3. the correct articulation of each sound is associated with its corresponding letter-symbol, which is written in cursive script;
4. expression is used as the foundation or starting point in building language; and
5. systematic sensorimotor association is used.

   Initially, the phonologic aspects of language are taught as a means of developing the semantic and syntactic systems of language. Correlative programs in the McGinnis approach include attention-getting exercises, writing exercises, speech training activities, and number work, so that it includes a complete academic program for the neurologically impaired child.

Kirk and Kirk's ITPA Remediation Approach. Samuel and Winifred Kirk (1971) have been leaders in the development of a remediation approach for psycholinguistic learning disabilities based on an instructional model derived from the Illinois Test of Psycholinguistic Abilities (ITPA). Basic to developing a language remediation program for a given child is careful administration and intepretation of the ITPA. It should be noted that the mental age range of the ITPA is 2-1/2 years to 9-1/2 years and that the profile of a child's abilities and disabilities is most reliable between the ages of three and 8-1/2 years. The ITPA profile will establish a basis for selecting remedial instructional areas that need attention in the child with linguistic and/or learning disabilities.

   Kirk and Kirk provide general guidelines for a psycholinguistic remediation program. They believe that training generally should be directed at deficit areas rather than strong areas, because most deficits are currently not considered innate or unalterable. These strong areas may be used as channels through which knowledge may be acquired. In general, multisensory and cross-modality approaches to stimulation in learning are advocated by Kirk and Kirk. They assert that most learning is intersensory but advise that the success of multisensory approaches versus unisensory approaches must be determined by the remedial teacher through careful assessment of the tolerance levels of the individual child.

   Kirk and Kirk contend that prerequisite deficits must be remediated first, and that it is the responsibility of the diagnostic-remedial teacher to determine whether one deficit is basic to another. They also believe that teaching should use feedback to promote learning. Three types of feedback can be used: (1) feedback that the teacher receives from a child when questions are answered or a lesson is completed; (2) feedback the teacher provides when a child's response is confirmed or corrected; and (3) external or internal feedback the child receives from actual and covert responses, either vocal or motor. In addition, stress is placed on early intervention programs for the psycholinguistically disabled, with individual instructional programs involving the itinerant diagnostic-remedial teacher, the resource room, the individualized class, and the two-teacher classroom.

The authors provide a task analysis of each of the ten functions assessed by the Illinois Test of Psycholinguistic Abilities to aid the teacher in determining the reason for the child's failure. A breakdown of reasons for failure in each of the functional areas indicates that some of the abilities fall into a developmental sequence and others represent various aspects of the task and contain varying degrees of attainment in the task. By using this task analysis of the ten function area, the teacher is able to make a further diagnosis of the child's functioning and can select particular activities and materials to improve the child's performance in the specific task in question.

On the basis of their task analyses, Kirk and Kirk provide an extensive list of activities and techniques that can be used to remediate performance in each of the task breakdowns that they have identified in the ten function areas. Several other writers have also developed activity and material programs that use the ITPA functional areas as a basis for an instruction model for children with language and learning handicaps. Bush and Giles (1969) have grouped activities and materials according to grade level in grades one through six. Karnes (1972, 1977) has developed a program called GOAL (Game Oriented Activities for Learning) for helping the preschool culturally different child (1972). GOAL II (1977) is a language development for children in grades two through junior and senior high school. Minskoff, Wiseman, and Minskoff (1971) have produced an extensive and detailed program called the MWM Program for Developing Language, and Rupert (1971) has categorized commercial instructional materials under each function tested by the ITPA.

The Bloom-Lahey Approach. Bloom and Lahey (1978) have emphasized the necessity for careful linguistic description and analysis of the language performance of the child with a developmental language disorder before a language intervention program is initiated. They argue that categorical classifications of language-disordered children, such as neurologically impaired, emotionally disturbed, mentally retarded, aphasic, or hearing impaired, offer the clinician little information for planning an intervention program for an individual child. Likewise, they argue that basing therapy programs on test results that describe language disorders in terms of clusters of cognitive and perceptual abilities and disabilities that correlate with language dysfunction also may have limited usefulness. They maintain that the widely postulated specific deficits in auditory sequential memory, comprehension of rapid auditory information, and ability to process multisensory inputs have not yet been proved as causative factors in language disorders. In addition, they conclude that there is very limited evidence that programs designed to remediate specific deficits as currently defined on tests such as the ITPA improve general language functioning.

In the light of these conclusions, they assert that a careful analysis of actual language performance in terms of linguistic processing will provide a more fruitful approach to language dysfunction than tests aimed at isolating specific perceptual and cognitive disabilities. This linguistic analysis will reveal language dysfunction in three areas: content, form, and use. *Content* of language refers to the child's ideas about objects and events in the world that are coded into language. *Form* is the system of signals of language including sounds and words, along with rules for combining these items in phrases and sentences. *Use* refers to the contexts in which language can be used and the functions for which it can be used. Dysfunctions may occur in any one of the three areas or in any combination of the three. Bloom and Lahey believe language learning occurs in therapy through an induction process in which the child extracts the relationships important to language from both the linguistic and the nonlinguistic world. The speech-language pathologist, therefore, is not a teacher of language but a facilitator of the induction process necessary for acquiring language. The role of the facilitator is to arrange external events in the child's life to enhance the induction of relationships between content, form, and use in language. Language facilitation should take place in as natural a setting as possible, and parents should be given the role of facilitators as frequently as possible. An individual child's needs for high or low structure in a language learning situation may vary; generally the child's attention level will determine the degree of structure required.

Bloom and Lahey suggest several techniques that may be employed to maintain an appropriate level of language response. These include modeling of language responses, imitation of language responses, and reinforcement of these responses. They believe that both comprehension and production must be taught in the language facilitation process and that emphasis on one over the other is inappropriate for effective intervention.

Certain processes help to facilitate the learning of interactions between the form and content aspects of interaction. The process of timing is particularly important in this interaction since the child must see and hear the appropriate linguistic forms at the same time that the concept to be comprehended or expressed is experienced. The process of repetition is also important because repeated instances of concept and linguistic form together will establish a conceptual relationship. The intensity, prosody, and rate of linguistic input must be varied systematically to make the linguistic signal salient for the child. Lexical items must be short, nonhomophonous, frequently used, and efficient.

In addition, attention should be paid to non-language input in facilitating language. Demonstration, rather than pictures, should be used, and a wide range of examples of single concepts should be employed. The child should become an active participant in manipulating objects and in expressing actions to code linguistically. For children for whom language use is a problem, enhancing interaction between content and form is not as important as facilitating the use of language. Communication with others must be stressed, and these children must be taught to use language for comment and other interpersonal functions.

Interactive Language Development Teaching. Interactive Language Development Teaching (Lee, Koenigsknecht, and Mulhern, 1975) uses the naturalness of storytelling to provide a clinical presentation of grammatical structure. This method grew out of the authors' extensive research with language-disordered children at Northwestern University and was developed for children whose primary problem was the learning of appropriate grammatical structure. The children they studied had a thirty- to forty-word expressive vocabulary and were beginning to produce two-word utterances. However, their use of sentences was greatly below the expected norms for their age group. Because of the young age of these children, the length of the therapy sequence (one to two years), and the intensive nature of the therapy program, it was necessary to find a method of teaching which would maintain the children's interest and enjoyment as well as be effective. This technique, if placed on a continuum, lies between simple language stimulation methods and the highly structured language drills. It provides language stimulation in a controlled manner, while preserving the nature of the parent-child interchange. The language sessions are usually fifty minutes long. Approximately thirty to thirty-five minutes are used for each story, and another three to five minutes are spent on some routine activity such as calendar work at the beginning of each session. The final ten to fifteen minutes are used in group activities which reinforce the story material, such as art work.

Interactive Language Development Teaching is based on Lee's developmental grammatical model, as described in Developmental Sentence Analysis (DSA) (1974). Developmental Sentence Scoring (DSS) (see table 2–10) is the aspect of DSA which presents the developmental sequence used in Interactive Language Development Teaching. Within the DSS, the developmental order of the eight grammatical structures is presented in the following sequence: indefinite pronouns or noun modifiers, personal pronouns, main verbs, secondary verbs, negatives, conjunctions, interrogative reversals, and wh- questions. A weighted score, as shown in table 2–10, is assigned to items in each of the eight categories, according to their early or late onset of acquisition. Words of similar meaning or grammatical function are grouped together. All of these categories resulted from the authors' experience with the normal developmental patterns in young children.

Interactive Language Development Teaching has largely been used with children of normal intelligence and normal hearing. Although the method can be adapted for other populations, such as the developmentally delayed or the hearing-impaired child, the normative data were derived from normal hearing language-delayed children. An adaptation of the method has been constructed for developmentally disabled children by McGivern, Rieff, and Vender (1978). Their approach, Language Stories: Teaching Language to Developmentally Disabled Children, is listed in table 2–9.

The Wiig-Semel Approach to Language-Disabled Children. Wiig (1980) characterized language-disabled children as a subgroup of the broader category of learning-disabled children. Children who are language-disabled, according to Wiig, show a disturbance in the understanding or use of spoken or written language, despite having intellectual capabilities in the normal range. Usually, these children do not show primary emotional or sensory deficits. Their disabilities are not often detected in early childhood, but upon entering school these children begin to have difficulty with academic subjects. It is usually then that these children are diagnosed as being language-disordered.

Learning-disabled (LD) children, on the other hand, constitute a group who may have a variety of psychosocial and academic problems from the early developmental years throughout the adult years. According to Wiig and Semel (1976), these children are often those whose prenatal history was marked by high-risk factors, have had complicated birth and medical histories, and present a series of perceptual and motor problems. If parents respond in a negative manner, Wiig and Semel suggest that "nonadaptive emotional reactions or secondary emotional problems" may develop which will interfere with effective interpersonal relations and thereby enlarge the specific disorder of learning.

Wiig (1980) reviews three subgroups of learning-disabled children into which 80 percent of all learning-disabled children would be classified. These are: (1) the language-disabled syndrome, (2) the articulatory-grapho-motor syndrome, and (3) the visual-spatial-perceptual syndrome. The language-disabled syndrome occurs in 40 to 60 percent of all learning-disabled children. This syndrome is characterized by difficulties in the areas of comprehension, expression, and discrimination of language and speech. The articulatory-grapho-motor syndrome accounts for behaviors in 10 to 40 percent of all learning-disabled children. Characteristics of this syndrome are those associated with developmental apraxia in all its forms, including oral apraxia and motor apraxia. The visual-spatial-perceptual syndrome manifests itself in 5 to 15 percent of learning-disabled children. This syndrome is associated with problems in the areas of visual motor functioning, visual discrimination, and spatial discrimination. Wiig (1980) believes that children within this group usually have the most favorable prognosis. After mastering the "psycholinguistic guessing game," the child's increased performance in language-related areas more accurately predicts success in those academic subjects which are interrelated with language.

Wiig notes that a child may have combinations of two of these syndromes and still be considered a learning-disabled child. Approximately 4 to 8 percent of all learning-disabled children have a combination of the language disorders and the articulatory-grapho-motor syndromes. Another 10 to 12 percent have a combination of the language disorders and the visual-spatial-perceptual syndromes. She points out that if a child has all three syndromes, identification as multiply handicapped, aphasic, or mentally retarded is apt to occur very early. Such children are very different from those who have only one or two of the syndromes.

Wiig and Semel (1976) present an approach to language remediation which focuses on three aspects supported by research. These include the improvement of auditory memory for words, phrases, and sentences; the improvement of convergent and divergent aspects of language production; and the improvement of the productive control of syntax.

They stated that memory is directly related to the processing and production of language. Similarly, since auditory memory deficits and a reduced ability to retain verbal stimuli characterize LD children, Wiig and Semel emphasize that such training should be provided in the remediation program. Both short-term and long-term auditory memory are stressed since "remedial procedures emphasizing immediate recall may result in improved performances on tasks requiring recall from long-term memory" (1976, p. 262).

Convergent language production is demonstrated by the ability to name a picture, to verbally provide the name of an opposite, to complete analogies, and to complete sentences or paragraphs from which words have been deleted. Language-disabled children often show delayed development in this area. Specific behaviors previously observed in LD children also include word substitutions when defining verbal opposites or when trying to retrieve words while discussing a topic and preservation of various responses. Wiig and Semel state that remediation should be focused on facilitating the identification and correct retrieval of a target within a series of related words and inhibiting the retrieval of similar words within a set of probable words.

Divergent language production is demonstrated when one can easily produce a

Table 2–10. The Developmental Sentence Scoring (DSS) Chart

Score	Indefinite Pronouns or Noun Modifiers	Personal Pronouns	Main Verbs	Secondary Verbs
1	it, this, that	1st and 2nd person: I, me, my, mine, you, your(s)	A. Uninflected verb: I *see* you. B. Copula, is or 's: *It's* red. C. is + verb + ing: He *is coming.*	
2		3rd person: he, him, his, she, her, hers	A. -s and -ed: *plays, played* B. Irregular past: *ate, saw* C. Copula: *am, are, was, were* D. Auxiliary *am, are, was, were*	Five early-developing infinitives: I wan*na* see (want *to see*) I'm gon*na* see (going *to see*) I got*ta* see (got *to see*) Lemme [to] see (let me [*to*] *see*) Let's [to] play (let [us *to*] *play*)
3	A. no, some, more, all, lot(s), one(s), two (etc.), other(s), another B. something, somebody, someone	A. Plurals: we, us, our(s), they, them, their B. these, those		Non-complementing infinitives: I stopped *to play.* I'm afraid *to look.* It's hard *to do* that.
4	nothing, nobody, none, no one		A. can, will, may + verb: *may go* B. Obligatory do + verb: *don't go* C. Emphatic do + verb: I *do see.*	Participle, present or past: I see a boy *running.* I found the toy *broken.*
5		Reflexives: myself, yourself, himself, herself, itself, themselves		A. Early infinitival complements with differing subjects in kernels: I want you *to come.* Let him [*to*] *see.* B. Later infinitival complements: I had *to go.* I told him *to go.* I tried *to go.* He ought *to go.* C. Obligatory deletions: Make it [*to*] *go.* I'd better [*to*] *go.* D. Infinitive with wh-word: I know what *to get.* I know how *to do* it.

Negatives	Conjunctions	Interrogative Reversals	WH-Questions
it, this, that + copula or auxiliary is, 's, + not: It's *not* mine. This is *not* a dog. That is *not* moving.		Reversal of copula: *Is*n't *it* red? *Were they* there?	
			A. who, what, what + noun: *Who* am I? *What* is he eating? *What book* are you reading? B. where, how many, how much, what . . . do, what . . . for *Where* did it go? *How much* do you want? *What* is he *doing?* *What* is a hammer *for?*
	and		
can't, don't		Reversal of auxiliary be: *Is he* coming? *Is*n't *he* coming? *Was he* going? *Was*n't *he* going?	
isn't, won't	A. but B. so, and so, so that C. or, if		when, how, how + adjective *When* shall I come? *How* do you do it? *How big* is it?

Score	Indefinite Pronouns or Noun Modifiers	Personal Pronouns	Main Verbs	Secondary Verbs
6		A. Wh-pronouns: who, which, whose, whom, what, that, how many, how much I know *who* came. That's *what* I said. B. Wh-word + infinitive: I know *what* to do. I know *who(m)* to take.	A. could, would, should, might + verb: *might come, could be* B. Obligatory does, did + verb C. Emphatic does, did + verb	
7	A. any, anything, anybody, anyone B. every, everything, everybody, everyone C. both, few, many, each, several, most, least, much, next, first, last, second (etc.)	(his) own, one, oneself, whichever, whoever, whatever Take *whatever* you like.	A. Passive with *get*, any tense Passive with *be*, any tense B. must, shall + verb: *must come* C. have + verb + en: *I've eaten.* D. have got: *I've got it.*	Passive infinitival complement: With *get:* I have *to get dressed.* I don't want *to get hurt.* With *be:* I want *to be pulled.* It's going *to be locked.*
8			A. have been + verb + ing had been + verb + ing B. modal + have + verb + en: *may have eaten* C. modal + be + verb + ing: *could be playing* D. Other auxiliary combinations: *should have been sleeping*	Gerund: *Swinging* is fun. I like *fishing.* He started *laughing.*

Negatives	Conjunctions	Interrogative Reversals	WH-Questions
	because	A. Obligatory do, does, did: *Do they* run? *Does it* bite? *Did*n't it hurt? B. Reversal of modal: *Can you* play? *Won't it* hurt? *Shall I* sit down? C. Tag question: It's fun, *isn't it?* It isn't fun, *is it?*	
All other negatives: A. Uncontracted negatives: I can *not* go. He has *not* gone. B. Pronoun-auxiliary or pronoun-copula contraction: I'm *not* coming. He's *not* here. C. Auxiliary-negative or copula-negative contraction: He was*n't* going. He has*n't* been seen. It could*n't* be mine. They are*n't* big.			why, what if, how come, how about + gerund *Why* are you crying? *What if* I won't do it? *How come* he is crying? *How about* coming with me?
	A. where, when, how, while, whether (or not), till, until, unless, since, before, after, for, as, as + adjective + as, as if, like, that, than I know *where* you are. Don't come *till* I call. B. Obligatory deletions: I run faster *than* you [run]. I'm *as big as* a man [is big]. It looks *like* a dog [looks]. C. Elliptical deletions (score 0): That's *why* [I took it]. I know *how* [I can do it]. D. Wh-words + infinitive. I know *how* to do it. I know *where* to go.	A. Reversal of auxiliary have: *Has he* seen you? B. Reversal with two or three auxiliaries: *Has he been* eating? *Could*n't *he have* waited? *Could he have been* crying? *Would*n't *he have been* going?	whose, which, which + noun *Whose* car is that? *Which book* do you want?

number of varied words, phrases, or sentences to describe events, ideas or objects. The specific abilities which support divergent language production are verbal fluency, originality, flexibility, and elaboration. Wiig and Semel (1976) provide information and specific techniques for enhancing the LD child's performance in this area. Among the techniques used are verbal description of familiar objects in direct response to questions about details, formulation of sentences when given a series of words, and formulation of cause-effect relationships. Wiig and Semel (1980) provide an interpretation of their method for the classroom teacher and other professionals who provide services to LD children.

Goldman-Lynch's Auditory Program. Goldman and Lynch (1980) view listening ability as a crucial skill in overall language development. They suggest that the abilities to understand speech, to speak, to read, and to spell are closely related to the ability to listen. They also assert that learning is fostered by listening. Despite this mutual influence, Goldman and Lynch believe that listening as a basic skill has been a neglected one in most academic programs. They point out that the school-age child spends approximately 57 percent of the total class time in listening.

The Listening to the World Program (Goldman and Lynch, 1980) consists of a series of ninety developmental lessons in listening. This program deliberately teaches listening skills for children in the kindergarten and early primary grades. As such, the program may be used as a prereading tool in a total language arts program.

Little Tune is the program's central character "who is heard but never seen" throughout the program. This character helps young children understand why listening is important and presents the different skills to be learned in the program. A wide array of visual materials, including stories, pictures, and posters, is used to supplement the auditory information taught in the program. The auditory materials consist of fifty audio-cassette stories and a "sound" book of sounds and songs.

The following skills are taught in Listening to the World:

1. Auditory discrimination of non-speech sounds, of words, and of sentences. This training is provided in quiet and in noise contexts.
2. Selective auditory attention. The following subskills are stressed: recognizing the presence or absence of sound; listening to speech while hearing a competing noise; concentrating on important aspects of a message; and ignoring distracting stimuli.
3. Auditory vigilance. This requires the listener to be on alert for a special sound or word.
4. Hypothesis testing. Students determine words which have been camouflaged by competing sounds or which are missing from a sentence.
5. Auditory memory. This fosters mastery of a number of strategies such as visualization, rehearsal, grouping, and linking.

Adler's Approach to Teaching Culturally Different Children. Adler (1979) provides a comprehensive view of the culturally different child in the areas of theory, testing and evaluation, and bidialectal education. He states:

Billions of dollars have been expended in compensatory education programs; yet, poor children still remain undereducated when compared to their middle-class peers. We believe that proper motivational models are lacking in our schools for a variety of reasons, one of the most important being the communication barrier between teacher and pupil. We urge teachers, particularly those in the preschool or early grades, to interface with the speech-language pathologist in promoting effective bidialectal-bicultural programs in their class-room. . . . This is particularly indicated since our research suggests that standard English is learned more effectively when taught by a bidialectal method rather than through the conventional language arts curriculum. (p. xiv)

Adler contends that a new type of professional in speech pathology and education is needed. He suggests that this new type of individual should have the ability to identify and train the child to use equivalent linguistic forms in standard and nonstandard English. Adler believes that intervention programs for culturally different children must be designed "to teach children to use standard English in appropriate context while respecting and maintaining the native dialect." He espouses a functional bidialectal approach for children of culturally different backgrounds. Use of such an approach results in (1) the development of competence in standard English while continuing the use and development of Black English; (2) the capability to adjust speech according to the situation; and (3) competence in using either standard English or a nonstandard form of English.

Specifically, Adler recommends use of a contrast and comparison approach to standard English. The child is given practice in hearing the standard English form and in comparing this form to the form routinely used by the child. Drill is provided in the areas of discrimination, identification, translation, and response.

SUMMARY

Children who are routinely seen by speech-language pathologists show clinical pictures in which there is a delayed development of the use of linguistic structures and a dependence on less well-formed sentences than normal children use. It is clear that these children with mild-to-moderate language impairment are distinct from those who have language impairment because of a gross and obvious neurological defect, mental retardation, deafness, severe emotional disturbance, or language delay that is environmentally induced. Current language remediation programs center on syntactic, semantic, and pragmatic aspects of language, recognizing that attention to linguistic functions and deficits provides a solid source of information for planning a management program.

Increased attention has also been focused on the child who presents a different linguistic pattern because of cultural heritage. Speech-language pathologists are becoming aware of the specific language differences apparent in black and Hispanic populations and are preparing tests and linguistic programs that will aid these children in adapting, when necessary, to the standard English patterns used by the majority of Americans.

An abundant number of screening and diagnostic tests of language have become available to the speech-language pathologist who wishes to assess and study the linguistic patterns of the children seen in school, hospital, and clinic programs. A particularly potent technique is language sampling, in which a body of spontaneous speech is submitted to linguistic analysis.

The widespread study of linguistically impaired children has prompted several theoretical speculations concerning the possible cause of language delay in those children in whom obvious physical etiology is not present. Speculation has centered on possible perceptual deficit, cognitive deficit, and linguistic deficit in the child. It is clear that a single cause theory is not sufficient for explaining the wide variety of language delay and disorder seen in the majority of the language-impaired population, where neurologic impairment, deafness, emotional disturbance, or environmental causes are not obvious.

Diagnosis and remediation of language disorders in children is finally being recognized as a well-defined discipline. There are now available in the literature both methods for accurately assessing the child and an abundance of remedial techniques that will help the child who is faced with problems in linguistic expression.

BIBLIOGRAPHY

Abernathy, J., Meaningful language curriculum. *Instructor*, **79,** 64 (1970).

Adler, S., Pluralism, relevance, and language intervention for culturally different children. *Asha*, **13,** 719–723 (1971).

Adler, S., *Poverty Children and Their Language: Implications for Teaching and Treating.* New York: Grune & Stratton, Inc. (1979).

Ammons, R., and Ammons, H., *Full Range Picture Vocabulary Test.* Missoula, Mont.: Psychological Test Specialists (1948).

Aram, D. M., and Nation, J. E., Patterns of language behavior in children with developmental language disorders. *J. Speech Hearing Res.*, **18,** 229–241 (1975).

Bangs, T. E., *Vocabulary Comprehension Scale.* Austin, Tex.: Learning Concepts (1975).

Banks, J. A., Issues and trends in American education. *Peabody Journal of Education*, **54,** 73–78 (1977).

Bankson, N. W., *Bankson Language Screening Test.* Baltimore: University Park Press (1977).

Baratz, J. C., Teaching reading in an urban Negro school system. In F. Williams (Ed.), *Language and Poverty.* Chicago: Markham Publishing Company (1970).

Bauman, R., An ethnographic framework for the investigation of communicative behaviors. *Asha*, **13,** 334–340 (1971).

Beard, R. M., *An Outline of Piaget's Developmental Psychology for Students and Teachers.* New York: Basic Books (1969).

Bereiter, C., and Englemann, S., *Teaching Disadvantaged Children in the Preschool.* Englewood Cliffs, N.J.: Prentice-Hall (1966).

Berko, J., The child's learning of English morphology. In S. Saporta (Ed.), *Psycholinguistics.* New York: Holt, Rinehart and Winston (1961).

Blakeley, R., *Screening Test for Developmental Apraxia of Speech.* Tigard, Ore.: CC Publications (1980).

Bloom, L., and Lahey, M., *Language Development and Language Disorders.* New York: John Wiley (1978).

Bountress, N. G., The Ann Arbor decision: Implications for the speech-language pathologist. *Asha*, **22,** 543–544 (1980).

Bronfenbrenner, U., *A Report on Longitudinal Evaluations of Preschool Programs* Vol. 2—Is early intervention effective? DHEW Publication No. (OHD) 76–30025. Washington, D.C. (1974).

Brown, J., Darley, F., and Gomez, M., Disorders of communication. *Ped. Clin. N. Am.*, **14,** 725–748 (1967).

Brown, R., *A First Language: The Early Stages.* Cambridge, Mass.: Harvard University Press (1973).

Bush, W. J., and Giles, M. T., *Aids to Psycholinguistic Teaching.* Columbus, Ohio: Charles E. Merrill (1969).

Bzoch, K., and League, R., *Receptive-Expressive Emergent Language Scale.* Gainesville, Fla.: Tree of Life Press (1971).

Carrow-Woolfolk, E., *Austin Spanish Articulation Test.* Hingham, Mass.: Teaching Resources (1974a).

Carrow-Woolfolk, E., *Carrow Elicited Language Inventory.* Hingham, Mass.: Teaching Resources (1974b).

Carrow-Woolfolk, E., *Screening Test for Auditory Comprehension of Language, English/Spanish.* Hingham, Mass.: Teaching Resources (1974c).

Carrow-Woolfolk, E., *Test for Auditory Comprehension of Language, English/Spanish.* Austin, Tex.: Learning Concepts (1974d).

Chomsky, N., *Syntactic Structures.* The Hague: Mouton (1957).

Chomsky, N., *Aspects of the Theory of Syntax.* Cambridge, Mass.: MIT Press (1965).

Chomsky, N., *Language and the Mind*. New York: Harcourt-Brace-Jovanovich (1972).

Chomsky, N., *The Logical Structure of Linguistic Theory*. New York: Plenum Press (1975).

Chomsky, N., *Reflections on Language*. New York: Pantheon (1976).

Chomsky, N., and Halle, M., *The Sound Pattern of English*. New York: Harper & Row (1968).

Cohen, D. J., Caparulo, B., Shaywitz, B., Primary childhood aphasia and childhood autism: Clinical, biological, and conceptual observations. *Journal of the American Academy of Child Psychiatry*, **15**, 604–645 (1976).

Cole, L. T., Racial and ethnic enrollment of training institutions with communicative disorders programs. *Asha*, **22**, 545–549 (1980).

Compton, A., *Compton Speech and Language Evaluation*. San Francisco: Carousel House (1978).

Compton, A., and Hutton, J., *Compton-Hutton Phonological Assessment*. San Francisco: Carousel House (1978).

Crabtree, M., *Houston Test of Language Development*. Houston: Houston Test Company (1963).

Cromer, R. F., The basis of childhood dysphasia: A linguistic approach. In M. A. Wyke (Ed.), *Developmental Dysphasia*. New York: Academic Press (1978).

Cruickshank, W., *A Teaching Method for Hyperactive Children*. Syracuse: Syracuse University Press (1961).

Crystal, D., Fletcher, P., and Garman, M., *The Grammatical Analysis of Language Disability: A Procedure for Assessment and Remediation*. New York: Elsevier (1976).

Darley, F. L. (Ed.), *Evaluation of Appraisal Techniques in Speech and Language Pathology*. Reading, Mass.: Addison-Wesley Publishing Company (1979).

Darley, F. L., Aronson, A., and Brown, J., *Motor Speech Disorders*. Philadelphia: W. B. Saunders (1975).

Darley, F. L., and Spriestersbach, D. C., *Diagnostic Methods in Speech Pathology*. (2nd ed.) New York: Harper & Row (1978).

DiSimoni, F., *The Token Test for Children*. Hingham, Mass.: Teaching Resources (1979).

Doll, E. A., *The Vineland Social Maturity Scale*. Circle Pines, Minn.: American Guidance Service (1965).

Dore, J., Holophrases, speech acts and language universals. *J. of Child Lang.*, **2**, 21–40 (1975).

Dreifuss, F. E., The pathology of central communicative disorders in children. In D. B. Tower (Ed.), *The Nervous System, Vol. 3: Human Communication and Its Disorders*. New York: Raven Press (1975).

Dunn, L., *Peabody Picture Vocabulary Test*. Circle Pines, Minn.: American Guidance Service, Inc. (1958, 1965).

Dunn, L., *Peabody Picture Vocabulary Test, Revised*. Circle Pines, Minn.: American Guidance Service, Inc. (1980).

Dunn, L. M., Horton, K. B., and Smith, J. O., *Peabody Language Development Kits, Level P, Revised*. Circle Pines, Minn.: American Guidance Service, Inc. (1981).

Dunn, L. M., Smith, J. O., Dunn, L. M., and Smith, D. D., *Peabody Language Development Kits, Levels 1, 2, and 3 (Revised)*. Circle Pines, Minn.: American Guidance Service, Inc. (1981).

Eimas, P., Speech perception in early infancy. In L. Cohen, and P. Salapatek (Eds.), *Infant Perception: From Sensation to Cognition*, Volume II, *Perception of Space, Speech and Sound*. New York: Academic Press (1975).

Eisenberg, R. B., The organization of auditory behavior. *J. Speech Hearing Res.*, **13**, 453–471 (1970).

Eisenberg, R. B., *Auditory Competence in Early Life*. Baltimore: University Park Press (1976).

Ferry, P. G., Culbertson, J. L., Fitzgibbons, P. A., and Netsky, M., Brain function and language disabilities. *International Journal of Pediatric Otorhinolaryngology*, **1**, 13–24 (1979).

Fisher, H. B., and Logemann, J. A., *Fisher-Logemann Test of Articulatory Competence*. Boston: Houghton-Mifflin (1971).

Flavell, J. H., *Cognitive Development*. Englewood Cliffs, N.J.: Prentice-Hall (1977).

Foster, R. J., Giddan, J. J., and Stark, J., *Assessment of Children's Language Comprehension*. Palo Alto, Calif.: Consulting Psychologists Press (1973).

Friedlander, B. Z., Receptive language behavior in infancy. *Merrill Palmer Quarterly*, **16**, 7–51 (1970).

Ginsburg, H., and Opper, S. *Piaget's Theory of Intellectual Development: An Introduction*. Englewood Cliffs, N.J.: Prentice-Hall (1969).

Goldman, R., and Fristoe, M., *Goldman-Fristoe Test of Articulation*. Circle Pines: Minn.: American Guidance Service, Inc. (1969).

Goldman, R., Fristoe, M., and Woodcock, R. W., *The Goldman-Fristoe-Woodcock Test of Auditory Discrimination*. Circle Pines, Minn.: American Guidance Service, Inc. (1970).

Goldman, R., and Lynch, M. E., *Listening to the World*. Circle Pines, Minn.: American Guidance Service, Inc. (1980).

Gruber, H. D., and Vonéche, J. J. (Eds.), *The Essential Piaget: An Interpretative Reference and Guide*. New York: Basic Books, Inc. (1977).

Halliday, M., Learning how to mean. In E. Lenneberg and E. Lenneberg (Eds.), *Foundations of Language Development: A Multidisciplinary Approach*, Vol. 1. New York: Academic Press (1975).

Hammill, D. D., Brown, V. L., Larsen, S. C., and Wiederholt, J. L. *Test of Adolescent Language (TOAL)*. East Aurora, NY: Slosson Educational Publications (1982).

Hedrick, D. L., Prather, E. M., and Tobin, A., *Sequenced Inventory of Communication Development*. Seattle: University of Washington Press (1975).

Hutchinson, B., Hanson, M., and Mecham, M., *Diagnostic Handbook of Speech Pathology*. Baltimore: Williams and Wilkins (1979).

Johnson, D., Darley, F. L., and Spriestersbach, D. E., *Diagnostic Methods in Speech Pathology*. New York: Harper and Row (1963).

Johnson, D., and Myklebust, H., *Learning Disabilities—Educational Principles and Practice*. New York: Grune and Stratton, Inc. (1967).

Johnson, O., and Smith, R. H., *Developmental Language Stories Parts 1 and 2*. Hingham, Mass.: Teaching Resources (1980).

Johnston, J. R., Personal communication, October, 1980.

Karnes, M. B., *Goal Program: Language Development*. Springfield, Mass.: Milton Bradley Company (1972).

Karnes, M. B., *Goal II: Language Development Program*. Springfield, Mass.: Milton Bradley Company (1977).

Kaufman, A. S., and Kaufman, N. L. *Kaufman Assessment Battery for Children (K-ABC)*. Circle Pines, MN: American Guidance Service (1983).

Kirk, S. A., and Kirk, W. D., *Psycholinguistic Learning Disabilities: Diagnosis and Remediation*. Urbana, Ill.: University of Illinois Press (1971).

Kirk, S. A., McCarthy, J. J., and Kirk, W., *Illinois Test of Psycholinguistic Abilities*. Urbana, Ill.: University of Illinois Press (1968).

Krashen, S., The critical period for language acquisition and its possible basis. In D. Aaronson and R. W. Reiber (Eds.), *Developmental Psycholinguistics and Communication Disorders, Annals of New York Academy of Science, 263*, 211–224 (1975).

Labov, W., *Language in the Inner City*. Philadelphia: University of Pennsylvania Press (1972).

LaPointe, L. L., Neurologic abnormalities affecting speech. In D. B. Tower (Ed.), *The Nervous System Vol. 3, Human Communication and Its Disorders*. New Raven Press (1975).

Lassman, F. M., Fisch, R. O., Vetter, D. K., and LaBenz, E. S. (Eds.), *Early Correlates of Speech, Language and Hearing*. Littleton, Mass.: PSG Publishing Co. (1980).

Lee, L. L., *Northwestern Syntax Screening Test*. Evanston, Ill.: Northwestern University Press (1971).

Lee, L. L., *Developmental Sentence Analysis*. Evanston, Ill.: Northwestern University Press (1974).

Lee, L. L., Koenigsknecht, R. A., and Mulhern, S., *Interactive Language Development Teaching*. Evanston, Ill.: Northwestern University Press (1975).

Lenneberg, E., *Biological Foundations of Language*. New York: John Wiley (1967).

Lenneberg, E., On explaining language. *Science, 164*, 635–643 (1969).

Leonard, L. B., Language impairment in children. *Merrill Palmer Quarterly, 25*, 205–232 (1979).

Leonard, L. B., Prutting, C. A., Perrozzi, J. A., and Berkley, R. K., Nonstandard approaches to the assessment of language behaviors. *Asha, 18*, 371–379 (1978).

Lerea, L., Assessing language development. *J. Speech Hearing Res., 1*, 75–85 (1958a).

Lerea, L., *Michigan Picture Language Inventory*. Ann Arbor: University of Michigan (1958b).

Lillywhite, H., and Bradley, D. P., *Communication Problems in Mental Retardation*. New York: Harper & Row (1969).

Longhurst, T., and Schrandt, T., Linguistic analysis of children's speech: A comparison of four procedures. *J. Speech Hearing Dis., 38*, 240–249 (1973).

Love, R. J., Oral language behavior of older cerebral palsied children. *J. Speech Hearing Res., 7*, 349–362 (1964).

Lund, N. J., and Duchan, J. F. *Assessing Children's Language in Naturalistic Contexts*. Englewood Cliffs, NJ: Prentice-Hall (1983).

Macaluso-Haynes, S., Developmental apraxia of speech: Symptoms and treatment. In D. F. Johns (Ed.), *Clinical Management of Neurogenic Communicative Disorders*. Boston: Little, Brown (1978).

MacDonald, J., *Environmental Language Inventory*. Columbus: Charles E. Merrill Publishing Company (1978).

McCarthy, D., Language development in children. In L. Carmichael (Ed.), *Manual of Child Psychology*. New York: John Wiley (1954).

McGinnis, M., *Aphasic Children: Identification and Evaluation by the Association Method*. Washington, D.C.: The Alexander Graham Bell Association for the Deaf, Inc. (1963).

McGivern, A. B., Rieff, M. L., and Vender, B. F., *Language Stories: Teaching Language to Developmentally Disabled Children*. New York: The John Day Company (1978).

McNeill, D., *The Acquisition of Language*. New York: Harper & Row (1970).

McReynolds, L., and Engmann, D., *Distinctive Feature Analysis of Misarticulations*. Baltimore: University Park Press (1975).

Mecham, M. J., *Verbal Language Development Scale*. Circle Pines, Minn.: American Guidance Service, Inc. (1971).

Mecham, M. J., Jex, J. L., and Jones, J. D., *Utah Test of Language Development*. Salt Lake City: Communication Research Associates (1978).

Menyuk, P., Comparison of grammar of children with functionally deviant and normal articulation. *J. Speech Hearing Res.*, **7**, 109–121 (1964).

Menyuk, P., *Sentences Children Use*. Cambridge, Mass.: MIT Press (1969).

Menyuk, P., Linguistic problems in children with developmental dysphasia. In M. A. Wyke (Ed.), *Developmental Dysphasia*. New York: Academic Press (1978).

Menyuk, P., and Looney, P., A problem of language disorder: Length versus structure. *J. Speech Hearing Res.*, **15**, 264–279 (1972).

Minskoff, E. H., Wiseman, D. E., and Minskoff, J. G., *The MWM Program for Developing Language Abilities*. Ridgefield, N.J.: Educational Performance Associates (1972).

Morehead, D., and Ingram, D., The development of base structure in normal and linguistically deviant children. *J. Speech Hearing Res.*, **16**, 330–352 (1973).

Morehead, D., and Morehead, A., From signal to sign: A Piagetian view of thought and language during the first two years. In R. Schiefelbush and L. Lloyd (Eds.), *Language Perspectives, Acquisition, Retardation and Intervention*. Baltimore: University Park Press (1974).

Morley, M., *The Development and Disorders of Speech in Childhood*. Baltimore: Williams and Wilkins (1965).

Muma, J. R., Language assessment: The co-occurring and restricted structure procedure. *Acta Symbolica*, **4**, 12–29 (1973).

Muma, J. R., *Language Handbook: Concepts, Assessment, Intervention*. Englewood Cliffs, N.J.: Prentice-Hall, Inc. (1978).

Mumm, M., Secord, W., and Dykstra, K., *Merrill Language Screening Test*. Columbus: Charles E. Merrill (1980).

Myers, P. I., and Hammill, D. D., *Methods for Learning Disorders*. New York: John Wiley (1969).

Naremore, R. C., Language variation in a multicultural society. In T. J. Hixon, L. D. Shriberg, and J. H. Saxman (Eds.), *Introduction to Communication Disorders*. Englewood Cliffs, N.J.: Prentice-Hall (1980).

Nation, J. E., and Aram, D. M., *Diagnosis of Speech and Language Disorders*. St. Louis, Mo.: C. V. Mosby Co. (1977).

O'Neill, J. J., and Oyer, H. J., *Applied Audiometry*. New York: Dodd, Mead and Co. (1966).

Osser, H., Wang, M. D., and Zaid, F., The young child's ability to imitate and comprehend speech: A comparison of two cultural groups. *Child Development*, **40**, 1063–1075 (1969).

Piaget, J., and Inhelder, B. *The Psychology of the Child*. New York: Basic Books (1969).

Poag, L., A comparison of the grammar abilities of Negro and White children. Unpublished master's thesis, Vanderbilt University (1968).

Porch, B., *The Porch Index of Communicative Abilities*. Palo Alto, Calif.: Consulting Psychologists Press (1969, 1971).

Porch, B., *The Porch Index of Communicative Ability in Children*. Palo Alto, Calif.: Consulting Psychologists Press (1975).

Rees, N. S., Auditory processing factors in language disorders: The view from Procrustes' bed. *J. Speech Hearing Dis.*, **38**, 304–315 (1973).

Riley, G., *The Riley Articulation and Language Test*. Los Angeles: Western Psychological Services (1971).

Rodgers, W., *Picture Articulation and Language Screening Test*. Salt Lake City: Word Making Productions (1976).

Rupert, H. A., *A Sequentially Compiled List of Instructional Materials for Remedial Use with the ITPA*. Washington, D.C.: Council for Exceptional Children (1971).

Sabatino, D., The construction and assessment of an experimental test of auditory perception. *Exceptional Children*, **35**, 729–736 (1969).

Sameroff, A. J., and Chandler, M. J., Reproductive risk and the continuum of care-taking casualty. In F. D. Horowitz (Ed.), *Review of Child Development Research* Vol. 4. Chicago: University of Chicago Press (1975).

Sanders, D. A., *Auditory Perception of Speech: An Introduction to Principles and Problems*. Englewood Cliffs, N.J.: Prentice-Hall (1977).

Schachter, F. F., *Everyday Mother Talk to Toddlers: Early Intervention*. New York: Academic Press (1979).

Semel, M., and Wiig, E., *Clinical Evaluation of Language Functions*. Columbus: Charles E. Merrill Publishing Company (1980).

Shriberg, L., and Kwiatkowski, J., *Natural Process Analysis (NPA): A Procedure for Phonological Analysis of Spontaneous Speech Samples*. New York: John Wiley (1980).

Stewart, W. A., Toward a history of American Negro dialect. In F. Williams (Ed.), *Language and Poverty*. Chicago: Markham Publishing Company (1970).

Strauss, A., and Lehtinen, L., *Psychopathology and Education of the Brain-Injured Child*. New York: Grune & Stratton (1947).

Subcommittee on Human Communication and Its Disorders, *Human Communication and Its Disorders—An Overview*. Bethesda: National Institute of Neurological Diseases and Stroke (1969).

Tallal, P., and Piercy, M., Defects of auditory processing in children with developmental aphasia. In M. A. Wyke (Ed.), *Developmental Dysphasia*. New York: Academic Press (1978).

Taylor, O. L., Recent developments in sociolinguistics: Some implications for ASHA. *Asha*, **13**, 341–345 (1971a).

Taylor, O. L., A psycholinguistic background for the study of urban language. Paper presented at the Institute on Urban Language and the Training of Personnel in Communication Disorders, Federal City College, Washington, D.C. (August 20, 1971b).

Taylor, O. L., ASHA: A black report card. *Asha*, **22**, 584–589 (1980).

Templin, M., and Darley, F. L., *The Templin-Darley Tests of Articulation*. Iowa City: The University of Iowa Bureau of Education Research and Service (1969).

Toronto, A., *Southwest Spanish Articulation Test*. Austin: Academic Tests (1977).

Tyack, D., and Gottsleben, R., *Language Sampling, Analysis, and Training: A Handbook for Teachers and Clinicians*. Palo Alto, Calif.: Consulting Psychologists Press (1974).

U.S. Bureau of the Census, Projections of the population of the United States: 1982 to 2050 (Advance Report), *Current Population Reports*, Series P-25, No. 922 (1982).

Vane, J., *Vane Evaluation of Language Scale*. Brandon, Vt.: Clinical Psychology Publishing Co. (1975).

Wechsler, D., *Wechsler Preschool and Primary Scale of Intelligence*. New York: The Psychological Corporation (1967).

Wechsler, D., *Wechsler Intelligence Scale for Children, Revised*. New York: The Psychological Corporation (1974).

Weiner, F., *Phonological Process Analysis*. Baltimore: University Park Press (1978).

Weiner, P. S., Cognitive functioning of language deficit children. In J. Hellmuth (Ed.), *Cognitive Studies II. Deficits in Cognition*. New York: Brunner/Mazel, Inc. (1971).

Weiner, P. S., Developmental Language Disorders. In H. Rie and E. Rie (Eds.), *Handbook of Minimal Brain Dysfunctions*. New York: John Wiley (1980).

Wepman, J. M., *Auditory Discrimination Test*. Chicago: Language Research Associates (1958, 1973).

Wepman, J., Jones, L. V., Bock, R. D., and Van Pelt, D., Studies in aphasia: Background and theoretical formulations. *J. Speech Hearing Dis.*, **25**, 323–332 (1960).

Wetherby, A. M., and Gaines, B. H. Cognition and language development in autism. *J. Speech Hearing Disorders*, **47**, 63–70 (1982).

Wiig, E. H., and Semel, E. M., *Language Disabilities in Children and Adolescents*. Columbus, Ohio: Charles E. Merrill Publishing Company (1976).

Wiig, E. H., and Semel, E. M., *Language Assessment and Intervention for the Learning Disabled*. Columbus, Ohio: Charles E. Merrill Publishing Company (1980).

Williams, F., Some preliminaries and prospects. In F. Williams (Ed.), *Language and Poverty*. Chicago: Markham Publishing Company (1970).

Williams, R., and Wolfram, W., *A Linguistic Description of Social Dialects*. Prepared for the Committee of Communication Problems of the Urban and Ethnic Populations, American Speech and Hearing Association (1974).

Wolfus, B., Moscovitch, M., and Kinsbourne, M., Subgroups of developmental language impairment. *Brain and Language*, **10,** 152–171 (1980).

Wolski, W., and Lerea, L., *The Michigan Picture Language Inventory*. Ann Arbor: University of Michigan (1962).

Worster-Drought, C., Suprabulbar paresis. *Dev. Med. Chil. Neurol.*, **16,** supplement 30, 1–33 (1974).

Yoss, K. A., and Darley, F. L., Developmental apraxia of speech in children with defective articulation. *J. Speech Hearing Res.*, **17,** 339–416 (1974).

Zachman, L., Huisingh, R., Jorgenson, C., and Barrett, M., *Oral Sentence Imitation Screening Test*. Moline, Ill.: Linguistic Systems (1977).

Zigmond, N. K., Disorders of auditory learning. In N. K. Zigmond and R. Cicci (Eds.), *Auditory Learning*. San Rafael, Calif.: Dimension Publishing Company (1968).

Zimmerman, I. L., Steiner, V. G., and Evatt, R. L., *Preschool Language Scale*. Columbus, Ohio: Charles E. Merrill Publishing Company (1979).

3 Nature and Remediation of Functional Articulation and Phonological Disorders

Ronald K. Sommers

INTRODUCTION: FUNCTIONAL ARTICULATION AND PHONOLOGICAL DISORDERS

The material presented in this chapter relates to both preschool and young school-age children who make multiple phoneme errors and show other forms of linguistic impairment such as syntactical weaknesses, and to older children who make one or two phoneme errors but have normal linguistic abilities. The latter group of children's defects may not include significant disabilities regarding language understanding and use, but often do include errors of /s/, /r/ or /l/ production. These may be best described as articulatory defects, rather than phonological disorders. Such conditions can be described as phonetic errors rather than phonemic ones, and, as we shall see, may have stronger links with certain perceptual and memory deficits than linguistic ones, particularly as children grow older and maintain misarticulations.

The incidence of the phonetic types of speech errors would probably be far greater than the phonemic type if all school children were accounted for in the population. By far, the speech-language clinician employed in school settings provides the greatest amount of therapy for children's articulatory and phonological disorders. Many of the children in kindergarten, first, and second grades in the United States who are not treated by school speech-language clinicians are likely to have single misarticulations of consonants, often /s/ or /r/. As they grow older, some portion of them probably are entered into articulation therapy groups in school programs, while those who make multiple phonemic errors and have accompanying difficulties with language on a rather broad linguistic front are likely to gain service much earlier. This service may be directed toward the language problem while it ignores the phonological component. Recent national survey data of school clinicians' caseloads showed that, on the average, in 14.9 percent of the caseloads the primary emphasis was on training

118

children in other aspects of linguistic deficiencies rather than defective phonology. On the other hand, respondents reported that 19.1 percent of the caseloads contained children having rather general linguistic deficiencies, but for whom the therapy emphasis was on their defective phonology. Also, there continues to be a significant emphasis in school therapy programs on providing articulation therapy to children who have been reported to be free of linguistic impairments and require only correction of defective speech sounds, a nationwide average of 48.9 percent (Sommers and Hatton, 1979).

Although far less commonly used as a clinical descriptor, the term "articulation disorder" may be useful. As mentioned earlier, perhaps this term should continue to be used to describe speech sound production defects which do not include linguistic involvement of any significance. The term "phonological disorder," on the other hand, perhaps should be used to describe speech sound production defects that are accompanied by general and/or specific linguistic defectiveness and for which there is certain evidence linking the occurrence of phonological production errors with other linguistic elements. For example, a phonological disorder may be indicated by the presence of certain types of phonological errors in a child's speech that are dependent upon factors such as the level of meaningfulness of the spoken message or other aspects of its linguistic complexity, particularly syntactical ones (Panagos, Quine, and Klich, 1979).

Although the writings of some authorities imply that children's phonological disorders are free from obvious organic components and thus can be categorized as "functional," the author feels that such a set of assumptions is untenable and that some young children who have delayed development of speech and language will also show evidence of perceptual, memory, and motor-skill weaknesses. It does not seem necessary to specify that no such problems can exist to justify the use of the terms "phonological disorder."

These distinctions imply that intervention strategies for correcting articulation and phonological disorders should be different in some important ways. Interest is rising in investigating phonological disorders and developing linguistic strategies for their correction, while interest in developing new intervention strategies for correction of traditional articulatory disorders is waning. We shall see the long, historical interest and subsequent development of basic therapy technique for the articulatory-disordered child and the emergence of the phonological disorder concept and its implications for therapy as we move almost chronologically through a review of some very old, not-so-old, and rather recent approaches to the correction of children's speech sound production errors.

THE MEANING OF FUNCTIONAL ARTICULATION AND PHONOLOGICAL DISORDERS

One of our first tasks is to clarify what we mean when speaking of functional articulation and phonological disorders, particularly as a diagnostic category distinct from organic articulation and phonological disorders. Because there is an important difference between the labels, and yet some overlapping of meaning, confusion can arise in attempts to apply them. Speech pathologists, like others engaged in the scientific investigation of human behavior, encounter this problem in their attempts to attribute cause. Indeed, the question of whether learning disorders, neuroses, psychoses, and perceptual difficulties are attributable to psychological or to physiological factors is perennial, and, in attempts to resolve it, pathologists tend to pigeonhole disorders as functional or organic, respectively. This has been described by Perkins and Curlee (1969):

> Speech pathologists are applied behavioral scientists. We often show greater respect, however, for physiological than for psychological data. We tend to be relatively critical in the ways we think about behavioral explanations of communicative disorders, but when organic disabilities—that are so "obvious"—can be related to these problems, our rigor slips. At this point, we often trap ourselves in the functional-organic dichotomy.

A more discriminating use of the word *functional* is needed if it is to clarify, rather than obscure, the etiology of articulation disorders. Presumably borrowed from medical literature, *functional* typically has denoted disorders for which no evidence of organic etiology or pathology could be found. For this reason, as Powers (1957) has observed, *functional* has become associated with, and possibly a synonym for, *nonorganic*; in a discussion about the circumstances governing the legitimate use of the word *functional*, she stated:

> Still another issue arises in the *organic* versus *functional* dilemma. Many *functional articulation* cases are so labeled unjustifiably through what this writer likes to call "diagnosis by default," meaning that an assumption is made that a speech defect must be functional if no obvious organic deviations are found to account for it. The term *functional* is used as a catchall for speech problems which cannot be explained in other terms. This is not a legitimate procedure. It is necessary for the speech diagnostician to demonstrate positive evidences of functional etiology as well as to eliminate negative evidences (p. 709).

To summarize, the writers quoted appear to have concluded that *functional* is appropriately applied to inadequate performance of the articulatory forms within a language, irrespective of etiology, when there are no obvious signs of structural and neurological deviations. It should carry no inference of either organic or nonorganic cause, but by that we are not suggesting that cause is unimportant; on the contrary, the more we learn about the determining factors in given problem areas, the more effective will be our remedial efforts.

The heterogeneity of articulatory development complicates the problem of determining what factors may have contributed to functional articulation disorders. In the first eight years of life articulation development is influenced by a mix of neurological, emotional, and environmental factors. It is conceivable that one or more disruptions could occur in each of these three categories and have a deleterious effect on the development of articulation. At present we do not understand as much as we might wish about these influences and their possible interactions, but there is reason to think that the development of functional articulation disorders often follows a recognizable pattern. Research into the development of articulation difficulties, reviewed below, may throw some light on the relationships between the variables, as well as on their relationships with specific kinds of problems. It is necessary first, however, to discuss in somewhat general terms the varying emphases and approaches shown in a review of the research.

VARIATIONS IN THEORETICAL PERSPECTIVES

Two questions underlying any discussion of articulation and phonological disorders are concerned with (1) the nature of the process of articulation and (2) the application of phonetic or phonemic analysis to articulation differences. The proponents of a phonemic orientation to articulation have recently been increasingly more vocal than those who have maintained that it is chiefly a phonetic process.

Articulation as Process or Language

We commonly identify six parameters of speech production—articulation, prosody, resonance, phonation, respiration, and cerebration—of which articulation seems to be the most variable and complex. It has overlapping functions with all of the other five, with one of its chief functions being the production of speech sounds in proper sequence. The exact nature of its relationships with the other parameters is unclear, although some relationships are apparent. For example, the nasality of cleft-palate speakers demonstrates the interaction between resonance and articulation, and the prosody of speech depends heavily on the articulatory function in a number of ways, such as the rising and falling of stress patterns on particular sounds as they initiate or arrest syllables. Speech scientists are constantly contributing new information about interactions between the various parameters, and linguists have theorized about the relative roles of each in communication. In fact, in view of the intricacies of the total speech process, it is legitimate to question whether it can be so easily divided into six parameters. Perhaps the one that we call "articulation" is only a man-made convenience.

We can run into problems if we try to explain the articulatory function as only a mechanical act performed by specific muscles, for it is more than that. The speech behaviors of aphasic adults, brain-injured children, and children with cerebral dysfunction indicate that cortical malfunction can impair the "programming" of articulation. Such programming from some area of the cerebral cortex is needed if the cranial nerves are to innervate the articulators and supply them with the coded messages to ensure their coordinated movement in the appropriate sequence and speed. When the information fails to be supplied, apraxic or dyspraxic speech is thought to result. Evidence to support this notion has been presented by Russian and American investigators interested in coarticulation (see, particularly, Moll & Daniloff, 1968).

Studies and speculation about the encoding and decoding of speech and the transformation from the phone of the speaker to the sound of the listener have convinced some researchers (Mattingly and Liberman, 1968, and others in association with Haskins Laboratories) that articulation is and must be a language function. A related view has been expressed by Chomsky and Miller (1963) and Chomsky and Halle (1968) who, on the assumption that a universal phonetics underlies speech production, maintain that speech is perceived not only as a function of the acoustic properties of the signal, but also as a function of the listener's knowledge of and sophistication with the language, plus a number of extragrammatical factors. The key idea here is that speech perception is a heuristic process, wherein the listener samples cues in the speech signal to achieve a hypothesis about the speaker's utterance. Even the simplest linguistic units, the phones, generate meaning within the listener.

A popular explanation of articulation as language is the generative grammar theory expressed by Chomsky (1957, 1965) and Chomsky and Miller (1963), which has been applied to articulation therapy by a number of speech pathologists. This theory postulates that there are different linguistic levels—a "deep" and a "surface" level. The smallest unit of cognitive information is the kernel sentence which makes up the basic part of the deep structure. Through syntactic and lexical alterations which do not change the essence of the deep structure, the kernel sentence can be "transformed" into slightly different surface structures.

Other attempts to relate linguistic theory to articulation competence include those by Compton (1968) and Crocker (1969). Using generative analysis to explain the occurrence of consonantal misarticulation in a child, Compton reported in a convention address that:

1. seemingly inconsistent sound productions are actually quite predictable and systematic when described by means of phonological rules of sound change; and
2. many of the misarticulations are relatively independent of ability to discriminate and produce the appropriate sounds.

Crocker, whose study was more comprehensive, cited distinctive-feature theory (as proposed by Jakobson, Fant, and Halle, 1951) in describing how the development of specific sounds in children's speech follows a logical pattern. He stated that a phonological model based on distinctive-feature theory accurately predicts the various types of articulation errors that children have been found to make. Sound substitutions, for example, can be predicted from an observation of the sounds that appear early in, and along the line of, the child's development; and failure to apply a rule (presumably a phonological rule) at a certain time in the development of a sound will result in another sound being substituted for it.

The Use of Phonetic or Phonemic Analysis

Traditionally, the study and description of articulation disorders have centered upon the sounds of speech as the units for discussion, without regard to the language in which they occur—the word *phone* often used synonymously with *sound* to refer to the smallest unit of articulation, which carries no meaning. Lately, however, this emphasis by speech pathologists on phonetics has been somewhat overshadowed by an increasing interest in linguistics, and hence on the meanings of the sound units (phonemics).

McDonald (1964) has explained the distinctions between phonetics and phonemics as follows:

"Phonemic" means that a given articulatory change of the syllable affects the meaning [whereas] "phonetic," "sound," "articulation," refer to articulate processes of speech without regard to meaning. The articulations and their variations and combinations when identified in a given vernacular constitute the basis for phonetics (p. 13).

Both types of analysis contribute to our knowledge of the etiology, maintenance, and remediation of articulation disorders. It is good, however, in reading any discussion, to ascertain whether its framework is phonetic or phonemic. Despite the trend toward the phonemic approach, the literature on articulation has contained more studies by persons interested in phonetics—acoustic phonetics in particular—than by persons interested in phonemics. Researchers who have focused on phonemic aspects have often been interested in differences in the articulation of socially and culturally deprived persons, as well as persons with the kinds of articulation differences traditionally dealt with by speech pathologists. Chapter 2 describes the articulation differences found in different cultural environments. Currently, we see a tendency to relate the two overlapping areas—a type of interdisciplinary trend between motor and acoustic phonetics and phonological construct.

RESEARCH INTO THE FACTORS RELATED TO CHILDREN'S ARTICULATION AND PHONOLOGICAL DISORDERS

Studies extending back to the 1930s on articulatory acquisition and behavior have been reviewed by Winitz (1969), and the reader is urged to consult pages 139 through 237 of his book for pertinent information on these topics. In general, early investigations were directed at seeing whether correlation existed between articulation—normal and defective—and such developmental variables as IQ, mental and chronological age, socioeconomic status, and sex. These early investigations did not focus on articulation defects per se.

It should also be observed that in keeping with an early review of literature on developmental variables, thought by some to relate to levels of children's articulatory/phonological development, Winitz (1969) reported that, of the many variables studied, chronological age was the most potent predictor of children's articulatory/phonological development while "obvious" factors such as children's IQ's, mental ages, and socioeconomic status were either nonsignificantly related to such development or related to a statistically significant but slight degree. Winitz's review also makes it clear that conflicting findings about developmental variables are the rule rather than the exception, although this is not the case with respect to intelligence and mental age.

Even the notion that females develop articulatory/phonological skills before males at preschool age is not heavily supported by research data. Norms on the *Templin-Darley Test of Articulation*, for example, frequently show females exceeding males in the numbers of correct responses by six-month age groups, yet when the author applied *t* tests to many of these comparisons, most females failed to reach a .05 level of statistical significance. While the trend was for females to be superior by age, the mean differences were small and the variance in performance great enough to destroy reliable statistical differences in favor of females at many age levels. This same notion, that across age levels in early development females exceed males generally on linguistic skills, is likely an overgeneralization of the status of the condition and probably relates to which linguistic ability is being examined at an age level.

Various investigators have shown that certain developmental skills separate the articulatory/phonologically impaired child from peers with normal speech. These factors are classified under the rubrics of: (a) linguistic weaknesses, (b) auditory skill impairments, (c) fine motor skill deficiencies, and (d) inferior oral discrimination and recognition skills and related ones such as diadochokinesis. This material is not intended to be complete, but it has been chosen to represent a cross-section of the older and newer literature on possible developmental correlates of articulatory/phonological defectiveness.

Auditory Discrimination for Speech Sounds

It has long been the opinion of certain speech pathologists that some functional articulation disorders are caused by deficiencies related to accurate discrimination of the sounds of language. Others believe this concept is still conjectural. Some speech-language pathologists show their indifference to the issue by ignoring attempts to improve speech sound discrimination training in the corrective process, working largely and intentionally upon models of therapy that focus solely upon accurate production of defective consonants, while other pathologists stress the importance of first determining the extent (if any) of speech sound discrimination difficulties and then including in therapy an adequate amount of training to minimize the problem and its possible influence upon the correction of defective speech. Which of these approaches seems best and in keeping with knowledge concerning the existence of speech sound discrimination problems in articulatory/phonologically impaired persons?

General, External Sound Discrimination. Early authoritative opinions (Powers, 1957) maintained that the issue of a weakness in the articulatory defective's abilities to discriminate speech sounds was very controversial in light of both negative and positive findings. Subsequently, perhaps as a result of a decade of additional research and some important findings related to earlier investigations, both Weiner (1967) and Winitz (1969) independently reviewed the issue and concluded that a link could be rather impressively established, for children eight years old or younger, between the existence of articulatory problems and defective speech sound discrimination skills. Additional reports after the Weiner and Winitz reviews supported this relationship by using general speech sound discrimination tests of various types (Gilmore, 1969; Sommers, Meyer, and Furlong, 1969; Stitt and Huntington, 1969). Additional evidence to support the belief that speech sound discrimination is more difficult for those having articulation or phonological disorders was gathered later by many investigators, some of whom viewed the essential elements of the speech sound discrimination process to be different from those involved in the traditional task of discrimination of minimal paired words (identical except for one phoneme, an example being the *Wepman Sound Discrimination Test*, 1959) or minimal paired nonsense syllables (also identical except for one phoneme, an example being the *Templin Test*, 1943). In such tasks, many consonants are paired against each other to test overall discrimination ability; thus the task involves having the subject listen to a person present the minimal pairs live or on tape and decide whether each pair is the same or different. Using this type of procedure, the examiner is often asking an individual to make discriminations across consonant pairs on which he has perfectly normal speech production. These procedures may describe *general, external* speech sound discrimination tasks.

Historically, the literature has shown that this general, external type of sound discrimination is not particularly troublesome for some children who are articulatory defectives. In particular, the ability of those having less severe defectiveness appears often to be equal or near-equal to that of normal-speaking children. The early studies that influenced the later, controversial literature were those of Kronvall and Diehl (1954) and Cohen and Diehl (1963), who reported that the more severely defective were those often showing significant deficiencies on the general, external form of discrimination tasks, while the milder defectives were similar in skill to normal speaking children. Confirmation for this set of findings came from evidence supplied by Farquhar (1961), Sherman and Geith (1967), and Sommers, Meyer, and Furlong

(1969). It is of interest, particularly in light of newer multivariate approaches to such investigations, that these studies focused on severely defective children whose sound discrimination scores approximated the milder defective and normal subjects, and all studies relied upon average or mean differences to substantiate their findings. More recently, using factor analysis and other forms of multivariate technique, investigators McNutt and Hamayan (1982) have demonstrated that subgroups of articulatory defective children may exist in the population, some of whom are normal on certain linguistic, cognitive, perceptual, and memory tasks. The data of these investigators show that certain subgroups do have normal speech sound discrimination performances on general, external tasks, while others do not. We await confirmation of the existence of the subgroups to sort out the older and newer findings about links with overall severity to show that sound discrimination problems may be part of a larger constellation of strengths and weaknesses in the areas studied by McNutt and Hamayan.

Specific, Internal Sound Discrimination. Some investigators believe that other types of speech sound discrimination skills beside the general, external one are related to defective articulation. As early as 1949, Anderson reported that children having defective /s/ productions had significantly greater numbers of /s/ discrimination errors. Related evidence to support a link between specific sound production errors and errors of discrimination was provided by Aungst and Frick (1964), who observed that /r/ defective children eight to ten years of age showed poorest discriminations of forms of /r/ in phonetic contexts in which they misarticulated it. Findings from this important study also suggested that the discrimination problems of children defective in /r/ were largely related to inabilities to discriminate their own accuracy of production of /r/ in various contexts rather than a general, external discrimination disability. As such, these findings were revealing in both ways. More recent investigations of children's speech sound discrimination performances (Wolfe and Irwin, 1973; Monnin and Huntington, 1974) support the notion that sound discrimination errors under certain conditions relate to phonetic contexts in which misarticulations occur.

Other investigators, who approached the issue from somewhat different strategic positions, provided additional support for the belief that internal- or self-detection of error discrimination deficiencies characterize certain articulatory/phonologically impaired children. For the most, evidence supplied by them seemed to imply that weakness in self-monitoring of speech, particularly related to phonetic contexts in which production errors occurred, was a common malady. Problems in accurate self-monitoring of errors were observed, for example, by Schiefelbusch and Lindsey (1958), Aufricht (1959), Smith (1965), and Hutter (1966). Thus, it would appear that good reasons to suspect a *specific, internal discrimination problem* may exist in a certain portion of the population of defectives, especially under the condition that only one phoneme or so is in error; however, under the condition of having many misarticulations, children may tend to show a more obvious, general, external discrimination problem. All such conclusions may await further evidence, but it does appear that many investigators have independent evidence for something akin to these stated relationships.

We can find additional evidence showing the interest of some investigators in identifying relationships between speech sound discrimination and speech sound production. To accomplish this, some have relied upon application of distinctive feature concepts. For example, Prins (1963), Lewis (1974), McReynolds, Kohn, and Williams (1975), and Waldman, Singh, and Hayden (1978) have looked for correspondence between feature discrimination and feature use. Evidence from the Waldman, Singh, and Hayden (1978) study that children were able to discriminate features that they could not produce well in certain phonemes seemed to support the findings of others (Lewis, 1974; McReynolds, Kohn, and Williams, 1975), but identification of exact relationships between feature discrimination and accuracy of use seems to have escaped researchers at this time.

Training Sound Discrimination. Documentation for the value of discrimination training to facilitate correct sound production has been supplied by Winitz and some of his colleagues. For example, Winitz and Bellerose (1962) proposed that discrimination between a target and error sound may be impeded by the learning of the phonetic nature of the error sound. Subsequently, Winitz and Preisler (1965, 1967) supplied evidence to show that sound discrimination pretraining, involving the error sound and the target sound, facilitated the learning of the correct sound. Finally, Winitz and Bellerose (1967) concluded that articulatory errors and discrimination errors are positively correlated.

Views like that of Winitz and his colleagues, based on experiments involving sound discrimination and sound learning, provided support for the early writings of some authorities in speech pathology. Van Riper (1938, 1972), for example, was an early advocate of ear training that included discrimination of the nature of the target and error sounds in early stages of articulation therapy—a view endorsed to a degree by Berry and Eisenson (1956), Cohen and Diehl (1963), Powers (1957), and Sherman and Geith (1967). Over a span of many years, Van Riper detailed comprehensive steps for training individuals to become highly knowledgeable about the phonetic nature of their error sounds and target sounds. Writings in the more recent research and therapy literature indicate that a covert disclaimer for the need for discrimination training characterizes the views of some individuals, the emphasis perhaps being on phonemic production gained and modified by using linguistic contexts and measures. As we shall discover later in this chapter, however, some of the more modern approaches to articulatory correction call for training the child to perceive accurately differences between the error and target sounds, and some portion of this training appears to be auditory discrimination.

Motor Skills

There are also reasons for believing that children with more severe articulation defects perform differently on other tasks, and many studies have been reported comparing articulatory defective children with normal speaking children on the basis of fine and general motor skills, eye-hand coordination, physical strength, and endurance, through tests such as tapping, tracing, rail- or tandem-walking, jumping and reaching, and hopping on one foot.

In a 1969 review of the motor skill literature, Winitz maintained, "Sufficient evidence is . . . lacking to support the hypothesis that articulatory defectives demonstrate a general retardation in motor skills" (p. 155). While there is a basis for that view in the lack of agreement among the older investigations—that is, those predating the use of the Oseretsky Tests—some tentative conclusions may be reached as a result of a review of the tests and tasks used in these early studies:

1. Although tests of general body control, strength, and speed seem to detect the fewest differences—as, for example, in the studies by Mase (1946) and Albright (1948), who used a rail-walking test, Bitlo's (1941) results using the Brace Motor Ability Test and the jump-and-reach test found that two thirds of the subjects with articulation defects were inferior to normal speakers in these areas.
2. Tests of hand speed and reaction time have usually had negative or inconclusive results, as noted, for example, by Albright (1948), who measured writing rate, hand steadiness, and tapping, and Carrell (1937) and Reid (1947), who measured tapping performance.
3. The four early studies by Albright (1948), Bitlo (1941), Carrell (1937), and Wellman (1926) found the performance of the subjects with articulation defects on tasks involving eye-hand coordination, rather than strength or steadiness, to be significantly inferior to that of normal speakers. Prins (1962), on the other hand, did not find that subjects with articulation defects were inferior on a task that presumably is somewhat dependent on eye-hand coordination.

Some investigators believed that a more sensitive and comprehensive set of fine motor tasks might provide a better test of the hypothesis that articulatory defective children's skills are poorer than comparable normal speaking children. In 1964 Jenkins and Lohr attempted to improve upon earlier studies by selecting *The Oseretsky Test of Motor Proficiency* (Sloan, 1950) as their tool. Studying a group of thirty-eight articulatory defective first-grade children having many misarticulations and thirty-eight normal speaking first-grade control subjects, they reported significant differences in favor of the control group subjects on all but one of the five subscales studied and overall as expressed in motor quotients. Support for their findings was found by Paul (1971) who replicated the Jenkins and Lohr study. Paul's results were identical in every way to those reported originally by Jenkins and Lohr (1964).

Further evidence that children's severity of articulatory defectiveness relates to their motor skills as measured using *The Oseretsky Test of Motor Proficiency* came from an investigation by Sommers, Moore, Brady, and Jackson (1976). They reported a moderate negative correlation of statistical significance between subjects' performances on the Oseretsky test subscale involving speed and accuracy of coordinated hand movements (Dynamic Manual Coordination), and articulation errors. In effect, as articulation severity tended to increase, performance scores on this motor task decreased—a finding that appears to support the hypothesis that severity of articulatory defectiveness increases the likelihood for inferior fine motor skills on some tasks.

A link between the maintenance of articulation defects in some children and performances on *The Oseretsky Test of Motor Proficiency* was established by Dickson (1962) who found that kindergarten and first grade children who retained errors at the end of an academic year tended to have poorer fine motor skills.

In summary, while very early findings from studies of articulatory defective children's fine motor skills were characterized by inconsistencies, more recent ones, using *The Oseretsky Test of Motor Proficiency*, have yielded positive findings. Obviously, the issue remains unresolved, but the evidence tends to support the belief that as articulatory defectiveness increases, a greater likelihood for poorer fine motor skill increases, at least in some portions of the population.

Oral Sensation and Related Abilities

Early in the clinical literature related to the diagnosis and treatment of articulation problems, one can find references to possible deficiencies of oral sensation and perception as etiological in such disorders. Oral motor control via oral sensory feedback systems has served as a pivotal concept in theories of speech production and is of long standing (Fairbanks, 1954; Mysak, 1959). As early as 1942, Patton maintained that without the "kinesthetic sense, . . . the conditioned reflex of speech could probably never be established or maintained." He further maintained that conscious or unconscious memory of motor acts for speech must exist prior to learning how to produce speech sounds. In essence, the kinesthetic sense assists an individual to develop an awareness of muscle tension and articulator positions at the moment speech sounds are produced. Its importance may be greater early in life when the child is first developing speech sounds.

One of the earliest tasks that investigators used to study the articulatory defective child's performances against normal speaking children was one involving the rapid assessment of imitated speech production. Termed "diadochokinesis," this task often required the rapid production of CV syllables, usually /pʌ/, /tʌ/, /kʌ/, or /pʌ, tʌ, kʌ/. Norms were provided by early researchers, but were sparsely gathered (Fairbanks and Spriestersbach, 1950).

Most of the early literature concerning the abilities of articulatory defective children to perform such tasks was conflicting (see, for example, Hixon and Hardy, 1964); however, some investigators reported that significant relationships exist between certain articulatory skills and this type of oral motor activity (see, for example, Prins, 1962a and 1962b). That some portion of articulatory defective children are inferior on diadochokinetic tasks seems more apparent at this time in view of findings in more recent research of poorer abilities to articulate syllables rapidly while maintaining accuracy of speech production (Shelton, Arndt, Krueger, and Huffman, 1966; McNutt, 1977).

The ability of some articulatory defective children to identify accurately small objects of various size and shape placed in their mouths and their skills in performing certain diadochokinetic rate tasks may be related. In a study of sixty elementary school children who reportedly had mild articulatory defectiveness, Hardesty (1975) determined that a significant relationship existed between children's diadochokinetic rates and their oral form identification skills.

Various procedures have been developed for the investigation of oral sensory skills (Ringel, Saxman, and Brooks, 1967; Aungst, 1965; Wegener, 1966), and some researchers have successfully tied performances on many such tasks to the presence or absence of articulation errors in children's speech. For example, Aungst (1965) found that the ability to produce /r/ correctly was more dependent upon accuracy of oral form identification than was the ability to produce other consonants. This finding was supported by the results of an investigation by Weinberg, Liss, and Hollis (1970) and by findings reported by McNutt (1977). In the former investigation "persistent" /r/ defective teenage subjects were found poorer in their abilities to identify oral forms than normal speaking controls. In the McNutt (1977) study the performances of teenage /r/, /s/, and normal speaking controls were compared using an oral form discrimination task. McNutt reported that only the /r/ defectives' performances were significantly poorer than those of the control subjects.

Some evidence, however, does link inferior oral form identification and discrimination to more homogeneous groups of articulatory defective children. Wegener (1966), for example, evaluated the oral form discrimination skills of a heterogeneous sample of articulatory defective children and found their performances significantly poorer overall than normal speaking control group subjects. Severity of articulator defectiveness was found related to oral form discrimination by Ringel, House, Burk, Dolinsky, and Scott (1970). Only children having severe forms of defectiveness were inferior on their task to the normal speaking subjects. Using exactly the same oral forms and identical testing and scoring procedures used by Ringel and his colleagues (Ringel and Ewanowski, 1965; Ringel and Fletcher, 1967); Sommers, Cox, and West (1972) found that children ages five and six having superior articulatory skills were significantly better in oral form discrimination than those judged to be deviant or defective in articulation development.

Related evidence came from a study reported by Fucci and Robertson (1971), who studied older misarticulating children, ages twelve to sixteen, and a control group of normal speakers. Using different tactics, these investigators used twenty geometric plastic forms to complete intersensory matching tasks which purported to measure perceptual discrimination at various loci, that is, eye to picture, fingertip to picture, tongue tip to picture, and tongue blade to picture. The number of errors across all related tasks was found to be significantly greater for those subjects having articulation errors.

In summary, the great weight of the evidence suggests that some portion of articulatory defective children in an age range from approximately five to sixteen years may show evidence of reduced skill in the identification and discrimination of oral forms. Rather strong and consistent evidence shows that the /r/ defective is particularly susceptible to this problem, but as Ringel et al. (1970) found, there also may be a more general type of difficulty that becomes associated with more severe forms of articulatory defectiveness. Rather interestingly, the oral form identification and discrimination task literature seems rather consistent in its reporting of differences—a development that is refreshing in the maze of conflicting reports and data that has characterized research of children's articulatory performances in the past.

Linguistic Factors

Although linguists and psycholinguistics have been able to relate the phonological aspects of language to its other elements, namely, syntax, semantics, and morphology, using logic and theory, a strong data base to explain such relationships has been slow in developing. What is probably the first study of certain relationships between normal developing and phonologically impaired children was made in 1964 when Menyuk provided information concerning the language skills of ten normal speaking subjects three to five years old, and a group of ten children defective in articulation.

She reported that evidence from analyses of a spoken language sample and a sentence repetition test showed that the misarticulating children had primitive and very general rule systems in contrast to normal speaking subjects. Structural complexity differences were also reported by Vandermark and Mann (1965), who studied fifty articulatory defective children and fifty normal speaking ones. In contrast to the control subjects, the fifty defectives suffered from weaknesses in grammar and in the complexity of their verbal responses.

Of the elements thought to comprise language, syntax seems to have shown the strongest link to articulation proficiency, as seen in a number of investigations. Severe articulatory defectiveness was found to reflect inferior syntactical skills in a study by Shriner, Holloway, and Daniloff (1969). Using spoken language samples, they concluded that grammatical usage of thirty children, ages six to nine, was inferior to that of thirty normal speaking ones of the same ages. They hypothesized that children having severe degrees of articulatory defectiveness may not talk as much as others and, thus, fail to practice and experiment with new syntactical forms.

Using different assessment strategies, Whitacre, Luper, and Pollio (1970) also found a pattern of general linguistic weakness characterized by the performances of subjects having a wide range of articulatory defectiveness. Children six to seven years old were tested on word association, sentence repetition, and implicit phonology tests. The investigators concluded that articulatory defective children are impaired in their knowledge of phonological rules, form, class, use, and in their sentence structure.

Additional evidence for a rather general display of linguistic weakness related to the degree of articulatory defectiveness was gathered by Jackson and Sommers (1971), who studied the skills of twenty-five children, ages 6–10. Five of the subjects were normal in articulation, five mildly impaired, five moderately impaired, five severely impaired, and five learning disabled. On tests measuring psycholinguistic abilities, sentence repetition skills, and syntax, the five subjects having the poorest articulation were far poorer than the others. Even the subjects from the moderately-impaired group showed average delays in skill development of only one year. Interestingly, errors on the *McDonald Deep Test of Articulation* (McDonald, 1964) were predictive of children's scores on each of the three language tests, the best prediction (with subjects' chronological ages controlled statistically) was a strong correlation between the number of phonetic contexts in error and the sentence repetition error score, the partial correlation coefficient being a highly significant .810.

Insight into the phonological errors and presence of impairments in syntax was provided by Dukes and Panagos (1973), who studied the sentence repetition skills of nine children, ages four to six, all of whom had serious delays in the development of phonological abilities. They observed that the nature of the syntactic rule was capable of predicting some phonological errors, that syllable complexity related to the presence of phonemic errors, and that errors of consonant omission could be interpreted to imply that the subjects' transformation skills were weak.

In summary, more evidence has been gathered and is being obtained to delineate much more specifically the nature of the relationships between other elements of children's linguistic abilities and their phonology. Most reports show that as the numbers of phonemic errors increase, other elements tend to be primitively developed, the strongest affected being those involved in syntactical rule systems and spoken language complexity.

THE REMEDIATION OF FUNCTIONAL ARTICULATION AND PHONOLOGICAL DISORDERS

Relevant to the remediation of functional articulation disorders are a number of additional questions which have served as topics for professional investigation. In this section, we shall discuss factors related to remediability and concepts underlying analyses of articulation change, as well as the implications for therapy using linguistic and psycholinguistic theories.

Factors Affecting Remediability

Investigations into the variables affecting the amount of improvement achieved by subjects over time have focused upon both speech and non-speech factors.

Speech Factors. The three measurable variables of articulation—stimulability, severity, and consistency—are known to be related to articulatory improvement. The stimulability and consistency factors have been found to relate most meaningfully to changes in young children's misarticulations.

Stimulability has been defined as ability of a person to articulate a defective speech sound correctly under stimulation from a speech clinician since attention was directed to its importance in an early publication by Snow and Milisen (1954). In a series of independent studies by researchers who tested the power of this phenomenon to predict articulation changes, evidence was gathered that, indeed, some important degree of prediction could be achieved. Prediction of change was found possible for untreated subjects of kindergarten age by Farquhar (1961), Haws (1969), Kisatsy (1966), and Sommers et al. (1967). The earliest investigation, one by Carter and Buck (1958), probably inspired much of the research that followed, because it presented a stimulability test that allowed examiners to identify somewhat accurately first grade children requiring speech therapy. Additional support for the use of their test and findings on first grade children was subsequently reported by Stoia (1961), Sommers et al. (1961), Sommers et al. (1967), and Gilmore and Bowz (1975). Positive findings have also been observed for second grade children's misarticulations in experiments reported by Irwin, West, and Trombetta (1966) and Sommers et al. (1967). Further analysis of the data from the 1967 Sommers et al. experiment showed that stimulability effects for children in kindergarten, and grades one and two, are related to which speech sound was being tested and to the grade level of the subject and made predictions on some speech sounds affected by the grade (or age) and speech sound interaction. Thus, stimulability influences appeared to be variable and complex.

Consistency of misarticulation has been viewed as a vital sign in children's speech over many years. Investigators have studied the influence of consistency of misarticulation over spans of time as brief as one year. Brungard did so in 1961 and determined that first grade children defective in /s/ appeared to show correction or significant improvements without therapy if their percentages of inconsistency of /s/ errors was high, while those with low percentages did not self-correct or show large improvements. Longitudinal investigations of consistency of misarticulation of certain consonants, studying as many as one thousand children, have been reported (McDonald and McDonald, 1974; McDonald and McDonald, 1976; Ryan, 1969). Results from the earlier two investigators show that measures of consistency of error based on the use of the *Screening Deep Test for Articulation* (McDonald, 1964) can be used to predict the articulatory status of children throughout the five-, six-, and seven-year age span, with the most revealing prediction being improvements on /s/, /r/, /tʃ/, /ʃ/, and /θ/. These results also reaffirm those observed earlier for the power of stimulability factor: effects are phoneme specific and tend to vary by age. Such specific information is more useful to the practitioner, than general statements of average influences of a prognostic factor, regardless of age or speech sound under discussion.

Severity appears to be a macrovariable, and its impact on prognosis is general and diffuse. For example, some children's misarticulations are many, but they tend to be largely inconsistent and show good stimulability testing effects. Other children may have fewer errors, largely of the consistent and poor stimulability type. Overall, it does appear that children having many single consonant sounds defective, as a group, will often show some residual errors when evaluated a few years later after a period of no treatment. One of the prognostic articulation tests, *The Predictive Screening Test of Articulation* (Van Riper, 1968), is a valuable test for predicting who, among first grade children with misarticulations, will spontaneously outgrow them by the time they reach third grade, because it serves as a general measure of the severity of the child's problem (Miller and Sommers, 1980). The influence of severity of articulatory defectiveness appears to influence the outcome of articulation therapy, as well as to relate to the changes children make without it (Sommers et al., 1966, 1967); however, its influences may be misleading and unsuitable to guide therapy decisions for individuals unless stimulability, consistency, and other relevant factors are taken into consideration.

Nonspeech Factors. Consistent with the findings mentioned on page 123, the so-called organismic factors, such as mental age (MA), IQ, and socioeconomic status, do not appear to be related to normal or induced articulation changes in children. Socioeconomic status, for example, has been studied by Andersland (1961) and Sommers (1962), and their data failed to demonstrate significant differences in articulation improvement between children from higher and lower socioeconomic groups. Sommers (1967), in a review of experiments in which he and his associates had engaged, reported a strong correlation between MA, IQ, and socioeconomic status and the changes effected by treatment. In only one of these studies (Sommers, 1962) could IQ be related to articulation improvement, and in that study slow learners (IQs of 75 to 90) were contrasted to normal children. The mean IQs of the subjects in the two groups differed by more than twenty points (80 and 102). Under such deliberately contrived experimental conditions, IQ may show an effect upon articulation improvement, but when IQ scores fall within the so-called normal range of 90 to 110 or above, there has been no demonstrated effect.

Concepts in Analyzing Articulation Change

Three learning concepts crucial to analyzing the remediation of functional articulation disorders are acquisition, habituation, and response generalization. They figured in studies describing and measuring articulation change by Chisum (1966), Chisum, Shelton, and Arndt (1969), and Elbert, Shelton, and Arndt (1967)—all of which represent important contributions to the understanding of articulation therapy.

Acquisition and Habituation. The basic unit of analysis is acquisition, which relates to the individual's use of a corrected phoneme in different phonetic contexts, in utterances of various lengths, in imitatively produced responses, in spontaneous responses, and under a variety of speaking conditions. Typically, the therapy process for an articulation error is thought to be complete only when the individual produces consistently correct responses under all of these conditions and when so-called carry-over is attained.

Chisum (1966) and Chisum, Shelton, and Arndt (1969), when introducing motor learning concepts into a description of the therapy process for articulation disorders, regarded acquisition as the first level of therapy. They defined it as the process of learning to produce a phoneme in practice material and in articulation responses elicited with test items; and the second level of therapy, habituation, they defined as the correct usage of a phoneme in the absence of deliberate or conscious effort. Many clinicians would accept the term *carry-over* as synonymous with *habituation*.

Some important differences between the acquisition and habituation of phonemes were described by Elbert, Shelton, and Arndt (1967). Studying articulation defects in a sample group of children, they measured articulation changes from lesson to lesson by means of sound production tasks. While the tasks permitted measurement of the acquisition of the skill required to produce a sound, they shed no light on the automatization of sound productions in connected speech. However, carry-over may depend on the clinician's recognizing when an adequate degree of acquisition has been achieved, for at that point, the authors maintained, the clinician should use techniques to ensure consistent use of the correct sound in automatic speech. The discreteness of their division between the acquisition and habituation stages suggests the need for a closer scrutiny of the two stages. While textbooks (Berry and Eisenson, 1956; Van Riper, 1978) have for some time divided the therapy process for articulation disorders into sound production and carry-over phases, there are troublesome and perplexing degrees of overlapping, which may occur by phoneme, age of the individual, and degree of acquisition.

The measurement of articulation change on a continuum from acquisition to habituation has rarely been made, perhaps because such studies were not felt to be important, or because many speech clinicians and researchers have assumed that habituation occurs automatically after some degree of acquisition has taken place. The latter assumption seems questionable—particularly for certain types of articulation errors on some phonemes—in light of tentative evidence that certain types of articulation errors were not well habituated in the speech of children dismissed from speech therapy (Sommers, Gerber, and Leiss, 1969). Of 177 school children studied who failed to gain carry-over, those having interdental sigmatisms on /s/ were least successful, whereas carry-over was found to occur much more successfully for those having errors on /r/. Other less dramatic phonemic differences were also noted.

Studies comparing performances on a sound during acquisition and during or after habituation have been reported. Some evidence that sound acquisition does, in fact, result in habituation without effort on the clinician's part—at least for certain individuals under certain conditions—was presented by Sommers, Gerber, and Leiss (1969). They used an articulation task developed by Gerber (1966) to measure the spontaneous speech of 131 children with articulation defects; it "forced" speech responses across six allophones of /r/ in an "interview" supposedly designed to elicit preferences for TV shows. To test their hypothesis that children of certain ages with errors on certain phonemes may not require total correction (habituation) before they can be dismissed from therapy, the authors dismissed sixty children at random and kept the other seventy-one. The results tended to validate the usefulness of test items measuring acquisition of allophones of /r/ as predictors of their correct articulation in spontaneous connected speech, since both groups performed as predicted, irrespective of continued therapy.

The variables affecting habituation have not been explored extensively, although Gerber (1966) did compare the efficacy of traditional carry-over techniques and automated learning based on feedback principles. From a population of sixteen school-age children with /r/ defects, all of whom were considered to have achieved acquisition (on the basis of responses to questions concerning their TV preferences, as described above), she randomly selected eight for the experimental group. They participated in individual, self-administered therapy using an automatic speech feedback device, the Echorder, while the eight control subjects remained in regular articulation therapy classes for carry-over training.

Gerber programmed the Echorder so that the tape carried a prerecorded stimulus followed by space for the child to record his or her imitation. The children judged their own performance and compared immediate and delayed feedback. As they improved, they moved to new material requiring faster judgments and more difficult speech productions. The goal was to advance each child's speech production toward the facility typical of rapid and continuous speech. Tasks ranged from highly structured ones to relatively spontaneous opportunities for response, and included the production of nonsense syllables, words, sentences, and sections of connected speech. The clinician monitored each child's activities, issued new material, and occasionally asked the child to repeat a task.

The control group's carry-over training consisted of reading, spontaneous conversation, skits, and reports. It was part of the therapy plan for members to detect each other's /r/ errors.

A comparison of results with responses elicited initially in the "interview" of TV preferences was based on 105 productions of /r/. Gerber found that her experimental subjects improved significantly in their mean change scores, as compared with the controls. But most important, four of the eight experimental subjects gained total habituation of /r/, while none of the controls did. Consequently, she concluded that carry-over for /r/ may be facilitated by a systematic program of self-listening and self-evaluation devised to intensify simultaneous auditory feedback.

Response Generalization. As applied to the sound learning process by Elbert, Shelton, and Arndt (1967), the concept of response generalization holds great promise for increasing the efficiency and effectiveness of articulation therapy. Response generalization occurs when a formerly incorrect response that has been correctly learned in some phonetic contexts is also produced correctly in similar, yet different, contexts for which there has been no specific therapy. The definition has been further extended to include the situation where the correction of some phonemic errors causes improvement in similar ones (usually along distinctive-feature lines) without direct intervention or teaching by the clinician. This latter hypothesis, not new clinically, has been the subject of a number of investigations. It has also formed the basis for the "Wedge Approach" to articulation therapy (see pp. 168–169).

Elbert, Shelton, and Arndt studied response generalization in seven children, aged 6–4 to 8–2, who were defective in the production of /s/, /z/, and /r/. They were given therapy for /s/ errors only and, as hypothesized, generalization to /z/ (which is only one distinctive feature different) occurred, but not to the phonetically dissimilar /r/. Six children with /r/ defects, two of whom also misarticulated /θ/, and one who misarticulated /s/, underwent a similar series of procedures. Improvements in the /r/ sound were not reflected in improvements in either /θ/ or /s/, which are markedly dissimilar to /r/ and have a number of distinctive-feature differences.

Information concerning the likelihood of generalization in various stages of training will be of much use to the clinician. With that end in mind, Powell and McReynolds (1969) divided a training program for four children consistently defective in /r/ into four phases, and tested them at the end of each phase to see whether they generalized the correct response to words that had not been used in training. The four phases consisted of isolated sound training, initial position training in nonsense syllables, final position training in nonsense syllables, and medial position training in nonsense syllables. Generalization from nonsense syllable training to untrained words occurred to some degree in all of the subjects, as shown by testing at the end of each phase. Two children generalized completely from nonsense syllable training to untrained words, while the other two demonstrated lesser degrees of generalization.

Also bearing on the subject of generalization was an earlier study (Winitz and Bellerose, 1963), the results of which supported the belief that response generalization can be demonstrated for speech sounds and maintained with reinforcement. The authors had samples of normal-speaking school children perform selected sound learning tasks, and explored how generalization was affected by such factors as syllables versus words and phonetic similarities in initial consonants of training and test items. Citing the phonetic similarities in initial consonants as factors contributing to generalization, the authors spoke of the initial consonants in terms of distinctive features. In still another study, McLean (1965) demonstrated that correct articulation shifted to untrained words if the sound was in the initial position, but not to words where the sound assumed other positions.

As the foregoing review has shown, research findings have corroborated clinical impressions about the generalization of speech sounds under therapy. Through work done on similar phonemes, phonemes with only one or two changes in distinctive features can be improved even if no direct effort is made to remediate them.

With the increasing emphasis on the application of linguistics and psycholinguistics to the study of articulation, researchers have been trying to determine how their theories can be more meaningful and helpful in both remediation and diagnosis.

The generative grammar theory of Chomsky and his associates, mentioned earlier in this chapter (p. 121), has been applied in therapy by Lee (1968), who used simple kernel sentences to make language suitable for young language-disordered children. Another therapy method used by Cooper (1968) is based on meaningful minimal contrasts; the system, which uses paired words and sentences, is based on learning theory principles, for it is Cooper's view that children will alter their defective utterances if the utterances are conditioned to a new meaning (see pp. 159–162).

The following section, which deals with remediation techniques, will illustrate the incorporation of the various concepts and theories which we have described into specific treatment approaches.

A REVIEW OF REMEDIATION APPROACHES

Thirteen approaches to the remediation of defective articulation/phonology are included in this section. This is not intended to be a closed set of those available for review and discussion; rather, it represents some traditional views and some more recent attempts to devise strategies and techniques which might lead to more rapid and effective correction.

In light of the sparse research evidence supporting the efficacy of one approach over another, readers are urged to arrive at their own conclusions about merit, and it seems probable that what "fits" a clinician may have its own intrinsic value in settling the issue of which approach is most desirable and effective. Experienced clinicians have probably settled on approaches that suit them, that they have confidence in, and in which they have been carefully instructed. Hopefully, the needs of the individual client will have an important bearing upon the choice of a therapy approach.

Basis for the Selection of Therapy Approaches

In this section, we emphasize historically significant approaches that have been found useful over a considerable period of time and, thus, are used extensively by practitioners. Their impact on therapy practices can often be seen in the extent to which authors of textbooks and others have relied on their principles and therapy recommendations. Many of these can be termed "traditional" techniques. These examples cannot show all of the steps required to advance a client from acquisition to habituation of a correct response, but they reveal enough to allow one to apply some of the principles and practices of the method. These examples are not intended to fit any particular time structure, such as half-hour therapy sessions. Finally, it should be mentioned that when clear examples of sample lesson plans were not available from the authority whose work is being described, the author and his former associate, Ann Kane (Sommers and Kane, 1974), took the liberty of preparing plans. We earnestly hope that they reflect accurately and adequately what the authority might have prepared and disseminated as typical of his or her work.

For purposes of continuity, the sample sessions based on traditional methods assume a diagnosis of /s/ sound difficulty. The other methods that are discussed present different problems and do not follow this same format.

Framework Governing the Analyses

The framework used for analyzing these therapy methods is designed to identify the distinguishing characteristics of each method and to arrive at descriptive statements about their primary factors. In general, each of the methods is analyzed in terms of the management of the therapy session, its major sensory-perceptual emphasis, and its major articulation production emphasis.

Management of the Therapy Session. In these discussions, we shall focus attention on:

1. the time limits suggested for the session;

2. the use of individual or group structure, and suggestions for changing from one to the other;
3. the material and equipment required for the session;
4. the operational level or unit of articulated speech recommended for the practice sessions; and
5. suggestions for altering the method to account for the variable factors of sex, mental age, chronological age, socioeconomic status, and auditory discrimination ability.

Major Sensory-Perceptual Emphasis. In this area, we shall examine techniques for developing the client's ability to receive and interpret presented stimuli, for often these aspects of training are interwoven with actual training in the production of speech sounds. Receptive development, for example, is emphasized by provisions for using the client's visual, auditory, kinesthetic, and tactile abilities in identifying and discriminating speech sounds; appropriate techniques thus include ear training, training in auditory and visual discrimination, and so on. The elements of perceptual development have been identified by Carrell (1968) as grouping, or the ability to separate incoming stimuli into related units; closure, or the ability to recognize stimuli (such as words) even if they are incompletely presented; figure-ground effect, or the ability to perceive a figure (the word to which we attend) against a background (of noise or other competing stimuli); and constancy, or the ability to perceive things (such as words) as essentially the same despite differences in their occurrence or production.

Major Articulation Production Emphasis. Under this heading we shall analyze procedures by which the clinician helps the client acquire and habituate the correct speech sound. These techniques often are common to approaches, and they will generally be presented in chronological order.

Major Remediation Approaches

The major originators or proponents of remediation approaches reviewed along with their distinguishing perceptual or behavioral characteristics, are

1. Scripture (phonetic placement)
2. Stinchfield-Hawk and Young (motokinesthesis)
3. Van Riper (ear training; progressive approximations)
4. Backus and Beasley (group therapy)
5. McDonald (sensorimotor skills)
6. Mysak (feedback theory and practice)
7. Winitz (discrimination training; concept training)
8. Gerber (carry-over through nonsense material)
9. Holland, Matthews, and others (teaching machines).

Other approaches not so neatly tied in to much of the traditional history include some founded in psycholinguistic and quasi-psycholinguistic theory and practice. Those reviewed include some whose techniques are reminiscent of traditional corrective techniques:

1. Cooper (minimal pair contrasts)
2. McReynolds, Costello, and Bountress (distinctive feature approaches)
3. Ingram, Weiner, and Shriberg/Kwiatkowski (process systems) and Patrick and Wilcox (phonological process therapy)
4. Sommers (the wedge approach to multi-phonemic therapy).

Sample Session Structure. To keep the descriptions of therapy methods within reasonable bounds, structured sample sessions of the type developed by Backus and Beasley (1951) are presented wherever necessary to detail principles and a number of methodologies, and they may be grouped into the following categories:

1. *feedback training,* which provides the client with skills for monitoring and adjusting articulatory errors or movements;
2. *key word practice,* which features words in which the error sound is correctly produced by the client;
3. *minimal pairing* of defective and correct utterances to which the client can attach meaning or significance, as a means of establishing linguistic contrasts;
4. *motokinesthesis,* or the manipulation of the articulators or related areas to help the client acquire correct sound production;
5. *negative practice,* or having the client deliberately practice errors that have become habitual as a way of ending their automatic occurrence;
6. *phonetic placement* instruction, in which verbal explanations, mirrors, or diagrams are used to inform the client about the correct positioning and movement of the articulators in the production of specific sounds;
7. *progressive approximation* techniques, designed to help the client make the transitory movement from the error sound to the correct sound;
8. *psychotherapy,* directed at helping the client understand and deal with the articulation problem; and
9. *stimulus-response procedures,* in which the clinician demonstrates sounds for the client to imitate.

Sample sessions not presented here can be found in the writings of the proponents of each technique and in Sommers and Kane (1974).

Some evaluation of the following will also be undertaken:

1. the role of the clinician in the therapeutic process;
2. the nature of therapy—that is, whether it is structured or nonstructured, or whether it is direct, nondirect, or indirect; and
3. the basis of therapy—that is, whether it is basically phonetic, phonemic, or a combination of the two.

Scripture. Scripture, an exponent of the phonetic approach, introduced exercises for the rehabilitation of articulation disorders into the field of speech therapy. The manual she wrote in collaboration with Jackson (1927) recommends that therapy be structured into forty-five-minute sessions, with provision being made for carefully detailed phonetic placement techniques, breathing and relaxation exercises, and "mouth gymnastics"; and it suggests the use of mirrors, drawings, and other devices, such as a tongue depressor and a velar hook, to teach the client the required position of articulators.

Applying the term *mouth gymnastics* to exercises designed to improve articulatory movements, Scripture stated that:

> In order to articulate correctly—that is to say, in order to speak each sound clearly and distinctly—we must have perfect control of the mouth. We must be able to place [the articulators] in whatever position is necessary for each sound. (1927, p. 13).

The same document contains the "Ten Commandments of Speech":

1. Say to yourself, "I have no fear. I know that I can speak well."
2. Think before you speak.
3. Always speak quietly and calmly, with all the muscles relaxed.
4. Always speak slowly and carefully.
5. Sit or stand quietly and erect when speaking.
6. Before speaking, inhale quickly, deeply and without straining, with the mouth open.
7. Be very careful of the first two words in each sentence.
8. Always lengthen and strengthen the principal vowels.
9. Be especially careful to lengthen the short vowels.
10. Be honest with yourself. Do not try to avoid words that you think difficult. (p. 21)

Management of the Therapy Session. The structured sample sessions in Scripture's manual make it clear that the clinician should first work on the sound in isolation and then through all phonetic levels to prepared dialog. Not all of the 45-minute session need be spent on direct attention to the sound being treated, for other objectives can also be pursued with the extensive range of tools and materials Scripture has suggested. Her approach presupposes a clinician-client interaction, but it seems likely that the client could practice the exercises and drills alone. No techniques, however, are outlined for adapting the procedures to individual differences or for skipping practice on a particular phonetic level.

Major Sensory-Perceptual Emphasis. Scripture's approach does not stress any particular sensory avenue. Auditory identification is based on the clinician's presentation of speech sounds. The client is told of kinesthetic patterns, articulatory points of contact, and direction of air streams and is provided gross movement patterns in the general exercises. Correct visual identifications depend first upon the clinician's acting as a correct model, and second upon the client's study of his or her own articulatory movements in a mirror.

Major Articulation Production Emphasis. The only standard remediation method that can be found in Scripture's approach is phonetic placement, which is taught by means of descriptions of the placement of articulators and their movements and sensations. Drills on the isolated sounds proceed from verbal explanations and are essentially presented in a stimulus-response paradigm.

Subjective Analysis. The clinician using Scripture's approach presents stimuli, explains procedures, and acts as drillmaster and does not have to think up procedures, since therapy is completely structured. The clinician is given no recommendations for modifying direct therapy techniques or adapting them to individual needs. Similarly, he or she is given no advice for using therapy time to help the client adjust to the speech problem, but only for ways of directing attention to the defective articulatory pattern. Individual speech sounds, rather than meaning, receive the primary emphasis for acquisition.

Stinchfield-Hawk and Young. In 1938, Stinchfield-Hawk and Young first introduced the motokinesthetic method of articulation therapy, which stresses the development of correct movement patterns and requires the clinician to manipulate or stimulate the articulators.

Stimulation or manipulation of the speech muscles by the clinician is intended to help the client understand how the articulators work individually and in coordination in the production of sound. In initiating tongue action, the clinician touches the part of the tongue involved in the production of the target sound. The stimulation by touch stresses movement and pressure in an attempt to develop kinesthetic patterns. Auditory patterns are established when the clinician says the sound or word simultaneously with the manipulation. Observation of the clinician's productions provides visual cues. Interestingly, although in their 1938 book the authors included procedures for progressing past the acquisition of single sounds to a sequencing of the sounds into words and sentences, they deleted these in the second edition (Young and Stinchfield-Hawk, 1955). The arrangement of chapters in the newer book progresses from voiceless consonants to vowels to voiced consonants, suggesting that this is the order in which the sounds should be remediated.

The motokinesthetic method is not simple; the clinician should be thoroughly trained in the acoustic and articulatory aspects of sound before attempting to use it; and, in addition, the clinician should have an understanding of psychology and take care to orient his client properly.

Management of the Therapy Session. Although Stinchfield-Hawk and Young (1938) discuss the importance of altering some of the motokinesthetic methods for different age levels and etiologies, their basic approach is the same for all clients. The isolated sound is stimulated first as the basic unit of therapy, and only later are word and sentence patterns established. Other aspects of the therapy session are not specified, but it should be noted that the technique cannot be administered to groups.

Major Sensory-Perceptual Emphasis. The clinician's presentation of the sound is the only auditory stimulation in this approach, and the client's observation of the clinician is the only way he can perceive visual differences. No speech sound discrimination techniques are included.

Major Articulation Production Emphasis. The motokinesthetic method is based on the assumption that it is possible to establish positive kinesthetic and tactile feedback patterns through manipulation of the client's articulators. As a result of the feedback the client is helped to recognize and then complete the movements of speech production. Auditory stimulation is provided concurrently, and the client participates by attempting correct production of the sounds. Also underlying the approach is the belief that correct sensory-perceptual identification will eventually allow the client to produce the correct sounds independently. There are, however, no suggestions for assisting the client in this transition from passive to active sound acquisition and beyond to total habituation.

Rapport between the clinician and client is stressed, although no suggestions are offered for achieving it. Strategies for improving the psychological climate are left to the clinician's ingenuity.

Subjective Analysis. As noted above, the clinician who manipulates and stimulates articulatory movements must know how to present the correct patterns; since the motokinesthetic techniques are highly structured, he or she must be highly trained to be considered expert in their use. The method is probably most effective with clients having motor or neurological deficits related to speech production—therapy for many clients with functional articulation disorders may not require their use. There is also the possibility that some clients will object to having their articulators manipulated.

Van Riper. Van Riper first formulated what is often called the traditional approach to speech therapy in his book *Speech Correction: Principles and Methods* in 1939. There have been five subsequent editions, and this discussion is based on the 1978 edition.

Noting the importance of planning therapy, Van Riper suggests that the client must first be helped to recognize the articulation errors and need for assistance in correcting them. Second, any factor that is still contributing to the articulation defect should be corrected, or reduced as much as possible. Then, the following outline can guide the client's training to correct a defective sound:

- identifying the standard sound; discriminating it from errors through scanning and comparing
- varying and correcting the various productions of the sound until it is produced correctly; and strengthening and stabilizing it in all contexts and speaking situations (p. 179).

Since it is "most efficient to teach [correct production of a sound] first in isolation by concentrating on its motor and acoustic aspects" (p. 216), the training program begins at that level and works through succeeding levels of syllables, words, and sentences; at each of these levels the clinician guides the client from identification of the error production (ear training) through acquisition to automatization of the correct production. Ear training activities are subdivided, with the clinician being instructed to provide models of the correct production through isolation, stimulation, identification, and discrimination techniques.

Van Riper presents a variety of procedures for each level of training and for different age groups, and he provides enough material for planning many sessions with any client. In general, the sounds which should be worked on first are those that have the most key words and are the simplest to utter, are normally mastered at an early age, can be uttered correctly after a relatively short period of therapy, and have been especially penalized by others for incorrect utterance.

The sample session here demonstrates the first level of therapy (on the isolated sound), and it follows the four-step outline given above. Presumably, the young child and the clinician figuring in the session have discussed the error sound, and the clinician has determined that no concomitant problems are contributing to the client's articulation disorder. The success of this or any therapeutic relationship using the method depends on the clinician's ability to assess the client's needs, help the client understand the goals of therapy, model correct sounds, and create an atmosphere conducive to learning.

Sample session

Procedures	Notes
A. Ear training (identifying correct and incorrect sounds).	
Clinician: Close and cover your eyes and listen to these pairs of sounds. I'll tell you if they're the same or different. You just listen. /f/—/f/ /p/—/b/ /s/—/θ/ /s/—/s/	Several different combinations may be used.
Did you hear your error sound that sounds like a hissing radiator?	
Client: Yeth.	
Clin: Let's try it again and this time you put a marble in this box if the two sounds I say are the same.	This activity may be done with the clinician's face hidden from the client so that only auditory cues are used.
	Any number of combinations may be used—particularly several with the error sound and correct sound.
Cl: (Listens and places marble in box when sound pairs are the same).	No sounds are produced by the client at this level.
B. Self-hearing.	
Clin: Now I'd like you to say these sounds after me. If you think you're saying them correctly, put a marble in the box. (Produces /f/.)	Techniques at this level should help the client recognize error production after it occurs, when it occurs, and before it occurs.
Cl: (Produces /f/ and puts a marble in the box.)	
Clin: (Produces /θ/.)	
Cl: (Produces /θ/ and puts a marble in the box.)	
Clin: (Produces /s/.)	

Cl: (Produces /θ/ and does not put marble in box.)

Clin: That should have been /s/. Listen again. (Produces /s/ several times.)

This activity may be repeated several times, using other sounds, the error sound, and the correct /s/ sound, varying the timing on placing the marble in the box, either before, during, or after the error production.

C. Establishing the correct sound.

Clin: Please produce the /s/ sound for me.

Cl: (Produces /θ/. May comment on its incorrectness.)

Reliance here on previous training in discrimination and self-hearing.

Clin: Now did that sound right—like a hissing radiator? (Produces /s/ sound several times.) You try it again.

Cl: (Produces /θ/.)

Clin: Listen to how you just said that. (Produces /θ/.)

Cl: It doethn't thound right.

Clin: Now this time you try it with me. Only watch my tongue and we'll try to change its position and get a different sound.

A mirror may be used for visual clues with this activity.

Cl: (Attempts to imitate the clinician's production changes.)

This is repeated several times until a near or exact approximation is achieved.

Clin: That time you produced a /t/. Let's see if you can repeat that sound rapidly several times. (Demonstrates /t-t-t-t-/.)

If the approximation obtains a standard sound, there can be a modification of that sound if the distinctive features are similar.

Cl: (Produces /t-t-t-t-/.)

Clin: Can you feel where your tongue is touching when you produce that?

Cl: Yeth, behind my teeth.

If the client does not respond correctly, the clinician can explain the tongue's position.

Clin: Let's try that again.

Cl: (Produces /t-t-t-t-/ and possibly gets /s/.)

Close or exact productions of the /s/ should be reinforced or rewarded.

D. Stabilizing the correct sound.

Clin: (Writes /s/ symbol on the chalk-board.) Let's try /tttts/ again and this time when you hear yourself produce the /s/, you write the symbol on the board.

Cl: (Produces /ttts/ and writes /s/ on the board.)

Clin: Now just try the /s/ and write it each time you say it.

Cl: (Produces and writes.)

Clin: Now I'd like you to produce the sounds I'm saying: /f/—/θ/—/s/.

Purposeful introduction on the sub-stituted error sound.

Cl: (Repeats sounds.)

Clin: Let's continue practicing the /s/. (Provides a model.)

Cl: (Produces /s/.)

Management of the Therapy Session. Descriptions of Van Riper's therapy approach suggest that it is intended for individual rather than group sessions. It includes the use of such articulation therapy aids as stimulus objects, pictures, word cards, and special training devices. When the client achieves acquisition of an isolated sound, other levels of articulatory competence relating to the sound are introduced.

Major Sensory-Perceptual Emphasis. Ear training techniques, designed to help the client recognize and discriminate articulation errors in both the clinician's speech and the client's own, are given major emphasis. For example, to teach the client the acoustic properties of the defective sound utterance, Van Riper suggests simul-taneously presenting the incorrect sound to one ear and the correct one to the other. Investing sounds with "personalities," as by depicting the /s/ sound as a snake because of its hissing characteristic, can help the client identify and remember target sounds, as can the practice of using phonetic diagrams, palatograms, or models of articulatory positions—depending on the client's age and ability to understand.

Major Articulation Production Emphasis. The comprehensiveness of Van Riper's approach can be seen in his variety of suggestions for actual sound production training. The clinician is free to choose any of five different techniques according to the needs of the individual client. One of the five, auditory stimulation, is based on the assumption that stimulating an individual with a correct form of the defective sound will result in producing it correctly. All of the remaining techniques—progres-sive approximation, phonetic placement, modification of sounds already mastered, and use of key words—are predicted upon stimulus-response learning. One widely discussed technique, progressive approximation, appears related to the "shaping of a response" and, as such, it appears related to operant conditioning techniques.

While Van Riper's articulation therapy is designed to effect a behavioral change, its techniques are rarely aimed at anything but the modification of articulation *per se*. Van Riper does not describe psychotherapeutic techniques for use in articulation therapy.

Subjective Analysis. A clinician using the Van Riper approach is responsible for providing auditory and visual stimuli, correct forms of sound production, and drill at each stage of the process; the clinician also must establish procedures for reinforcing correct sound production. He or she is not supposed to alter the basic therapy stages but has flexibility in choosing or developing activities. Since a hierarchy of articulatory skills is the goal of therapy, Van Riper's approach may be classified as basically phonetic. The method does not employ meaning as a vehicle to correct production.

Clearly, the Van Riper approach has much to offer the clinician with its rich content and suggestions for teaching sound production, up to total habituation. It is questionable, however, whether application of some of the techniques is always necessary, and whether it is too comprehensive in requiring that each stage of therapy be experienced before correction is achieved.

Backus and Beasley. In 1951, Backus and Beasley presented an innovation in articulation therapy in their recommendation that clients with different kinds of speech problems, representing different degrees of severity, be grouped together for treatment. Their procedure is designed to minimize psychological problems accruing from being "labeled" with others of a certain type, or from feeling "different" in receiving individual attention. By organizing therapy classes around clients with various types of speech disorders, the clinician can use the ability of each one to contribute to the verbal interaction, to serve as a model for others, and to provide recognition for their achievements—all of which are thought to increase feelings of success within the group.

Grouping clients for therapy is not intended to free the clinician's time or save energy, but to increase the effectiveness of therapy. Within the group structure, the clinician must meet individual needs, help group members relate to each other and respect each other's rights, and establish limits to ensure an orderly flow of instruction while still developing individual attitudes of freedom, security, acceptance, and success. All of this demands a well-trained clinician whose perceptions of self are healthy, who is capable of assessing individual needs, and who is adept at applying learning principles flexibly.

An important principle of this approach is that teaching can revolve around and evolve from interpersonal relationships, thus allowing for an infinite number of communication situations. (For a chart of the kinds of interpersonal situations that can be used in therapy, the reader is advised to consult Backus, 1957.) Conversational speech is thus basic to therapy—it is consistent with the principle that "learning proceeds from the whole to the parts by a process of differentiation" (Backus and Beasley, 1951, p. 47). The conversational speech patterns used in the therapy sessions should be chosen for their phonetic simplicity and familiar vocabulary. Concerning the selection of sounds for treatment, the authors suggest that this be guided by the group's needs and the members' abilities to produce some sounds correctly. Since Backus and Beasley feel that the acquisition of speech sounds is best accomplished through connected speech patterns rather than by practice on individual sounds, they are of the opinion that if it is necessary to practice isolated sounds, these should be immediately practiced in connected speech.

Backus and Beasley have designed their sessions to include and be structured around five broad areas:

1. practice in interpersonal relationships, as expressed in the competitive situation of game-playing and in the cooperative situation of taking turns;
2. the speaking aspects of situations, such as greeting and guessing;
3. practice in particular speech patterns, such as the names of the other children in the group and such individually structured sentences as "I think it is ———" and "The ——— needs a ———";
4. the emphasis of the particular sounds each child has to correct, such as /s/, /z/, and /θ/; and
5. the use of equipment, such as a chalkboard, chalk, and /s/-sound-picture-word-sentence cards mounted on oak tags, to elicit appropriate responses.

Sample session

Procedures	*Notes*
Clinician: Good morning.	Before entering the room, the clinician has arranged the chairs in a semicircle facing the chalkboard.
Clients: (Exchange greeting with clinician and each other using the names of each.)	
Clin: Today we're going to play a guessing game for which you need a thinking sentence. I'll write it on the board: I think it is a ———.	An additional supplement to associative learning for the clients would be the use of imaginary thinking hats and listening ears.
Cls: (Read the sentence together.)	
Clin: (Directs attention of the children to the /θ/ sound in *think* and the /z/ sound in *is*.)	
Cls: (Each says the sentence.)	
Clin or *Cls:* (Comments on each verbalization.)	Successful verbalizations of words or vocal patterns should be noted. From previous lessons, the children may have learned to listen to and comment on each other's verbalizations.
Clin: (Begins drawing a picture on the board by parts, a sailboat, for example.)	
Cls: (Each one takes a turn at guessing, completing the sentence "I think it is a ———.")	As various objects are guessed, the clinician has the opportunity to work on the production of many sounds in word contexts.

Clin: (Adds additional parts to the drawing as the clients take turns using the "thinking" sentence.)

(This continues until the picture is guessed. When the object is guessed and if it still needs parts, the following activity can be introduced.)

Clin: (Presents the sentence structure "The sailboat needs a ———.")

Attention is called to the /s/ at the beginning of *sailboat* and the /z/ in *needs*.

Cls: (Each takes turns adding something to the picture.)

Clin: Make sure your tongue is touching on the mountain behind your top teeth and the air stream is coming out between your upper and lower front teeth.

The clinician can check each child and they can check each other on production. The children can be directed to feel the air stream with their fingers on the front teeth.

Clin: Sailboat is our listening key word for the /s/ sound. Who can give me a word with /s/ in the middle or /s/ at the end?

Cls: (Supply words that they can think of.)

The words can be written on the board under appropriate columns. If the children cannot think of words, the clinician can give clues through riddles. The clients are asked to identify the right column for the words they are supplying according to the position of the /s/ sound.

Clin: Now I'm going to read some sentences which contain words with the /s/ sound. Each of you will have a turn to tell me a word containing an /s/ sound. (Reads sentences one at a time.)

Cls: (Each in turn identifies an /s/ word from the sentence read.)

The clinician gives extra chances on the first round if a client needs help. If a client has continued trouble in listening, he or she is asked to repeat each word in the sentence and the original listening key word.

Clin: (Gives the picture-word-sentence card to the child if he or she identified the word correctly.)

(This may be repeated for several rounds as time permits.)

Production of the /s/ can be checked by the clinician and other clients.

Clin: Will you each count the number of cards you have?

Cls: (Each replies when asked the number.)

Opportunity here to check on production of other sounds, such as the /f/ and /t/.

Clin: Now I want you to think of a story for each one of your cards.

Cls: (Each in turn gives a sentence for one picture.)

Stress should be placed on not copying the clinician's sentence, thus encouraging the use and development of each child's own vocabulary.

Clin: (Praises successes. Helps each child individually with sound difficulties.)

Children also act as monitors of each other's stories, praising good aspects and telling what could be improved.

(Stories continue as time permits.)

Clin: Our session is over. What will you remember and try to work on from today?

Cls: (Respond with the listening key word *sailboat*, the "thinking" sentence, and other language patterns or areas of success.)

Management of the Therapy Session. Placement of clients within groups is not based on the type of speech disorder, as is customarily done, but is guided by motivation, adaptation, and goal setting. In their discussion of therapy, Backus and Beasley describe the materials or equipment necessary; and they include some techniques used by others, such as working on production of problem sounds in controlled conversational patterns. While they suggest no time limits for the sessions, half an hour would probably be sufficient for covering the material.

Major Sensory-Perceptual Emphasis. No specific plan for improving clients' auditory, visual, tactile, and kinesthetic perceptions is detailed by Backus and Beasley. Apparently, however, they regard the clinician as the principal model for correct auditory and kinesthetic patterns, abetted by the group members as they identify the correct patterns.

Major Articulation Production Emphasis. It is not part of the Backus and Beasley approach to suggest techniques for sound acquisition; nor do they give specific procedures for error detection. They suggest that the clinician direct a client's attention to correct forms that may be demonstrated by the clinician or a group member. After once having established the correct form of the sound, the client presumably is able to assimilate it by monitoring his or her own productions. The clinician controls the conversational patterns that are used to introduce and practice the sounds requiring correction but does not demand the repetition of certain forms. So long as the sound being worked on is produced correctly, the words and sentences of the conversation may be varied.

Broadly conceived, many of the techniques for assisting correct productions in the Backus and Beasley approach might be considered psychotherapeutic. The clinician reinforces correct aspects of individual utterances and verbalizes weaknesses of productions as needed improvements for the whole group. When the productions of individuals approximate standard utterance, the clinician uses verbal rewards. Since the therapy itself is structured from language-oriented interpersonal situations, the individual's feelings and reactions become an integral part of the total therapy process. The building of confidence and feelings of success are essential components of the clinician's approach to production difficulties. The Backus and Beasley approach may consequently represent articulation therapy through group dynamics and psychotherapy.

Subjective Analysis. The power of the Backus and Beasley approach is in its employment of group dynamics, coupled with patterned conversational language. This combination can provide incentive for clients to improve their articulation, and it may also facilitate carry-over. The degree to which the homogeneity of the group membership contributes to the effectiveness of therapy is not certain. And while the approach employs meaningful utterances to correct sound-production difficulties, it may not give enough attention to sound-production techniques.

On the surface, the care needed in structuring therapy sessions is not evident, but the process does involve planning along the lines of sound-production goals and specific speaking and social situations. Before feeling free to deviate from Backus and Beasley's sample sessions, a clinician needs considerable experience with group therapy. Adjusting the session's atmosphere and meeting the needs of individual members are probably the most difficult aspects of administering this type of therapy.

McDonald. McDonald (1964) is the formulator of sensorimotor articulation therapy, basing it on studies from phonology, acoustic phonetics, motor phonetics, experimental phonetics, and linguistics. It is McDonald's feeling that:

> The essential character of articulation cannot be comprehended if one attempts to study it as an isolated event. Even though it can be identified and described as a process, it is inextricably interrelated to the other processes involved in speech production. Similarly, speech is inseparably related to language. (p. 66)

McDonald thus defines articulation as a recognizable process within a total language concept:

> Articulation is a process consisting of a series of overlapping, ballistic movements which place varying degrees of obstruction in the way of the outgoing air stream and simultaneously modify the size, shape, and coupling of resonating cavities. (p. 87)

Functional misarticulations can be attributed to any disturbance or interference in the process—associated, for example, with the organism's inability to compensate for undetectable neurological abnormalities. Similarly, inadequate reception of stimuli might produce inadequate sensorimotor patterns; and insufficient learning, possibly due to environmental deprivation, might result in the habituation of immature sensorimotor patterns.

Phonetic contexts assume the greatest importance in McDonald's approach, for it is his purpose to increase the number of such contexts in which the client can correctly produce the error sounds. The responsibility for success is placed on the client as much as the clinician, in that therapy becomes a process of teaching the client to be self-directing and self-correcting. McDonald believes that guiding the client through changes in sensorimotor speech patterns should not involve the help of word lists and other materials and exercises, but rather should draw practice material (words and sentences for expanding correct phonetic production into new contexts) from the client's vocabulary needs and interests.

Therapy should begin at a level where the client achieves success (as indicated by McDonald's deep-testing technique), and every stage should provide opportunity for practice. These considerations are helpful in deciding what sounds to treat first: the client's own preference; quickness of habituation of correct production; simplicity of sensorimotor patterns; and correctness in at least one phonetic context of the deep test. On the other hand, sounds with high percentages of correct productions should be left until last, as they usually improve without primary attention.

Although his sensorimotor therapy is geared to the individual, McDonald does make suggestions for placing individuals in groups, for encouraging members' participation, and for attending to individual needs within the group structure. Throughout it all, however, the basic therapy procedures do not change.

Management of the Therapy Session. McDonald does not specify the time to be spent in either group or individual therapy sessions, nor does he discuss ways to vary his approach to account for such variables as age, sex, and IQ. His therapy techniques begin with the syllable as the unit of sound production, and advance to phonetic contexts and ultimately to sentences. Placing considerable emphasis on the fact that the clinician does not need to depend on word lists, exercises, or other materials usually associated with articulation therapy, he requires only that the individual be given a notebook for recording practice material during the procedures for the transfer of a correct production to other phonetic contexts.

Major Sensory-Perceptual Emphasis. The major emphasis in McDonald's approach is on correct articulatory movement patterns. Improving auditory discrimination and auditory memory span are secondary benefits. The client's attention is not directed to acoustic characteristics or differences; instead, he is asked to describe kinesthetic and tactile sensations in order to detect subtle differences in sound characteristics. Visual discriminations are not stressed.

Major Articulation Production Emphasis. To make the client increasingly responsible for correcting his articulation errors, the stimulus-response format is used, in which the clinician presents the verbal stimuli as bisyllables, trisyllables, phonetic contexts, and sentences, and the client responds by imitating the stimuli and describing them verbally. Through this continued repetition of the phonetic stimuli and the individual's description of kinesthetic and tactile sensations, positive feedback patterns may be established. Correctly produced phonetic contexts are used as a basis for practice. No other production techniques are incorporated into McDonald's approach.

Subjective Analysis. Viewed in the light of his discussion of articulation as an integral part of the total communication act, McDonald's suggestions for articulation therapy do not seem consistent. He discusses phonemics and phonetics at length, but he advocates articulation therapy techniques almost devoid of meaning at an awareness level.

Further, the highly structured and highly rewarded sensorimotor therapy makes absolute demands on the clinician to provide practice at every level of therapy whether it is needed or not. The procedures, based as they are on continuous drill and the client's imitation and description of movement patterns, seem tedious and cast the clinician in the role of a sensorimotor technician. The clinician must work to keep up the client's motivation, but he cannot be innovative other than with the stimuli presented and used. Finally, he is not told how to handle a client's misconceptions of incorrect production so as to obtain acceptable sensorimotor feedback patterns, and he is given nothing new in the way of techniques for achieving habituation of the correct sound. Carryover is once again left to the enterprising clinician.

Mysak. It has often been noted that speech therapy borrows principles and techniques from behavioral and other sciences. This is particularly true of Mysak's (1971) approach to speech pathology, which is discussed within the framework of cybernetics and feedback theory. Mysak considers the speaking process to be analogous to the working of an automated machine. The machine's operation and output are controlled by closed-loop mechanisms which continuously detect errors and effect corrections. Speaking, too, is a multiloop system, with internal processes, such as thought propagation, word formation, word production, and several comparative operations; and external processes, such as message transmittal and assessment of listener reaction to word production and word choice. In both internal and external systems, speaking is automatized if all feedback and feedforward operations are error-free.

Essentially, Mysak conceives of the speaking process as involving ten perceptual-linguistic operations, of which the five most important are the *receptor*, which includes all of the receiving sensory avenues; the *integrator*, which stores information, attaches and interprets meaning, and compares and corrects the content of a message; the *transmitter*, which stores word patterns, activates word signals and production operations, and similarly corrects and compares the end product; the *effector*, which controls and coordinates the individual output motor mechanisms of respiration, phonation, and articulation-resonance; and the *sensor*, or feedback device, which returns information on all aspects of the output or speech signal via the various sensory channels. A message can thus be traced from its mental conception through several feedback and feedforward patterns to the final error-free product.

In introducing his therapy concepts, Mysak acknowledged that they represented an extension—based on servosystem theory and on his own testing and clinical experience—of concepts discussed earlier in part by Fairbanks (1954) and Van Riper and Irwin (1958). In his approach there are two stages of therapy—the first designed to "activate error-sound sensitivity and error-sound measuring processes" and the second, to "activate correct-sound seeking and approximating and correct-sound tracking." Sometimes, only the first stage is needed; the speech corrector device may be activated and articulatory homeostasis may occur. Just how these principles are to be put into practice is not fully explained.

Sample session

Procedures	Notes
A. For activating error-sound sensitivity and error-sound measuring processes:	

Error-Sound Sensitivity

Clinician: Let's listen to these words. (Pronounces a list of /s/ words, some correctly, some using the error sound, but when the error sound is produced, an identification of the error is made.)

Introduction of therapeutic error signal (TES). The motivation for the goal of error-sound correction should be provided at this stage.

The error and correct sounds may also be introduced with a tape recorder.

Error-Sound Measuring

Clin: Listen carefully to the following phrase and identify the incorrectly produced word: *See the thky.*

Client: Thky.

Auditory sensory avenue being used for identifying an error in a model's speech pattern.

This type of activity may be continued with syllables, words, phrases, and sentences.

Clin: Thail the seven seas.

Cl: Thail.

Clin: As I say the next phrase, watch my tongue and tell me whether the mistake is on the first, second, or third word: *Thikth and seven.*

Visual sensory avenue is used in this activity.

Cl: Firtht word.

Clin: A silver star.

Provision for positive as well as negative visual feedback.

Activity may be repeated as necessary.

Cl: None.

Clin: As we say the following words, first feel my tongue and face, then feel your own. *Sun.*

(Client can have hands on face and teeth of clinician during the production.)

Tactile and kinesthetic sensation or error and correct productions are employed.

With both visual and tactile activities, auditory stimulation may or may not be present.

Cl: Thun. (Has hands on face and tongue and should feel the tongue protrusion.)

Clin: Let's try again. *Thoup.*

Cl: (Feels appropriate articulators of the clinician and then repeats the word while feeling his or her own articulators.)

Activity may be repeated as necessary.

B. For activating correct-sound seeking
and correct-sound tracking:

Sound-Seeking and Approximating

Clin: Now I'd like you to experiment with the production of the /s/ sound. Try it several different times.

Cl: (Produces /θ/, /tʃ/, /θ/, /s/.)

Close approximations should be praised and correct productions reinforced. The clinician should observe which sensory avenue is giving the client the most positive feedback for future practice.

Correct-Sound Tracking

Clin: Now I want you to try to make the /s/ sound. On the first try, listen carefully to your production and compare it to mine.

During these direct attempts at production, the clinician may use one or all or a combination of whichever sensory avenues have provided the greatest feedback for the client.

Cl: (Produces /s/ but slips back to /θ/.)

Varying the sensory avenue should continue until the correct production is attained.

Correct-Sound Automaticity

Clin: Now we'll practice the /s/ sound in some words: *six, save.*

Correct productions are praised and reinforced.

Cl: six, save.

Activities for carry-over may be structured with words, phrases, and sentences, and continue until automatized.

Management of the Therapy Session. Mysak gives few directions for establishing the therapeutic session or atmosphere, and no suggestions for the length of sessions, choice of material, or ways of adapting to developmental variants. The few activities that he proposes suggest that the approach is individualized. The unit of speech used for stimulus and practice material varies, but eventually the therapy involves conversational sentences.

Major Sensory-Perceptual Emphasis. The introduction of a "therapeutic error signal" (TES) during Mysak's first-stage activities allows the clinician to manipulate acoustic, visual, and proprioceptive sensory stimuli so as to increase the client's discrimination ability. Both negative and positive sensory feedback come into play in helping the client recognize errors and establish goals, with particular emphasis being placed on whatever sensory modality proves most beneficial in helping the client advance.

Major Articulation Production Emphasis. The first stage of Mysak's therapy, centering on sensory-perceptual reception and interpretation, may make the second stage—

directed at actual production—unnecessary. If the clinician has activated error feed-back signals to the point where the processing of speech is interrupted, the correction of error sounds may be automatic. This seems comparable to a statement by Van Riper (1972) to the effect that if ear-training is done well, the correction of error sounds can be accomplished without other techniques, such as phonetic placement.

In Mysak's approach, stimulus-response patterns between clinician and client are the means of strengthening positive auditory and kinesthetic feedback patterns. During the part of the second stage when the client is approximating the production of a model, the clinician is asked to reward successful approximations. Then, when the client is attempting direct production of a sound, the reinforcement is provided by his or her own feedback apparatus, for the client is asked to scan utterances and compare them with the clinician's, or with a tape-recorded model.

Subjective Analysis. Mysak's approach, concerned with feedback patterns and intended to assist the individual in monitoring and adjusting articulatory movements, depends on the clinician's providing a correct model for self-correction, which is then reinforced. However, Mysak presents few techniques for reaching these therapeutic goals.

Winitz: Discrimination and Concept Training.
Perhaps the strongest propo-nent for the use of discrimination training in the correction of defective speech sounds in children is Harris Winitz. In his book, *From Syllable to Conversation* (1975), he discussed several beliefs concerning the nature of the corrective process for such disorders, including ten discrimination-training principles. He has strong faith in the power of discrimination training to positively affect articulation changes:

> Training in speech production should not begin until discrimination can be made easily between the standard and the non-standard sound in sentences. Thus, not until a high degree of discrimination training is achieved, would articulatory training begin (Winitz, 1975, p. 61).

It appears that not since Van Riper's early writings has any authority taken such a positive and adamant position about the value and need for the discrimination model in the corrective process. The notion that production of target sounds not be under-taken until a child has developed good abilities to discriminate the error sound from the target sound was advocated by Van Riper, whose "four steps in ear training" were taught to many speech pathologists. A prominent ear training activity in this se-quence was the one advocated by Winitz—discrimination training.

Therapy for defective speech sound advocated by Winitz also included the recom-mendation that, for some children at least, an important adjunct was to teach them some principles, generalizations, and concepts. Thus, speech sound improvement appeared to involve two components: first, perceptual or auditory discrimination of the target sound and the error sound, and second, the concept or basic "idea" involved in certain of the phonological rule systems underpinning aspects of phonology. The second component, borrowed in part from learning theory and its literature, appears to be uniquely part of his recommended training and different from traditional approaches. In this section, examples of both components of his therapy will be illustrated in one therapy plan. The reader should note that the author prepared this material, not Harris Winitz.

Sample session: Goal is correction of /t/ for /s/ substitution

Procedures	Notes
Clinician: I have some toys here. We can have fun with them. Look at my seesaw, soldier, sandbox, and sink (shows child each object).	First step in discrimination training of /s/ in correct context and words.
Client: (Watches and listens.)	
Clin: Look, I have more toys for us to play with. See my top, tank, table, and TV (shows child each object).	Second step in discrimination training of /t/ in correct context and words.
Cl: (Watches and listens.)	
Clin: Let's make a house out of this paper. You help me make it. Now let's put things that belong in the house in it and put things that belong in the yard outside it.	Third step in discrimination training: association of words with familiar learning environment.
Clin: You help me. Where shall we put the table? What shall we put in the house next? What shall we put in the yard?	Child becomes responsible for the selection of items.
Clin: Tell me what other things should be put into the house?	Child names objects and asks the clinician for them.
Cl: Incessantly asks for /tink/.	Clinician waits five seconds and says "OK, here it is," and hands the child a different object such as a toy cat. Child indicates that this is not what he or she wanted.
Clin: OK, you meant "sink," not /tink/. You wanted "sink"; well, here it is. Let's put the sink in the house.	The child's attention and interest culminate in discrimination of the correct and incorrect word forms.
Clin: Now let's play another game. This time raise this arm (grasps child's right arm) when I say a word with /s/ in it and this arm (grasps child's left arm) when I say other words. Clinician begins: The first word is "spool." Now raise this arm (grasps child's right arm and lifts it). Good. Now the word is "pill" (grasps child's left arm and raises it). Now the word is "kite" (grasps child's left arm and raises it); now the word is "stove" (grasps the child's right	Later in therapy for the same child, when /s/ is developing and replacing the substituted /t/, cluster /s/ productions are stressed. Conceptualization using a sorting task is taught. Omissions of /s/ in clusters is a conceptualization problem requiring this type of training. Child learns concept of cluster as a result of this training.
	Winitz recommends this type of training if it can be determined that a child's

arm and raises it). This is followed by presentations of other words, e.g., book, pie, stop, spy, gate, story, etc. errors are rule-governed and not related to sound discrimination inadequacies per se.

Management of the Sessions. Although not explicitly stated in his writings, it appears from the training examples that Winitz (1975) has provided that young children receive individual rather than group therapy. No trace of any disinterest or lack of faith in group articulation therapy, however, can be found in his writings, and it may be that he considers that his principles of therapy are equally manageable and effective in either case. Additionally, he does not recommend a specified length of time for individual or group sessions.

Major Perceptual-Sensory Emphasis. The ten principles of auditory discrimination training suggested by Winitz attest to his strong emphasis on the auditory perceptual training needed to facilitate new sound learning. He particularly believes in gaining accurate discriminations between error and target sounds, and he recommends training so that phonetic differences between them are at first large and then gradually narrowed if discrimination is difficult for the child. Interestingly, based on some of his research on normal children's learning of non-English phones, Winitz recommends that initial training of sounds begin with the error sound, not the target sound—a recommendation that appears opposite to that often found in earlier, traditional approaches.

Major Articulation Production Emphasis. Winitz acknowledges that discrimination training is not the only approach and recommends that it be supplemented by production training. To guide production training activities he urges testing for sound stimulability and inconsistency. If the client's stimulability scores are poor and the sound is consistently defective, he recommends that phonetic placement procedures be used to establish some form of correct sound production. Winitz also recommends distinctive feature training if an important feature is missing from a child's repertoire of sounds, suggesting that a sound be taught which is easy for the child to produce and which contains the missing feature. Using the technique of shaping, he would attempt to transfer the particular feature to the target sound.

Winitz feels that nonsense words are very helpful in production training, because they minimize interference from the error sound and thus increase the rate of learning of the new target sound. He cites research evidence to support this view.

Subjective Analysis. Winitz's method of sound learning appears to be a complex set of interrelationships, much of which stems from research evidence and writings concerning auditory discrimination and its affects on sound learning, distinctive feature theory and applications, coarticulation evidence, knowledge of contextual influences on sound production, and concepts from learning theory related to interference and retention. The sound discrimination training and some of his recommended production activities (if needed) appear to be modifications of old tactics and techniques of the traditional therapies. Other strategies and principles that he expounds seem to embellish these older, fundamental aspects of the corrective process. As such, his recommendations are comprehensive, and, while not tested in many regards, some of his ideas are intriguing and provocative.

Gerber: Carry-Over Through Nonsense Materials. Gerber's (1970) program for habituating correct articulation patterns requires that the client produce nonsense syllables and words in all of the combinations and conditions of rapid connected speech at each of several levels of difficulty. Because of the strong bond between meaning and the habitual patterns of the error sound, she does not introduce meaningful units of speech until normal production and self-monitoring have been achieved at each level. Otherwise, the premature use of the newly acquired sound in words and phrases can result in an exaggerated production which distorts the natural rate and rhythm of speech.

The various activities of Gerber's program are oriented toward specific subgoals so that the child is fully aware of the dimensions of the tasks and the frameworks within which they may be accomplished. As the child completes each activity and sees progress toward the ultimate goal, the child gains a sense of concrete achievement, a strong internal motivation, which is a significant ingredient in the process of speech-behavior modification.

As the nonsense material becomes phonetically and syntactically more complex, it is more specifically related to the child's problem and level of achievement. For example, if a child has mastered production in vocalic environments and initial consonant clusters, but still has trouble with medial abutting consonants and final consonant clusters, he or she may be given practice on nonsense words built around the troublesome sound patterns and embedded in pseudocommunication units. The clinician must, of course, analyze the client's defective pattern and level of achievement constantly—and accurately—to be able to create appropriate material.

It should be noted that Gerber's program is recommended primarily for those who do not have maturation working in their favor—that is, for those who are past the speech development stage.

Management of the Session. Gerber suggests that therapy sessions be approximately 45 minutes long, and says that her method is applicable to both individuals and groups, children and adults. She recognizes, however, that her method may not be entirely desirable for children who are still developing speech.

Her approach differs from others chiefly in the amount of time spent on nonsense material before introducing meaningful material, although she states that other important distinctions are the specificity of the materials for each case, their "programmed" nature, and their intensive use to teach, and carefully refine, speech skills. The programmed materials that constitute the sequential steps of the therapy program are frequently supplemented by tape recorders, automatic speech playback devices, mirrors, straws, and signaling devices (such as clickers).

Major Sensory-Perceptual Emphasis. In order to help the client reach the goal of monitoring his own productions, the clinician teaches him to evaluate the speech of a model. As he then progresses from simple to more complex materials and from slow to rapid rates of production at each level, he is required to demonstrate a high level of precision in evaluating his productions. This evaluation, however, does not depend only upon auditory cues, for Gerber considers her therapy approach multisensory experience, with the emphasized modality varying with the sound being taught. She feels that perception is heightened by not embedding the sound in a meaningful unit.

Major Articulation Production Emphasis. In Gerber's method, the primary emphasis is on feedback, coupled with modified phonetic placement techniques, as required. Feedback is achieved through whatever modalities are appropriate, a premium being placed on a high degree of precision and specificity. Phonetic placement procedures take the form of vivid verbal imagery aimed at subvolitional movements, rather than the manipulation of the articulators. For example, if retraction of the tongue from an occluded position is desired, the clinician asks the child to show empty windows (spaces between the teeth) and no pink pillow (tongue between the teeth). These cues can then be used by the child in self-monitoring specific bits of behavior. The clinician may also try to make placement clear to the child by modifying another sound.

It should be noted that, like many other approaches, Gerber's method depends heavily upon a stimulus-response paradigm.

Subjective Analysis. Rather than assume that acquisition will automatically lead to carry-over, Gerber's approach suggests that carry-over requires a gradual buildup of articulation skills of increasing difficulty through programmed learning and the client's self-monitoring. Because the nonsense syllable is the vehicle for attaining articulatory skills, her approach assumes more readily than others that generalization to meaningful words will occur. Gerber's is thus a highly structured phonetic approach, in which meaning becomes important only in the final stage of learning. Taking nothing for granted and establishing special requirements for success at each level of articulatory efficiency, Gerber's materials for therapy reflect a high level of organization. The degree to which this organization contributes to the effectiveness of therapy might be questioned, however, by a clinician who prefers more freedom and to direct participation in the process.

Gerber's approach relies on some of the better-known therapies such as those of McDonald, Mysak, and Van Riper, for its basic principles and techniques. It is unique, however, in its deliberate effort to achieve carry-over, its great emphasis on nonsense syllables as training vehicles for articulatory skills, and its use of highly developed programmed materials.

Holland, Matthews, and Others: Teaching Machines.

Most studies concerned with the use of teaching machines in articulation therapy (such as those by Holland, 1960; Holland and Matthews, 1968; Mowrer, Baker, and Schutz, 1968; and Winitz, 1969) have been too narrowly conceived to produce any strong evidence for their effectiveness, most not even including control groups who received traditional therapy methods. The results have, however, been promising enough to justify some discussion of the basic method.

Teaching machines work on the principles of operant conditioning, that is, a person using one must respond to material that has been programmed to ensure success. Immediately reinforced for appropriate responses, the subject progresses gradually toward more complex responses, slowly loses stimulus support, and, while observing and echoic behavior is controlled, the subject develops discriminative abilities, even for abstract concepts (Holland and Matthews, 1968). These same authors point out that the advantages of using teaching machines include the chance to revise their programs in line with the feedback provided by the student, since the step-by-step record of progress in learning the material can point up the program's weaknesses and strengths. The paramount advantage, of course, is the machine's ability to progress at the student's own pace.

More generally, Winitz (1969) has spoken of teaching machines as instruments for eliciting selected, or terminal responses via events sequenced to increase the acquisition of a skill and to ensure retention of the skill and its generalization to other skills. Where the desired terminal response is a discrimination between the error and the correct sound, a response which he feels seems to "facilitate the learning of correct sound," Winitz favors beginning the training with maximum linguistic contrasts and later progressing to training on sounds with a number of distinctive feature similarities. He also observes that there is some evidence that early discrimination training should build on the substituted sound, developing a distinction between it and linguistically contrasting sounds, rather than on the target sound to be remediated. Other areas which Winitz feels can be handled on a teaching machine are successive approximation of responses, stimulus-response generalization, acquisition interference, motivation, extinction, delay of reinforcement, latency of response, and retention.

Mowrer, Baker, and Schutz (1968) also favor teaching machines over traditional speech correction techniques. Their own experiments with a program based on successive approximations and differential reinforcement suggested to them that external reinforcement facilitates the learning of correct articulation responses; that the client who responds actively in a teaching machine situation makes faster progress than by participating in group therapy, where the client would have to be a passive observer-listener at least part of the time; that facial cues from a clinician are not essential to articulation improvement; and that the teaching machine can be monitored and the client's responses can be evaluated by someone without the training of a speech clinician, thus freeing the clinician to cope more effectively with the more difficult problems of speech.

Only one study appears to have tested the effectiveness of an automatic teaching device against more "traditional" techniques for carry-over. Gerber (1966) used an automatic tape recording instrument, the Echorder, in therapy with four children with /r/ defects and contrasted their progress on all /r/ allophones with that of four matched control subjects. She reported highly significant relative improvements for the experimental subjects: three of the four achieved total carry-over, while none of the controls did so.

Most proponents of teaching machines in articulation therapy feel that they have particular value in supplementing the clinician's work and in challenging the clinician to provide programs that motivate the client toward self-improvement. Though their value has not been fully proven, these tools clearly deserve further consideration.

Psycholinguistic and Related Approaches

Cooper: Minimal Contrast Therapy. As mentioned on page 135, Cooper's (1968) Minimal Contrast Therapy is an approach to functional articulation therapy which stresses meaning in establishing minimal contrasts between paired words or sentences and thereby conditions a child to the correct utterance. It is best explained by Cooper's remarks that:

> This problem (articulation learning) is solved if: (a) to the defective utterance a meaning or significance is established; (b) the child can make the sounds required in the standard utterance; and (c) the child is confronted with the defective utterance and the standard utterance, both of which are now meaningful, and he is asked to name each one at a time. . . . In general, the method is based on the principle that in paired contrasts of the articulation of defective and standard utterances of words where the defective utterance is conditioned to a new meaning, children will tend to alter the articulation of the defective utterance.

He answers the problem of what is meant by "meaning" by examining several studies on meaning as a variable in the learning process and evolving a working, or operational, definition of the term as:

> the conditioning of a referent to an utterance so that the subject will reliably point to the referent with the utterance as a stimulus.

In this form of therapy, the clinician must first linguistically analyze the speech pattern of the client and identify defective utterances that are being used for correct ones. The clinician must then construct a *nonword* for one of the defective sound productions, using a picture or object to represent its meaning. Then the clinician assigns certain imaginary functions to the nonword for the purpose of developing meaning in the mind of the client, contrasting the nonword with a real one with real functions until the client achieves production discriminations. Then, "once one pair of contrasts is established, the child is ready for the second paradigmatic pair which will be completed more rapidly" (Cooper, 1970).

Cooper concluded the 1968 presentation of his method with a comment about its effects:

> . . . for certain types of clients where omissions and substitutions are prevalent, the method has cut down substantially on the time required to achieve correction, develops standard speech in accordance with natural language processes, prevents therapeutic boredom, and places the problem of correction on the child's conceptual ability rather than on mechanical and laborious drills, even if presented in the guise of speech play.

Sample session (Structured on an assumed t/s substitution.)

Procedures	Notes
A. Establishing associations between the real word and the nonword.	
Clinician: Today we're going to play a game. I'm going to show you some pictures and you tell me what they are. Each time you show me the right picture, you'll get one of these. (Points to rewards.)	Any type of reinforcement may be used depending on the needs of the individual and the demands of the situation.
Clin: This is soap. (Points to picture or object.) Now show me soap.	Presents nonsense picture or object to be associated with *toap* and real picture or object for *soap*.

Client: (Points to picture or object and is rewarded according to the rules of the game.)

Clin: This is toap. (Points to picture or object.) Show me toap.

Cl: (Points to toap and is rewarded.)

This activity may be continued with the clinician presenting stimulus words and pictures randomly and until there is sufficient evidence that the client is responding without error and with confidence.

B. Establishing the functions of the real word and the nonword.

Clin: This is toap. You can carry it in your pocket. You can play with it. You can throw it in the air. You can throw it to a friend.

The functions of the nonword are fabricated to provide a greater significance in addition to the name of the object or picture.

Cl: (May repeat the functions of toap as presented by the clinician. May contribute additional functions.)

Clin: This is soap. What is it for?

Cl: We wash with it.

Clin: What else do we do with it?

Cl: Mother washes dishes with it. We wash clothes with it.

This activity may be continued until the client shows an understanding of the different functions of the contrasting words through verbal answers to the clinician's questions or by acting out the functions.

C. Establishing contrasting productions of the real word and the nonword.

Clin: This is toap. Show me toap.

Cl: (Points to picture or object.)

Clin: What is it for?

Cl: (Responds with functions.)

Clin: (Points to toap.) What is this?

Cl: Toap.

Client is rewarded for his response.

Clin: This is soap. Show me soap.

Cl: (Points to soap.)

Clin: What is soap for?

Cl: (Responds with functions.)

Clin: (Points to soap.) What is this?

Cl: Toap.

Clin: (Points to contrast picture or object.) This is toap. (Points to soap.) This is soap. (Points to soap again.) What is this?

Cl: (Attempts varying productions in order to produce *soap*.)

Any attempt to change articulation is encouraged. The clinician may use any attempts at making the sound which will help the client come closer to the verbal production contrasts.

Management of the Session. Cooper's method of meaningful minimal contrasts is intended to be used with individual children, but it could be used with groups if all members had identical sound errors. Since errors of omission and substitution are most frequently seen in preschool and lower elementary-school-aged children, it is likely that the clients would belong to the younger age groups.

Major Sensory-Perceptual Emphasis. Cooper stresses no particular sensory-perceptual modality. Audition probably assumes the major role, however, because of the continued stimulation by the clinician. The visual modality, too, is expected to function, as suggested by the use of objects and pictures, but it is not challenged in any significant way. The use of tactile-proprioceptive cues to facilitate learning is not mentioned.

Major Articulation Production Emphasis. The interaction between concepts and auditory perception shapes the articulatory process, as the child is rewarded for correct identifications of visual and verbal stimuli and for productions which approximate the correct one. Cooper feels that the clinician can incorporate into the method any of the "usual" techniques for correcting production—the choice of any one in particular being guided by an assessment of the way the child attempts to change error productions.

Subjective Analysis. One possible difficulty in Cooper's approach is that articulation practice might be too limited for sound generalization to occur, for it is uncertain how many paradigmatic pairs would have to be mastered to completely correct each sound. The method is probably not necessary for all young children with functional articulation disorders, for a highly stimulable child would certainly do as well in another form of therapy. It might be most beneficial for older retarded or brain-damaged children, since the efficacy of the "traditional" articulation therapy approaches has not been established for these groups. Of course, a background in linguistic theory is required of the clinician using the minimal-contrast method.

McReynolds, Costello, Bountress: Distinctive Feature Orientations. Distinctive feature approaches to the correction of children's defective phonology were originated by a small number of investigators. By the mid-1970s, a number of prominent persons had taken the bold step of suggesting that both the efficiency and effectiveness of therapy could be enhanced if distinctive features were carefully assessed and then adroitly manipulated in the corrected process to allow features (and their most important underlying phonological rules) to generalize. Evidence to support the assertion that such feature training was valuable came largely from case studies which, unfortunately, most often did not show changes in untreated control subjects or in those for whom other corrective procedures were undertaken. Nevertheless, more progressive researchers actively promoted distinctive feature approaches. However, by the middle of the 1970s, articles and convention presentations concerning distinctive feature approaches to therapy had largely disappeared. This apparent decline in interest may have limited the thrust of the early '70s and its potential for the improvement of the condition of the phonologically impaired child.

In this discussion of distinctive feature applications, no sample lesson plan will be presented because many lesson plans have been published by advocates of the approach. One of the most detailed examples can be found in Costello and Onstine (1976), and other related, helpful, and detailed information about the strategies and requirements of feature therapy is abundant in articles by McReynolds and Bennett (1972) and Bountress (1982). While some of the specific steps in the programs written by these advocates differ, the basic thrust of the approach remains the same. The most important concept, of course, is that features adequately trained in one phoneme will generalize to other phonemes in which they were absent or misused.

The basic training strategy uses contrast to highlight differences in phonemes that contain the feature to be acquired with those which do not contain this feature. Almost all training includes sound discrimination, which typically enables the child to perceive the important differences between /p/ and /f/, for example, in the event that + stridency (high frequency sound energy, harsh in production) was the feature being trained. When stridency is heard on /f/ after some period of auditory training, the clinician probes other consonants, such as /s/, /ʃ/, and /v/, on which the child erred to see if stridency can now be detected in them.

Certain feature programs specify some production training as well as prior periods of auditory training, and they use operant learning tactics to advance the sound from isolation, to syllables, and finally to words. Most distinctive feature approaches that have been presented have specified therapy using the operant paradigm.

For the most part, feature training approaches offer us no new therapy techniques per se. Rather, feature concepts guide the choices of phonemes to be trained and phonemes to be left untrained and checked for feature generalization. The issue of whether features per se actually generalize appears unresolved, and it appears that, if they indeed do generalize to untrained phonemes, this condition may help explain the better-researched phenomenon of sound generalization.

Feature programs use traditional techniques: auditory discrimination, imitated production techniques, and the operant approach to learning. Even the choices of phonemes to contrast often appear to be the same as one might find in a non-feature approach, e.g., the child cannot produce + stridency in /f/ and uses the /p/ phoneme instead. The clinician "ear trains" /p/ against /f/ in the traditional way, using a contrastive type of technique. Still, this is not feature therapy, because the clinician does not know that + stridency has been trained and does not check to see if + stridency now begins to be used in other defective phonemes in which it was not present before. Perhaps many clinicians in the past have been training features and obtaining generalization without knowledge of the existence of features, phonological rules, and techniques for their manipulation.

Ingram, Weiner, Shriberg, and Kwiatkowski: Processes, Nature, and Testing. As study of distinctive features declined in popularity, phonological processing explanations and systems emerged in the late '70s and early '80s. These ideas appeared to stem from the work of Stampe (1969) who claimed that sets of phonological processes could explain children's sound substitutions. Stampe maintained that young children pass through stages of normal development in which they use certain types of processes to simplify their speech, presumably, to allow them to communicate effectively by decreasing the complexity of their phonology so as to encode other vital linguistic elements such as vocabulary, length of utterance, and syntax.

Subsequently, Ingram (1981), Weiner (1979), and Shriberg and Kwiatkowski (1980) developed and published systems for phonological analysis. Unfortunately, none of the published evaluative systems contained normative information concerning which phonological processes children use at specific age levels, and the developmental aspects of processing use in normal children remains to be ascertained.

While a lengthy discussion of the relative similarities and differences in the three processing analysis systems is not necessary here, some basic comparisons can be made which may be helpful to those choosing one analysis system over another. The reader can easily locate copies of the three systems for closer comparisons.

The basic categories in all systems are some version of those described by Ingram (1977). In the first category, syllable structure processes, there is a tendency to reduce all words to basic CV syllables. In the second category, assimilatory processes, sounds become influenced by other sounds within words. The third category, substitution processes, includes systematic replacement of one sound by another. The systems of analysis proposed by Weiner (1979) and Shriberg and Kwiatkowski (1980) also include these same concepts and categories stated in slightly different terms. To show some of the phonological processes that are included in all three approaches to analysis, the Shriberg and Kwiatkowski system will be briefly reviewed. This is the only system of the three that requires that processes be evaluated from a spoken language sample.

In the *Natural Process Analysis* system of Shriberg and Kwiatkowski eight processes are evaluated, and a description and examples of them can be gleaned from the following material. First, in the process of *final consonant deletion* there is a tendency for final consonants to be deleted in words, particularly in CVC syllables (e.g., *ball*→/ba/). In the *velar fronting process* replacement of the phonemes /k/ and /g/ by /t/ and /d/ (e.g., *kitty*→/dIti/) occurs. The process of *stopping* describes the replacing of fricatives and affricates with homorganic stops (e.g., *this*→/dIti/). The substitution of alveolars for the palatals /ʃ/, /ʒ/, /tʃ/, and /dʒ/ is referred to as the *palatal fronting process* (e.g., *chalk*→/tɔk/). Three stages of simplification of the phonemes /l/ and /r/ occur in the *liquid simplification process*. Initially, /l/ becomes a stop and the /r/ is replaced by a /d/. Then /l/ is replaced by a /w/ or /j/ and the /r/ is also replaced by a /w/. In the final stage, a liquid replaces another (e.g., *ride*→/laɪd/). *Regressive assimilation* accounts for the fact that consonants are affected by following consonants even though there is a vowel between them (e.g., *talk*→/kuk/), while *progressive assimilation* consonants are affected by preceding consonants although a vowel comes between them (e.g., *noisy*→/nɔ:ni/). The process of *cluster reduction* influences simplification of consonant clusters often by the deletion of the marked consonant in the cluster (e.g., *stop*→/tap/). The final process is *unstressed syllable deletion* and concerns the deletion of the unstressed syllable of adult words with more than one syllable (e.g., *apple*→/æp/).

Therapy Guidelines. General, preliminary recommendations have been advanced by some to aid the speech-language clinician in an attempt to use phonological process information and rules to guide therapy practices. For example, Ingram (1977) maintained that correction should stress processes, not specific phonemes, a statement akin to some made earlier by proponents of feature therapy. Again, the notion that working on a class of processing errors might allow generalization to occur to untreated others was the basic rationale for process therapy.

A hierarchy of processing errors was posited by Hodson (1978) and supported to a degree by some pilot data. Using this information, Hodson suggested that therapy initially stress establishment of word-final consonants that discourage the processing error of final consonant deletion. Following this step, she suggested that front/back contrasts need to be developed focusing on postvocalic /k/ and then prevocalic /g/ to eliminate the processing error of velar fronting. In the final stage of therapy, she suggested that development of an awareness of stridency be used to eliminate the occurrence of the processing error, stopping. It should be mentioned that Hodson's views of the order and priorities for therapy appeared to be based on the frequency of occurrence of certain processing errors in normal children's development and not on experimental therapy for children having delayed speech and language development. In spite of these limitations, they may prove to be helpful insights into processing therapy planning.

No specific therapy techniques are involved in process therapy at this time. Like feature therapy, the specific phases, steps, training models, and other basic elements of the corrective process appear to be rather traditional in nature. The major difference, as in feature therapy, is orientation, focus, planning, and testing specific phonemes that have certain types of processing errors to determine whether generalization is taking place.

A Successful Example: Patrick and Wilcox, A Process Approach to Remediation of Phonological Disorders: A Case Study (1981). Following Hodson's (1978) recommendations concerning the selection of certain types of processing errors for remediation, Patrick and Wilcox (1981) selected a child having large numbers of phonemic errors resembling delayed speech and systematically set out to eliminate certain processing errors. The *Natural Process Analysis* system was used to identify the frequency and types of processing errors in the connected speech of the four-year-and-four-month-old female subject. The subject has a mean length of utterance prior to therapy of 4.2 morphemes, normal hearing, normal intelligence, and no known medical, emotional, or neurological disorders.

The processing analysis revealed a pattern of errors consisting of: final consonant deletion /t,d,f,s,v,θ,ð,z,l,r/; stopping /d/ and /t/ for /ð/ and /θ/; velar fronting /t/ and /d/ for /k/ and /g/; liquid simplification of /w/ for /l/; and cluster reduction (all clusters reduced to one member). The percentages of processing error use were found to be (1) final consonant deletion, 50 percent; (2) velar fronting, 78 percent; (3) stopping, 100 percent; (4) liquid simplification (initial), 100 percent; and (5) cluster reduction, 100 percent. Based on these data, Patrick and Wilcox decided to train the processing errors of final consonant deletion and velar fronting, and the other three types of consistent processing errors were ignored.

The subject received processing therapy for thirteen weeks with two sessions provided weekly. She received fifty minutes of group therapy and thirty minutes of individual therapy weekly. While the individual therapy aimed at correcting the child's phonological targets in structured and unstructured activities, the group therapy gave the clinician (Patrick) an opportunity to facilitate generalization of therapy targets.

Patrick tried to eliminate the final consonant deletion error pattern using /t,d,k,g/ as key sounds. The /t/ and /d/ were selected as targets since other phonemes affected by the process (such as /f,v,s,z,l,r/) were also involved in errors of stopping and liquid simplification. Remediation of the velar fronting process error was to be accomplished using the /k/ and /g/ phonemes.

Therapy employed structured and unstructured activities, modeling of correct productions, and some phonetic placement, when required, to get correct production. Visual, kinesthetic, and articulatory cues were used to obtain correct productions. The unstructured activities featured role playing and parallel play to get generalization of target processes. The child's self correction of target processes was stressed in these activities.

The outcome of this small investigation was that final testing (thirteen weeks later) showed that final consonant deletion dropped from the original 50 percent to 15 percent while velar fronting errors dropped from the original percentage of 78 to 40. The untrained processing errors of stopping, liquid simplification, and cluster reduction remained at their 100 percent occurrence rates and thus showed no change or generalization to them.

A Second Example: Weiner, *Treatment of Phonological Disability Using the Method of Meaningful Minimal Contrast: Two Case Studies* (1981). The psycholinguistic method of Meaningful Minimal Contrast, described briefly earlier in this chapter, was used by Weiner (1981) as a basic phonological therapy technique to teach two four-and-a-half-year-old children to overcome certain of their phonological processing errors. Using his method of process analysis, Weiner found deficiencies in both subjects in deletion of final consonants, stopping, and word-initial fronting. Each child was trained, through the Meaningful Minimal Contrast approach, to correct these process errors. Weiner felt these particular errors reflected delayed development of speech sounds often produced normally by four-year-old children.

A game approach was used to eliminate process errors, and each subject was reinforced for a favorable response with stars which could be exchanged for a small toy. Each child was seen individually for one-hour periods three times weekly. Therapy for the first child continued over six sessions, and therapy for the second over fourteen sessions. In each case two subsequent sessions were used to test for generalization to non-trained instances of each of the three types of process errors.

Using a multi-response baseline treatment design, Weiner used five repetitions each of four target words within each minimal pair selected as training items for each of the three processes. For final consonant deletion the pairs were "bee-bead," "pie-pipe," "no-nose," and "tea-teeth." The pairs used for the training of the stopping process were "fin-pin," "vase-base," "zip-dip," and "see-tea." To train the process of fronting he used "can-tan," "key-tea," "gum-dumb," and "gate-date."

The progress of the two children varied considerably. The first child reduced many of his baseline errors on the processes of deletion of final consonants, stopping, and fronting after six one-hour training sessions. The second child reduced his processing errors to a lesser degree after fourteen sessions. After the training sessions ended, two subsequent sessions showed essentially little if any generalization to nontrained stimuli. Weiner concluded that even after phonological oppositions are trained in therapy, one cannot necessarily expect them to generalize rapidly throughout a child's speech.

In contrast to the first therapy study of processing training, that by Patrick and Wilcox, Weiner's data seemed to show much more rapid progress in his first child. His second subject's remediation of processes over a long span of training seemed to parallel the Patrick and Wilcox subject's degree of improvement. Perhaps Weiner's first subject was more stimulable across many defective phonemes, thus opening up many opportunities for reduction of phonological process errors. It would seem that information concerning how stimulable a child is for each defective phoneme (or even by type of process error) would help clinicians decide how effective any particular form of treatment might be for such disorders.

Subjective Analysis. Evidence to support an increased efficacy in therapy for phonological disorders because processes generalize has yet to be forthcoming. Such evidence may come from studies of longer duration than the few completed to date. The two case studies reviewed briefly here, while interesting and carefully conducted, cannot be construed as solid evidence that processes generalize. They indicate only that processes can be treated in therapy and errors diminished drastically when measured in terms of training stimuli. Unlike other programs or approaches to phonological training, these attempts to train processes measure success differently in that they do not require the child to use the exact phoneme correctly: they merely require that the process in error be eliminated, e.g., for final consonant selection in which "bow-boat" are minimally contrasted if the child says "boap" for "boat" it is scored correct since final consonant deletion no longer exists. Regardless of this difference, the existing evidence from these two case studies does show that targeted phonological processes can be reduced significantly, thus providing more evidence that specific intervention into children's defective phonology has some degree of effectiveness. We obviously do not have comparative research evidence to show that process therapy is superior, equal to, or less effective than feature therapy or more traditional therapy approaches. This type of evidence is in great demand but in very short supply.

Sommers: The Wedge Approach to Planning Articulation Therapy. One of the decisions the clinician must make when a client has more than one defective sound revolves around the best order for taking up the sounds, but he or she has rarely had any evidence to back up the clinical impression that the order chosen will increase the effectiveness of therapy. However, recent findings concerning sound generalization indicate that there are important interactions among different defective sounds, and therefore that decisions concerning the order in which sounds are worked on may be very important (see pp. 134–135). These findings have special significance for Sommers, whose wedge approach to planning articulation therapy suggests that generalization does occur and that it is an important determining factor in therapy planning. Sommers developed the wedge approach in 1960, initially applying it as a means of planning therapy with multisound defective children; subsequently he also applied it to severely defective preschool children.

The Wedge Concept. Basic to the wedge approach are the beliefs that patterns of defective sounds can be identified and can be classified in such a way that a "best" therapy program can be devised. The wedge approach therefore requires of the clinician a careful and thorough evaluation of the client's articulation before therapy is ever begun, classifies the results of this evaluation, and uses this classification as the basis of the therapy program. The wedge approach itself is only a plan for articulation therapy; it does not include new or different therapy procedures or techniques.

Although the wedge approach was conceived before most speech clinicians were aware of distinctive feature theory, principles of the latter can be seen operating in the wedge approach. Distinctive feature theorists have altered the older concepts of classifying speech sounds according to their manner and place of articulation in a way that allows for more exactness in defining the phonological system; that is, they identify phonemes according to their minimal contrastive sound units, regardless of the language in which they are used (Jakobson, Fant, and Halle, 1951).

The wedge approach does not take into account all of the ten distinctive features of language enumerated by Jakobson, Fant, and Halle: (1) vocalic/nonvocalic; (2) consonantal/nonconsonantal; (3) interrupted/continuant; (4) strident/mellow; (5) voiced/voiceless; (6) compact/diffuse; (7) tense/lax; (8) grave/acute; (9) flat/plain; and (10) nasal/oral. Instead, it considers only the articulatory aspects of those distinctive features that were part of the Miller and Nicely (1955) system: voicing, nasality, affrication, duration, and place. Similarities between pairs of sounds are based on the number of distinctive features they have in common, and similar sounds have a greater influence on each other than on dissimilar sounds. Accordingly, sounds which share distinctive features, such as /s/ and /z/, can be treated by attacking only one, the "wedge," in therapy.

(Distinctive feature analysis is not required in the use of the wedge approach—at least not at this point in its development—but a clear awareness of distinctive features as a basis for planning therapy *is* required. The reader is urged to consult the references cited in the bibliography, as well as recent psycholinguistic literature.)

The use of a "wedge" phoneme is intended to ensure a minimum of treatment effort, for a wedge, in effect, is designed to "open" the total defective articulatory pattern. The approach assumes that not all defective phonemes should need comprehensive attention and that some sounds may not require any direct therapy once some progress has been made. The key to this concept is the assumption that generalization can occur simultaneously across more than one sound, or even group of phonetically similar sounds, particularly in the case of preschool children. Thus, more than one wedge sound can be introduced into therapy at a time without confusing a young client so long as the wedges are very dissimilar in terms of distinctive features. Such an attack on vital points—those that facilitate sound generalization—is assumed to result in greater efficiency in articulation therapy.

The effectiveness of the wedge approach depends first and most importantly on a careful phonetic analysis to reveal the exact nature of the defective phonemes. It depends to a lesser extent on an assessment of the consistency of the defectiveness for each sound, for the less consistent articulatory errors may be more amenable to change.

Using the Wedge Approach. The clinician's responsibility is to complete the needed articulatory assessment, study the total pattern, make choices of where to begin, and plan the sequence of events. Factors that may bear on decisions concerning which phonemes to attack, how many wedges (phonemes) to use simultaneously, and how to sequence their introduction into the therapy process include the pattern of the defect, the age of the individual, and whether group or individual therapy is provided.

An example may help explain the nature of the task and the bases for the judgments to be made. The client in this case was Alex, age 5, who was diagnosed as having a severe functional articulation disorder.

Defective sound	*Error produced*
/s/	bilateral emission, all positions
/z/	bilateral emissions, all positions
/tʃ/	bilateral emission, all positions
/ʃ/	bilateral emission, all positions
/l/	w/l substitution in initial position; omissions in medial and final positions
/r/ initial prevocal	w/r initial substitution
/r/ consonantal blends	/r/ omission
/ɜ˞/	omitted in all positions
/ə˞/	omitted in all positions
t/k substitution	initial position (e.g., "Tristmas"); medial and final ok
d/g/ substitution	initial and medial positions, final ok (e.g., "dreat big hamburder")

Sounds introduced at the initial stage of therapy: /ʃ/ and /k/

(It was possible to introduce two sounds in the first session because the many distinctive feature differences between them would help avoid confusion in Alex's mind. Major emphasis was given to /ʃ/, but there was some production and ear training on the substitution of /t/ for /k/.)

Rationale

/ʃ/, one of the four errors of lateral emission (which were of the same type in terms of place and manner), was chosen for the first therapy session because it was the only one of the four to show any inconsistency on a deep test of articulation on which five of thirty phonetic contexts were correctly articulated, and also because it was easier to teach than /s/. Compared with /s/, /ʃ/ is mellow rather than strident, and it has rounding, which makes it easier to demonstrate and get lip positioning. Both sounds, however, have the common distinctive feature of continuant, and the plan calls for the correction of /s/ when the major (lingual) error of the /ʃ/ bilateral emission is corrected. No consideration was given to /z/ because, with only one distinctive feature different from /s/, generalization from the corrected /s/ could be expected to occur; nor was consideration given to /tʃ/, because of its number of distinctive feature differences.

Sounds introduced at the second stage of therapy: /s/ and /l/

(Again, two sounds are taught at the same time. Some degree of reinforcement and carry-over training is also required for the lateral /ʃ/ and the t/k substitution, their correction having now moved beyond acquisition, yet probably not totally habituated.)

Rationale

Establishing a correct lingual pattern for the /ʃ/ has improved the possibilities of correcting /s/. Working from a correct /ʃ/ position may allow the clinician to alter its mellow feature and move to develop the more strident one of /s/.

Correction of /l/ may generalize to the vocalic /r/ and ultimately to /ɚ/ and to the initial prevocalic /r/. It may also contribute to a tongue-up and broadened position for the stressed /ɝ/. The vocalic /r/ appears to have all of /l/'s distinctive features except compactness.

Additionally, when the problem is truly functional, the substitution of /w/ for /l/ is usually easier to correct than it is for /r/, possibly due to /l/'s greater visibility and the easier sound discrimination between /w/ and /l/.

Sound introduced at the third stage of therapy: /tʃ/

(For this sound, negative practice, self-hearing, and other techniques are used as appropriate. Carry-over training continues on /k/, /g/, and /l/, as well as placement of the fricatives, /ʃ/ and /s/. The parents become more involved, and assist in the carry-over stages.)

Correction of the bilateral emission pattern on /ʃ/ and concomitant correction of /s/ and /z/ permits introduction of /tʃ/. Having established a pattern of not dropping the sides of his tongue and emitting air laterally, Alex shows an ability to gain correct production of /tʃ/ quickly and easily. He will need to change the continuant feature of /ʃ/ to an interrupted one, and to alter his tongue pattern so as to modify the mellow feature of /ʃ/ to the more strident one of /tʃ/.

Sounds never formally introduced: /g/, /z/, /ɝ/, /ɚ/

Generalization of /g/ and /z/ occurred. The /ɚ/ and /ɝ/ were not formally introduced because conceivably the establishment of /ɚ/ would lead to automatic development of the sound in the initial prevocal position and in prevocalic blends. Similarly, with correct production of /ɝ/, the medial and final vocalic sounds would come with almost no effort.

Conclusions. It seems likely that the popular therapies of Van Riper, McDonald, and Gerber would be suitable for use with the wedge approach, since all three are based on the acquisition of correct sounds through increasing perceptual and motor skill. By its emphasis on the distinctive feature classification of defective sounds, the wedge approach takes into account the specific perceptual and motor experiences needed for speech correction and thus would seem to ensure appropriate stimulation of the client through the exercise of the feedback networks. After all, it seems logical that distinctive feature clusters for each phoneme have corollary clusters of sensory and motor feedback networks in all modalities—tactile, proprioceptive, auditory, and visual—so that emphasis on a feature from a distinctive feature cluster should produce a perceptual and motor learning which fosters and maximizes sound generalization.

The wedge approach has not been well researched, but it has been supported by clinical experience with multisound defective children. A number of studies support the contention that sound generalization learning does occur across therapy trials and that sounds having the greatest number of common distinctive features are most capable of being generalized. The degree to which a multiple attack on a client's pattern of articulation affects generalization is difficult to say.

With adults or older children who have more consistently defective sounds, the wedge approach may not be as effective as it is with young children because we have no evidence to indicate that sound generalization occurs in such populations. On the other hand, we have observed that using the wedge approach with adult cleft-palate cases has resulted in some success.

SUMMARY

Functional articulation disorders, characterized by inadequate articulation due to learning, personality, or perceptual problems, constitute a large part of the cases seen by the speech clinician. Those affected by them share associated difficulties with auditory memory and discrimination, motor skills, and oral sensation. Recent research emphases have focused upon the relationships of severity, consistency, and stimulability to treatment results, but firm conclusions must wait upon further studies.

Remediation has been shown to depend upon three things—acquisition, habituation (or carry-over), and response generalization—and accordingly all approaches to articulation therapy focus upon achieving one or all of these things. They achieve this focus through very different rationales and techniques, although in practice they have more in common than one might suspect. For example, most require that the client learn the correct sound in a brief utterance—a sound in isolation, in a nonsense syllable, or in a word. In most cases, the clinician presents a model of the correct sound and the client produces a version of it until some level of satisfactory performance results. In one approach the clinician finds a phonetic context in which the individual's production of the defective sound is correct and expands this demonstrated success to other related phonetic contexts rather than presenting a model of the correct sound. Rather predictably, the S-R learning paradigm prevails throughout the clinician/client relationship.

Since articulation therapy represents a learning experience for the client, it seems logical that the laws of learning are operative. It is therefore not too surprising that the specific techniques for therapy are more alike than different, regardless of the approach. Not unlike many teaching activities, articulation therapy is aimed at heightening the client's awareness of the nature of the defect and of the correct sound. As a result, techniques of ear training, "self-monitoring," phonetic placement, tactile stimulation, negative practice, and progressive approximations can be identified as common elements of the approaches reviewed, despite variations in theoretical orientation. Obviously, some approaches, such as the one using meaningful minimal contrasts or those with psychotherapeutic flavor, stress other types of learning experiences.

The choice of an articulation approach is not easy for the clinician. Which one should be used? Under what conditions is one more effective than another? To be considered "competent," how many approaches should a clinician master? Only opinions can be offered in reply, since there is little research on the comparative effectiveness of therapies. The speech clinician will have to make that choice alone.

BIBLIOGRAPHY

Albright, R. W., The motor abilities of speakers with good and poor articulation. *Speech Monog.*, **15**, 286–292 (1948).

Andersland, P. B., Maternal and environmental factors related to success in speech improvement training. *J. Speech Hearing Res.*, **4**, 79–90 (1961).

Anderson, P. W., The relationship of normal and defective articulation of the consonant /s/ in various phonetic contexts to auditory discrimination between normal and defective /s/ productions among children from kindergarten through fourth grade. Unpublished master's thesis, State University of Iowa (1949).

Aufricht, H., A comparison of listening skills of sixty-five children with articulation defects and a matched group of children with normal speech. Unpublished doctoral dissertation, Northwestern University (1959).

Aungst, L. F., The relationship between oral stereognosis and articulation proficiency. Unpublished doctoral dissertation, Pennsylvania State University (1965).

Aungst, L. F., and Frick, J. V., Auditory discrimination ability and consistency of articulation of /r/. *J. Speech Hearing Dis.*, **28**, 76–85 (1964).

Backus, O., Group structure in speech therapy. In L. E. Travis (Ed.), *Handbook of Speech Pathology*. New York: Appleton-Century-Crofts, Inc. (1957).

Backus, O., and Beasley, J., *Speech Therapy with Children*. Boston: Houghton Mifflin Company (1951).

Berry, M. F., and Eisenson, J., *Speech Disorders: Principles and Practices of Therapy.* New York: Appleton-Century-Crofts, Inc. (1956).

Bitlo, E. W., A comparative study of certain physical abilities of children with speech defects and children with normal speech. *J. Speech Dis.*, **6**, 187–203 (1941).

Bountress, N., Use of distinctive features in articulation training. In C. W. Bennet, N. G. Bountress, and G. L. Bull (Eds.), *Contemporary Readings in Articulation Disorders.* Dubuque: Kendall/Hunt Pub. Co. (1982).

Brungard, M., Effect of consistency of articulation of /r/ and /s/ on gains made with and without therapy. Doctoral dissertation, Pennsylvania State University (1961).

Carrell, J., The etiology of sound substitution defects. *Speech Monog.*, **4**, 17–37 (1937).

Carrell, J., *Disorders of Articulation.* Englewood Cliffs, N.J.: Prentice-Hall, Inc. (1968).

Carter, E. T., and Buck, W. McK., Prognostic testing for functional articulation disorders among children in the first grade. *J. Speech Hearing Dis.*, **23**, 124–133 (1958).

Chisum, L., Relationship between remedial speech instruction activities and articulation change. Unpublished master's thesis, University of Kansas (1966).

Chisum, L., Shelton, R., and Arndt, W., Relationship between remedial speech instruction activities and articulation change. *Cleft Palate J.*, **6**, 57–64 (1969).

Chomsky, N., *Syntactic Structures.* The Hague: Mouton Press (1957).

Chomsky, N., *Aspects of the Theory of Syntax.* Cambridge, Mass.: The M.I.T. Press (1969).

Chomsky, N., and Halle, M., *The Sound Pattern of English.* New York: Harper and Row (1968).

Chomsky, N., and Miller, G. A., Introduction to the formal analysis of natural languages. In R. D. Luce, R. R. Bush, and E. Galanter (Eds.), *Handbook of Mathematical Psychology.* New York: John Wiley and Sons, Inc. (1963).

Cohen, J. H., and Diehl, C. F., Relation of speech-sound discrimination ability to articulation-type speech defects. *J. Speech Hearing Dis.*, **28**, 187–190 (1963).

Compton, A. J., A generative analysis of articulatory deviations. Paper presented at the American Speech and Hearing Association convention, Denver (1968).

Cooper, R., The method of meaningful minimal contrasts in functional articulation problems. *J. Speech Hearing Assoc. Va.*, **10**, 17–22 (1968).

Costello, J., and Onstine, J., The modification of multiple articulation errors based on distinctive features. *J. Speech Hearing Dis.*, **41**, 199–216 (1976).

Crocker, J., A phonological model of children's articulation competence. *J. Speech Hearing Dis.*, **34**, 203–213 (1969).

Dickson, S., Differences between children who spontaneously outgrow and children who retain functional articulation errors. *J. Speech Hearing Res.*, **5**, 263–271 (1962).

Dukes, P., and Panagos, J., Reception of comprehensible sentences by children with deviant speech. *British J. Dis. Comm.*, **8**, 139 (1973).

Elbert, M., Shelton, R. L., and Arndt, W. B., A task for the evaluation of articulation change: I. Development of methodology. *J. Speech Hearing Res.*, **10**, 281–288 (1967).

Fairbanks, G., Systematic research in experimental phonetics: I. A theory of the speech mechanism as a servosystem. *J. Speech Hearing Dis.*, **19**, 133–139 (1954).

Fairbanks, G., and Spriestersbach, D. C., A study of minor organic deviation in "functional" disorders of articulation: I. Rate of movement of oral structures. *J. Speech Hearing Dis.*, **15**, 60–69 (1950).

Farquhar, M. S., Prognostic value of imitative and auditory discrimination tests. *J. Speech Hearing Dis.*, **26**, 342–347 (1961).

Fucci, D., and Robertson, J., Functional defective articulation: An oral sensory disturbance. *Percept. and Motor Skills*, **33**, 711–714 (1971).

Gerber, A., The achievement of /r/ carryover through intensification of simultaneous auditory feedback. *Pa. Speech Hearing Assoc. Newsletter*, **7**, 7–11 (1966).

Gerber, A., *Goal Carryover: An Approach to Articulation Therapy.* Philadelphia: Temple University Press (1970).

Gilmore, S. I., A study of the effects of age and articulatory adequacy on auditory discrimination. Paper presented at the American Speech and Hearing Association convention, Chicago (1969).

Hardesty, P., Oral motor abilities of speech defective children. Unpublished doctoral dissertation, University of Southern Mississippi (1975).

Haws, R. J., Predictive testing of functional articulation disorders among children in kindergarten by means of a stimulability test. Paper presented at the American Speech and Hearing Association convention, Chicago (1969).

Hixon, T., and Hardy, J., Restricted mobility of the speech articulators in cerebral palsy. *J. Speech Hearing Dis.*, **29**, 294–306 (1964).

Hodson, B. W., A preliminary hierarchical model for phonological remediation. *Language Speech and Hearing Services in the Schools*, **9**, 236–240 (1978).

Holland, A. L., and Matthews, J., Application of teaching machine concepts to speech pathology and audiology. In H. N. Sloane and B. D. MacAulay (Eds.), *Operant Procedures in Remedial Speech and Language Training*. Boston: Houghton Mifflin Company (1968).

Holland, J. G., Teaching machines: An application of principles from the laboratory. In A. A. Lumsdaine and R. Glaser (Eds.), *Teaching Machines and Programmed Learning*. Washington, D.C.: National Education Association (1960).

Hutter, G., Children's evaluations of their own articulation of selected words. Unpublished doctoral dissertation, Ohio State University (1966).

Ingram, D., *Phonological Disability in Children*. New York: Elsevier (1977).

Ingram, D., *Procedures for the Phonological Analysis of Children's Language*. Baltimore: University Park Press (1981).

Jackson, P., and Sommers, R., Performances of articulatory-defective and minimal cerebral-dysfunctioning children on selected language and speech tasks. Paper presented at the American Speech and Hearing Association convention, Chicago, Illinois (1971).

Jakobson, R., Fant, G., and Halle, M., *Preliminaries to Speech Analysis: The Distinctive Features and Their Correlates*. Cambridge, Mass.: The M.I.T. Press (1951) (2nd ed., 1963).

Jenkins, E., and Lohr, F. E., Severe articulation disorders and motor ability. *J. Speech Hearing Dis.*, **29**, 286–292 (1964).

Kisatsky, T. J., The prognostic value of Carter-Buck tests in measuring articulation skills of selected kindergarten children. *Pa. Speech Hearing Assoc. Newsletter*, **7**, 4–9 (1966).

Kronvall, E. L., and Diehl, C. F., The relationship of auditory discrimination to articulatory defects of children with no known organic impairment. *J. Speech Hearing Dis.*, **19**, 335–338 (1954).

Lee, L., Recent studies in language acquisition, *ASHA*, **2**, 272–274 (1968).

Lewis, F., Distinctive features confusions in production and discrimination of selected consonants. *Lang. and Speech*, **17**, 60–67 (1974).

McDonald, E. T., *Articulation Testing and Treatment: A Sensory-Motor Approach*. Pittsburgh: Stanwix House (1964).

McDonald, E., and McDonald J., Norms for the *Screening Deep Test of Articulation* based on a longitudinal study of articulation development from beginning kindergarten to beginning third grade. Altoona, Pa.: Appalachia Intermediate Unit (1974).

McDonald, E., and McDonald, J., Comparison of the longitudinal and cross-sectional norms of the *Screening Deep Test*. Altoona, Pa.: Appalachia Intermediate Unit (1976).

McLean, J., Shifting stimulus control of articulation responses by operant techniques. Unpublished doctoral dissertation, University of Kansas (1965).

McNutt, J., Oral sensory and motor behaviors in children who misarticulate /s/ or /r/. *J. Speech Hearing Res.*, **20**, 694–703 (1977).

McNutt, J., and Hamayan, E., Subgroups of older children with articulation disorders. In R. Daniloff (Ed.) *Position Papers in Speech Hearing, and Language*. Baltimore: College Hill Press (1982).

McReynolds, L., and Bennett, S., Distinctive feature generalization in articulation training. *J. Speech Hearing Dis.*, **37**, 462–470 (1972).

McReynolds, L., Kohn, J., and Williams, G., Articulatory-defective children's discrimination of their production errors. *J. Speech Hearing Dis.*, **40**, 327–338 (1975).

Mase, D. L., Etiology of articulatory defects. *Teachers College Contribution to Education*, No. 921. New York: Columbia University (1946).

Mattingly, I., and Liberman, A., The speech code and the physiology of language. *Status Report on Speech Research*. New York: Haskins Laboratories (1968).

Menyuk, P., Comparison of grammar of children with functionally deviant and normal speech. *J. Speech Hearing Res.*, **7**, 109–121 (1964).

Miller, G. A., and Nicely, P. E., An analysis of perceptual confusions among some English consonants. *J. Acous. Soc. Am.*, **27**, 338–352 (1955).

Miller, S., and Sommers, R., Performances of articulatory defectives on two prognostic tests. Paper presented to the annual convention of the American Speech-Language Hearing Association, Detroit, 1980.

Moll, K., and Daniloff, J., Coarticulation of lip rounding. *J. Speech Hearing Res.*, **11**, 707–721 (1968).

Monnin, L., and Huntington, D., Relationship of auditory defects to speech-sound identification. *J. Speech Hearing Res.*, **17**, 352–366 (1974).

Mowrer, D., Baker, R. L., and Schutz, R. D., Operant procedures in the control of speech articulation. In H. N. Sloane and B. D. MacAulay (Eds.), *Operant Procedures in Remedial Speech and Language Training.* Boston: Houghton Mifflin Company (1968).

Mysak, E. D., A servo model for speech therapy. *J. Speech Hearing Dis.*, **24**, 144–149 (1959).

Mysak, E. D., *Speech Pathology and Feedback Theory* (2nd ed.) Springfield, Ill.: Charles C. Thomas (1971).

Panagos, J., Quine, M., and Klich, R., Syntactic and phonological influences on children's speech. *J. Speech Hearing Res.*, **22**, 841–848 (1979).

Patrick, M., Wilcox, J., A process approach to remediation of phonological disorders: a case study. Unpublished paper, Kent State University (1981).

Patton, F. E., A comparison of the kinaesthetic sensibility of speech-defective and normal speaking children. *J. Speech Hearing Dis.*, **7**, 305–310 (1942).

Paul, B., A replication of the Jenkins and Lohr investigation of articulatory defectives' fine motor skills. Unpublished investigation, Kent State University (1971).

Perkins, W., and Curlee, R., Causality in speech pathology. *J. Speech Hearing Dis.*, **34**, 231–239 (1969).

Powell, J., and McReynolds, L., A procedure for testing position generalization from articulatory training. *J. Speech and Hearing Research*, **3**, 629–645 (1969).

Powers, M. H., Functional disorders of articulation-symptomatology and etiology. In L. E. Travis (Ed.), *Handbook of Speech Pathology.* New York: Appleton-Century-Crofts, Inc. (1957, 1971).

Prins, I. D., Motor and auditory abilities in different groups of children with articulation deviations. *J. Speech Hearing Res.*, **5**, 161–168 (1962a).

Prins, T., Analysis of correlations among various articulatory deviation. *J. Speech Hearing Res.*, **5**, 152–160 (1962b).

Prins, T., Relations among specific articulatory deviations and responses to a clinical measure of sound discrimination ability. *J. Speech Hearing Dis.*, **28**, 382–388 (1963).

Reid, G., The etiology and nature of functional articulatory defects in elementary school children. *J. Speech Hearing Dis.*, **12**, 143–150 (1947).

Ringel, R., and Ewanowski, S., Oral perception: I. Two point discrimination. *J. Speech Hearing Res.*, **8**, 389–398 (1965).

Ringel, R., and Fletcher, H., Oral perception: III. Texture discrimination. *J. Speech Hearing Res.*, **10**, 642–649 (1967).

Ringel, R., Saxman, J., and Brooks, A., Oral perception: II. Mandibular kinaesthesia. *J. Speech Hearing Res.*, **10**, 637–641 (1967).

Ringel, R., House, A., Burk, K., Dolinsky, J., and Scott, C., Some relationships between orosensory discrimination and articulatory aspects of speech perception. *J. Speech Hearing Dis.*, **35**, 3–11 (1970).

Ryan, B. P., The prediction of articulation proficiency of children in first grade. Paper presented at the American Speech and Hearing Association convention, Chicago 1969.

Schielfelbuch, R., and Lindsey, M., A new test for sound discrimination. *J. Speech Hearing Dis.*, **23**, 153–159 (1958).

Scripture, M. K., and Jackson, E., *A Manual of Exercises for the Correction of Speech Disorders.* Philadelphia: F. A. Davis Co. (1927).

Shelton, R., Arndt, W., Krueger, A., and Huffman, E., Identification of persons with articulation errors from observation of nonspeech movements. *Amer. J. of Physic. Med.*, **45**, 143–150 (1966).

Sherman, D., and Geith, A., Speech sound discrimination and articulation skill. *J. Speech Hearing Res.*, **10**, 277–281 (1967).

Shriberg, L. D., Kwiatkowski, J. *Natural Process Analysis.* New York: John Wiley and Sons (1980).

Shriner, T., Holloway, M., and Daniloff, R., The relationship between articulatory deficit and syntax in speech defective children. *J. Speech Hearing Res.*, **12**, 319–325 (1969).

Sloan, N., *The Lincoln Adaptation of the Oseretsky Test.* Lincoln, Ill.: State School and Colony (1950).

Smith, V., Self-perceptive and projective sound discrimination of children with defective articulation. Unpublished master's thesis, Ohio State University (1965).

Snow, K., and Milisen, R., The influence of oral versus pictorial presentation upon articulation testing results. *J. Speech Hearing Dis.*, Monog. suppl. No. 4 (1954).

Sommers, R. K., Factors in the effectiveness of mothers trained to aid in speech correction. *J. Speech Hearing Dis.*, **27**, 179–187 (1962).

Sommers, R. K., Problems in articulation research: Methodology and error. *Asha*, **7**, 405–408 (1967).

Sommers, R. K., Cockerville, C. E., Paul, C. D., Bowser, D. C., Fichter, G. R., Fenton, A. K., and Copetas, F. G., Effects of speech therapy and speech improvement upon articulation and reading. *J. Speech Hearing Dis.*, **26**, 27–38 (1961).

Sommers, R. K., Meyer, W. J., and Fenton, A. K., Pitch discrimination and articulation. *J. Speech Hearing Res.*, **4**, 56–60 (1961).

Sommers, R. K., Schaeffer, M. H., Leiss, R., Gerber, A., Bray, M. A., Fundrella, D., Olson, J. K., and Tompkins, E. R., Factors in the effectiveness of group and individual articulation therapy. *J. Speech Hearing Res.*, **9**, 144–152 (1966).

Sommers, R. K., Leiss, R., Delp, M., Gerber, A., Fundrella, D., Smith, R., Revucky, M., Ellis, D., and Haley, V., Factors related to the effectiveness of articulation therapy for kindergarten, first, and second grade children. *J. Speech Hearing Res.*, **10**, 428–437 (1967).

Sommers, R. K., Meyer, W. J., and Furlong, A. K., Pitch discrimination and speech sound discrimination in articulatory defective and normal speaking children. *J. Aud. Res.*, **9**, 45–50 (1969).

Sommers, R., Cox, S., and West, C., Articulatory effectiveness, stimulability and children's performances on perceptual and memory tasks. *J. Speech Hearing Res.*, **15**, 579–589 (1972).

Sommers, R., and Kane, A., Nature and remediation of functional articulation disorders. In S. Dickson (Ed.) *Communication Disorders: Remedial Principles and Practices.* (1st ed.) Glenview, Ill.: Scott, Foresman and Company (1974).

Sommers, R., Moore, W., Brady, W., and Jackson, P., Performance of articulatory defective, minimal brain dysfunctioning and normal children on dichotic ear preference, laterality, and fine-motor skills. *J. Special Ed.*, **10**, 5–14 (1976).

Sommers, R., and Hatton, M., School speech, language, and hearing programs: A survey of clinicians, programs, and services. *Ohio Journal of Speech and Hearing*, **14**, 274–293, Fall, 1979.

Stampe, D., The acquisition of phonetic representation. Paper presented at the 5th Regional Meeting of CLS, Chicago, Illinois. 443–454 (1969).

Stinchfield (Hawk), S. M., and Young, E. H., *Children with Delayed or Defective Speech.* Stanford, Calif.: Stanford University Press (1938).

Stitt, C., and Huntington, D., Some relationships among articulation, auditory ability, and certain other variables. *J. Speech Hearing Res.*, **12**, 576–594 (1969).

Stoia, L., An investigation of improvement in articulation in a therapy group and non-therapy group of first grade children having functional articulatory speech disorders. Unpublished doctoral dissertation, Columbia University (1961).

Templin, M., A study of the sound discrimination ability of elementary school pupils. *J. Speech Dis.*, **8**, 127–132 (1943).

Van Denmark, A., and Mann, M., Oral language skills of children with defective articulation. *J. Speech Hearing Res.*, **8**, 409–414 (1965).

Van Riper, C., *Speech Correction: Principles and Methods.* (6th ed.) Englewood Cliffs, N.J.: Prentice-Hall, Inc. (1978).

Van Riper, C., and Irwin, J. V., *Voice and Articulation.* Englewood Cliffs, N.J.: Prentice-Hall, Inc. (1958).

Van Riper, R., and Erickson, R., *Predictive Screening Test of Articulation.* Kalamazoo: Western Michigan University, Continuing Education Office (1968).

Waldman, F., Singh, S., and Hayden, M., A comparison of speech-sound production and discrimination in children with functional articulatory disorders. *Lang. and Speech*, **21**, 205–220 (1978).

Wegener, J., Stereognostic ability in articulatory defective children. Unpublished master's thesis, Indiana University (1966).

Weinberg, B., Liss, G., and Hollis, J., A comparative study of visual, manual, and oral form identification in speech impaired and normal speaking children. In J. F. Boxman (Ed.), *Second Symposium on Oral Sensation and Perception.* Springfield, Ill.: Charles C. Thomas (1970).

Weiner, Frederick F., *Phonological Process Analysis.* Baltimore: University Park Press (1979).

Weiner, F., Treatment of phonological disability using the method of meaningful minimal contrast: Two case studies. *J. Speech Hearing Dis.*, **46**, 97–103 (1981).

Weiner, P., Auditory discrimination and articulation. *J. Speech Hearing Dis.*, **32**, 19–29 (1967).

Wellman, B. L., The development of motor coordination in young children: An experimental study in the control of hand and arm movements. *University of Iowa Studies in Child Welfare*, **3**, 1–93 (1926).

Wepman, J., Relationship of auditory discrimination to speech and reading difficulties. Paper presented at the American Speech and Hearing Association convention (1959).

Whitacre, J., Luper, H., and Pollio, H., General language deficits in children with articulation problems. *Lang. and Speech*, **12**, 231–239 (1970).

Winitz, H., *Articulatory Acquisition and Behavior*. New York: Appleton-Century-Crofts, Inc. (1969).

Winitz, H., *From Syllable to Conversation*. Baltimore: University Park Press (1975).

Winitz, H., and Bellerose, B., Sound discrimination as a function of pretraining conditions. *J. Speech Hearing Res.*, **5**, 340–348 (1962).

Winitz, H., and Bellerose, B., Relation between sound discrimination and sound learning. *Commun. Dis.*, **1**, 215–235 (1967).

Winitz, H., and Priesler, L., Discrimination pretraining and sound learning. *Percept. Motor Skills*, **20**, 905–916 (1965).

Winitz, H., and Priesler, L., Effect of distinctive feature pretraining on phoneme discrimination learning. *J. Speech Hearing Res.*, **10**, 515–530 (1967).

Wolfe, V., and Irwin, R., Sound discrimination ability of children with misarticulation of the /r/ sound. *Percept. Motor Skills*, 415–420 (1973).

Young, E. H., and Stinchfield-Hawk, S., *Moto-Kinaesthetic Speech Training*. Stanford, Calif.: Stanford University Press (1955).

4 Stuttering: A Clinically Related Overview

Gene J. Brutten
M. N. Hegde

A MATTER OF DEFINITION

Stuttering may be said to be what a stutterer does. This is a purely operational definition. It carries with it the implication that in some way and to some extent, what the stutterer does is different from what the non-stutterer does and that this difference is measurable. If this were not the case the term stuttering and thus the category stutterer would have no meaning. Neither term would, in a definable way, be distinctive from its opposite, normally fluent speech and non-stutterer.

An operational approach does not involve explanation. What differences there may be between what stutterers and non-stutterers do are important in their own right. It is left to the theoretician to offer an understanding as to whether it reflects, for example, breakdown, repression of need, or anticipatory struggle (Bloodstein, 1981). Therefore, the operational approach to stuttering avoids theoretical entanglements and controversies. As a result, it differs markedly from that embodied in the seemingly similar definition of stuttering as "what a speaker does trying not to stutter again" (Johnson, 1956, p. 216). If we were to adopt this latter definition we would be faced immediately with two fundamental issues. One of these is associated with the definitional implication that stuttering is volitional, that it is a purposive act. The other revolves around the matter of the original stutter. Where did it come from? And how can we define stuttering as the avoidance of stuttering? It would seem questionable at best to take this seemingly circular position.

To avoid controversies associated with theoretically based definitions, like the one we have just discussed, let us return to an operational framework and strive to see what if anything objectively differentiates what the stutterer does from that which the non-stutterer does. Maybe then we will be able to understand what separates those who fall into one or another of these categories.

The onset of stuttering is typically during childhood. Some place onset as being predominant during the ages of two to four; others say it is between three and five. The difference matters little. Clearly, it is generally associated with the development of speech and language. But more important are its visible characteristics. What does it look like at onset and how does it differ from speech that is considered normal? What is the topography of the speech of stutterers that differentiates it from the speech of nonstutterers? To find answers to these questions we must turn to the reports of parents, those who considered their children to be stutterers and those who viewed their offspring as non-stutterers. The descriptions of the speech of the children given by these two groups of parents differed markedly. When the parents of the stutterers imitated and described the speech of their children at onset they highlighted the presence of syllable repetition and prolongations that were oral and silent (i.e., a non-audible block). When the parents of non-stutterers were asked to report about the kinds of behaviors they observed when their children were first dysfluent, they gave a very different picture. Their dysfluencies were characterized by silent intervals or pauses, interjections, and phrase repetitions—behaviors that may well be indicative of editing activities.

Parental reports can be questioned, of course. Parents are not bias-free observers. Moreover, time tends to cloud memory. Lack of reliability could have resulted from the fact that, for example, the parents of the stutterers were interviewed about their children's dysfluencies some eighteen months, on the average, after onset. However, there is little reason to dispute the data. There is no reason to believe that unreliability is more likely to be evidenced by the parents of stutterers than the parents of non-stutterers. Moreover, the separate reports of the fathers and mothers in both groups were quite similar. This provides face validity to the finding.

The differing reports of the two groups of parents about the types and extent of dysfluencies that they observed are consistent with the results from normative studies of children who do and do not stutter. One such study involved forty-two stutterers and a like number of non-stutterers whose age ranged from two to eight years (Johnson, 1956). As might be expected the stutterers turned out to have more overall fluency failures than did the non-stutterers. Much more important, however, was the finding that the real difference between the groups was in part word (sound and syllable) repetition and sound prolongation.[1] The stutterers averaged 5.7 of these two forms of dysfluencies per 100 words, on the average, while the non-stutterers displayed these behaviors on less than one half of one percent (.45) of the words spoken. This is a meaningful disparity, whether one looks at the difference in the totals for these two forms of dysfluency or attends to the singular fact that the stutterers emitted an average of 4.2 part word repetitions and 1.5 prolongations per hundred words while the non-stutterers displayed, respectively, averages of only 0.4 and 0.15 of these behaviors relative to the same number of words. Even if the miniscule counts of part word repetitions and prolongations evidenced by the non-stutterers are real and not representative of measurement error, they essentially indicate that normal-speaking children rarely display these behaviors. This finding has been confirmed recently when the speech of 108 nursery school children was investigated (Bjerken,

---

[1] Whole word repetition was also emitted to a considerably greater extent by stutterers than by the normal speaking control group. However, this category of dysfluency was a contaminated one. Both single and multisyllable whole word repetitions were counted as equivalent events. Yet the repetition of a single syllable word is akin to syllable repetition and the latter was counted as a part word repetition. Since the latter category notably separated stutterers from non-stutterers, it is likely that it served in the same way to inflate the difference among the subject groups for whole word repetition.

1980). Part word repetitions and prolongations, silent and oral, were virtually absent from the sampled speech.

The importance of the differences in the extent to which particular dysfluencies are displayed by stutterers and non-stutterers goes well beyond the fact that the differences are reliable. To be sure, replication adds support to what we can say about the findings, as does the fact that the differences are statistically significant, and not likely a chance result (Johnson and Associates, 1959). However, the real import resides in the fact that the differences that we have been discussing may be used as a part of an objectively based means for distinguishing the stutterer from the non-stutterer: for all practical purposes the average child is devoid of part word repetitions and prolongations when speaking. In contrast, other forms of dysfluency, such as revisions, interjections, and incomplete phrases are emitted by stutterers and non-stutterers to an extent that is quite similar. These and other forms of what has been called normal dysfluencies are not, therefore, clinically significant in helping to distinguish stutterers from non-stutterers. They differ, that is, from part word repetitions—particularly those of rapid rate—and tension prolongations, both of which appear to be differentially significant behaviors.

Issue can and has been taken with the contention that for certain forms of dysfluency, a behavioral dichotomy exists between children who stutter and those who do not. With respect to the preceding data, it has been pointed out that part word repetitions, for example, do occur in the speech of normal youngsters. Indeed, as many as 20 percent of the non-stutterers studied displayed more of these dysfluencies than did those who were considered to be stutterers. This suggests that an overlap exists and that any attempt to use this behavior as a means of categorizing individuals is risky. The implication is that relative to part word repetitions, the categories of stutterers and non-stutterers are somewhat blurred. But the ambiguity pointed to has not been consistently evidenced. A study of the syllable repetitions of preschool stutterers and non-stutterers makes this evident (Floyd and Perkins, 1974): in this investigation the individual stutterer who had the lowest percentage of dysfluent syllables (7.28) still differed markedly from the non-stutterer who had the highest percentage (2.58). Moreover, the distribution of this behavior for the two groups showed little variance and a notable separation. As a result, the investigators concluded that the stutterers and non-stutterers that they studied were "discretely different" in their display of syllable repetitions.

If, as our review has suggested, part word repetitions and prolongations are characteristic stuttering behaviors, it is likely that people would generally view these behaviors as *different from normal*, while in contrast, they would classify as *normal* those forms of fluency failure that are as likely to be displayed by non-stutterers as stutterers. This appears to be the case. The research indicates that listeners tend to categorize the former behaviors as stuttering and the latter ones as normal dysfluencies, ones that are not representative of disordered speech (Williams and Kent, 1958; Schiavetti, 1975).

The judgment of the *severity* of stuttering also appears to be tied to type of dysfluency. Young (1961) found a moderately high positive correlation of .87 between judges' ratings of severity and the frequency with which repetitions, sound prolongations, silent prolongations (broken words), and signs of word-specific tension were present; thus, there was a communality of 76 percent between these dysfluencies and severity judgments. It follows, then, that only about 24 percent of the severity judgments were not accounted for by the frequency with which these forms of dysfluency were displayed. These figures make it apparent that there is a remarkable relationship between severity, as listeners judge it, and part word repetitions and prolongations. However, the relationship was not perfect. As a result, the frequency of part word repetitions and sound prolongations can only be used by the clinician to get a *general* picture of listener reactions. It will not provide a highly accurate prediction of judged severity.

The specific forms of dysfluency that are highly prevalent among stutterers are not a very precise predictor of severity, in part because such judgments are subjective and thus rather variable. Morever, elements other than the frequency of these forms of dysfluency appear to contribute to the judgment of severity. The rapidity with which a sound is repeated, the tension involved, the length of the prolongation, and the extent to which rate is affected are but some of the additional elements that also seem to affect severity judgments.

It should come as no great surprise that many of the same factors that affect judgments about the severity of stuttering are involved in the *identification* of stuttering. For example, people are more likely to indicate that stuttering is being displayed by a speaker if the dysfluencies take the form of part word repetitions and prolongations and if they are frequent and of long duration (Lingwall and Bergstrand, 1979; Sander, 1963). But there are some additional factors, possibly unique ones, that go into the identification of dysfluent speech as stuttering. A longer—a multiple unit— repetition of a sound is more likely to be viewed as stuttering than a sound that is repeated just one time. But even single unit word repetitions, behavior considered to be a form of normal dysfluency, will be judged as stuttering if they occur frequently enough. Hegde and Hartman (1979a; 1979b) found that a majority of their listeners made this determination when single unit word repetitions occurred more than 15 percent of the time. They also found that yet another so-called normal dysfluency can lead some to decide that the speaker is stuttering if it occurs often enough. Some 39 percent of their listeners judged speech samples to be stuttering when interjections occurred on 20 percent of the words spoken. Thus, when interjections are present at approximately ten times their usual frequency some listeners will label the behavior as stuttering.

Though Hegde and Hartman's listeners showed considerable restraint in labeling whole word repetitions and interjections as stuttering, the fact that some ultimately did, when they occurred frequently, raises again the question as to whether there is any real diagnostic difference between particular forms of dysfluency. If whole word repetitions and interjections can be considered stuttering, is it appropriate to call them normal dysfluency and to limit stuttering to rapid part word repetitions and tension prolongations? There are those who would say no. They would point to the fact that all children are dysfluent, that fluency failures of one kind or another occur on about 6.5 percent of the words that children speak. They would thus say either that stuttering and dysfluency are not the same (Johnson, 1956) or that stuttering is dysfluency that is severe and chronic (Bloodstein, 1981). The former would say that dysfluency is a normal event, the frequency of which will vary somewhat from person to person, while stuttering is a result of the attempt to *avoid* normal dysfluency; they indicate that it is not the *magnitude* of dysfluency that is significant. Members of the second camp would point out, as we have, that certain types of dysfluencies reportedly predominate at onset and that these were rarely reported by the parents of non-stutterers. They would, therefore, reject the avoidance hypothesis. Instead, they would stress the fact that dysfluencies are found in the speech of *both* stutterers and non-stutterers. Stuttering, they would contend, is dysfluency that occurs more frequently, is chronic rather than sporadic, and is more severe in its nature. Stuttering and the dysfluency of normal speakers would not, then, be viewed as fundamentally different. Stuttering is merely dysfluent behavior that occurs more often. A continuum is said to exist such that, at some point, normal dysfluency shades into stuttering. The *crossover point* is thus of great import. Measurable standards need to be provided for differentiating the non-stutterer from the stutterer. A fundamental issue is whether an agreed upon operational definition of stuttering can ever be provided when a continuum is proposed. What one person calls stuttering another may call normal dysfluency. Johnson made this point long ago when he asked—*how much is much?* Hegde and Hartman's research may ultimately serve to put this issue to rest. As we have seen, their investigations have shown that it is possible to determine the amount of specific forms of dysfluency that will lead listeners to judge speech as stuttered.

It should be clear by this time that almost all frameworks, in one way or another, indicate that stuttered speech is characterized by sound repetition, and/or sound prolongations. To be sure, those who see stuttering as avoidance of normal dysfluency say that the two are different; fluency failures are not stutterings. But it is instructive that most pathologists view the particular repetitions and prolongations that are relatively prevalent in the speech of stutterers as *primary, kernel, or factor I behaviors* (Brutten, 1975; Van Riper, 1963; Wingate, 1964). As we have seen, other forms of dysfluency are generally considered to be normal. This is the case for non-stutterers. But stutterers may employ these forms of dysfluency as a mechanism by which they can attempt, as unobtrusively as possible, to avoid anticipated stuttering or cope with its occurrence. They may, for example, interject a sound or word or repeat an already spoken phrase if they expect that they are going to stutter. They may revise what they have said already to bypass a word that is giving them difficulty. When this happens, these behaviors are considered *secondary, accessory, or factor II responses*. Dysfluencies of this sort are not the only features that are accessory or secondary to stuttering. Voluntary behaviors of any kind may be used by the stutterer to adjust to anticipated or ongoing failures of fluency. The speaker may look away from the listener, pause as if thinking, take a deep breath, move in any of innumerable ways. Any bodily activity over which voluntary control is exerted can become a factor II behavior (Brutten and Shoemaker, 1967), and can be used adjustively.

Not all stutterers display these accessory behaviors. It follows that the presence or absence of factor II responses cannot be used as a diagnostic tool. They can't be used to differentiate stuttering from non-stuttering. Yet, most people who stutter evidence a goodly number of these coping strategies. However, the adjustive tactics are not the same from stutterer to stutterer. The differences are partly a reflection of the speakers experiential history. The responses that a particular stutterer employs appears to depend on those that have, for one reason or another, been associated with successful avoidance or escape. They also depend, in part, on the loci of concern and difficulty. If a stutterer typically has difficulty with *certain sounds*, if anticipation of dysfluency is *word specific*, the adjustments will generally be quite different than if some aspect of the speech *situation* is regarded as negative. Word-specific concern might well lead to omission, rehearsal, circumlocution. Situational fears may, on the other hand, lead to refusal to use a phone, go to a restaurant, or ask a question in class.

Most stutterers anticipate and have difficulty that relates to both words and situations. One or the other may predominate but it is quite rare to find a stutterer whose difficulty is exclusively associated with words or situations. As a result, a mix of adjustive behaviors is likely. Most of these will be directly involved with the act of speech. Articulatory, phonatory, and respiratory maneuvers will predominate. Adjustive behaviors involving movements of the extremities are less likely to occur (Bakker and Brower, 1982). But, as has already been pointed out, voluntary actions of any kind and involving any muscle group might be used adjustively.

Clearly, the stutterer may display a number of different behaviors. Some of these we have pointed to as being kernel. One or another of these disruptions of fluency is evidenced by all individuals who are called stutterers. Other behaviors are adjustive. Though often very frequent and attention-getting they are not necessarily evidenced by stutterers. They are not, therefore, characteristic of stuttering or definitive of this disorder of speech.

The distinction between those behaviors that are fundamental to stuttering and those that are accessory aspects of the disorder has not always been made. Factor I behaviors, ones that are characteristic of stuttered speech, and Factor II behaviors, the adjustive responses stutterers tend to make, have generally been lumped together into a molar category called a *moment* of stuttering. Moments have reference to those instances when a judgment is somehow made that something called stuttering has occurred. Moments appear to have come about both because of the clinical and research need to count stutterings and the absence of full agreement among pathologists as to which of the behaviors that stutterers emit are characteristic. The result was a relatively inclusive and nonspecific category.

Moments do not reflect the presence of a particular behavior or a specific combination of behaviors. Moments are best seen as a mixture of separate behaviors that tend to be independent of each other. The moments evidenced by a stutterer are quite likely to differ from each other in their constituent elements and in the order in which they appear (Krych, 1978). Moreover, the composition of stuttering moments are likely to differ in a possibly notable way from one stutterer to the next. In other words, a moment of stuttering is anything but a constant and stable event. This fact and the ambiguity created by the absence of behavioral boundaries seems to have contributed heavily to disagreement in the identification of where and when stuttering occurred (Tuthill, 1940).

Stuttering has traditionally been measured in terms of moments. But as we have seen, moments represent an ever-changing scene in which various kernel and accessory features may or may not be present at any particular instance in time. It would seem wise, then, not to rely too heavily on results based on this molar measure, and prudent to move in the direction of clinical measurement that is limited to a more precisely defined event. It would appear to be more useful, in other words, to carefully measure the frequency of a factor I sound prolongation or a factor II interjection than it would be to keep a precise count of imprecise moments.

The molecular approach to measuring the behaviors emitted by stutterers appears to have recently gained favor (Brutten and Shoemaker, 1967; Adams, 1976; Wingate, 1977). However, some clinicians still prefer to use moments, because, in their view, stuttering is a perceptual phenomenon. A test of sorts has recently been conducted to compare this molar position with the stand that stuttering refers to "a group of specific speech dysfluencies" (Martin and Haroldson, 1981, p. 59). Toward this end, two groups of *untrained* subjects were asked to listen to tapes and identify the words on which stuttering occurred. One group was given no instructions as to what stuttering was. The other group of subjects was told that stuttering was sound repetition, syllable repetition, repetition of single-syllable whole words, silent prolongation and/or audible prolongation. This definition did not enhance *reliability*. As a matter of fact the uninstructed group showed greater intra and inter observer consistency in identifying stuttered words. It should be noted here that we are talking about reliability and not validity. Moreover, it must be pointed out the instructed group was not asked to identify a particular form of dysfluency. The subjects were instead given a definition of stuttering that included five different behaviors. The words were counted as stuttered if any one or combination of these behaviors was thought to be present. As such, the reliability of another kind of molar event was being tested. To be sure, these moments had reference to behaviors that are characteristic of stuttering. But the molar use of these behaviors means that measurement was confounded. Response specific precision was missing even though the definition excluded normal dysfluencies and factor II responses, behaviors that are not the cardinal features of stuttering.

Precision is a critically vital aspect of an operational definition. In its absence there is ambiguity and confusion. To avoid these in defining the constituent elements of stuttering, we have limited ourselves to those *distinctive* features that characterize the speech of stutterers. We have pointed to measures of what stutterers do when speaking that distinguishes them from non-stutterers. Identification of the stutterers from the non-stutterers was made possible by measurement procedures that are molecular rather than molar and objective rather than subjective. Within this frame, stuttering is considered an objectively palpable event rather than a perceptual phenomenon. It is viewed as observable behavior rather than as something to be found in the ear of the listener.

But to define, even precisely, is not to explain. The purpose of an operational definition is to assure the *consistency of measurement*. For, if we all do the same thing in the same way we will find the same thing. Operationism is not designed to deal with the issue of *why* something happens. Thus, an operational definition of stuttering is not one that deals with the cause of stuttering. The fact that we can, for example, reliably measure the audible repetitions or prolongations of stutterers does not at all illuminate their cause. Various conditions and circumstances may be antecedent to these and the other disorganizations that typify stuttering.

THE QUESTION OF CAUSE

The cause of stuttering, like the etiology of a number of other human disorders, is not presently known. This should not be taken to mean that we are not knowledgeable about stuttering or the stutterer. We have accumulated a considerable amount of reliable information over the years. These data have permitted us to describe, with increasing accuracy, the behaviors involved and the conditions under which they are more likely to occur and be maintained. They have not as yet, however, fully enabled us to come to grips with the issue of causality. Though we have some ideas about the variables that are causally related to stuttering we do not currently know with certainty those that lead to the onset of this disorder.

The presence of data, as well as the desire to understand the fundamental relationship among events and to explain why things happen as they do, have led scientists throughout the ages to theorize and to test their theories. Those who are interested in stuttering are no different. Like their colleagues they have promulgated theories. Indeed, a rather large number of theories about the cause of stuttering have been set forth over the years. These explanatory models have varied remarkably. Given some license, we can classify them as *organismic, environmental,* and *interactional* in nature.

Organismic models have reference not only to clearly defined organs of the body but also functional organizations such as neurological processes. The models proposed may or may not suggest that stuttering is genetically determined. Constitutional factors that are nongenetic also have been set forth to explain the cause of stuttering. Inherent in all of these models, however, is the concept of a weakness, a liability, or an insufficiency of the organism that in one way or another leads to the disruption of speech performance. Sampling these models we see that stuttering has, at one time or another, been attributed to such different factors as inordinate tongue length, metabolic imbalance, interhemispheric conflict, tetany, and a type of epilepsy (Bloodstein, 1981).

The view that stuttering is caused by organic factors gave way, in time, to concepts that were purely environmental. The move away from organismic positions was a result of the inability to uncover any physical evidence of differences between stutterers and non-stutterers that were consistent and that could be used to explain occurrences of stuttering. A dysphemia or organismic weakness was not at all apparent. In addition, the fact that some people, at least, recovered from the disorder—whether naturally or as a result of therapy and without known physical intervention—appeared to belie the contention that a weakness existed. Another, powerful argument against an organismic position was the fact that, at certain times and in certain conditions, the stutterer could speak for a considerable period in a normally fluent manner.

The *environmental* models that have been proposed are far from homogeneous. All that they share is the belief that stuttering is caused by some element or elements present in an individual's past experiences. The organism is merely a vessel through which these determining experiences pass. The organism is seen as a clean slate, and behavior, disordered or normal, is seen as a result of the events of life. Stuttering, then, could come about because speech habits are incorrectly learned or inappropriate attention is paid to the dysfluencies that all speakers evidence. Hostility, the repression of unconscious needs, speech-associated conflicts, and phobias about speech, speech sounds, and the act of speaking have also been considered to be possible causes of stuttering (Van Riper, 1982). Indeed, it has been suggested that stuttering can be caused by any of a set of events that lead the individual to believe that speech is difficult, that special precautions need to be taken, and that unusual effort is required to produce it (Bloodstein, 1981).

The environmental models have been anything but wholly successful in dealing with the issue of causality. Certain concepts about the environmental circumstances that set the occasion for onset seemed to defy either naturalistic or experimental observation. The contention, for example, that at onset the speech of stutterers is not different, in terms of dysfluency, from that of the non-stutterer could not be scientifically tested (Johnson and Associates, 1959). It follows, therefore, that the position that stuttering was caused by the inappropriate reaction to and labeling of normal dysfluency could not be directly supported (Bloodstein, 1981). Other constructs of potential value led to predictions that were not confirmed. Still others were not researched. Sometimes this was because it was more than a little difficult to operationally define the concepts that were basic to a particular theory.

Environmental theories sparked considerable research. Data about various aspects of stuttering accumulated at a heady pace. Undoubtedly, it was this steady increase in knowledge about stuttering that led many of the explanatory models to be removed from consideration. Sometimes the data served to support, at least for a time, a particular position. But often the findings required the theory to be refined or eliminated from consideration. The theories, then, served their purpose. They stimulated research that in turn led to changes in our understanding of stuttering.

Change in the way behavior is viewed has marked all of the behavioral sciences in recent years. Both increased sophistication in design and statistical inference and the explosion in research productivity have led to enormous changes in our understanding of various forms of human behavior. As a result, theoretical postures have moved from those that emphasize the organism to those that stress the environment to those that recognize the *interplay* between the two. What became apparent, ultimately, is that human behavior—normal or disordered—is best understood if organismic and environmental variables are not seen as mutually exclusive. A nature-nurture dichotomy was not consistent with the facts; the data made it evident that behavior is a product of the interplay or interaction between organismic and environmental events.

The clinician should note in this respect that learning does not occur in a void. Stimulation that sets the occasion for and controls the occurrence of behavior impinges on an organism. And, organisms differ in their reactivity to these stimuli. To be sure, some of these differences are environmentally determined. But the distribution of a myriad of genetic elements also affects responsivity. There is an enormous potential for differences that determine, in some part, such behaviorally important attributes as response thresholds, arousal levels, conditionability, and stimulability (Brutten and Shoemaker, 1967).

Behavioral genetic elements undoubtedly affect and interact with environmental events. However, they are not in themselves sufficient to explain all human behavior. This fact is clear. Yet, equally clear is the fact that genetic elements contribute to the occurrence of behavior. Though the many ramifications of this statement are not yet fully understood, behavioral scientists no longer accept a purely environmental view of behavior. The organism is no longer seen merely as a vehicle to be shaped as a result of the causative relationship between events. On the other hand, a purely physical explanation of behavior, like stuttering, has not been shown to be viable either. No organismic variables have been uncovered that are necessary and sufficient to explain the occurrence of this behavior. Furthermore, as we have and will see, stuttering varies with environmental events.

Because human behavior is complex and interactively determined, and because it is simplistic to suggest otherwise, obviously does not mean that human behavior is outside the realm of study. The data available are not consistent with such a position. Similarly, the fact that we are not currently able to specify the particular variables that are causally related to stuttering does not mean that we lack knowledge or the ability to achieve remediation. Much is known about the circumstances that are associated with this behavior. Stated differently, we are aware of many of the variables that are covariant with stuttering. These are predictively related to its occurrence, maintenance, and behavioral progression. We need to explore some of the more important of these predictor variables. They are vital to our understanding of stuttering and those who stutter. We will also bring these variables to your attention because their relationship with stuttering is suggestive—though not indicative—of causality: some of these variables are likely to be ones that are determinative. In other words, some of these variables are probably ones that cause the initial and continued occurrence of stuttering behaviors. They are therefore important to the clinician.

Organismic Factors and Their Indicators

Recently those concerned with stuttering have taken another look at the evidence that non-environmental factors are, in some way, causally related to stuttering. The data that was previously looked at as being of historical interest only was dusted off and reevaluated in light of current technological advances. Genetic models that, for example, were statistically beyond our scope a relatively few years ago are now being used to see if we can still assume that heredity does *not* play a causative role in stuttering.

The issue of heredity has its basis in a number of facts about stutterers and their families. Many of these pieces of information have been known for quite some time. Others have been suspected, and still others are just now coming to the fore. Early on it became apparent to speech therapists that males were more prone to this disorder than were females. School-aged stutterers were about three times as likely to be males than females. This difference between the sexes is not limited to particular ages, however. Almost exactly the same incidence is revealed whatever the clients age (Kidd, Kidd, and Records, 1978).

The finding that a *sex ratio* exists among those who stutter has been consistently uncovered in studies that have spanned time and cultures (Eisenson, 1966). Consequently, some theorists have come to the conclusion that a sex-limited or sex-modified genetic predisposition, susceptibility, or liability exists that makes males more likely to become stutterers (Kidd, Kidd, and Records, 1978; West, 1958). Others, however, have held that the sex ratio is merely a reflection of the way society reacts to male and female children and the dysfluencies in their speech (Johnson and Associates, 1959; Schuell, 1946). In the past, this environmental viewpoint was given considerable credence despite cross-cultural findings of male proneness. Indeed, it was considered the most meaningful explanation of the sex ratio until recently.

The sex ratio was not, however, the only evidence that pointed to the relationship between heredity and stuttering. The influence of genetic factors was suggested, also, by reports that there were proportionately more stutterers in the families of stutterers than in the family of non-stutterers. A composite of some of the earliest studies indicated that the relatives of stutterers were about four times as likely to have a history of stuttering than were the families of non-stutterers (Bryngelson and Rutherford, 1937; Wepman, 1939; Bryngelson, 1939). Similar findings have resulted from more recent studies though the proportion is slightly lower: these investigations of reported family incidence suggest that the relatives of stutterers are three times as likely to have a history of stuttering (Darley, 1955; Martyn and Sheehan, 1968;

Porfert and Rosenfield, 1978). No matter. The fact remains that the proportion is notably higher for stutterers than non-stutterers. Moreover, there is evidence that the incidence of stuttering in the family increases as the relationship to the stutterer becomes closer (Andrews and Harris, 1964; Johnson and Associates, 1959).

The tendency for there to be a greater history of stuttering in the family of stutterers than non-stutterers can, of course, result from cultural transmissions. The presence of a family history does not ensure genetic control. After all, religion and the language spoken at home also runs in families. But it is reasonable to assume that these would remain relatively constant, among the members of the immediate family. It is relatively unlikely, that is, that relatives would differ markedly in the proportional extent to which these and similar socially determined "traits" occur. With this in mind, it is instructive to look at the *frequency* of stutterers in the immediate family of stutterers. When we look at the first-degree relatives of stutterers we find that the incidence of stutterers increases. The incidence of those with a history of stuttering exceeds that found in the general population to a still greater extent than when the family unit includes a wider range of relatives. In addition, when the sex of both the stutterer and that of the members of the immediate family are considered it becomes clear that sex is an active variable. This conclusion flows from the fact that the incidence of stutterers among the first-degree male relatives (i.e., fathers, brothers, and sons) of male stutterers was 20 percent, while for the first-degree female relatives it was about 5 percent. When, on the other hand, we look at the immediate family of the female stutterer we find that their mothers, sisters, and daughters show an average incidence of about 13 percent while the male members of the immediate family have an incidence of 20 percent (Kidd, Heimbuch, and Records, 1981). It seems clear, then, that maleness in some way adds to the risk of being a stutterer. Whether stutterers are males or females, they have a greater proportion of affected male relatives in their immediate family.

The *risk factor* has been evaluated in a number of ways. One way involves analyzing the extent to which stuttering appears in the immediate family of an adult male stutterer when neither parent ever stuttered, when the father is or was a stutterer, and when the mother is or was a stutterer. When neither parent stuttered, the brothers and sons of the stutterer nevertheless were considerably more likely to stutter than their sisters and daughters. The percent of stutterers among these four members of the immediate family was 17, 21, 2, and 9, respectively. The risk was increased when the father stuttered. Now, 24 percent of the brothers and 35 percent of the sons of the male stutterer were also stutterers, and 10 percent of the sisters and daughters stuttered. When the adult stutterer was a female, similar results were obtained. Males in the immediate family were more likely to stutter than females. Moreover, if the father and his daughter stuttered, the risk to the rest of the immediate family was likely to be increased (Kidd, 1980).[2]

The risk data we have just been discussing can be looked at descriptively to get a general impression as to whether there is a meaningful difference in the percentage of stutterers in the immediate family of males and females who stutter. The data suggests that the difference is notable. For whether or not the parents stuttered, there

---

[2] Stuttering among the mothers of either males or females occurred too infrequently for a similar analysis to be made of the family risk factor.

was a greater percentage of siblings and children who stuttered in the family of the female stutterer than in that of the male stutterer. Approximately 24 percent of the immediate members of the female stutterers' family stuttered compared to 16 percent for the male stutterers. This tendency appears to be a reliable one; it is consistent with the findings that have shown that a significantly greater proportion of the immediate relatives of female stutterers are or have been stutterers than is the case for the immediate relatives of male stutterers (Kidd, Kidd, and Records, 1978).

The fact that there is *less* likelihood of stuttering among the relatives of male than female stutterers suggests differential susceptibility. It indicates that the male is more at risk and, therefore, more prone to genetic influences than is the female. This inference is supported by the fact that males have a higher probability of being stutterers. Taken together, these data have led to the conclusion that sex-modified inheritance plays a role in determining whether or not one becomes a stutterer. Specifically, it has been proposed that there is a genetically determined threshold for stuttering that is lower for males than females. It follows that because males have a greater liability, it takes less in the way of negative environmental factors for this threshold to be crossed. This theory exemplifies the way that genetic and environmental variables seemingly interact in determining whether or not one is likely to become a stutterer (Kidd, Kidd, and Records, 1978).

Using the differential threshold concept, two genetic-environmental models have been tested to see if they can help explain the family concentration of stuttering and the susceptibility to stuttering. Both models, ones that have been used in psychiatric genetics, fit the data well. Relative to the data we have been discussing, they met all of the criteria for sex-modified transmission. They also provided genetic correlations that were quite high. A multifactorial-polygeneic model fit the data particularly well. The model assumes that many genes contribute a small amount to the underlying susceptibility to stuttering. Interestingly, it "predicts that about 86 percent of the variation (measured as a variance) among individuals in whether or not they ever stutter is due to genetic variation . . . ." (Kidd, 1980, p. 197). Nongenetic influences, therefore, seem to account for but 14 percent of individual variability.

The fact that familial susceptibility seems to correlate more highly with genetic than nongenetic variables should not be overemphasized. The relative difference in the role that these variables appear to play may seem to be greater than it actually is. This is because the familial incidence data are confounded; environmental and genetic similarity could not be separated. Environmental factors may, as a result, have been inappropriately attributed to genetic control. This would, of course, lead to an overestimation of the genetic contribution to transmission. Conversely, cultural transmission to the risk of stuttering would be underestimated.

To a great extent, the confounding effect of familial similarity can be randomized out and so put aside by investigating the extent to which stuttering occurs in the families of adopted children who become stutterers. For these children there is no reason to believe that the family environments will be similar. We are, therefore, free to compare the incidence of stuttering in the families of adopted stutterers with the incidence in that of stutterers brought up in their own family. Of the twelve adopted stutterers who have so far been studied, only three have a history of stuttering in the adoptive family. Since about one to two thirds of the family members of non-adopted stutterers are likely to stutter, it appears evident that genetic elements do indeed affect transmission. However, the data make it equally clear that cultural elements play a meaningful role, and "that both heredity and environmental factors make their contribution to the familial incidence of stuttering. . . ." (Bloodstein, 1981, p. 102).

Still another way of determining the specific contribution of heredity to stuttering has been to control for rather than to randomize out environmental influences. If we can assume that the environment is essentially the same for both members of a twin pair this variable is taken care of. Environment is no longer a confounding variable. Now if we look at stutterers who are identical or fraternal twins and at the other member of the twin pairs we have the opportunity to assess more fully the impact of heredity. After all, identical twins share all their genes while, on the average, fraternal twins share only half of them. Thus, if the transmission of stuttering were totally dependent on genetic factor we would expect that both members of an identical pair would stutter, if one does. Among fraternal twins we would anticipate different results. The fact that one member of the twin pair stuttered would not necessarily mean that the other would. Indeed, if the transmission were polygenic it is likely that less than half would evidence stuttering.

The earliest published study involving both twin types showed that among identical pairs both members stuttered in nine out of the ten cases sampled. In contrast, among the thirty fraternal twins, stuttering was displayed by only two twin pairs. In twenty-eight of the pairs, the presence of stuttering in one member did not mean that the other also stuttered (Nelson, Hunter, and Walter, 1945). This finding does not stand alone, though the extent of concordancy among identical and fraternal twins does differ somewhat from study to study. Averaging across these studies, we find that among 78 percent of the identical twins, both members stuttered (concordancy) while for the fraternal twins discordancy was predominant. For the fraternal twins concordancy was present for only 9 percent of the pairs (Howie, 1981). Taken together, then, these studies suggest that genetic factors play a rather important role in stuttering. It must be pointed out, however, that stuttering in one member of an identical pair did not necessarily mean that stuttering would be displayed by the other member. In other words, whether or not one becomes a stutterer was not fully determined by genetic factors. They are necessary but not sufficient to explain the presence of stuttering. This conclusion rests, of course, on the accuracy with which the twins were classified as identical or fraternal and the validity of speech evaluation that led some speakers to be called stutterers and other non-stutterers. In early studies, for example, twin classification was often made by the so-called instantaneous identification method. The twins were compared with respect to observable features like hair color and texture, eye color and iris pattern, hand formation, skin color and texture. Sometimes, in addition, the twins' fingerprints were examined to see if the ridge patterns were alike or different (Nelson, Hunter, and Walter, 1945). Moreover, subjective means were used to determine if the members of the twin pairs were or were not stutterers. In addition, these determinations were not made in a way that was independent of knowledge about twin type (identical or fraternal) and were not based on specific diagnostic criteria. Thus, the findings could have been affected by experimental bias. These and other concerns have led to the conclusion that "little confidence can be placed in the results of the early studies" (Howie, 1981) and that the genetic issue revealed by studying twins needed to be reinvestigated. This has recently been done and with considerable care. Blood and tissue typing were among the means used to distinguish identical from fraternal twins. The diagnosis that the speaker was or was not a stutterer was made from listening to randomly ordered audio tapes, a standard definition of stuttering was utilized, and the diagnosis was checked against the mothers' reports about their children's speech. These efforts to achieve accuracy undoubtedly served to dampen whatever biasing effects might have been present in the previous studies. Nonetheless, the findings were similar. There was a considerably higher likelihood that both members of an identical twin pair stuttered, if one did, than was the case for fraternal twins. This difference among the twin groups was statistically significant. Moreover, the data indicated that the estimated risk of stuttering was .77 for the identical co-twin of a stutterer and .32 for a fraternal co-twin. Clearly, this is meaningful evidence of the import of genetic factors in transmission. But, probably as a result of the care taken to put aside biasing effects, the difference between the identical and fraternal twin groups was somewhat less imposing than before. The genetically identical co-twin of a stutterer did not necessarily stutter. This fact makes it evident that nongenetic factors also play a meaningful role in the etiology of stuttering. This conclusion flows from the fact that genetic factors were not, in themselves, sufficient to determine the presence of stuttering. Once again, then, the clinician must see that stuttering is best understood as a result of the interplay between genetic and environmental factors.

The Role of the Environment

We have seen that environmental factors of one kind or another must play a determinative role in the presence of stuttering. If they did not, the prevalence of stuttering would be essentially the same from culture to culture and era to era. It would also be relatively consistent from one socioeconomic level to another. But, as we shall see, this does not appear to be the case.

Observations make it evident that the prevalence of stuttering does vary, sometimes considerably. It differs among people, like those who are members of Western cultures and who therefore are thought to have at least certain similarities. It differs, too, among those whose cultures are widely different. Studies show that school age children in various European countries show a prevalence that ranges from a low of about .55 percent to a high of about 1.82 percent (Bloodstein, 1981). Studies involving more diverse cultures show an even greater disparity. For example, there is a marked difference in the prevalence of stuttering reportedly found among the Ute Indians, Malayans, and Polynesians, on the one hand, and the Idoma, Ibo, Kwakiutl peoples on the other. There appears to be little or no evidence of stuttering among the former while among the latter it is reportedly quite prevalent. Among the Idoma of West Africa, it has been said that stuttering is practically a mass phenomenon. Among the Ibo, another West African people, 2.67 percent of the school children were found to stutter. The Kwakiutl, like some other coastal Indians from the Pacific Northwest, also seem to have an inordinate number of stutterers in their tribe (Lemert, 1953).

It seems likely that the aforementioned differences in prevalence are, at least in part, related to environmental differences, since there were relatively few reports of stutterers in permissive and supportive societies. In contrast, the presence of stuttering was more likely to be observed in those societies in which there was marked competition, achievement motivation, conformity and/or communicative pressure (Lemert, 1953; Stewart, 1960).

The evidence that stuttering varies from one point in time to another and with socioeconomic variables is best considered circumstantial. Yet, clinical reports and some naturalistic observation suggest that they create at least some variability: It would seem, that is, that the prevalence of stuttering is not constant.

In sum, as we have seen, both heredity and environmental factors appear to interact in determining whether or not an individual will stutter. The specific heritable and environmental elements that are causative are, as we have said, not fully known. But, the clinician needs to keep in mind the risk-related factors we have discussed in this section. That is not to say that a person should be viewed as a stutterer merely because fluency failures are displayed and stutterers are numerous in the immediate family, or because he or she comes from a culture or subculture that appears to be associated with an increased likelihood of stuttering. But it does say that the clinician should be attuned to various speech and speech-associated variables that may serve to increase the accuracy of assessment. After all, probability is involved when the clinician indicates that one is or is not a stutterer and that therapy designed to enhance fluency will or will not be beneficial. It follows that the speech pathologist should use all available information to enhance prediction whether it deals with type of disorder or therapy recommendations. The hereditary and environmental elements that we have discussed will serve this purpose. So, too, do the data points provided by the various other variables that have been discussed throughout this chapter.

STUTTERING: NEUROPHYSIOLOGICAL ASPECTS

The hypothesis that people who stutter may be different from those who do not in terms of their neurophysiological structure and/or function has a long history. In fact, the so-called organic theories of stuttering are older than those that have suggested environmental causation for the disorder. A variety of structural anomalies have been thought to cause stuttering, involving organs such as the tongue, the hyoid bone, tonsils and uvula, hard palate, and brain. One of the ancient beliefs (held by Hippocrates in the fourth century, B.C.) was that stuttering was due to an accumulation of "black bile." That stuttering was either a form of aphasia or epilepsy was also a notion held in the not-too-distant past.

Although most of these beliefs are now discarded, research efforts to find organic causes, or at least bases of stuttering, have continued, and for justifiable reasons. First, there are a number of neurophysiological phenomena associated with stuttering, and a valid theory must explain them. Second, the fact that a given organic hypothesis has been abandoned does not mean that the hypothesis was necessarily false or that a more valid hypothesis of the same kind cannot be formulated. Third, development of sophisticated scientific instruments makes it possible to measure more complex and subtle neurophysiological processes, ones that may lead to startling new information. Indeed, the current surge of interest in the neurophysiological aspects of stuttering is partly a result of the opportunities provided by space-age technology. This is because it is now possible to observe more directly the functioning of long-suspected laryngeal and central neural structures.

Advances in methods of observation have resulted in refinements in the organically based hypotheses concerning stuttering. Few, if any, think that stuttering is due to some gross structural deviation in any of the mechanisms that are associated with speech. Current thinking focuses on subtle differences in the way some of the speech-related neurophysiological mechanisms seem to function differently for stutterers and nonstutterers under specific environmental conditions.

A thorough discussion of information resulting from neurophysiological research is outside the reach of this chapter. However, we will point out some of the current research trends and major findings that have resulted from the study of: (1) phonatory behaviors and laryngeal muscle activity; (2) neuromotor mechanisms; (3) cerebral dominance and hemispheric processing; (4) coordination among neuromotor systems; and (5) auditory mechanisms.

Phonatory Behaviors and Laryngeal Muscle Activity

When a sound is prolonged, repeated or abruptly stopped, as in stuttering, one can intuitively sense that the larynx is behaving in some abnormal manner. Laryngeal deviations have been a matter of speculation for a long time, but in recent years a number of investigators have tried to isolate specific types of deviations. Studies designed to determine if there are specific laryngeal deviations associated with dysfluent speech have been concerned with, among other things, *phonatory reaction time* and *laryngeal muscle activity*.

Phonatory reaction time. *Phonatory reaction time* refers to the shortest duration of time required to initiate and terminate phonation upon a given signal. Some studies have shown that *on the average*, adult stutterers take more time than normal speakers to initiate and terminate phonation, even when the utterance is fluent. On the other hand, there is some evidence that young children whose only speech problem is stuttering may not show delayed phonatory reaction time (Cullinan and Springer, 1980). Normal reaction time in stuttering children, if supported by additional research, would not support the hypothesis that slow phonatory reaction *causes* stuttering. Rather, it would suggest that phonatory slowness may be an *effect* of stuttering.

Laryngeal Muscle Activity. *Laryngeal muscle activity* is another area of investigation which has produced some new information in recent years. That stuttered speech might involve abnormalities of certain laryngeal muscles has been suspected for a long time. In recent years development of sophisticated instruments, such as a fiberscope that allows a direct superior view of the larynx, has made it possible to observe laryngeal activity. Other techniques used in the analysis of the laryngeal muscle activity include cineradiography and electromyography. These techniques have made it possible to verify the long-held view that the laryngeal muscle behaviors during the production of fluent and dysfluent speech are different. Some of the earlier studies have shown that stuttering is associated with irregular vocal fold vibration, inconsistent and unpredictable glottal openings, absence of voicing during glottal activity, and tight closure of the laryngeal opening (Chevrie-Muller, 1963; Fujita, 1966; Ushijima et al., 1965; Freeman, 1974). A number of other deviations have been described recently. For example, Freeman and Ushijima (1978) using electromyography to pick up, amplify, and record the electrical activity of muscles, found that during stuttering laryngeal muscles are unusually active. Electromyographic tracings suggested that stuttering was associated with excessive tension in the laryngeal muscles. They also observed that sometimes muscles that have opposing actions were active simultaneously. A laryngeal abductor (posterior cricoarytenoid), for example, which pulls the two vocal folds *apart* and a laryngeal adductor (thyroarytenoid) which pulls them *together* may both be active at the same time. During production of fluent speech, however, these muscles were found to be active in a more normal, reciprocal manner.

As can be expected, a question often raised is whether such laryngeal abnormalities are a cause of stuttering. Although some investigators are inclined to think that abnormal laryngeal muscle activities may cause stuttering, it may be more appropriate to consider them as part of the *effect* we call stuttering. Excessive muscle tension and stuttering are evidently simultaneous. Both tension and stuttering seem to be part of a single event, dysfluent speech production. As pointed out by Freeman (1974), abnormal laryngeal behaviors may be considered a disrupted physiological aspect of stuttering.

Neuromotor Mechanisms

Since normal speech production is a neuromotor phenomenon, the hypothesis that there might be something wrong with the neuromotor mechanisms or functions of people who stutter has often been investigated. This hypothesis has been put to test with respect to general motor performance and speech-specific neuromotor systems.

Many of the early investigators analyzed the general motor ability of stutterers and non-stutterers. A variety of motor tasks, including foot tapping, card sorting, bean bag tossing, and gymnastic exercises have been investigated (see Bloodstein, 1981, and St. Louis, 1979 for reviews). The results of these studies have been contradictory. While some have found that people who stutter are less proficient in executing certain motor tasks, other studies have found them to be more proficient than those who do not stutter.

Many studies have simply not uncovered a significant difference in the performance of those who stutter and those who do not. Moreover, it can be argued that motor tasks such as bean bag tossing, carrying a full glass of water, or foot tapping are not relevant to a meaningful analysis of stuttering and non-stuttering behaviors. An analysis of the neuromotor functions directly involved in the production of speech seems to be particularly relevant, however. That appears to be why, at this time, investigators are analyzing speech-related aspects of the neuromotor systems of stutterers. We will summarize the major findings concerning two speech-related neuromotor functions: *respiration and aerodynamics*, and *neuromotor articulatory dynamics*.

Respiration and Aerodynamics. *Respiration and aerodynamic* studies have analyzed the way stutterers manage their breath stream when they are fluent and dysfluent. These initially resulted from the simple observation that during stuttering there is often improper management of the breath stream. Since the 1930s various pneumographic investigations have made it evident that abnormal *respiratory* behaviors, such as a lack of rhythmic reciprocity between inhalation and exhalation, attempts to speak on residual air, inhalations and exhalations interrupted by each other, simultaneous and opposing movements of abdomen and thorax, spasms and tremors of the speech musculature, lower vital capacities, reduced air volumes, and shallow breathing may be associated with stuttering. Some stutterers may not show any of these abnormalities. Others may show most of them.

More recent investigations of the breath stream management of stutterers for the purposes of speech production have often been described as *aerodynamic* studies. Some of these studies have shown that stutterers may not be able to modulate intraoral air pressure during speech production. Production of different speech sounds and sylla-bles in different phonetic contexts require frequent, quick, and subtle adjustments of air pressure in the oral region. Stutterers may be slow in making such adjustments or they may be unable to make certain kinds of adjustments. A common finding of a few studies is that stutterers tend to have a very high intraoral air pressure during the production of dysfluencies. In other words, they seem to impound more air than is required to produce speech within the oral region. There is also some indication that different forms of dysfluency may be associated with deviations in intraoral air pressure that are different (Hutchinson and Brown, 1978).

Neuromotor Articulatory Dynamics. *Neuromotor articulatory dynamics* refer pri-marily to the movement of the various organs and mechanisms involved in speech production. Studies of articulation (movement) have also been undertaken in order to analyze the possible neural controls involved in such movements. When a stutterer repeats a sound, a syllable or even a word, or when he or she prolongs a sound, it would appear that there is a difficulty in moving on to the next target sound, syllable, or word. Therefore, several investigators have tested the hypothesis that people who stutter may be slower than the normal speakers in executing efficient movement of the articulators in rapid succession. Studies in the past have examined stutterers' ability to produce certain speech sounds or syllables (such as /t/ or pa-ta-ka) repeatedly and rapidly, and have compared their rate to that of the normal speakers. In addition, the speed with which rhythmic movements of jaw, tongue, and lips are achieved has been analyzed. In general, a number of studies have shown that stutterers are slower than the normal speakers on tasks such as these.

Articulatory performance studies in recent years have become more sophisticated. These studies have involved an analysis of both the movement patterns of the peripheral speech organs and the integrity of the higher neuromotor systems involved in the control of speech. Techniques such as cineradiography, which provides motion pictures of the behaviors of the speech mechanisms through X-rays, have been used to follow complex movement patterns. As a result of studies of this kind, it has become apparent that even the perceptually fluent productions of stutterers involved different neuromotor organizations than the fluent production of non-stutterers (Zimmerman, 1980a). The stutterers were found to be slower than the normal speakers in initiating movement of the speech organs. After the movement was initiated, they took more time to move on to the next target, resulting in longer transition times. Perhaps as a result, stutterers showed longer steady states (lack of movement). It was also apparent that even though some speech organs had begun their motion, voice onset lagged behind. Stutterers also showed lower peak velocities and smaller displacement when compared to nonstutterers. In addition, the lip and jaw movements were uncoordi-nated. The magnitude of such articulatory deviations were small, but they do suggest that the spatio-temporal organization of movement necessary for speech is deviant in speakers who stutter. More importantly, such deviations may be found even when stutterers produce what appears to be fluent speech. It has been suggested, therefore, that stuttering is basically a disorder of movement (Zimmerman, 1980b). It is hypoth-esized that an unstable neuromotor system can induce oscillations, fixations, and tonic behaviors.

It must be noted that the articulatory deviations that we have just described are not necessarily the causes of stuttering. Though deviations in movement factors appear to be present it is not yet fully clear whether they are the cause of or concomitants of stuttering. In addition, the fact that there are movement deviations does not minimize the possible importance of environmental, emotional, and conditioning factors which might play a role in the etiology of stuttering.

Cerebral Dominance and Hemispheric Processing

One of the major theories of the first few decades of this century held that stuttering was due to a lack of clear-cut cerebral dominance for speech (Orton & Travis, 1929). It was partly based on the then-current belief that speech is controlled by the left hemisphere of the brain for most right-handed and some left-handed persons. In other words, for the purposes of speech, the left hemisphere is typically dominant. If, for whatever the reason, the left hemisphere is not dominant, the right hemisphere might interfere with the normal regulation of speech functions and thus cause stuttering. In the past, a person's handedness was considered a sure sign of cerebral dominance. Right-handedness indicated the presence of left cerebral dominance for speech. This was considered typical. Left-handedness, on the other hand, suggested that motor control for speech was determined by the right hemisphere.

In recent years, it once more seems possible that cerebral dominance for language may play a role in the etiology of stuttering, a result of the flow of data from procedures that have recently been devised to determine cerebral dominance for language. Prominent among these are dichotic listening, the Wada, and the assessment of the hemispheric alpha wave activity. In addition, investigators are currently analyzing hemispheric processing of linguistic and nonlinguistic material: it seems likely that most right-handed individuals whose speech is normal process language in the left hemisphere, while the right hemisphere appears to process nonlinguistic material such as music.

When dichotic listening is employed to test for dominance, different verbal stimuli are simultaneously presented to the left and right ear and the individual is asked to report what is heard. Most normal speakers seem to hear what is presented to the right ear better than what is simultaneously presented to the left ear (Sommers, Brady, and Moore, 1975). This fact suggests that, for the normal speakers, the left hemisphere is dominant in the processing of linguistic information. Some stutterers, on the other hand, heard the word that was presented to the left ear (Sommers et al., 1975; Hall and Jerger, 1978), which implies that they were processing the linguistic information in the right hemisphere.

Both linguistic and nonlinguistic stimuli have been used in dichotic listening studies. However, a difference between the performance of stutterers and non-stutterers was more likely to emerge when the stimuli were meaningful linguistic material. It must be noted, however, that in almost every dichotic listening study, there were some stutterers who performed essentially as the non-stutterers did. There was not a clean separation in the performance of subject groups in several other studies (Slorach and Noehr, 1973; Brady and Berson, 1975).

The relative extent to which hemispheric alpha wave activity is present gives an indication of the degree to which the two hemispheres are involved in processing speech. An electroencephalographic (EEG) procedure for recording the electrical activity of the brain has been used by a few investigators to analyze the relative amounts of alpha wave activity in the right and the left hemispheres when verbal and nonverbal stimuli are presented. The results suggest that stutterers might process *both* linguistic and nonlinguistic stimuli in their right hemisphere (Moore and Haynes, 1980). Since most non-stutterers process linguistic information in their left hemisphere, this would seem to indicate that stutterers process linguistic material in their "wrong" hemisphere.

In sum, it seems as if there is some evidence that language processing for stutterers and non-stutterers differs. For stutterers, the right hemisphere may be involved to a greater extent than the left hemisphere. In interpreting these results, one should exercise some caution. Even if these data are reliable, they do not necessarily suggest a purely neurophysiological interpretation of stuttering because it is now known that there are individual differences in hemispheric processing strategies, which appear to be a result of an individual's experience history. For instance, there is some evidence that professional musicians are unlike most people. They process musical information in their left hemisphere (Gates and Bradshaw, 1977). Sex difference in hemispheric processing is also known to exist. It seems likely, then, that a person's history and background have at least some influence on where the linguistic and nonlinguistic information is processed.

Coordination Between Different Neuromotor Systems

Another line of neurophysiologically oriented research has led to still a different perspective on stuttering. Some studies by Perkins and his associates have indicated that if an organic deviation does exist among stutterers, it may *not* be found in any particular neurophysiological system or function (Perkins, et al. 1976, 1979). In other words, the laryngeal, phonatory, or respiratory function of stutterers by itself may be perfectly normal. In fact, analysis of isolated neurophysiological systems have not produced convincing evidence of pathology among stutterers. Nevertheless, when different systems have to function in a smoothly coordinated fashion, problems might arise.

Evidently, speech production is an activity that requires a very high degree of coordination between different but highly complex neuromotor functions. Furthermore, such coordinations have to be achieved rapidly, continuously, and in a sequence where different actions shift and converge in quick succession. To begin with, the speaker needs to manage the breathstream with proper flow and pressure characteristics for the purposes of generating phonation. Then, the laryngeal mechanism must respond with appropriate abductory, adductory, and vibratory actions. Moreover, certain properties of mass, elasticity, and viscosity must be present for adequate phonatory behaviors to result. Finally, the phonation so generated must be modulated with subtle but rapid intraoral air pressure changes and the movements of the articulators such as the tongue, the lips, and the jaw. Thus, normal fluent speech is not a function of any single neurophysiological system; it is a product of coordinated action of different systems. This observation inevitably raises the question as to whether or not there is some central involvement associated with stuttering. Different neurophysiological processes are regulated by the central nervous system and, therefore, any hypothesis of discoordination would necessarily suggest an as yet unspecified dysfunction in the central control of speech mechanisms.

The observation that stutterers are relatively fluent when they speak in a very slow rate appears to support the hypothesis that it is the rapidity with which different neuromotor systems need to be coordinated that can create problems. More specifically, Perkins and his associates have shown that when the process of speech production is systematically simplified, there is progressively greater fluency. In one study (Perkins et al., 1976), stutterers were observed under three different production conditions: normal voice, whispered speech, and articulation without phonation. In the last condition, where the stutterers simply "lipped" the words without phonation, the need to coordinate phonation with respiration was eliminated. Both whispered and "lipped" speech contained significantly less stuttering than was present in the voiced speech condition. However, the stutterers were most fluent in the lipped condition where the simplest form of output was required. In a subsequent study, Perkins et al. (1979) showed that slowing down the rate at which phones (sounds) are produced results in much greater fluency than a rate in which individual words spoken per unit of time is slowed. From results such as these, Perkins et al. (1976, 1979) have concluded that when the complexity of coordinations between different functions increases, stuttering also increases.

The evidence concerning the discoordination of speech-related neuromotor systems, like other kinds of evidence on possible organic dysfunctions, does not necessarily imply exclusive organic causes of stuttering. They may not even suggest any kind of organic cause at all, since many of the neurophysiological dysfunctions or discoordinations that are seemingly present may be a part of the stuttering itself. Specifically, it has been pointed out that "discoordination of elements of speech does not cause stuttering, it is the stuttering" (Perkins, et al., 1976, p. 510). There is as yet no evidence to rule out the possibility that neuromotor dysfunctions and discoordinations may be learned behaviors or that they are a result of conditioned anxiety reactions that are disruptive of the complex speech production process. Other possibilities cannot be ruled out, either. Some causal factors might emerge when research studies address the question as to why stutterers display neuromotor deviations and discoordinations.

Auditory Mechanisms

The hypothesis that stuttering may somehow be related to the hearing mechanism is an old one. Early on, it was reported that congenitally deaf persons do not stutter (Bluemel, 1913). However, it is not clear whether the deaf persons observed were even capable of oral communication. Clearly, a certain level of oral communicative skill would have to be present before dysfluencies could be exhibited. Whether or not these skills were present, the belief that the deaf do not stutter prevailed for a number of years. Some years later, however, it became evident that stuttering does indeed exist among the deaf who are capable of oral communication. Investigators who sent out questionnaires to various schools for the deaf found out that in each school there were at least a few stutterers (Voelker and Voelker, 1937; Harms and Malone, 1939). These studies on the prevalence of stuttering among the deaf once more raised the question as to whether or not there is some link between the hearing mechanism and stuttering.

Over the years several different lines of investigation have seemed to show a relationship between the auditory mechanism and stuttering. The current interest in this relationship has nothing to do with deafness or hearing impairment, however. Investigators are now trying to analyze subtle differences in the way the hearing mechanism functions for stutterers and non-stutterers. Studies have been designed to investigate whether or not some aspect of the auditory mechanism plays a role in the etiology of stuttering. The major findings of these studies will be summarized.

Delayed Auditory Feedback. It is usually assumed that not only normal hearing is required for the acquisition of speech and language but that instantaneous feedback of speech is needed for efficient self-monitoring of speech production. We normally hear our own speech instantaneously. Immediate feedback helps us regulate our speech so that we can, for example, correct occasional errors of articulation and prosody. There is plenty of research evidence which shows that a delay in auditory feedback, introduced mechanically, has certain effects on the speech of stutterers as well as non-stutterers. In the beginning it was thought that DAF (delayed auditory feedback) produces stuttering in normal speakers and fluency in stutterers. This suggested the possibility that the auditory feedback mechanism of stutterers was making an error that somehow was corrected by a delayed feedback. The result was fluency. Recent research has shown that disruptions found in the speech of normal speakers under DAF are not exactly the same as those observed in stutterers.

The possibility exists that the fluency enhancement that stutterers' tend to experience under DAF may be a function of the fact that it generates a slower rate of speech. This seems to be the case. Without the help of DAF, stutterers' rate of speech can be slowed down. This usually results in a more deliberate production of speech and somewhat increased fluency. DAF also produces an increase in pitch and loudness and it is known that when stutterers alter these vocal aspects (with or without DAF) fluency is improved to some extent. Thus, although it is evident that DAF has some beneficial effect on stuttering, the exact mechanism of that effect is still a matter of controversy.

The White Noise Effect. The possibility that the auditory mechanism is somehow involved in stuttering was suggested by the finding that when stutterers' hearing is masked by high intensity noise they tend to be rather fluent (Shane, 1955; Cherry, Sayers and Marland, 1955). Initially, it was thought that under masking noise, stutterers were unable to hear their own speech. Subsequent studies have shown that stuttering decreases even when the noise levels are low enough to permit auditory perception of speech (Maraist and Hutton, 1957). In more recent years, it has been suggested that an increase in vocal intensity, which is typically associated with speech under masking noise, may be responsible for fluency (Adams and Hutchinson, 1974). But some studies have shown that a mere increase in vocal intensity in the absence of noise does not produce fluency (Garber and Martin, 1977). There is some evidence that in under masking noise, stutterers tend to increase their syllable durations, which in turn may reduce stuttering (Brayton and Conture, 1978). There are other hypotheses, but none appear to be fully supported by evidence.

The Metronome Effect. When stutterers pace the utterance of syllables or words to the beat of a metronome, they are remarkably fluent. Since the metronomic beats are obviously rhythmic, it has been proposed that an externally imposed rhythm is the basis of this effect. There is some evidence which suggests that rhythmicity is at least partly responsible for reduced stuttering. Some studies have shown that rhythmic beats have a greater effect on stuttering than arhythmic beats (Azrin, Jones, and

Flye, 1968). It must be recognized that the metronome effect may not have anything to do with the auditory mechanism at all. After all, tactile and visual rhythmic stimuli can also reduce stuttering (Azrin, Jones and Flye, 1968). In fact, any manner of speaking that is unusual for a given stutterer can reduce stuttering. Like many other phenomena associated with stuttering, the metronome effect is yet to be fully explained.

Central Auditory Functions. Another line of investigation has led some to suggest that while the auditory mechanism of stutterers may be normal, the central auditory mechanism may not be (Hall and Jerger, 1978). In other words, it may be the cortical functions involved in auditory perception that may be abnormal. Central auditory problems are usually not evident on pure tone hearing tests which might reveal normal thresholds. In recent years, a series of special tests have been devised to assess central auditory functions.

Many of these tests involve perceptual processing of distorted and competing speech stimuli. The results of investigations of the central auditory functioning in stutterers are somewhat contradictory. While some studies have indicated a possible central auditory dysfunction, others have failed to find such dysfunction (Gregory, 1979; Karr, 1977; Hall and Jerger, 1978). It should be noted that the dichotic listening studies that we have previously discussed do suggest the involvement of the central auditory mechanism in stuttering. Most investigators have emphasized that whatever the involvement of the central auditory mechanism, it is very subtle. There is no evidence of any gross cortical pathology relative to the perceptual processing of complex auditory stimuli in stutterers. In fact, on a number of tests, some stutterers have performed just as well as non-stutterers. Those stutterers who did not perform as well as non-stutterers have done so only on particular central auditory tests.

Other Variables

There are a few other conditions that may or may not be auditory in nature that affect stuttering frequency. It is known that stutterers are usually fluent while they sing in a chorus or by themselves. Stuttering is also reduced when stutterers "shadow" another person reading aloud. That is, when stutterers read aloud, but slightly after, the reading of another person, they are usually more fluent. Why this is the case, why singing and shadowing reduce stuttering has been a matter of speculation for a long time. Evidently, both are novel forms of speech. Stuttering is typically not acquired in the context of singing or shadowing. Singing involves rhythm, and we know that rhythm induces fluency. In addition, singing refers to a highly "rehearsed" form of behavior and there is some suggestion that rehearsal induces fluency. Shadowing, on the other hand, involves both cueing and a certain degree of masking. When someone reads aloud with the stutterer, cues are provided that in some way serve as an aid. It is possible that these two elements, along with others, are responsible for fluency in shadowing.

STUTTERING: LINGUISTIC PROPERTIES

An early line of investigation was concerned with the loci of stutterings in the speech sequence and the structural-linguistic properties of words typically stuttered. Research studies concerning the loci of stutterings were designed to determine where in the sequence of continuous speech or oral reading stutterings were more likely to occur. Several other studies were designed to analyze the phonological and grammatical characteristics of stuttered words. Some studies were also concerned with meaning in language and how it affected stuttering frequency. Evidently, all of these studies were concerned with one or the other aspect of language and its relation to stuttering.

One of the earliest studies on the loci of stuttering was made by Johnson and Brown (1935). Subsequently, a series of reports on various linguistic aspects of stuttering was published by Brown (1937, 1938a, b, 1945). In more recent years, additional studies have been reported by speech pathologists, psychologists, and linguists. The results of most of these studies are fairly consistent. We will highlight the major research findings on the phonological, morphological, grammatical, and semantic properties of stuttering.

Phonological Properties

Research has shown that stuttering is more likely to occur on the initial sounds of words. Even young children's stutterings tend to occur on the initial sounds. Most investigators have found 92 to 100 percent of stutterings occur on the initial sounds of words (Johnson and Brown, 1935; Hahn, 1942; Sheehan, 1974). This phonological property was evident even when stutterers read nonsense words or single words one at a time. Thus, stutterers are far more likely to say *"stu, stu, stuttering* than *stuttering, ring, ring."* Similarly, prolongation of an initial sound such as the /f/ in the word "fall" is very common, but the prolongation of a final sound in any word is very rare.

Another phonological property of stuttering is referred to as the *consonant-vowel* distinction. On the average, stuttering tends to occur on consonants rather than vowels (Sheehan, 1974; Silverman and Williams, 1967; Taylor, 1966). However, stuttering does occasionally involve vowels, and, for some stutterers, a majority of their fluency failures are on vowels. Thus, as a phonological property, the consonant-vowel distinction is not as strong as the initial sound property described above. Furthermore, it must be noted that no particular set of consonants has been found to be consistently associated with stuttering in a majority of stutterers. An individual stutterer, however, may typically stutter on certain consonants, but consistently stuttered consonants can be different from stutterer to stutterer (St. Louis and Martin, 1976).

Morphological Properties

The term morphological is used here to describe factors relating to the structure of individual words. Are there structure-related properties of words that increase the frequency of stuttering? From a subjective standpoint, most stutterers feel that some words are more difficult than others. Research in this area has shown that the length of words is significantly associated with a higher frequency of stuttering. Generally speaking, longer words tend to be stuttered more frequently than shorter words (Brown and Moren, 1942; Oxtoby, 1955; Trotter, 1951; Soderberg, 1967). This tendency seems to hold for oral reading as well as for conversational speech. It holds for elementary school children as well as for adults (Williams et al., 1969).

It has been suggested that longer words are stuttered more often because they are more difficult to articulate than shorter words (Bloodstein, 1981). It has also been hypothesized that longer words may carry more information or meaning which may somehow increase the probability of stuttering (Schlesinger et al., 1965). It is also known that sound durations are shortened in multi-syllabic words. This places on the speech mechanism added demands for speed and coordination of movements.

Word frequency, the extent to which a word occurs, is also known to be a significant linguistic aspect of frequently stuttered words. This is not strictly a morphological variable. Instead, it refers to the fact that some words are used more frequently in language than others. Generally, studies have indicated that words that are used less frequently are stuttered more often than those that are used more frequently. It should be noted, however, that there is a high positive correlation between the probability of stuttering on various parts of speech and their frequency of usage in the English language (Wischner, 1950), indicating that the relationship between frequency of usage and stuttering is anything but simple. Indeed, it suggests that the relationship is curvilinear: in other words, both infrequently used words and words which have a greater probability of being spoken dysfluently because of their frequent use, are more likely to be stuttered.

A note of caution is in order since the linguistic properties of stuttering that we have been discussing are hard to separate. If two properties cannot be separated, or simply were not separated in a given study, then the effect observed may be due to either one of them, or both of them. We cannot be sure about their independent effect, so confounding occurs. Take, for example, the two observations that longer words and words of low frequency are stuttered more often than shorter and high frequency words. It is known that longer words tend to be used less frequently and vice versa, indicating that most of the times when the effect of longer words are analyzed, the effects of low frequency of usage are also involved. Thus, longer words may be stuttered more frequently because they are used less frequently, or low frequency words are stuttered more often because they are just longer. This type of confounding is common with regard to several linguistic variables.

Grammatical Properties

Various grammatical properties have been analyzed to see if some induce more stuttering than others. Research has demonstrated that word position, grammatical class, and grammatical complexity constitute significant linguistic aspects of frequently stuttered words.

The position of a word in a given sentence seems to affect whether or not a word is stuttered. In general, studies have shown that the first three words of a sentence tend to be stuttered more often than the subsequent words (Brown, 1938a; Oxtoby, 1955; Trotter, 1951; Silverman and Williams, 1967). The probability of stuttering is highest for the first word of a sentence and lowest for the very last word. Although this trend seems to be fairly consistent when the task is oral reading, there is some question as to whether it holds for conversational speech. Some investigators have failed to notice a position effect when they analyzed the conversational speech of stutterers (Hejna, 1955).

Word position is an active variable for children as well as adults. Indeed, it has been shown that stuttering as well as non-stuttering young children tend to have more dysfluencies on the initial words (Williams et al., 1969). It has been reported, also, that words at the beginning of a grammatical clause are more likely to be stuttered than those at the end of clauses (Bloodstein and Gantwerk, 1967).

The grammatical class to which words belong seems to be a factor of some importance in the occurrence of stuttering. Two grammatical categories have been researched frequently. The first category of words, called *content* words, includes adjectives, nouns, adverbs, verbs, etc. The second is the *function* category which includes pronouns, conjunctions, prepositions, articles, and so on. A number of early studies led to the finding that, for adults, content words are stuttered more often than function words (Brown, 1945; Hahn, 1942; Oxtoby, 1955; Trotter, 1951). The validity of this observation was questioned because careful analysis made it clear that there are more content words that start with consonants than with vowels and that there are more function words that start with vowels than with consonants. In addition, more function words are found in the initial position of sentences and clauses. Therefore, the reported differences among the categories that were reported early on may be more apparent than real. The observed differences in stuttering frequency on content and function words may be due either to the consonant-vowel distinction, to the position factor, or even to some other variable (Taylor, 1966).

Very young stutterers do not appear to experience more fluency failures on content words than on function words. In fact, young stutterers have been shown to be more dysfluent on function words, particularly conjunctions and pronouns, than on content words (Bloodstein and Gantwerk, 1967; Fisher, 1977). Non-stuttering young children also experience more dysfluencies on pronouns and conjunctions (function words). However, adult non-stutterers, like adult stutterers, seem to be more dysfluent on content words than on function words. This has led to a speculation that as both stutterers and non-stutterers grow older, there is a shift in the pattern of their dysfluencies as it relates to the content-function distinction. For the very young, dysfluencies tend to occur on function words. For adults, they tend to occur on content words.

The grammatical complexity of sentences appears to be another variable that affects the probability of stuttering. There is a tendency for stuttering to be more likely on sentences that are grammatically more complex than on those that are less complex (Hannah and Gardner, 1968). In addition, there is some evidence which suggests that more stuttering occurs on negative sentences (e.g., "the kindergarten teacher didn't help the seven new children") than on simple declarative sentences (Ronson, 1976). Still, more stuttering occurs on sentences that involve the passive form (e.g., "the seven new children were helped by the kindergarten teacher").

Semantic Properties

Early on it was theorized that meaning plays a determinative role in the occurrence of stuttering. It was suggested that the greater the responsibility to communicate meaningful speech, the higher the probability of stuttering (Eisenson, 1975). This position was probably prompted by a number of observations that relate to the variability of stuttering in different situations. It is well known that stutterers typically exhibit more stuttering in some situations than in others. For example, most stutterers are relatively fluent while talking with small children and close friends. They can also be very fluent while talking to their pet animals or to themselves. The same persons can be very dysfluent while talking before a group of people and to their bosses or persons in any kind of authority. It has been assumed that situations that are associated with a high degree of dysfluencies demand a high degree of communicative responsibility and propositional (meaningful) speech (Eisenson, 1975).

Specific studies designed to test the hypothesis that meaning is a significant factor in stuttering have produced inconsistent results. One study has shown that stutterers exhibit more dysfluencies while reading a meaningful passage than a selection of nonsense syllables (Eisenson and Horowitz, 1945). Another has shown no significant difference in the frequency of dysfluencies evoked by meaningful and meaningless passages (Hegde, 1970). It now appears doubtful that meaning as such is an important variable associated with dysfluencies.

Information theory has led to a different line of investigation into the possible relationship between meaning in language and the frequency of stuttering. Information theory, as it is applied to language in general, holds that both in written and verbal communication some words carry more meaning than others. Words that carry less meaning are redundant. Through sophisticated statistical procedures, it is possible to determine the relative amounts of information (or meaning) carried by individual words. A few studies have shown that words with a relatively high information load are stuttered more often than those that have a low information load (Quarrington, 1965; Schlesinger et al., 1965; Taylor, 1966). The picture is complicated, however, by the fact that high information words are typically longer than low information words. It is also known that longer words are used less frequently in communication than are shorter words. It is possible, therefore, that some words are stuttered more frequently than others not because they carry more meaning or information, but because they are relatively long and are used less frequently.

To summarize, words that are stuttered more frequently have certain structural-linguistic properties: stuttered words are usually found in the first few positions in a sentence; they are more likely to begin with a consonant than with a vowel; it is the initial sound of a word that is stuttered more frequently than are subsequent sounds; stuttered words are predominantly function words for very young stutterers and content words for adults who stutter; and they may also be longer and less frequently used words.

THERAPY: A CHANGING VIEW OF BEHAVIOR CHANGE TACTICS

As we have seen, the cause of stuttering is not known. This does not mean that there are not theories about the cause of stuttering. The contrary is true. Explanations about how stuttering comes about abound. Moreover, these theoretical frameworks are often quite different from each other. It follows that they tend to suggest therapeutic strategies and specific tactics that differ in kind. This is not always the case. Sometimes therapeutic procedures develop a popularity that cuts across theoretical positions and underlying assumptions. But more frequently, the clinical procedures that therapists use have a rather fundamental relationship to the theoretical position to which they subscribe. As Johnson has pointed out, "the particular theory we favor does influence us in the decisions we make as to what to do. . . ." (1967, p. 291). It follows, therefore, that we need to know the assumptions that are basic to a theory and that serve to guide therapeutic decision making.

Johnson: A Semantic Framework

As we have seen, Johnson did not view stuttering as synonymous with dysfluency. All people, he observed, are dysfluent. Some display more dysfluencies than others just as some are better or poorer at dancing, golf, tennis, or bowling. The important issue, from his point of view, was that there is no form of dysfluency that the stutterer displays that is not also evidenced by the non-stutterer. Indeed, Johnson stressed that stutterers and non-stutterers show considerable overlap in both total amount of dysfluency and in each of the various forms of fluency failure. As a result, he concluded that dysfluency and stuttering are not one and the same.

What, then, did Johnson consider to be stuttering? It was, from his point of view, an avoidance of normal dysfluency that results from the inappropriate reactions and judgments made by overly sensitive listeners. The negative reactions from parents, teachers, family, friends, and relatives, serve to motivate the child to avoid the very same behaviors that non-stuttering peers tend to display. It is this avoidance, then, and not dysfluency that distinguishes the stutterer from the non-stutterer. Normal speakers don't avoid dysfluency. They take it in stride. It is not a notable event.

Stuttering then is a particular kind of avoidance behavior. Stuttering is an "anticipatory, apprehensive, hypertonic, avoidance reaction" (Johnson, 1956, p. 217). In other words, stuttering is what the stutterer does when expecting difficulty in a particular speech situation or on a specific word or sound: he or she becomes concerned and tenses the respiratory, phonatory, and/or articulatory musculature that play a role in the act of speaking. What the stutterer does, then, to avoid difficulty *is* the difficulty. It leads to abnormal speech production.

Certain assumptions underlie the Johnsonian definition of stuttering, and these gave form to his approach to therapy. A basic notion of his was that dysfluency is normal and that it should not be confused with stuttering. It follows that therapy was not directed at dysfluencies. Another is that the heart of the problem, the motive force for avoidance, is the anticipation of speech interruption. Because of the overly sensitive reactions of listeners, the speaker develops inappropriate concerns about dysfluencies. An important aspect of therapy, then, is the reduction of concern that stutterers have about dysfluency and their ability to speak normally.

Dysfluency related concern was dealt with, in part, by having the client carefully observe the speech of normal speakers. This tactic served to make it apparent that dysfluencies are not something that only stutterers display; it is not their sole property. Normal speakers display dysfluencies, too. It followed that dysfluency is normal and not something to be feared or avoided.

Another element of Johnson's approach to the perceptual and evaluative reorientation of the stutterer involved the purposive display of dysfluency. For a number of years, stutterers were asked to practice being dysfluent in various circumstances. This served a dual function. It made evident the fact that listeners were not as concerned about dysfluency as the stutterer had anticipated and it reduced the drive to avoid dysfluencies.

The stutterers' worry that they are not able to speak normally, that they speak in a disorganized way because there is something physically wrong with their speech mechanism or because heredity dictates it, was also attacked by Johnson's clinical procedures. The concern about the ability to speak normally was directly dealt with by demonstrating that they were indeed able to speak without stuttering. To accomplish this, it was pointed out that stutterers tend to be fluent when they speak aloud while alone, talk in a rhythmic way (for example, to the beat of a metronome or the swing of an arm), sing, and whisper or talk in the presence of masking. Their ability to speak normally in these and other circumstances was used to dispel the clients' belief that normal speech is a physical impossibility. It served to provide stutterers not only with confidence in their ability to speak normally but also with the motivation to begin work on those things they do that interfere with speech.

It was Johnson's position that stuttering is purposive, that it is the misguided attempt to avoid dysfluency. It was his contention that stutterers would be normal speakers if they were not concerned about dysfluencies and would not try to avoid them. From his point of view, stutterers had to learn that stuttering is not something that happens to them but something *they* do. They had to understand that their behavior is not a condition. They had to come to know precisely what it was that they did when they stuttered. They had to learn their role in undoing these maladaptive habits. Toward these ends stutterers, whose habit patterns were well established, were required to observe and carefully analyze what it is they did when they stuttered. They were given support as they faced up to their struggle behaviors and learned to speak with less and less tension and effort. The stutterers learned to contrast what it was that went on when their speech was fluent and what occurred when stuttering was displayed. This aided the stutterer in problem-solving; it gave the direction needed for modifying what was done so that "the benevolent spiral of smoother and easier speech leading to speech still smoother and more easy . . . is attained" (Johnson, 1967, p. 310). The object was to reduce and simplify the tension reactions, the struggle behaviors, that interfere with speech. Awareness was a fundamental aspect of these endeavors. And it was the awareness that stuttering was not uncontrollable, that it was something that one does, that it was modifiable, that led to a decrease in the anticipation of difficulty. Speech associated anxiety, the force that motivated avoidance, decreased as the stutterer learned to speak with less and less struggle. In a stepwise fashion the stutterer, it was hoped, would thus learn to speak as the normal speaker does, as he or she did when not stuttering. It all depended on learning that "if he does not tense at all, he does not experience anything that he is used to recognizing as stuttering" (Johnson, 1967, p. 317). This was the ultimate goal of therapy.

Van Riper: An Eclectic Viewpoint

As we have seen, Johnson's therapeutic program was designed to bring the stutterer to the point where he or she was a dysfluent normal. Van Riper, a contemporary of Johnson, sought to make the speaker a fluent stutterer. Thus, though both have stressed the need to reduce anxiety and to modify stuttering through behavioral observation and analysis, they differed in the tactics they employed to bring about behavior change.

Van Riper's view of stuttering, its nature, cause, and treatment differs from that held by Johnson in a number of notable ways, in part, because Van Riper's framework seems to have been more of an outgrowth of clinical experiences than of experimental manipulation or theoretical posture. This is not to suggest that Van Riper's stance on various issues is not data bound. On the contrary, he has been able to *see the clinical meaningfulness* of experimental data.

The evidence that all speakers are dysfluent and that no form of dysfluency displayed by the stutterer is not, to some extent, shown by non-stutterers led Johnson to define stuttering as an avoidance reaction. However, Van Riper, looking at the very same data, saw that with respect to certain forms of dysfluency there was a considerable difference between stutterers and non-stutterers. Furthermore, he took note of the fact that not all stutterers are avoidant. Avoidance could not, therefore, be seen as characteristic of stutterers. Moreover, if avoidance was present it often differed remarkably from stutterer to stutterer. To be sure, avoidance behaviors are often present to a considerable extent, especially among older stutterers. Moreover, these behaviors interfere with communication and draw attention away from what is being said to the way it is being said. Because of this, Van Riper has distinguished primary stuttering from secondary stuttering. From his point of view, the primary aspect of stuttering is defined by the presence of excessive part word repetitions and sound prolongations. Secondary stuttering, on the other hand, is evidenced by the occurrence of escape and avoidance behaviors. Major differences thus exist between Van Riper and Johnson. Van Riper saw stuttering, at least as it is initially evidenced, in terms of speech disruptions of a particular kind. It follows that what Johnson viewed as normal dysfluencies might well be called primary stutterings by Van Riper, because the presence of avoidance is not necessary for Van Riper to say that an individual is a primary stutterer. Van Riper's distinction between primary and secondary stuttering, then, served to point out the developmental nature of stuttering. For Van Riper, stuttering is a disorder, the form of which may worsen as a result of learning.

Though the primary-secondary distinction has been fundamental to Van Riper's position, he amended it somewhat over the years. First he added a transitional period because the categories were not truly dichotomous. There were children who seemed to be on the way from one category to the next. Then, he described the course of stuttering in terms of four stages, the first and fourth of these corresponding roughly to primary and secondary stuttering. These and other changes are consistent with Van Riper's statement that "stuttering occurs when the flow of speech is interrupted abnormally by repetitions or prolongations of a sound or syllable or posture, or by avoidance and struggle reactions" (1963, p. 311).

Van Riper's definition of stuttering encompasses the overt speech disruptions and the stutterer's attempts to deal with them and their anticipated occurrence. The covert features of stuttering, ones not explicitly included in his definition, include feelings associated with penalty, frustration, anxiety, and guilt. These factors according to Van Riper, when added to situational concerns, word fears, and communicative stress, are the numerator of a formula that can be used to determine the frequency and severity of an individual's stuttering. The denominator is ego strength and the extent to which smoothly flowing fluent speech is present in the non-stuttered speech of the stutterer. The latter factor, to the extent that it is present, provides a measure of the individual's confidence in his speech mechanism and the ability to learn to speak in a more adequate manner. It also reflects on the extent to which they will need to be taught to improve their non-stuttered speech. For if their fluent speech lacks smoothness this problem will need to be dealt with also.

It should be clear from the above discussion that the numerator of the formula has reference to those factors that are potential disruptors and the denominator to those that serve to facilitate fluency. The extent to which these factors are present determines, to some extent, whether or not a particular individual will come to be a stutterer. For Van Riper, unlike Johnson who posited that the *sole* cause of stuttering is the inappropriate concern about and misdiagnosis of normal dysfluency, there are many different ways that stuttering can come about. From his point of view the belief that there is a single cause for stuttering has created confusion and has interfered with the progress of therapy.

Van Riper posits that for some, a marked minority, stuttering is the result of neurosis. Stuttering is symptomatic of an inner conflict. For others, stuttering is learned behavior. The child learns to speak with the excessive disruptions indicative of stuttering because, for example, the dysfluencies he displays while learning to speak are penalized, the fluency standards that need to be achieved to attain approval are set too high, he is in a setting where his speech is often interrupted, the speech competencies of those in the speech environment put him at a constant disadvantage. Stuttering, within this multi-causal framework, may also result from some sort of neuromuscular weakness that is set off by stress. In the absence of stress, when the speech setting is positive, coordination may well be adequate and speech production relatively fluent. Under stress, however, the neuromotor impulses will be more poorly timed and stuttering will result. For dysphemic individuals, ones who have a lower threshold, it takes less stress to create the emotional flooding that disrupts fluency.

Because the etiology of stuttering can differ from one person to the next and differentially affect the factors that can disrupt fluency, assessment must precede therapy. However, from Van Riper's point of view assessment would precede therapy even if there were only one cause for stuttering, because the factors that contribute to the frequency and severity of stuttering change as a function of the experience the speaker has as a stutterer. Learning takes place and alters the ratio that gives direction to therapy. He does describe four phases comprising the therapeutic sequence. They are the identification phase, a desensitization phase, a modification phase, and a stabilization phase (Van Riper, 1973).

The overall strategy of Van Riper's therapy is multi-dimensional. It is directed at both the emotional factors and the maladaptive adjustments that can disrupt speech. Fundamental to his strategy is the assumption that a "many pronged therapy" is needed if stutterers are to be helped. From this point of view, therapy directed at one or another of the factors that determine the occurrence and severity of stuttering will help only a special few, since stuttering is under the control of many factors.

The specific tactics employed to modify the emotional quotient, that is, to decrease the disruptive factors and to enhance those that support fluency, differ with the developmental stage that the stutterer is in, in part because stage one and stage two stutterers tend to have little in the way of fear of speech situations and words. For Van Riper, this is particularly true of stutterers whose etiology is dependent on either constitutional elements or speech learning that has been associated with excessive demands and pressures. Therapy, then, is directed at the following: reducing penalties placed on the child—particularly those contingent on speech disruptions; reducing the frustrating experiences that are associated with acculturation and the occasional realization that speech production has been difficult; reducing anxiety, guilt, and hostility by positive regard; promoting acceptance and the reassurance of love and support from the family; reducing the standards of fluency that are acceptable, the requirement of speech in circumstances that are needlessly demanding, and the occurrence of negative reactions when stuttering is evidenced. These changes are brought about predominantly through parental counseling, play therapy, creative dramatics, and an interaction among parents of children who stutter.

Children who are in the first or second developmental stage are also toughened so that they can face greater dosages of frustration without it bringing about a breakdown in the fluency with which they speak. This toughening is reportedly accomplished by a desensitization procedure that is aimed at keeping the child fluent while ever-increasing amounts of stress are applied. When correctly used, the pressure is withdrawn when signs of impending dysfluency become evident. In this way, fluency is less and less affected by communicative stress. Associated with this approach are other tactics designed to promote an increase in the net amount of fluency. Speech is encouraged during periods of fluency. In addition, circumstances are arranged that are likely to promote fluency. For example, games involving rhythm and speaking in unison are played. During the time that fluency is less in evidence than usual, when dysfluency is on the rise, things are arranged so that the stutterer talks less. More physical or mental activities are engaged in than are those that involve verbal behavior.

According to Van Riper, the third developmental stage is marked by an awareness of speech difficulty, frustration, longer prolongations, repetitions of greater duration and force, and escape behaviors. In the fourth stage, situational and word fear are present, avoidance of anticipated difficulty replaces the stutterer's struggle to escape from the occurrence of dysfluency, and shame and guilt about the inability to speak adequately come to the fore.

As stage four (secondary) stuttering is approached and reached, more and more attention is given to tactics for *directly* modifying those things that the speaker does when stuttering. The emotional component is not overlooked, however. Attempts are made to reduce frustration, provide for the ventilation of this feeling, increase emotional security, and desensitize the stutterer to communicative stress. Speaking situations of graduated difficulty are faced up to as part of a toughening procedure that also enhances the client's ego strength. But importantly, the speaker's manner of stuttering is now brought under scrutiny. It is analyzed, varied, and brought under control so that the goal of more fluent ways of stuttering can be achieved.

The absence of stuttering is not sought since only by stuttering can the behaviors involved be studied and identified so that changes to a less abnormal way of speaking can be achieved. According to Van Riper, stuttering moments are stereotypic. The response pattern is consistent to the point of being compulsive. And, the stutterer tends to view his behavior as something over which he has no control. It is necessary, then, to make the stutterer aware that other speech behaviors are possible, that there are different ways of stuttering, that there are ways that involve less tension and effort and that are more like fluent speech. Awareness of this depends on experience, which is provided by having the stutterer voluntarily repeat the first syllable of non-feared words, use an avoidance behavior that is not part of the speaker's response repertoire, use a breathing pattern that is the opposite of the one typically used when stuttering. The stutterer who closes his eyes when stuttering might, for example, be asked to open them or to blink them. It is not that new avoidance behaviors are being taught. It is that the stutterer in this way learns that it is not necessary to talk in one particular way.

When variation has made it apparent that change is possible, that different responses can be made, that responses modeled by the therapist can replace those that have been habitually used, the stutterer is ready to learn how to cancel, pull-out, and initiate speech in an easier fashion. He is ready to begin the steps that will aid him in becoming a more fluent stutterer.

Cancellation *follows* the occurrence of a stuttering moment. The word is to be stuttered again but now in a less complex, less hypertensive way. The change modeled by the clinician, be it a reduction in force or the absence of a head turn or an arm swing is now incorporated into the cancelled production of the stuttering moment. Speech, which is stopped when a stutter occurs, is continued only after cancellation has taken place. In this way the stutterer begins to learn how to replace the old pattern of stuttering with one that is less aberrant.

After the ability to cancel a specific behavior has been acquired, the stutterer is called upon to use this ability *during* stuttering. That is to say, when a stuttering moment occurs, the client is to *pull-out* of the block the behavioral element that has been worked on in cancellation training. In this way, the moment is made less severe as it occurs. Through the pull-out the stutterer learns that he can take control of his stuttering behavior and make the moment less complex.

The lessons learned during the cancellation and the pull-out training sessions serve the stutterer well when the behavior change is brought into the period that *precedes* stuttering. Specifically, the stutterer is instructed to stutter without the target behavior when stuttering is expected. When expectancy is present, the stutterer is to rehearse so that the word is produced in the more simple fashion. According to Van Riper, this is done because the preparatory motor plan determines the behaviors that are likely to be displayed during moments of stuttering.

Element by element, the behaviors that comprise the stuttering moment are cancelled, pulled-out, and finally eliminated by proper rehearsal during the anticipatory period. In this step-wise way, fluent stuttering is fashioned. The stutterer learns to control speech, to speak in a way that is more normal. The result is speech that is less likely to call attention to itself, interfere with communication and cause the stutterer and the listener concern.

Bloodstein: A Sociomotor Approach

Bloodstein has been affected by both Johnson and Van Riper. He was a student of Johnson, and he has carefully studied the clinical reports and theoretical statements of Van Riper. But, over the years, he developed his own framework. He has integrated certain of their key ideas into his thinking and rejected others.

Bloodstein, like Johnson, contends that stuttering is not an organic or a neurotic disorder. He views stuttering as a disorder that results from speech specific doubts. These doubts cause the speaker to do things that interfere with the motor performance that is intrinsic to speech. For Bloodstein stuttering is a sociomotor disorder. The doubts that the speaker has acquired, the belief that speech is difficult, lead to responses that disrupt the skilled motor performance that is speech. Because of mal-attitudes and beliefs, stutterers tense the speech-related muscles and break up or fragment the speech attempt. The doubts they acquire about their ability to speak adequately leads them to try too hard and to approach speaking in a piecemeal way. Fundamentally, then, stuttering is what speakers *do*; it is *not* something that happens to them. Stuttering is not involuntary. It is a consequence of the speakers' actions and these interfere with the motor planning necessary for fluent speech performance.

Bloodstein points out that even though stuttering is the consequence of struggle that is motivated by the anticipation of difficulty, this does not mean that it is due to anxiety. He does not view stuttering as due to anxiety about speech or stuttering. Moreover, he does not believe that stuttering is the anxiety motivated avoidance of normal dysfluencies. For Bloodstein, the learned belief that speech is difficult, that one has to do certain things when speaking so as to be able to cope, does not mean that the speaker is anxious. It merely reflects the presence of preconceptions and superstitions.

Bloodstein rejects anxiety as being basic to stuttering because fluency failures occur even when physiologic arousal, expressed concern, and avoidance responses are absent. Moreover, he points out that stuttering has not been greatly or consistently reduced by tranquilizers, desensitization, and various forms of psychotherapy. He suggests, then, that anxiety is not a necessary condition for the occurrence of stuttering.

Traditionally, anxiety has been defined as the anticipation of difficulty. And, as we have seen, Bloodstein contends that stuttering results from the expectation that speech will be difficult. But for Bloodstein, anticipation does not necessarily reflect anxiety. Stutterers are merely making an objective report. They are aware of their past speech experiences and these shape their anticipations. Consistent with this is the fact that the predictions of adult stutterers are relatively accurate. Unlike young stutterers they have a considerable experience history to call upon in deciding when and where they are likely to have difficulty. As a result, they tend to be more knowledgeable about the cues of past difficulty, the ones that set the occasion for stuttering.

Children who stutter tend to express an anticipation of difficulty that is usually more general than that evidenced by adult stutterers. Their concerns are about speech and speaking rather than about specific words, sounds, or situations. But, once again, the anticipation does not reflect anxiety. It is the objective result of a variety of experiences that fundamentally shake their "faith in their ability to speak" (Bloodstein, 1975, p. 40). They expect difficulty in communicating and they anticipate speech failure when they try to speak. The anticipation of failure may result from the presence of delayed speech, defective articulation, cluttering and/or difficulties in oral reading. These are not the only factors that can lead to tense and fragmented speech, however. A large number of conditions and events can set the occasion for the speech-associated doubts of stutterers.

Bloodstein has been quick to point out that a history of speech failure and the presence of doubt are necessary but not sufficient to cause stuttering. Speech pressure is also a necessary condition, and it may have any number of sources. It may arise from cultural, social, and/or parental attitudes and practices that stress the importance of speech and the need to meet stringent standards. The speech-related pressure combines, in a singularly destructive way, with the doubts that speech failures create. The pushes and pulls of these elements produce a crucially disruptive blend. And, from Bloodstein's point of view, these doubts and pressures are to some extent present in the world of all children. They do not exist only for those who are called stutterers. This is why all children exhibit dysfluencies and some degree of tension and fragmentation. They all tend to evidence some part word repetitions and prolongations, dysfluent behaviors that are generally seen as characteristic of stuttering. This has led Bloodstein to state that there is no clear-cut distinction between those children who are called stutterers and those who are not. From his point of view, most young children will stutter sometime. Those who are eventually called stutterers are those who stutter severely and persistently. It follows that diagnosis "is a futile and meaningless exercise" (Bloodstein, 1975, p. 51). There are not stutterers and non-stutterers. There are those for whom tension and fragmentation create a problem and those for whom it does not.

The treatment for those who seek help varies with the symptom display. Stuttering changes over time. Its form is modified, new behaviors are evidenced, the frequency and severity of the stuttering tends to increase, and its occurrence, which is initially episodic becomes chronic. These developmental changes have been described by Bloodstein (1981) in terms of phases.

Simple repetitions at the beginning of syntactic units typify phase 1 stuttering. Frustration may be evidenced but usually speech is not avoided and there is no outward evidence of concern. Therapy for those who are in phase 1 is aimed both at keeping the stuttering from taking a more advanced form and at preventing the child from developing a self-concept as a defective speaker. Toward these ends, the parents are given a basic understanding about their child's speech difficulties, are told about the need to remove speech pressure, and are helped to bring about changes in the way they deal with their child so that these pressures are eliminated. They are also shown ways that take advantage of their child's fluency and utilize the conditions under which fluency prevails so as to enhance the anticipation of fluency. Successful speech experiences are utilized to instill a positive belief system about the ability to speak in a normal fashion.

Phase 2 stuttering is reportedly characterized by a chronic fragmentation of words. Fragmentation is no longer specific to the beginning of syntactic units. Moreover, the phase 2 stutterer now views himself as a defective speaker.

The main thrust of therapy for phase 2 stutterers is directed at modifying the perception of being a defective speaker. Therapeutic attention is not directed at particular aspects of the speech symptomatology. Fragmentation has not led to a concern about speaking, and the child does not avoid speech. Since therapeutic tactics that are specific to minute aspects of speech might trigger these unwanted responses, they are not employed.

The phase 2 stutterer's self-concept is dealt with by procedures additional to those prescribed for phase 1 stutterers. They are designed to increase the child's general feelings of self-worth. This is achieved by developing new abilities and improving existing assets so as to increase the positive regard with which the child is held by his peers. Though no attempt is made to increase fluency, therapy is aimed at improving the child's communication skills (e.g., voice and diction).

The phase 3 stutterer is said to have become aware that certain speech situations and words or sounds are difficult. Expectation of stuttering is now clearly present. The tension and fragmentation of stuttering is fully in evidence. At this juncture, it is unlikely that therapeutic attempts to eliminate the individual's speech doubts by reducing environmental demands and negative reactions will have much of an effect. The stutterer's self-concept and belief system is relatively well established. As a result, therapy emphasizes the modification of stuttering. Many of the procedures that Bloodstein suggests to bring this change about are like those that have been set forth by Johnson and Van Riper. They are designed to promote objectivity, knowledge of the stuttering symptomatology, and an awareness that stuttering is alterable and not something that is an uncontrollable event.

The stutterer who is in phase 4 reacts emotionally to speech and stuttering. The expectation of difficulty triggers affective reactions. Words and sounds are feared. Speech situations are avoided. The presence of chronic anxiety significantly handicaps the phase 4 stutterer. It also tends to interfere with clinical activities designed to bring about the modification of stuttering. At this developmental stage, then, anxiety reduction is a major goal of therapy.

Various clinical procedures are set forth by Bloodstein as a means of bringing about a reduction in anxiety. These include tactics that are traditional to mental hygiene. The stutterer is helped to bring the speech problem into the open, accept its presence, admit its existence to others, and discuss it objectively and openly with others. In addition, stutterers learn that normal speech contains dysfluencies and that it is an unrealistic goal to seek speech that is free of all dysfluency. They learn, too, that their inferences about the reactions of listeners to their stuttered speech is often inaccurate. Training is undertaken so that the inferences are replaced by objective descriptions of the listeners' actual responses.

Bloodstein indicates that once the stutterer becomes better able to face speech disruption in a more objective way and speech-associated anxiety is reduced, the therapist can help the stutterer overcome his fluency problem. Therapy should be aimed at modifying stuttering rather than at an acceptance of the condition. It should focus on reducing tension in the vocal tract. This is because the prolongations and repetitions of stuttering are seen as resulting from laryngeal and buccal constriction. Hypertension in these areas critically interferes with the air flow that is basic to adequate speech production. It follows that the stutterer must determine the locus of the tension points and learn, through practice, to speak with less and less of the constriction that is disruptive of speech.

Fragmentation, like tension, is viewed as a struggle reaction that interferes with the normal flow of speech. Fragmentation and tension are not, therefore, truly separable actions. They both serve to create the symptomatology of stuttering. The tendency of stutterers to fragment their speech is evidenced by the presence of inappropriate rhythm, pausing, phrasing, and word production. The fragmentation of the movements of speech needs to be corrected. The stutterer must learn to eliminate fragmentation and to restore normal movement, so as to restore the normal flow of speech. Normal speech is smoothly forward moving. Its production is integrated and wholistic rather than broken into segmented units.

According to Bloodstein the avoidance and escape behaviors that are associated with the integral symptoms of stuttering (i.e., part word repetition and prolongation) will tend to be stripped off as the stutterer learns to speak in a less effortful and more forward-moving manner. He suggests that this occurs because many of the clinical procedures that lead to a reduction in tension and fragmentation serve also to eliminate the extraneous secondary responses.

Wischner: An Avoidance Construct

Starting sometime in the middle forties the views and clinical tactics of people like Johnson and Van Riper were translated into the terms of the then-current learning theories. Probably the first person to do this was George Wischner (1950), who was Johnson's assistant and a disciple of Hull. Utilizing Hullian's learning theory he undertook a research program that led him to conclude that stuttering is an anxiety motivated avoidance *response*. According to Wischner, anxiety, the expectancy of difficulty specific to words and situations, probably has its origin in parental rejection of normal dysfluency. Stuttering is the avoidance of speech-associated punishment, and it is reinforced by the anxiety reduction that follows its occurrence. In other words, the release that follows stuttering is a reward that increases the likelihood of its occurring again.

Wischner stressed research and the theoretical implications of his findings. He did not offer a therapeutic program that was specifically designed for those who stutter. Yet, his framework carried with it the implication that it would be therapeutic to reduce speech specific anxiety and the avoidance of words and situations. After all, anxiety is the motive force that impelled avoidance, and avoidance is behaviorally maladaptive since words and speech situations are not objectively dangerous; they cannot truly hurt one.

Clearly, Wischner's approach to stuttering and, by implication, its modification, is consistent with the stance taken by Johnson. Despite this, there was a fundamental difference between the two. For Wischner, stuttering is a learned response. As such it should obey the laws of learning. For example, it should behave in a way that is consistent with the law of effect; it should be increased by a consequence that is reinforcing and decreased by one that is punishing. Johnson, in contrast, viewed stuttering as a *reaction* and not as a response. Partly as a result of this he did not condone behavior change tactics that involve the direct manipulation of avoidance behaviors.

Sheehan: An Approach-Avoidance Model

At about the same time that Wischner began thinking of stuttering in learning terms, Sheehan was too. However, Sheehan appears to have been more influenced by Van Riper and by those learning theorists who attempted to bring together the clinical insights of psychoanalysis and the more precise behavioral approach required for laboratory-based research (Dollard and Miller, 1950). These and other learning theorists helped create behavior therapy. Behaviorism was no longer confined to the animal laboratory. Experimental findings had clinical implications; they could give direction to therapeutic maneuvers.

Miller's (1944) research into the effect on behavior of opposing response tendencies led him to propose conflict models and to study their relationship to fear. Sheehan adopted an approach-avoidance model because it served to explain both the stutterers' speech-associated fears and their symptoms. For Sheehan, the fears displayed by stutterers are symptomatic of speech-associated conflict, and their poor self-concept results from their lack of normal speech fluency.

For Sheehan the fear-inducing conflict has its basis in words, speech situations, emotional content, interpersonal relationships, and role expectations. Conflict at any of these levels can affect speech; it can lead to the behavioral vacillation or fixation that is displayed as sound or syllable repetition and sound prolongation. These speech behaviors characterize the defect side of stuttering. The emotional and attitudinal aspects of the conflict are, for Sheehan, the handicap element of stuttering.

The approach-avoidance model that Sheehan employs allows him to encompass both the defect and handicap aspects of stuttering. The conflict not only elicits fear, it creates the overt symptomatology of stuttering. Because there is both an approach and avoidance to speech and silence, speech is disrupted. The conflict is externalized. There is an emotional cost, however. The stutterer feels guilty about avoiding, ashamed by the speech disruption, and frustrated by the inability to communicate.

The start-stop vacillation in speech that occurs when the approach and avoidance tendencies near equality and the blocking of speech that occurs when an equilibrium is achieved are, according to Sheehan, momentarily terminated by the occurrence of stuttering. Because stuttering, the response that was being avoided, has occurred, the conflict has momentarily been resolved and speech is released.

It should be clear from the above discussion that Sheehan's approach to therapy involves procedures that are designed to reduce and ultimately eliminate those factors that cause the speaker to be conflicted. At whatever level the conflict exists (e.g., word, situational), the object of therapy is to reduce the avoidance of speech and the act of speaking and to increase the approach drive until there is no longer an equilibrium that adversely affects speech. But, either decreasing the avoidance of speech or increasing the approach tendencies brings the speaker closer to the feared goal. Both, that is, lead to an increase in the fear that motivates avoidance. This response will occur to a lesser degree if the clinical procedures are aimed at decreasing the stutterer's avoidance prior to enhancing the approach to speech. As Sheehan points out, "avoidance reduction is the major vehicle to therapy" (Eisenson, 1975; p. 145).

Sheehan excludes from therapy any and all procedures that are designed to (1) achieve control over stuttering so as to make speech more closely approximate that of the fluent speaker, (2) create circumstances under which fluency will occur since these experiences are unreal; (3) suppress the occurrence of stuttering because the changes that take place are temporary, and can be destructive. They can lead the stutterer to a false sense of improvement.

The avoidance reduction therapy procedures that Sheehan uses with adults, adolescents, and older children are aided by group therapy. From his point of view, the group serves as a powerful supportive and therapeutic force; it aids the individual in the understanding and utilization of procedures that are designed to reduce avoidance and thus stuttering.

Various tactics are employed by Sheehan to reduce speech-associated avoidances. The client is trained to maintain eye contact with the listener, whether or not stuttering occurs. To look away, to avoid eye contact, implies shame and it serves to increase such feelings. For Sheehan, stuttering is not to be hidden. The fact that one stutters should be openly discussed with listeners, be they friends or acquaintances. Trying to hide one's stuttering from the listener is an avoidance, and it increases the fear and tension that is basic to stuttering. In contrast, openness about stuttering reduces both avoidance and fear. They are reduced, also, when the stutterer faces up to his own stuttering. The stutterer should not hide what he does from himself. The stutterer needs to explore and learn about the things that he does when stuttering, and to learn that he does not have to stutter in one particular way. What he sees are not things that happen to him, they are instead things that he does. The stutterer must learn that he is responsible for his stuttering behaviors. When this occurs, they can be monitored and altered.

The avoidance responses of stutterers are not the only ones that can be altered. Fears can also be modified by using the word that you fear and by entering the speech situation that you have avoided. By taking the initiative, by "fear-seeking" maneuvers of this kind, it is assumed that the grip that emotion has on the stutterer and his speech will be lessened. It can be decreased, too, by practice in open stuttering. That is stuttering without avoidance, struggle, hurry, and concomitant shame and guilt.

Open stuttering is a step forward in the improvement process. Open stuttering, stuttering that is not associated with attempts to shorten its occurrence, stuttering that is allowed to take its course with ease and without concealment, is a key to success. So, too, is practice in smoothly initiated voluntary stuttering on non-feared words. This is because it ultimately leads to a slide that can be used "as an alternative method of stuttering on *feared* words" (Sheehan, 1975, p. 168, italics added). Fundamental to these procedures is the position that through open stuttering one can learn that there are other ways of stuttering, ways that are easier, non-avoidant, and fear reducing.

The therapies we have so far described have been directed at reducing the anticipation of speech difficulty and the avoidance it supposedly engenders. None of the therapies are aimed at either the instatement of fluency or the suppression of stuttering. This is because the theoretical positions of the clinicians reviewed and their past experiences with such techniques argue against such tactics.

Johnson, as we have seen, viewed stuttering as an avoidance reaction. Because of this, his therapy was designed to reduce the speaker's avoidance of words and situations. It was not an approach that was directed at reducing dysfluency since he considered dysfluency to be normal. It was not directed at creating fluency since dysfluency was exhibited by all. Van Riper also shied away from therapy that was designed to achieve fluency. His procedures were aimed at achieving control so that the adult stutterer could speak with as much ease as possible. The goal of therapy was fluent stuttering not stutter-free speech. In part, this was a result of Van Riper's belief that an adult stutterer would always stutter. It was necessary, then, to rid the adult of the unnecessary tension and struggle that accompanied stuttered speech. Sheehan has been particularly adamant about therapy that attempts either to directly promote fluency or to suppress dysfluency. Like Johnson and Van Riper before him, he pointed out the deleterious effects of the fluency procedures used in years past. At one time or another, each of these clinicians has pointed out that the tactics used to achieve fluency have produced only temporary improvement. They noted that fluency is easily achieved by various means, but the devices that produce it often remain long after stuttering has returned. Moreover, these devices can be more distressing to the listener, interfere more with communication, and be more behaviorally bizarre than the stuttering they were designed to cure. In addition, the fluency that occurs is often temporary. This can have a serious effect on the stutterer who momentarily achieves it. It is debilitating, at best, to have reached longed-for fluency, only to lose one's grip on it.

Sheehan has pointed out that it is a farce to propose the use of procedures the aim of which is the instatement of fluency. He asserts that stutterers do not need to learn how to speak fluently. They are fluent most of the time. Stuttering does not predominate, fluency does. This being the case, he contends that one does not need to develop a therapy program that is designed to teach one how to speak fluently.

Sheehan views stuttering as a problem that the individual must face and conquer. As a result, he contends that therapy should not be directed at speech alone. It should be psychotherapeutic and global. Moroever, he says that it should not utilize procedures that serve to achieve fluency by hiding stuttering. Such procedures appeal "to the worst in the stutterer: his tendency to deny the problem, to cover up to conceal" (Sheehan, 1975, p. 148). Sheehan goes on to say that it is inappropriate to suppress stuttering behaviors or use "any procedure (such as the phony 'establishment' of fluency via distractive or disruptive stimuli. . . .)" (Sheehan, 1975, p. 145). From his point of view such methods increase avoidance and thus enhance the conflict over speech that produces stuttering.

Shames: Operant Technology

Shames is fully aware of the concerns of traditionalists, those who view stuttering as a symptom of an underlying condition or who avoid direct intervention designed to affect fluency. But Shames views stuttering as operant behavior and not as a symptom of some underlying condition. His position is that stuttering can be reduced and fluency can be increased by the use of operant tactics. An operant is behavior that is modifiable by its consequences, and that can be increased or decreased when particular stimuli are made contingent upon its occurrence.

Shames, unlike a Johnson or Van Riper, makes no attempt to define stuttering. He does not define fluency, either. Though the goal of his therapeutic approach is stutter-free speech he does not suggest that *his* goals are necessarily those of *all* clinicians. What he says, instead, is that clinicians can use operant procedures to modify whatever they select as the target or targets that need to be modified to bring about improvement.

Because Shames views speech and the behaviors displayed by stutterers as operants it is apparent that their occurrence must have been shaped by environmental consequences. At one time, in a way somewhat reminiscent of Johnson, he did suggest that stuttering is a changed form of dysfluency. He suggested that it could be brought about by the avoidance of threatened punishment of dysfluency (Shames and Sherrick, 1963). He pointed out, however, that stuttering can come about in different ways and that the circumstances that shape and maintain it are many and varied.

Currently, Shames is far more concerned with the way operant procedures can be successfully employed to modify stuttering than in theorizing about the conditions under which it came about. He is essentially an atheoretical practitioner of the operant mold. He posits that it is far better to deal directly with the observable world, applying basic operant methods so as to achieve behavior change, than it is to be sidetracked by assumptions and concepts. He finds that there is no need for concepts like apprehension and unconscious conflict.

Shames, as we have said, views stuttering as an operant and has suggested that a number of the other behaviors displayed by stutterers are also operants. Among these are various attributes of their speech that are associated with fluency. In addition, he has indicated that the attitudes and emotional responses of stutterers should be considered operants if they can be brought under the control of consequent stimuli. If so, they too can become the targets of therapy. All that is necessary is that the targets are observable and specifiable so that when they occur they can be consequated in a scheduled manner.

Measurement is a fundamental aspect of operant methodology. After all, if one proposes that an operant response is one that can be brought under stimulus control it is necessary to evidence this fact. More important, from a clinical point of view, is evidence that the targeted behavior is being affected in the way desired. After all, clinicians are concerned with increasing fluency and reducing stuttering and not with the mere demonstration that behaviors can be manipulated. As a first step, the clinician must determine the base-rate of the targeted behavior. That is to say that, prior to therapeutic intervention, it is necessary to determine the stable rate with which the response to be changed is emitted. Only then is it appropriate to begin delivering contingent stimulation, for only then can the clinician know its effect. Indeed, it is the on-line measurement of the target behavior that informs the clinician as to the effectiveness of the therapy procedure being utilized.

Shames has pointed out that operant tactics can help traditionally oriented therapists more readily achieve their goals. He has shown that the cancellation, pull-out, and easy initiation procedures of Van Riper can be put into an operant program involving oral reading and conversational speech. He contends, however, that though stuttering can be reduced by such form-modifying procedures there is no carry-over. He suggests that this is a result of the fact that these procedures do not support the establishment of a changed way of behaving for those stutterers who display relatively few fluency failures.

Shames has applied consequences, also, to the way stutterers talk about their speech. For, as Johnson and his students have pointed out, they are more likely to regard stuttering as something that happens to them than something they do to avoid dysfluency. Ridding stutterers of the belief that "it" happens to them is thus therapeutic. It helps put aside their feeling of helplessness. It enables them to deal with their maladaptive avoidances. Johnson's view seems to have been supported. Shames found that reinforcements of statements that are desirable (e.g., "I substituted a word," or "I don't have to turn my head when I talk") led to an increase in their frequency. In contrast, disapproval of comments indicative of speech-associated helplessness led to a decrease in their number. Moreover, these changes were reportedly associated with some decrease in stuttering (Shames, Egolf, and Rhodes 1969).

As the more traditional therapists have suggested, attempts to suppress stuttering moments are considerably less successful. Shames found that though the aversive stimulation of stuttering occasionally produced a decrease in their occurrence, this was not always the case. More importantly, strongly aversive consequences like shock were less effective than mild consequences. These findings were not consistent with the law of effect and the operant position. The stronger the consequence the greater the stimulus control should have been.

But Shames does not contend that all of the procedures that operant therapists use are equally advantageous. He has pointed out that both the tactics we have described and those that are designed to establish fluency by reinforcing its occurrence and by modifying speech rate all have certain advantages and limitations. No one procedure works for all who stutter. No single procedure meets the needs of establishing self-responsibility, a fluent belief system, and fluent speech behavior in clinical and real life situations.

Shames points out that fluency is readily and quickly achieved when delayed auditory feedback (DAF) or instructions are used to produce a change in manner of speaking. By one or the other of these two means, stutterers learn to prolong and slow down their speech production. When DAF is used, slowed and prolonged utterances lead to negative reinforcement (escape from DAF). When instructions are used, often in association with modeling by the clinician, positive reinforcement is made contingent on slowed and prolonged speech. When speech is produced in this manner it tends, for whatever reason, to be stutter-free. The resulting intervals of fluent speech can then be reinforced by a gradual reduction in the presumably aversive DAF or by the delivery of positive reinforcement. The length of these fluent intervals, as they occur in different speech situations, can also be increased by reinforcement. In addition, the speech can ultimately be shaped so that its production approximates normal rate and duration. Over time, the responsibility for therapy targets, like slowed and prolonged speech, is transferred to the stutterer. So, too, is the delivery of reinforcements. As a result, stutterers become responsible for their own behavior and its modification. This is an important aspect of the therapy procedure that Shames, among others, utilizes. It is advantageous because it facilitates change that carries over to real-life settings.

One of the fundamental aspects of responsibility is self-monitoring, because recognition that the target behavior has or has not occurred is a necessary precursor of self-reinforcement. In order for the stutterer to reinforce the occurrence of a desired behavior, its presence must be recognized. Self-monitoring serves, also, to enhance the speaker's awareness that speech can be stutter-free. Monitoring makes obvious the fact that the speech produced is indeed fluent. The burgeoning recognition of this fact apparently serves to change the speaker's self concept and to support the presence of fluency. Slowly, it also brings about a change in the belief system. Self-monitoring, then, serves to help change the attitudes that interfere with the instatement and maintenance of fluency.

Brutten: A Two-Factor Multi-Modal Methodology

Brutten also makes use of operant procedures. However, he does not ignore the responses that have been called respondents (Skinner, 1938). Respondents have also been called problem-making behaviors and have been contrasted with the problem-solving responses that operants represent (Mowrer, 1947).

Brutten, like Skinner and Mowrer, has taken the position that two different conditioning procedures are involved in learning. Like them, he is a two-factor theorist. As a result, the targets of therapy for Brutten include both the negative emotional respondents that may disrupt speech and create the factor I behaviors that define stuttering, and the maladaptive operant adjustments or factor II behaviors that are motivated by speech specific concerns.

Brutten contends that factor II operant responses are not the only behaviors that should be the target of therapy. Consistent with this position is the implication that operant tactics are neither the only means nor necessarily the most efficient means of affecting each of the various behaviors that are in need of modification. Indeed, Brutten has taken the stance that the use of operant procedures may not be appropriate. This is because factor II or operant responses are not universally displayed by all who stutter. On the other hand, he has stressed that operant tactics are appropriate for eliminating the adjustive responses that many stutterers employ to avoid anticipated dysfluency or to escape from the actual occurrence of fluency failure.

Brutten's position that factor I and II behaviors reflect different forms of conditioning and that this should be taken into consideration when planning therapy deserves attention. This is because it suggests that the incorrect matching of tactics and conditioning history is inefficient and even potentially harmful. Indeed, he has indicated that punishment, especially that involving strongly negative stimuli, is contraindicated for use with factor I behaviors (Brutten, 1970, 1980).

As we have seen, Brutten makes a distinction between stuttering and the operant adjustments that stutterers tend to make. Stuttering, from his point of view, is the *involuntary* repetition and prolongation of simple and compound phones that result when speech is disrupted by the presence of conditioned negative emotion. Within this framework, speech is normally fluent. Negative emotion interferes with the fluent state. The respondent reduces the accuracy of the motor response. In operational terms it is this decrease in the fluency or accuracy of performance that defines anxiety.

The position that the behaviors displayed by those called stutterers may include both involuntary and voluntary or purposive elements rests on the self-reports of stutterers, personal observation of their behaviors, and experimental studies involving contingent stimulation. This data bank has shaped the diagnostic, assessment, and therapy procedures that are basic to the two-factor approach to stuttering (Brutten and Shoemaker, 1967; Webster and Brutten, 1974; Brutten, 1975).

As the therapists reviewed have pointed out, stutterers rather consistently maintain that their fast repetitions and tension prolongations are involuntary. They scoff at the contention that these behaviors are purposive. Stutterers refer to these particular forms of dysfluency as ones that are out of their control (Bloodstein, 1981; Williams, 1957). They say things like, "it happens to me." They do not feel responsible for their occurrence. When it is suggested that they initiate these behaviors they are incredulous and say, "Why would I want to do that?" In contrast, they are generally quite candid in pointing out their operant adjustments. Though they may not be fully aware of all of the devices that they are currently using, they rather readily point out their voluntary attempts to deal with anticipated and actual speech difficulties. But they do not typically view these behaviors as akin to their involuntary repetitions and prolongations. Moreover, they do not generally view these adjustive responses as stutterings. Stutterers generally distinguish factor I from factor II behaviors.

It should be apparent that Brutten does not disregard the distinction that stutterers make between involuntary fluency failures and voluntary coping strategies. He has paid attention to the separation they make between stuttering, on the one hand, and efforts to avoid or escape difficulty, on the other hand. Brutten is aware, of course, that the stutterers' self-reports may not be accurate. Their reports may not be any more valid than are the theoretical judgments that all of the stutterers' behaviors are avoidances, that all are voluntary acts for which the stutterer is fully responsible, or that all stuttering behaviors are operant responses that can be manipulated by contingent stimulation. These positions may also be invalid. They may represent nothing more than an attempt to force the reportedly different behaviors into one category for the sake of theoretical or clinical convenience.

To help resolve the question of response class, that is, to help determine if the behaviors displayed during the stuttering moment were all of the same kind, Brutten and his associates undertook the molecular analysis of stuttering moments. They filmed stutterers during speech activity and separately scored each occurrence of a number of different behaviors: those that were supposedly involuntary and those that were reported or observed to be adjustive devices (Brutten and Shoemaker, 1969; Webster and Brutten, 1972; Krych, 1978). What they found was that moments were not behavioral constants. They involved mixtures of behaviors whose composition and order generally differed from instance to instance. More importantly, they found evidence that supported the contention that the behaviors were categorically different. This conclusion was a necessary result of the fact that though the measured stuttering behaviors correlated significantly with each other, and the operant responses did likewise, there was not a significant inter-correlation between the behaviors in these two separate groups (Webster and Brutten, 1972). Consistent with these data were the independent findings of a factor analysis study conducted at another laboratory (Prins and Lohr, 1972). What was evidenced again was that the behaviors displayed by stutterers factored into separate classes. Once more, factor I behaviors like fast repetition of a sound or syllable and tension prolongation separated out from factor II responses. The behaviors that fell into the latter category were clearly concomitant responses, ones that were secondary to stuttering. They were adjustive in nature rather than speech disruptions characteristic of stuttering.

Further support for the distinction that Brutten has made between factor I and II behaviors has come from a number of studies in which the effect of contingent stimulation has been observed. In these investigations, unlike in some others, specific molecularly defined behaviors were punished. Molar moments were not contingently stimulated. The results were instructive. Response-contingent negative stimuli (punishment) significantly affected factor II responses but did not reduce the frequency of factor I behaviors. In other words, factor II responses responded to punishment as operants do, but factor I behaviors did not. To test the robustness of this difference, a number of studies have been run in which response contingent positive stimulation (reinforcement) was utilized to investigate the modifiability of factor I behaviors. Once more, the behaviors that Brutten defined as stuttering were not manipulated by contingent stimulation (Kohout, 1974; Oelschlaeger and Brutten, 1975). It follows from these results, then, that neither punishment nor reinforcement produced the kind of change that would lead one to say that fast repetitions and tension prolongations are operant responses.[3]

The presence of fundamental differences between factor I and II behaviors is of considerable clinical import for Brutten. These differences gave shape to the assessment procedures he employs and the decision-making that is basic to two-factor therapy (Brutten, 1970; 1973; 1975).

Two-factor therapy requires individual determination of the stimuli that set the occasion for negative emotion and the operant responses that it typically motivates. The clinician must determine the word and situational stimuli that cue-off the conditioned emotional responses that disrupt fluency and must ascertain the discriminative stimuli that lead to maladaptive adjustive responses. Often, though not always, these are the very same stimuli. It is the therapist's responsibility, also, to specify the particular operant adjustments that the client employs. To the extent possible, these determinations should precede therapy. Clearly, then, assessment is a vital precurser to therapy. What this means is that therapy is tailored to individual needs. Therapy is not the same for all who stutter because all who stutter are not concerned about the same speech sounds or situations. Moreover, they do not cope with their speech difficulties in the same way. Each stutterer is *unique* from Brutten's point of view. It follows that he is critical of clinical procedures that are employed without recourse to assessment and that disregard the client's particular behavioral display. This does not mean that two-factor tactics cannot be programmed. It means only that the tactics programmed must be made client-specific. The overall strategy of two-factor therapy is to interactively eliminate unobjective speech concerns and maladaptive adjustive

---

[3] A fuller review of such studies is not appropriate to the purpose of this chapter. It may be found elsewhere (see Brutten and Shoemaker, 1971).

behaviors. In a dovetailed fashion it is designed to make speech a positive emotional experience, one that is approached rather than avoided, one that the individual is skilled at and not concerned about. Though these are the general goals of therapy, the specific targets and the particular tactics used to bring about the needed behavior change can vary from client to client.

In the respondent-operant therapy that Brutten employs, two tactics are basic to all the behavior change procedures that follow. The first of these has been termed *reality training* and the second *awareness training*. Reality training is a tactic that lays the groundwork for the subsequent use of respondent procedures. The various respondent procedures available to the therapist are designed to eliminate the stutterers' speech-associated concerns. Reality training aids this process by making stutterers accurately aware of their speech behaviors and that of non-stutterers. Reality training can serve, therefore, to bring about a cognitive-perceptual restructuring. This is often needed because stutterers have a tendency to overestimate the extent to which they are dysfluent and to underestimate the occurrence of fluency failures in the speech of their non-stuttering peers. They have a tendency, also, to believe that they alone have speech-associated concerns.

Reality training involves objective count procedures and reinforcement for accurate determinations. Through these means stutterers come to learn that they are not inherently incapable, that they too speak fluently, that stuttering is not ever-present, and that the speech of non-stutterers is not error-free. Stutterers learn that concerns about speech situations are not totally absent among those who are non-stutterers; non-stutterers, too, have concerns about a variety of speech situations. They learn, therefore, to be objective about their behaviors and those of non-stutterers. They learn to understand that the goal of being a non-stutterer does not mean that they should anticipate either perfect fluency or the total absence of concern. They learn, that is, to face reality as it relates to the task before them and the end result to be achieved.

Awareness training is specific to operant behaviors. It precedes the use of both those tactics that are designed to increase and those that are employed to decrease the frequency of a particular response. Awareness training is used because it has been found that behavior change is more efficiently achieved and maintained if the stutterer is fully aware of the targeted factor II response and the times when it occurs. There is the need, therefore, to train the stutterer in response identification and discrimination. Through the use of video tapes the stutterer is trained to identify past occurrences of the response to be modified. When, through reinforced experiences, accuracy is achieved the stutterer learns to discriminate the occurrence of the target response in live speech of graduated length. After this has been achieved, the response to be consequated is dealt with by any of a rather large number of tactics that have been designed for use with operant responses (Kanfer and Goldstein, 1975).

In two-factor therapy various respondent techniques are utilized to reduce significantly the individual stutterer's concerns about specific sounds, words, or speech situations. These deconditioning, counterconditioning, and desensitization tactics tend to vary in their power efficiency (Rimm and Masters, 1979). However, clinicians should be cautioned to keep their therapeutic options open since (1) individuals differ in the way they respond to and are affected by specific therapeutic procedures, and (2) the techniques that are appropriate to a particular behavioral class are not mutually exclusive. When used conjointly the tactics appropriate to a particular behavioral class may well produce an additive effect, one that is greater than is achieved by any one of the tactics alone (Brutten, 1975). These comments are appropriate, also, for those procedures that are designed to decrease maladaptive operant responses and enhance adaptive ones. The first caution is given because what is true for most who stutter may not be so for a particular stutterer. In relation to the second caution, it has been demonstrated that clinical procedures can have a limited effectiveness. They may not be able to carry change to its ultimate point. As a result, the effect of therapy needs to be measurably monitored so as to cue the clinician of the need for a change in tactics or a broadening of the procedures used (Bastijens, Brutten, and Stés, 1978).

With respect to the manipulation of operants, two-factor therapy stresses the use of consequences that are reinforcing and response enhancing. Punishment procedures, ones designed to suppress particular factor II responses, are *not* employed. They can produce detrimental side effects. Though they undoubtedly can bring about a significant reduction in instrumental responses like a tongue thrust or an arm swing they can, at the same time, lead to an increase in negative emotion and factor I dysfluencies (Brutten, 1970; Brutten and Shoemaker, 1971). This dual effect has been attributed to the so-called respondent-operant overlap. Essentially, this refers to the fact that there are separate operant and respondent effects when a factor II response is consequated. This is a result of the fact that when a response is contingently stimulated (R-S conditioning) so too is the situation in which it occurs (S-S conditioning).

The respondent-operant overlap also occurs when reinforcement is employed, which is one of the reasons why reinforcement is a frequently utilized aspect of two-factor therapy. Reinforcement of an adaptive speech or speech-associated skill not only increases its occurrence, but also enhances the positive emotional responses that support fluency. There are other reasons why reinforcement of speech skills are employed. For one, these skills predominate even in the speech of adult stutterers. This is evidenced by the fact that fluency characterizes their speech production. Moreover, the abundance of these responses means that they are much more available for contingent stimulation than are the maladaptive responses. In turn, this means that there is an increased opportunity for speech practice that is adaptive and emotional experiences that are positive. There is, thus, an increased likelihood that the improvement achieved will be maintained. This contrasts rather sharply with those techniques designed to produce suppression. Because maladaptive factor II responses may occur less frequently, carryover of the punishment effect can be rather limited. This has concerned clinicians in recent years, though procedures have been developed to reduce this difficulty (Boberg, 1981).

Another reason that reinforcement procedures are stressed is that they serve to give the speaker direction. They teach the speaker what to do and how to do it. The conditioning procedures are not designed to deal with what should not be done. It thus provides the client with adjustive speech skills and not admonitions. This should not be taken to mean that in two-factor therapy procedures are not utilized, the purpose of which is the reduction of maladaptive factor II responses. Various tactics are employed that serve this purpose. But they are not ones that involve response suppression through the delivery of aversive consequences. Instead, various means are employed through which reinforcement is provided for the omission of undesirable responses. Their occurrence is met by the absence of reinforcement. Undesirable responses may also be consequated. However, the contingent stimulus used is informing rather than painful, intense, or negative. They are client-defined as neutral stimuli and are used to notify. They serve to highlight the presence of a response that the client and the clinician, together, have targeted for elimination. The informing stimuli aid in this change process and they do so without negative side effects. They remind the client to monitor what it is that he does when speaking so that he will increasingly be able to omit the undesirable factor II response being worked with. They are not punitive.

The various tactics employed by two-factor therapists to modify maladaptive respondents and operants have only been alluded to. Two-factor therapists have available to them all of the behavior change procedures that are appropriate to these different response forms. It is this fact that makes it a multi-modal and multidimensional approach to modifying the various factor I and factor II responses displayed by those who stutter (Brutten, 1970).

Fluency Inducing Techniques

As we have seen stuttering therapies have often been based on certain theoretical viewpoints concerning the origin and nature of stuttering. In recent years, however, a number of techniques, with theoretical bases that are not clear, have gained the acceptance of clinicians. Many of these techniques are not new. Some flow from research which has shown that stuttering frequency is systematically reduced under certain conditions of stimulus manipulation. Others involve older techniques that have been refined and modified to increase their clinical effectiveness. Evidently, these techniques have gained the acceptance of clinicians because of their utility rather than because of their well-understood and fully validated theoretical base.

Most of the current therapeutic packages combine several different procedures. The different therapeutic packages generally contain some unique components, but most of them share a few elements. In this section, we will review some of the tactics that are a part of the various therapeutic packages used by research clinicians.

Rate Control and Speech Prolongation Procedures. Two of the tactics that are currently in wide use are rate control and speech prolongation. It has been known for some time that stutterers tend to be relatively fluent when they speak slowly (Van Riper, 1971, 1973). Parents of young stuttering children often insist on slow rate as a means of ensuring fluency. Adult stutterers, too, sometimes report that they slow their rate in order to control their dysfluencies. Not surprisingly, experts have long advocated slow speaking as a method of treatment (Van Riper, 1973).

In the past, slow speaking was clinically induced mainly through instructions to slow down. Stutterers were asked to slow their speech rate down to a level that seemed to be necessary to speak fluently. Even though its immediate results were encouraging, the procedure proved disappointing in that it failed to induce lasting and generalized fluency. Stutterers were simply unable to maintain a rate which was slow enough to speak fluently in everyday situations (Van Riper, 1973). Besides, it is known that stutterers' speech rate is typically slower than that of normal speakers (Bloodstein, 1944, 1981). Therefore, in order to speak fluently, most stutterers would have to slow their rate to an unnatural degree. Such a rate would likely be socially unacceptable because it would be devoid of normal prosody.

The effectiveness of slowed speaking has been considerably enhanced by modern developments. Most of the difficulties initially associated with this procedure have been overcome by the combined use of delayed auditory feedback (DAF) and operant shaping techniques. As pointed out earlier, DAF typically reduces the rate of speech. Generally speaking, the greater the delay, the slower the rate. Research clinicians have found that a delay of about 250 msec reduces the speech rate to about thirty words or fifty syllables per minute. They have also found that most stutterers are able to maintain fluency at that rate of speech (Goldiamond, 1965; Perkins, 1973a, 1973b; Ryan and Van Kirk, 1974). With the help of DAF, it is thus possible to maintain a slow rate in which speech is practically fluent.

Once fluency is established and strengthened at a slow rate of speech, operant shaping has been used to increase the rate until it is within the normal range. This is done by reducing the amount of time by which the feedback signal is delayed, in gradual and carefully chosen steps. In a program designed by Perkins and his associates, for example, slow and fluent oral reading is first established with a 250 msec of delayed auditory feedback (Perkins, 1973a). Later on, slow and fluent conversational speech is established by the same means. In subsequent steps, however, the feedback delay is reduced to 200, 150, and 50 msec. If fluency is maintained as the speaker's rate is increased, the volume of DAF is reduced gradually. Next, the DAF unit is turned off. Finally, first the earphones and then the headset are removed. If the delayed feedback is reduced or removed abruptly, stutterers are not able to maintain either a slowed rate or fluency. Therefore, shaping is a crucial element of rate control procedures.

It must be noted that the rate control does not have as its final target a dramatically reduced speech rate. The target is a rate that at least comes close to normal. But what constitutes normal rate is highly variable. Studies by Bloodstein (1944) and Darley (1940) have shown that stutterers' mean oral reading rate is 123 words per minute whereas the normal speakers' rate is 167 words per minute. But the range for stutterers was 92 to 191 words per minute, and for the normal speakers it was 129 to 222 words per minute. Most research clinicians, therefore, have not indicated the specific rate to be achieved. Rate is probably allowed to vary within a subjectively acceptable range. Each stutterer is taught to maintain a rate that is necessary to speak fluently in a natural setting.

During the early stages of training, most clinicians prefer to have the clients *read* aloud at a rate slower than normal. A majority of clients find it easier to control the rate in oral reading. This is especially true when the clients are trying to reduce the rate under instructions only, without the help of DAF. The clinician can also better monitor fluency and other aspects of speech when the client reads aloud. Once the client has mastered slow and fluent reading, conversational speech is undertaken. DAF and/or instructions have been used to control word and phone rate in both oral reading and conversational speech.

Rate control has been an important component of several therapeutic programs. Goldiamond (1965) was one of the researchers who early on described a systematic procedure involving DAF to slow rate. In subsequent years Perkins and his associates (Curlee and Perkins, 1973; Perkins, 1973a, 1973b; Perkins et al., 1974; Perkins et al., 1979), Ryan and Van Kirk (1974), Webster et al., (1970), Ingham and Andrews and their associates (Ingham, 1975; Ingham and Andrews, 1973; Howie, Tanner and Andrews, 1981), among others, have described specific procedures involving rate control by means of DAF. Most have found it necessary to include other procedures in the attempt to achieve and maintain fluency. Though rate control by itself may not produce lasting and generalized fluency it seems fairly reasonable to conclude that it can help reduce stuttering in a relatively short period of time.

Some recent research indicates that the specific manner in which the speech rate is reduced is an important therapeutic consideration. Evidently, there are different tactics by which a speaker can reduce the rate of speech. One obvious tactic is to reduce the number of words spoken per minute by increasing the durations of pauses between words. The result is a dramatic reduction in rate even though more time is not taken to produce the individual words. When this tactic is used, stuttering is known to decrease. It is not always eliminated, however (Adams, Lewis, and Besozzi, 1973). In some cases, reduced word output may even result in increased stuttering (Ingham, Martin, and Kuhl, 1974).

Another tactic used to slow speech involves the manner in which *phones* are produced. The phone rate is slowed down. When this is done more time is taken to produce individual words. A rate reduction is achieved but not through increased inter-word pause durations. In fact, pauses in between words may actually be reduced or eliminated. One word may smoothly blend into the next, resulting in an uninterrupted flow of speech with no word boundaries. A study by Perkins, Bell, Johnson, and Stocks (1979) compared the number of dysfluently spoken syllables when stutterers were asked to say either one word every two seconds, or prolong the speech sounds of every word blending each word into the next word. The number of dysfluencies exhibited under these two conditions was compared with the number exhibited in a controlled condition. When this comparison was made it became evident that the number of dysfluently spoken syllables decreased by a little more than 2 percent under the reduced word rate condition. But when the stutterers reduced the rate by prolonging sounds of words, there was a further reduction in rate and a dramatic decrease in dysfluencies. This finding led Perkins and his associates (1979) to suggest that slowing the phone rate is a more effective way to control stuttering than is reducing the word rate.

A slow rate, achieved by prolonging phones, results in time-stretched speech in which there is slow and continuous phonation. Most research clinicians who have developed rate reduction procedures involving DAF have emphasized that prolonged speech is an important component of their therapeutic package (Goldiamond, 1965; Perkins, 1973a, 1973b; Ryan and Van Kirk, 1974; Ingham and Andrews, 1973). Prolonged speech can be induced without DAF, however. In both oral reading and conversational speech, stutterers can be instructed to prolong speech sounds. Initially, the clinician models the prolonged speech, and closely monitors the client's performance throughout the therapy sessions. Procedures described by Howie, Tanner, and Andrews (1981) and Webster (1974) are designed to achieve reduced rate by prolonged speech but without the help of DAF.

Rhythm Based Procedures. Several treatment procedures are based on the basic observation that stutterers are usually fluent when some kind of rhythmic signal is associated with the production of every syllable, word, or phrase. Rhythmic or timing devices are often a part of the response display of stutterers. Just before an utterance is initiated a stutterer might, for example, evidence a head jerk, foot tap, eyebrow movement, or finger swing. These behaviors have been described by some as "timing devices" (Van Riper 1971, 1973). They have also been viewed as deviant motor behaviors that are learned through coincidental reinforcement.

Modern clinical interest in rhythmic speech has been sustained mainly by research on the metronome effect. In the past, desk metronomes were used to induce rhythmic speech. In recent years, however, many treatment programs involving rhythmic speech have utilized electronic metronomes. Probably the most popular of these is the miniature, behind-the-ear type of electronic metronome. The unit can deliver beats whose frequency and volume can be changed. Initially, a slow beat at a level that is comfortably loud is maintained. The stutterer is asked to time a syllable or a word with each of the beats. Gradually, the number of beats per minute is increased while the intensity is decreased. This type of shaping procedure is needed because the initial slow beats, which may be necessary to produce fluency, result in an unusually slow rate of speech. The rate is then increased, in gradual steps, so that a normal rate is approximated. The intensity of the beats is gradually decreased also. It is hoped that eventually the unit can first be turned off and later removed so that fluency does not depend on the metronome.

An advantage of the miniaturized electronic metronome is that it can be used in everyday situations in which the stutterer can control the number and intensity of the beats. The Pacemaster, a behind-the-ear model of this type, was used by Brady in conjunction with what is called the Metronome-Conditioned Speech Training (MCSR) program. Brady (1971) has published data on 26 stutterers who went through his training program. He has reported follow-up information gathered both six months and over four years after the completion of treatment. The data indicated that a majority of the stutterers showed improved fluency that was sustained. The results have not been supported by the findings of a number of subsequent studies (Berman and Brady, 1973; Adams and Hotchkiss, 1973; Ost, Gotestam, and Melin, 1976; Trotter and Silverman, 1974). It is now evident that some stutterers do not gain significant fluency with the Pacemaster. Others simply do not like to wear the unit. Furthermore, there is no assurance that the treatment results in speech that approximates rate and intonational patterns that are normal. Finally, the long-term effect of using the metronome has not been established. The self-report of a researcher who has used the Pacemaster continuously for a period of three years suggests that the effect gradually decreases to a point where it has very little effect on the frequency of stuttering (Silverman, 1976).

By and large, it seems evident that rhythm-based procedures have not been proven effective in producing normal and lasting fluency in a majority of stutterers treated. Generally speaking, rhythmic speech, whether generated by a metronome or by syllable-timed procedure, does not sound "natural." The speech output does not flow in a natural rhythm; words and phrases stand alone. Because it does not lead to normal intonational patterns, the speech sounds monotonous. Partly because of these reasons, the technique is often not acceptable to stutterers. This problem is not unique to rhythmic speech procedures, however. As we have seen, rate control procedures, including those that involve prolonged speech, also generate speech that may not be socially acceptable. The importance of shaping normal rate and prosody is well recognized by those who use rate control procedures (Perkins, 1973a, 1973b; Ryan and Van Kirk, 1974). That is why carefully planned shaping procedures are considered an important part of current rate-control procedures. It is possible that with the use of shaping and fading techniques the effectiveness of rhythmic procedures can be increased. A well-planned program of generalization might also help sustain fluency without the aid of a metronome.

Masking and Related Procedures. The laboratory studies by Shane (1955), Cherry, Sayers, and Marland (1955) and others that were reviewed earlier in this chapter have demonstrated that stutterers are relatively fluent under masking. It is not surprising, therefore, that a series of treatment procedures have been developed that are based on the auditory masking effect. Even before laboratory studies were conducted on the effect of masking it had been observed that stutterers were relatively fluent when they spoke in noisy environments (Van Riper, 1971, 1973). Indeed, attempts to cure stuttering by reducing the hearing acuity of stutterers temporarily or permanently were made long before the effect of white noise was described in the '50s. In Europe, one of the disconcerting therapy procedures recommended in the '20s was to simply deafen stutterers (Froeschels, 1962). Other, more humane treatment procedures such as beating of drums while stutterers read aloud were also suggested.

Modern treatment procedures based on auditory masking began with the use of desk model noise-generators. The procedure became more practical and flexible with the development of portable masking units. The first of the portable units was developed in Russia. They were called Derazne correctophones (Derazne, 1966) and were relatively heavy. Modern electronic maskers are lighter and more utilitarian. The currently available masking units can be turned on or off as desired, and the intensity of the noise can be increased or decreased.

Van Riper (1965) was one of the early researchers who developed a hand-held masking unit. He conducted extensive clinical trials with this unit over a number of years. Van Riper quickly found out that most stutterers were reluctant to accept this form of treatment. The continuous masking noise was an annoying stimulus which often resulted in headaches. The sight of the unit with its double earphones was suggestive of hearing loss. As a result, listeners tended to treat stutterers wearing these instruments as deaf or hard of hearing. In addition, stutterers felt that their hearing acuity was reduced in social situations by the fact that they had to wear earmolds. Still more important was the fact that stutterers were fluent only as long as they used the masking unit. The fluency that resulted from using a masking unit showed little tendency to generalize.

More recently, the Edinburgh Masker, a voice-activated electronic masking device, has been clinically tested by a few investigators. One advantage of the voice-activated unit is that the noise gets turned on as the stutterer begins to speak, and stays on only as long as the client continues to speak. Since the unit remains off during periods of silence, there is neither the annoyance nor the reduction in listening acuity that stutterers report when masking noise is continuously present. Nonetheless, the double earphones result in some reduction in hearing, and the unit is conspicuous.

Even though some of the advantages of a voice-activated masking unit over traditional devices are clear, its usefulness in establishing generalized fluency is not. We do not have many studies on the long-range effects of masking noise. There is some evidence which suggests that the effect of masking noise wears off over a prolonged period of use (Hedge, 1971b; Garber and Martin, 1974). A clinical study by Dewar, Dewar, and Barnes (1976) contains more positive findings. Using the Edinburgh

Masker, they treated fifty-three stutterers, ages nine to fifty-six, with the voice-activated masking unit and reported significant reductions in "speech errors" when the stutterers performed various speech tasks. The effectiveness of the Edinburgh masker has been recently investigated again by a different experimenter (Janssen, 1982). Thirty stutterers, whose factor I and II behaviors were separately analyzed during oral reading and extemporaneous speech, were the subjects of this study. Masking resulted in an average reduction of 44 percent in stuttering frequency. Though the reduction in factor I behaviors was statistically significant the results did not support the claim that the Edinburgh masker reduces dysfluency 90 to 100 percent.

In sum, studies involving masking noise do not suggest that it is an impressive procedure for modifying stuttering. In addition to the fact that most stutterers find masking unpleasant and the use of earphones socially unacceptable, there is no evidence that noise is permanently effective in enhancing fluency. Moreover, there does not appear to be any real evidence that the positive effect of masking is maintained when the earphones are removed.

Aerodynamic Procedures. As our overview of clinically related findings has shown, several studies have indicated that stutterers exhibit difficulties in managing the breathstream for the purposes of speech production. Although particular breathing abnormalities have been associated with dysfluent speech, only some have received therapeutic attention. Of these, the tendency for stutterers to speak without sufficient air pressure seems to have received the most attention from clinicians. Other difficulties for which modification procedures have been designed in recent years include disrupted air stream during the attempted production of a phrase or a sentence and the sudden stoppage of airflow at the level of the glottis that is associated with a hard vocal attack.

Since some of the breathing abnormalities are relatively easy to observe, exercises to teach "correct" breathing were popular in years past (Van Riper, 1973). Somehow it was assumed that stutterers need to learn how to breathe properly. Despite the fact that their vegetative breathing was perfectly normal, breathing exercises were prescribed. Generally, the effects of such exercises were negligible at best. Occasionally, the only clear-cut result was hyperventilation. As Van Riper reports (1973), some stutterers simply fainted during therapy sessions. Even though it is well known that speech is normally produced while air is being exhaled, a therapy procedure that was once strongly recommended taught stutterers to speak on inhalation (Van Riper, 1973). At one time, diaphragmatic breathing was also prescribed (Reichel, 1964). Probably the most common technique recommended in years past was for the stutterer to take a deep breath before saying something.

Most researchers now agree that stutterers do not generally need lessons in correct breathing. In fact, breathing exercises have been rarely used during the past several years. Nevertheless, some clinicians currently find it useful to deal with stutterers' breathing responses in their fluency modification programs (Zaliouk and Zaliouk, 1965; Perkins, 1973a, 1973b; Azrin, Nunn, and Frantz, 1979). We will briefly review some of these therapy tactics. But first, a brief comparison will be made between the older breathing exercises and the recent breathstream management procedures.

The newer approaches, which involve modifying the breathing patterns of stutterers, are different from the traditional breathing "exercises." While the latter exercises were designed to teach correct breathing per se, the newer approaches emphasize appropriate ways of managing the breathstream so as to attain fluent speech. Breathing responses themselves were the focus of the older techniques, while fluent speech production is the target of the newer procedures. It should be noted, also, that the breathstream management procedures are rarely used as exclusive therapy techniques. They are often one component of a more comprehensive therapeutic program (Perkins, 1973a, 1973b; Perkins et al., 1974).

Perkins (1973a, 1973b) has described a therapeutic program which includes a breathstream management procedure. The procedure is based on the assumption that the "smooth, easy flow of breath from the initial to the final syllable of each phrase will necessarily exclude abnormal dysfluency" (Perkins, 1973a, p. 287). Additional justification for this procedure has come from some research studies which have shown that stutterers experience difficulty in achieving smooth coordination between respiratory, phonatory, and articulatory processes. Purely from a clinical standpoint, it is evident that during speech stutterers are often unable to maintain exhalation that is smooth and easy. Sudden stoppages during exhalation disrupt fluency. Moreover, the release of excessive subglottic air pressure can result in a hard vocal attack. For smooth, continuous phonation, and for easy speech transitions, exhalation needs to be even and relaxed. Fluent speech production also requires that the lungs provide sufficient air pressure that is released in controlled exhalation. In addition, the speaker must pause at appropriate junctures to inhale so that an exhalation pattern conducive to smooth, fluent speech can be maintained. Most breathstream management procedures take these needs into consideration.

Generally speaking, a majority of breathstream management procedures involve some or all of the following components. Initially emphasized is the need to have an adequate air supply before speech is attempted. Stutterers are trained to inhale proper amounts of air at the beginning of words, phrases, sentences, and at other appropriate junctures. As soon as a proper amount of air is inhaled, stutterers are asked to begin a smooth, relaxed exhalation. It is impressed upon the stutterer that the inhaled air should not be held in the lungs since this would create excessive tension in the muscles of the chest and larynx. After an even flow of exhalation has been initiated, gentle onset of phonation is encouraged. With this step, stutterers are taught to avoid hard vocal attacks, "blocks" at the laryngeal level, speech production that is sudden, explosive, and tense. Finally, the stutterer is required to keep the exhalatory flow going until the end of the utterance. Properly mastered, this last step helps the stutterer avoid the inefficient ways of speaking that result when there is not enough air pressure in the lungs.

The maintenance of a relaxed posture appears to be another aspect of breathstream programs. Occasionally, the stutterer is given special training in deep muscle relaxation. During the initial stages of therapy, only one or two words are read aloud on each exhalation. As the stutterer begins to gain control over the coordinated processes of respiration, phonation, and articulation and fluency results, the length of utterance is increased in gradual steps. Breathstream management during conversational speech is initiated as soon as the client is able to maintain fluency at the sentence level while reading aloud. Here, too, the number of words spoken per exhalation is gradually increased.

The therapy programs described by Perkins (1973a, 1973b) and Cooper (1979) involve more than breathstream management. As we noted earlier, DAF-induced, slow, prolonged speech is a major aspect of the Perkins program. The Cooper program also includes slow speech but is achieved without the aid of DAF. Only one of the recently published treatment programs relies heavily on breathing techniques (Azrin, Nunn, and Frantz, 1979). But, even this "regulated breathing" procedure involves rate reduction.

Although only a few studies have demonstrated the effectiveness of breathstream management (Perkins, 1973a, 1973b; Perkins et al., 1974; Azrin et al., 1979), it appears to be a promising technique. The exact mechanism underlying this procedure needs a careful analysis, however. The process of breathstream management seems to affect practically every other aspect of speech production. When the client begins to have deep, slow, smooth and even inhalation and exhalation patterns, the resulting speech rate typically becomes slower than normal. Concomitantly, the movements of the articulators are also slowed down. Moreover, deep and slow breathing induces a relaxed neuromuscular state. Soft, gently phonatory onset is promoted by the slow and even exhalation. It is for these reasons, then, that breathstream management procedures may result in speech production that is fluent.

Other Treatment Procedures. There are several other clinical tactics worthy of mention. Some of these are not typically employed by speech-language pathologists. Other techniques are of recent origin. Their effectiveness needs to be assessed. Both of these types of procedures will be described briefly.

Therapy involving one drug or another has a long history of use with stutterers. The results have been mixed. Even when improvement has occurred, it has tended to be limited in nature. Recently, interest has been renewed by the development of psychotropic drugs. These drugs act on various subsystems and mechanisms of the nervous system in a way that produces behavior change. Stimulants, sedatives, and tranquilizers are probably the most widely known and frequently used drugs that change various aspects of behavior. These drugs are typically used in psychiatric settings where behavior disorders of wide range and severity are treated.

Throughout the world, various types of stimulants, sedatives, and tranquilizers have been used and are being used to treat stuttering. Vitamin therapy and carbon dioxide inhalation therapy have also been used. At the present time, drugs are more commonly used in Europe than in the United States (Van Riper, 1973). To some extent, the use of medication has continued despite the fact that studies have not generally indicated that drugs can produce consistently favorable results. Stutterers who undergo drug therapy are not able to maintain whatever improvement has occurred once the medication is removed. Even while the stutterer is using the drug, there may not be a significant decrease in the frequency of stuttering. The only outstanding effect of drugs has been the reduced severity of individual stutterings.

Psychotherapy is another of the treatment approaches that are not typically employed by speech-language clinicians. There are many psychotherapeutic techniques and schools of thought, and some of these are inconsistent with each other. Yet, psychotherapies have in common the fact that they were devised to treat various disorders such as those involving anxiety, phobia, and hysteria. These disorders are often described as neurotic reactions. Clinicians who would recommend psychotherapy for stutterers do so because they consider stuttering to be a form of neurotic reaction. Most psychotherapists probably agree that neurotic reactions are "symptoms" of an underlying psychological disturbance. Following this medical model of behavior, they would suggest that the underlying psychopathology *must* be treated if the neurotic symptoms are to be eliminated. The well-known Freudian psycho-analysis illustrates a basic approach to psychopathology and psychotherapy.

Psychoanalytically oriented psychotherapy for stuttering has a long history. Freud himself is reported to have treated stuttering with psychoanalysis, though without much success (Glauber, 1958; Froeschels, 1951). As a result, Freud did not recommend the use of psychoanalysis for stutterers. Despite this, his followers have treated stutterers. Unfortunately, the reports of such treatment tend to be neither systematic nor encouraging. The reports usually do not include such measures of speech as the frequency of stuttering. Also lacking in these studies are the controls that would appropriately enable one to reach supportable conclusions. Most psychoanalysts who recommend psychotherapy to stutterers do so on the basis of their clinical impressions and not on objective data (Coriat, 1928, 1943; Fenichel, 1945; Glauber, 1958).

An offshoot of psychotherapy is known as attitudinal therapy. This form of therapy is somewhat similar to psychotherapy, although the focus is on the faulty attitudes of stutterers. Disordered speech can affect the social, personal, emotional, and occupa-tional life of people who stutter. As a result, stutterers are said to have faulty attitudes and bad "self-images." Some clinicians believe that unless these maladaptive attitudes are changed, any fluency they may gain by direct treatment will not be permanent (Williams, 1957, 1968, 1979; Cooper, 1968, 1979).

The need for attitudinal therapy has been questioned by a number of clinicians, however (Ryan, 1979; Webster, 1979; Ingham, 1979). These clinicians have devel-oped and used therapy programs that work directly on stuttering. Their programs do not contain procedures that focus on the attitude and belief systems of stutterers. It is argued that faulty attitudes and beliefs that stutterers hold are a result of the stuttering. It follows that the most effective way of changing them is to achieve a significant reduction in stuttering. When the treated client begins to speak fluently the unfavorable attitudes and beliefs associated will dissipate.

It must be noted that most of those who advocate attitudinal change also work directly with stuttering. The results of therapy are thus confounded. The effect of attitudinal therapy, if any, cannot be separated from that of the other clinical procedures that were also utilized. As a result, we do not have controlled evidence to show that attitudinal therapy is either needed, or effective. A few studies that have been reported in this area have not produced convincing evidence supportive of the need for attitudinal therapy (Guitar, 1976; Guitar and Bass, 1978; Guitar, 1981).

Recently, biofeedback has been increasingly used as a treatment procedure for controlling various kinds of neurophysiological processes. The essence of biofeedback is that the client is given information about neurophysiological activity, such as heart rate or muscle tension, so that a desired change can be brought about.

The use of biofeedback in the treatment of stuttering is not widespread, in part, because the application of biofeedback is relatively new, the information sparse, and the long-term effects have not yet been established. The technique may prove to be useful, however. This hope is based on the fact that unusually high levels of muscular tension, especially in the muscles that are involved in the production of speech, often accompany stuttering. Biofeedback makes it possible to train stutterers to reduce this muscle tension. A few clinical reports that suggest that this can have a positive effect on speech have been published (Hanna, Wilfling, and McNeill, 1975; Lanyon, Barrington, and Newman, 1976; Cross, 1977). Specifically, modification of tension levels in the muscles of the face, neck, and larynx have led to improved levels of fluency. More experimental evidence is needed to assess the overall effectiveness of this procedure, however.

SUMMARY

Times have changed dramatically. Not many years ago, the clinician who sought to deal with the speech and speech-associated difficulties of those who stutter had relatively few available tactics. Moreover, the power-efficiency of these procedures was not truly known. Their value could only be surmised since outcome studies were not run. Yet, their limited clinical utility was implied. Therapies were designed to produce controlled stuttering, reduced severity, improved attitudes, or an acceptance of dysfluency. These goals were partly a result of the restricted data bank and partly a function of theoretical viewpoints.

As we have seen, the last few years have produced an explosion in the data that bear on the dimensions of stuttering and fluency. These data have had an understandably remarkable effect on our knowledge about fluency and fluency failure. They have led to a reevaluation of the constituents that define the disorder. They have made apparent the role of genetic risk in the onset of stuttering and its determinative interactions with triggering environmental elements. They have clarified neurophysiologic and linguistic issues. These and other advances in knowledge have affected clinical decision-making. The data have led many to a revised view about the goals of therapy. As a result, the targets and the tactics of behavior change have been altered, sometimes considerably, from what they were just a few years ago. Therapy has tended to become programmatic and focused on the development of normally fluent or stutter-free speech. Outcome studies have shown that clinical procedures are not equally powerful. They have also highlighted the strengths and limitations of particular therapeutic tactics and approaches. The data have made it clear that improvement is easier to achieve than it is to maintain. This has brought considerable attention to the matter of carry-over. Indeed, maintenance has come to the fore as a major clinical problem.

The fact is that some rather fundamental changes in clinical principles and practices have resulted from the recent outpouring of both basic and applied research studies. And, the pace is quickening. Research that is immediately or ultimately applicable to clinical endeavors is coming forth at a heady pace. Clinical viewpoints and tactics are likely, therefore, to show continued and considerable change in the years ahead. Clinicians need to be attuned to this and to avoid a hardening of their thinking about stuttering. They need to remain open to the innovations in diagnosis, assessment, and therapy that are undoubtedly on the way.

BIBLIOGRAPHY

Adams, M. R., Some common problems in the design and conduct of experiments in stuttering. *Journal of Speech and Hearing Disorders*, **41**, 3–9 (1976).

Adams, M. R., and Hotchkiss, J., Some reactions and responses of stutterers to a miniaturized metronome and metronome-conditioning therapy: Three case reports. *Behavior Therapy*, **4**, 565–569 (1973).

Adams, M. R., and Hutchinson, J., The effects of three levels of auditory masking on selected vocal characteristics and the frequency of disfluency of adult stutterers. *Journal of Speech and Hearing Research*, **17**, 682–88 (1974).

Adams, M. R., Lewis, J. I., and Besozzi, T. E., The effect of reduced reading rate on stuttering frequency. *Journal of Speech and Hearing Research*, **16**, 671–75 (1973).

Andrews, G., and Harris, M., *The Syndrome of Stuttering*. Clinics in Developmental Med., No. 17, London: Spastics Society Medical Education and Information Unit in Association with Wm. Heinemann Medical Books (1964).

Azrin, N., Jones, R. J., and Flye, B., A synchronization effect and its application to stuttering by a portable apparatus. *Journal of Applied Behavior Analysis*, **1**, 283–95 (1968).

Azrin, N. H., Nunn, R. G., and Frantz, S. E., Comparison of regulated breathing versus abbreviated desensitization on reported stuttering episodes. *Journal of Speech and Hearing Disorders*, **44**, 331–339 (1979).

Bakker, K., and Brower, C., Nonverbale stotterge draqinqeu. *Loqopedie en Foniatrie*, 1982 (in press).

Bastijens, P., Brutten, G. J. and Stés, R., The effect of punishment and reinforcement procedures on a stutterer's factor two avoidance response. *Journal of Fluency Disorders*, **3**, 77–85 (1978).

Berman, P. A., and Brady, J. P., Miniaturized metronomes in the treatment of stuttering: A survey of clinician's experiences. *Journal of Behavior Therapy and Experimental Psychiatry*, **4**, 117–119 (1973).

Bjerkan, B., Word fragmentations and repetitions in the spontaneous speech of 2–6-year old children. *Journal of Fluency Disorders*, **5**, 137–48 (1980).

Bloodstein, O., Studies in the Psychology of Stuttering: XIX. The relationship between oral reading rate and severity of stuttering. *Journal of Speech Disorders*, **9**, 161–73 (1944).

Bloodstein, O., Stuttering as tension and fragmentation. In J. Eisenson (Ed.), *Stuttering: A Second Symposium*. New York: Harper and Row (1975).

Bloodstein, O., *A Handbook of Stuttering*. Chicago, Ill.: National Easter Seal Society (1981).

Bloodstein, O., and Gantwerk, B. F., Grammatical function in relation to stuttering in young children. *Journal of Speech and Hearing Research*, **10**, 786–89 (1967).

Bluemel, C. S., *Stammering and Cognate Defects of Speech*. New York: G. F. Stechert (1913).

Boberg, E. (Ed.), *Maintenance of Fluency· Proceedings of the Bauff Conference*. New York: Elsevier North-Holland (1981).

Brady, J. P., Metronome-conditioned speech retraining for stuttering. *Behavior Therapy*, **2**, 129–50 (1971).

Brady, J. P., and Berson, J., Stuttering dichotic listening, and cerebral dominance. *Archives of General Psychiatry*, **32**, 1449–52 (1975).

Brayton, E. R., and Conture, E. G., Effects of noise and rhythmic stimulation on the speech of stutterers. *Journal of Speech and Hearing Research*, **21**, 285–294 (1978).

Brown, S. F., The influence of grammatical function on the incidence of stuttering. *Journal of Speech Disorders*, **2**, 207–15 (1937).

Brown, S. F., Stuttering with relation to word accent and word position. *Journal of Abnormal and Social Psychology*, **33**, 112–20 (1938a).

Brown, S. F., The theoretical importance of certain factors influencing the incidence of stuttering. *Journal of Speech Disorders*, **3**, 223–30 (1938b).

Brown, S. F., The loci of stutterings in the speech sequence. *Journal of Speech Disorders*, **10**, 181–92 (1945).

Brown, S. F., and Moren, A., The frequency of stuttering in relation to word length during oral reading. *Journal of Speech Disorders*, **7**, 153–59 (1942).

Brutten, G. J., Two factor behavior theory and therapy. In *Conditioning in Stuttering Therapy*. Memphis, Tenn.: Speech Foundation of America (1970).

Brutten, G. J., Behavior assessment and the strategy of therapy. In Y. Lebrun and R. Hoops (Eds.), *Neurolinguistic Approaches to Stuttering*. The Hague: Mouton (1973).

Brutten, G. J., Stuttering: Topography, assessment, and behavior change strategies. In S. Eisenson (Ed.), *Stuttering: A Second Symposium*. New York: Harper and Row (1975).

Brutten, G. J., The effect of punishment on a factor I stuttering behavior. *Journal of Fluency Disorders*, **5**, 1–10 (1980).

Brutten, E. J., and Gray, B. B., Effect of word cue removal on adaptation and adjacency: A clinical paradigm. *Journal of Speech and Hearing Disorders*, **26**, 385–89 (1961).

Brutten, G. J., and Shoemaker, D. J., *The modification of stuttering*. Englewood Cliffs, N.J.: Prentice Hall (1967).

Brutten, G. J., and Shoemaker, D. J., Stuttering: The disintegration of speech due to conditioned negative emotion. In B. B. Gray and G. England (Eds.), *Stuttering and the Conditioning Therapies*. Monterey, Calif.: Monterey Institute of Speech and Hearing (1969).

Brutten, G. J., and Shoemaker, D. J., A two-factor learning theory of stuttering. In L. Travis (Ed.), *Handbook of Speech Path. gy and Audiology* (1971).

Bryngelson, B., A study of the laterality of stutterers and normal speakers. *Journal of Speech Disorders*, **4**, 231–34 (1939).

Bryngelson, B., and Rutherford, B., A comparative study of laterality of stutterers and non-stutterers. *Journal of Speech Disorders*, **2**, 15–16 (1937).

Chase, R. A., Effect of delayed auditory feedback on the repetition of speech sounds. *Journal of Speech and Hearing Disorders*, **23**, 583–90 (1958).

Cherry, C., Sayers, B., and Marland, P. M., Experiments on the complete suppression of stammering. *Nature*, **176**, 874–75 (1955).

Chevrie-Muller, C., A study of larnygeal function in stutterers by the glottalgraphic method. In Proceedings VII, Congress de la societé Francaise de Medicinc de la Voixe et de la Parole, Paris (1963).

Cooper, E. B., A therapy process for the adult stutterer. *Journal of Speech and Hearing Disorders*, **33**, 246–60 (1968).

Cooper, E. B., Intervention procedures for the young stutterer. In H. H. Gregory (Ed.), *Controversies About Stuttering Therapy*. Baltimore: University Park Press (1979).

Coriat, I. H., Stammering: A psychoanalytic interpretation. *Nervous and Mental Disorders*. Monograph, Ser. No. 47, 1–68 (1928).

Coriat, I. H., The psychoanalytic conception of stammering. *Nervous Child*, **2**, 167–71 (1943).

Cross, D. E., Effects of false increasing, decreasing, and true electromyographic biofeedback on the frequency of stuttering. *Journal of Fluency Disorders*, **2**, 109–16 (1977).

Cullinan, W. L., and Springer, M. T., Voice initiation times in stuttering and non-stuttering children. *Journal of Speech and Hearing Research*, **23**, 344–60 (1980).

Curlee, R. F., and Perkins, W. H., Effectiveness of a DAF conditioning program for adolescent and adult stutterers. *Behavior Research Therapy*, **11**, 395–401 (1973).

Darley, F. L., A normative study of oral reading rate. M. A. Thesis, University of Iowa (1940).

Darley, F. L., The relationship of parental attitudes and adjustments to the development of stuttering. In W. Johnson and R. R. Leuteuegger (Eds.), *Stuttering in Children and Adults*. Minneapolis: University of Minn. Press (1955).

Derazne, J. L., Speech pathology in the U.S.S.R. In R. W. Rieber and R. S. Brubaker (Eds.), *Speech Pathology*. Amsterdam: North Holland (1966).

Dewar, A., Dewar, A. D., and Barnes, H. E., Automatic triggering of auditory feedback masking in stammering and stuttering. *British Journal of Disorders of Communications*, **11**, 19–26 (1976).

Dickson, S., Incipient stuttering and spontaneous remission of stuttered speech. *Journal of Communicative Disorders*, **4**, 99–110 (1971).

Dollard, J., and Miller, M. E., *Personality and Psychotherapy*. New York: McGraw-Hill (1950).

Eisenson, J., Observations of the incidence of stuttering in a special culture. *Asha*, **8**, 391–394 (1966).

Eisenson, J., Stuttering as perseverative behavior. In J. Eisenson (Ed.), *Stuttering: A Second Symposium*. New York: Harper and Row (1975).

Eisenson, J., and Horowitz, E., The influence of propositionality on stuttering. *Journal of Speech Disorders*, **10**, 193–97 (1945).

Fairbanks, G., Selective vocal effects of delayed auditory feedback. *Journal of Speech and Hearing Disorders*, **20**, 333–46 (1955).

Fenichel, O., *The Psychoanalytic Theory of Neurosis*. New York: W. W. Norton (1945).

Fisher, C. H., A study of the main and interactive effects of audience size and parts of speech on the part-word repetitions of pre-school non-stutterers and stutterers. Unpublished dissertation, Southern Illinois University (1977).

Floyd, S., and Perkins, W. H., Early syllable dysfluencies in stutterers and non-stutterers: A preliminary report. *Journal of Communication Disorders*, **7**, 279–82 (1974).

Freeman, F. J., Fluency and phonation. In M. Webster and L. Furst (Eds.), *Vocal Trait Dynamics and Dysfluency*. New York: Speech and Hearing Institute of New York, 229–266 (1974).

Freeman, F. J., and Ushijima, T., Laryngeal muscle activity during stuttering. *Journal of Speech and Hearing Research*, **21**, 538–562 (1978).

Froeschels, E., Stuttering and psychotherapy. *Folia Phoniatrica*, **3**, 1–9 (1951).

Froeschels, E., A survey of european literature in speech and voice pathology. *Asha*, **4**, 172–81 (1962).

Fujita, K., Pathophysiology of the larynx from the viewpoint of phonation. *Journal of the Japanese Society of Otoyhinolaryngology*, **69**, 459 (1966).

Garber, S. F., and Martin, R. R., The effects of white noise on the frequency of stuttering. *Journal of Speech and Hearing Research*, **17**, 73–79 (1974).

Gates, A., and Bradshaw, J., The role of cerebral dominance in music. *Brain and Language*, **9**, 403–431 (1977).

Glauber, I. P., The psychoanalysis of stuttering. In J. Eisenson (Ed.), *Stuttering: A Symposium*. New York: Harper and Row (1958).

Goldiamond, I., Stuttering and fluency as manipulatable operant response classes. In L. Krasner and L. P. Ullmann (Eds.), *Research in Behavior Modification*. New York: Holt, Rinehart and Winston (1965).

Gregory, H. H., Controversial issues: Statement and review of literature. In H. H. Gregory (Ed.), *Controversies in Stuttering Therapy*. Baltimore: University Park Press (1979).

Guitar, B., Pretreatment factors associated with the outcome of stuttering therapy. *Journal of Speech and Hearing Research*, **19**, 590–600 (1976).

Guitar, B., A correction to "a response to Ingham's critique". *Journal of Speech and Hearing Disorders*, **46**, 440 (1981).

Guitar, B., and Bass, C., Stuttering therapy: The relation between attitude change and long-term outcome. *Journal of Speech and Hearing Disorders*, **43**, 392–400 (1978).

Hahn, E. F., A study of the relationship between stuttering occurrence and phonetic factors in oral reading. *Journal of Speech Disorders*, **7**, 143–51 (1942).

Hall, J. W., and Jerger, J., Central auditory function in stutters. *Journal of Speech and Hearing Research*, **21**, 324–37 (1978).

Hanna, R., Wilfling, F., and McNeil, B., A biofeedback treatment for stuttering. *Journal of Speech and Hearing Disorders*, **40**, 270–73 (1975).

Hannah, E. P., and Gardner, J. G., A note on syntactic relationships in non-fluency. *Journal of Speech and Hearing Research*, **11**, 853–60 (1968).

Harms, M. A., and Malone, J. Y., The relationship of hearing acuity to stammering. *Journal of Speech Disorders*, **4**, 363–70 (1939).

Hegde, M. N., Propositional speech and stuttering. *Journal of the All India Institute of Speech and Hearing*, **1**, 21–24 (1970).

Hegde, M. N., The effect of shock on stuttering. *Journal of the All India Institute of Speech and Hearing*, **2**, 104–10 (1971a).

Hegde, M. N., The short and long term effects of contingent aversive noise on stuttering. *Journal of the All India Institute of Speech and Hearing*, **2**, 7–14 (1971b).

Hegde, M. N., Stuttering adaptation, reactive inhibition and spontaneous recovery. *Journal of The All India Institute of Speech and Hearing*, **2**, 40–47 (1971c).

Hegde, M. N., and Hartman, D. E., Factors affecting judgments of fluency: I interjections. *Journal of Fluency Disorders*, **4**, 13–22 (1979a).

Hegde, M. N., and Hartman, D. E., Factors affecting judgments of fluency: II word repetitions. *Journal of Fluency Disorders*, **4**, 13–22 (179b).

Hejna, R. F., A study of the loci of stuttering in spontaneous speech. Ph.D. dissertation, Northwestern University (1955).

Howie, P. M., Concordance for stuttering in monozygotic and dizygotic twin pairs. *Journal of Speech and Hearing Research*, **24**, 317–21 (1981).

Howie, P. M., Tanner, S., and Andrews, G., Short and long term outcome in an intensive treatment program for adult stutterers. *Journal of Speech and Hearing Disorders*, **46**, 104–109 (1981).

Hutchinson, J. M., and Brown, D., The Adams and Reis observations revisited. *Journal of Fluency Disorders*, **3**, 149–54 (1978).

Ingham, R. J., A comparison of covert and overt assessment-procedures in stuttering therapy outcome evaluation. *Journal of Speech and Hearing Research*, **18**, 346–54 (1975).

Ingham, R. J., Comment on "stuttering therapy: The relation between attitude change and long-term outcome." *Journal of Speech and Hearing Disorders*, **44**, 397–400 (1979).

Ingham, R. J., and Andrews, G., Stuttering: The quality of fluency after treatment. *Journal of Communicative Disorders*, **4**, 279–88 (1971).

Ingham, R. J., and Andrews, G., Behavior therapy and stuttering: A review. *Journal of Speech and Hearing Disorders*, **38**, 405–41 (1973).

Ingham, R. J., Martin, R. R., and Kuhl, P., Modification and control of rate of speaking by stutterers. *Journal of Speech and Hearing Research*, **17**, 489–96 (1974).

Janssen, P., De Edinburgh Masker: eeu welkom geluid voor de stotteraar? *Logopedie eu Fouiatrie*, **54**, 54–62 (1982).

Johnson, W., and Brown, S. F., Stuttering in relation to various speech sounds. *Quarterly Journal of Speech*, **21**, 481–96 (1935).

Johnson, W. (Ed.), *Speech Handicapped School Children*. (2nd ed.) New York: Harper and Row (1956).

Johnson, W., Ed., *Speech Handicapped School Children*. (3rd ed.) New York: Harper and Row (1967).

Johnson, W., and Associates, *The Onset of Stuttering*. Minneapolis: University of Minnesota Press (1959).

Johnson, W., and Leutenegger, R. R. (Eds.), *Stuttering in Children and Adults*. Minneapolis: University of Minnesota Press (1955).

Kanfer, F. H., and Goldstein, A. P., *Helping People Change*. New York: Pergamon Press (1975).

Karr, G. M., The performance of stutterers on central auditory tests. *South African Journal of Communicative Disorders*. **24**, 100–09 (1977).

Kidd, K. K., Genetic models of stuttering. *Journal of Fluency Disorders*, **5**, 187–201 (1980).

Kidd, K. K., Heimbuch, R. C., and Records, M. A., Vertical transmission of susceptibility to stuttering with sex-modified expression. *Proceedings of the National Academy of Sciences*, **78**, 606–610 (1981).

Kidd, K. K., Kidd, J. R., and Records, M. A., The possible causes of the sex ratio in stuttering and its implications. *Journal of Fluency Disorders*, **3**, 13–23 (1978).

Kohout, B. M., *The Contingent and Non-Contingent Effects of Positive Verbal Stimulation on Selected Aspects of the Stuttering Moment*, M.S. thesis, Southern Illinois University (1974).

Krych, D. K., *An Audio-Visual Analysis of Behavioral Sequences Evidenced During Moments of Stuttering*. M.S. thesis, Southern Illinois University (1978).

Lanyon, R. I., Barrington, C. C., and Newman, A. C., Modification of stuttering through EMG biofeedback: A preliminary study. *Behavior Therapy*, **7**, 96–103 (1976).

Lechner, B. K., The effects of delayed auditory feedback and masking on the fundamental frequency of stutterers and non-stutterers. *Journal of Speech and Hearing Research*, **22**, 343–53 (1979).

Lee, B. S., Effects of delayed speech feedback. *Journal of the Acoustic Society of America*, **22**, 824–826 (1950).

Lee, B. S., Artificial stutter. *Journal of Speech and Hearing Disorders*, **16**, 53–55 (1951).

Lemert, E. U., Some Indians who stutter. *Journal of Speech and Hearing Disorders*, **18**, 168–74 (1953).

Lingwall, J. B., and Bergstrand, G. G., Perceptual boundaries for judgments of "normal," "abnormal," and "stuttered" prolongations. *Asha*, **21**, 733, 1979 (abstract).

Maraist, J. A., and Hulton, C., Effects of auditory masking upon the speech of stutterers. *Journal of Speech and Hearing Disorders*, **22**, 388–89 (1957).

Martin, R. R., and Haroldson, S. K., Stuttering identification: Standard definition and moment of stuttering. *Journal of Speech and Hearing Research*, **24**, 59–63 (1981).

Martyn, M. M., and Sheehan, J., Onset of stuttering and recovery. *Behavior Research and Therapy*, **6**, 295–307 (1968).

Miller, M. E., Experimental studies in conflict. In J. McVicker Hunt, (Ed.), *Personality and the Behavior Disorders*. New York: Ronald Press (1944).

Moore, W. H., Jr., and Haynes, W. D., Alpha hemispheric asymmetry and stuttering: Some support for a segmentation dysfunction hypothesis. *Journal of Speech and Hearing Disorders*, **23**, 229–247 (1980).

Mowrer, O. H., The dual nature of learning—A re-interpretation of "conditioning" and "problem solving." *Harvard Educational Review*, **17**, 102–148 (1947).

Neelley, J. N., A study of the speech behavior of stutterers and non stutterers under normal and delayed auditory feedback. *Journal of Speech and Hearing Disorders, Monograph supplement*, **7**, 63–82 (1961).

Nelson, S. E., Hunter, M., and Walter, M., Stuttering in twin types. *Journal of Speech Disorders*, **10**, 335–43 (1945).

Oelschlaeger, M. L., and Brutten, G. J., Response contingent positive stimulation of the part-word repetitions displayed by four stutterers. *Journal of Fluency Disorders*, **1**, 10–17 (1975).

Orton, S., and Travis, L. E., Studies in stuttering: IV Studies of action currents in stutterers. *Archives of Neurology, Psychiatry*, **21**, 61–68 (1929).

Ost, L. G., Gotestam, K. G., and Melin, L., A controlled study of two behavioral methods in the treatment of stuttering. *Behavior Therapy*, **7**, 587–92 (1976).

Oxtoby, E. T., Frequency of stuttering in relation to induced modification following expectancy of stuttering. In W. Johnson and R. R. Leutenegger (Eds.), *Stuttering in Children and Adults*. Minneapolis: University of Minnesota Press (1955).

Panconcelli-Calyia, G., Die Bedingtheit des Lombardschen Versuches in der Stimm-und-Sprachheilkunde. *Acta Otolaryngology*, **45**, 244–51 (1955).

Perkins, W. H., Replacement of stuttering with normal speech: 1 Rationale. *Journal of Speech and Hearing Disorders*, **38**, 283–94 (1973a).

Perkins, W. H., Replacement of stuttering with normal speech: II Clinical procedures. *Journal of Speech and Hearing Disorders*, **38**, 295–303 (1973b).

Perkins, W. H., Bell, J., Johnson, L., and Stocks, J., Phone rate and the effective planning time hypothesis of stuttering. *Journal of Speech and Hearing Research*, **22**, 747–55 (1979).

Perkins, W., Rudas, J., Johnson, L., and Bell, J., Stuttering: Discoordination of phonation with articulation and respiration. *Journal of Speech and Hearing Research*, **19**, 509–22 (1976).

Perkins, W., Rudas, J., Johnson, L., Micheal, W. B., and Curlee, R. F., Replacement of stuttering with normal speech: III Clinical effectiveness. *Journal of Speech and Hearing Disorders*, **39**, 416–28 (1974).

Porfert, A. R., and Rosenfield, D. B., Prevalence of stuttering. *Journal of Neurology, Neurosurgery and Psychiatry*, **41**, 954–56 (1978).

Prins, D., and Lohr, F., Behavioral dimensions of stuttered speech. *Journal of Speech and Hearing Research*, **15**, 61–71 (1972).

Quarrington, B., Stuttering as a function of the information value and sentence position of words. *Journal of Abnormal Psychology*, **70**, 221–24 (1965).

Reichel, C. W., *Stop Stammering and Stuttering*. New York: Vintage Press (1964).

Rimm, D. C., and Masters, J. C., *Behavior Therapy*. (2nd ed.) New York: Academic Press (1979).

Ronson, I., Word frequency and stuttering: The relationship to sentence structure. *Journal of Speech and Hearing Research*, **19**, 813–19 (1976).

Ryan, B. P., Stuttering therapy in a framework of operant conditioning and programmed learning. In H. H. Gregory (Ed.), *Controversies in Stuttering Therapy*. Baltimore: University Park Press (1979).

Ryan, B. P., and Van Kirk, B., The establishment, transfer, and maintenance of fluent-speech in 50 stutterers using delayed auditory feedback and operant-procedures. *Journal of Speech and Hearing Disorders*, **39**, 3–10 (1974).

Sander, E. K., Frequency of syllable repetition and "stutterer" judgments. *Journal of Speech and Hearing Disorders*, **28**, 19–30 (1963).

Schiavetti, M., Judgments of stuttering severity as a function of type and locus of disfluency. *Folia Phoniatrica*, **27**, 26–37 (1975).

Schlesinger, I. M., Forte, M., Fried, B., and Melkman, R., Stuttering, information load, and response strength. *Journal of Speech and Hearing Disorders*, **30**, 32–36 (1965).

Schuell, H., Sex differences in relation to stuttering: Part I. *Journal of Speech Disorders*, **11**, 227–98 (1946).

Shames, G. H., Egolf, D. B., and Rhodes, R. C., Experimental programs in stuttering therapy. *Journal of Speech and Hearing Disorders*, **34**, 30–47 (1969).

Shames, G., and Sherrick, C. E., Discussions of non-fluency and stuttering as operant behavior. *Journal of Speech and Hearing Disorders*, **28**, 3–13 (1963).

Shane, M. L. S., Effect on stuttering of alteration in auditory feedback. In W. Johnson and R. R. Leutenegger (Eds.), *Stuttering in Children and Adults*. Minneapolis: University of Minnesota Press (1955).

Sheehan, J., Stuttering behavior: A phonetic analysis. *Journal of Communicative Disorders*, **7**, 193–212 (1974).

Sheehan, J., (Ed.), Conflict theory and avoidance-reduction therapy. *Stuttering: A Second Symposium*. New York: Harper and Row (1975).

Silverman, F. H., Long-term impact of a miniature metronome on stuttering: An interim report. *Perceptual Motor Skills*, **42**, 1322 (1976).

Silverman, F., and Williams, D. E., Loci of disfluencies in the speech of stutterers. *Perceptual Motor Skills*, **24**, 1085–86 (1967).

Skinner, B., *The Behavior of Organisms: An Experimental Analysis*. New York: Appleton (1938).

Slorach, N., and Noehr, B., Dichotic listening in stuttering and dyslalic children. *Cortex*, **9**, 295–300 (1973).

Soderberg, G. A., Linguistic factors in stuttering. *Journal of Speech and Hearing Research*, **10**, 801–810 (1967).

Sommers, R. K., Brady, W. A., and Moore, W. H., Jr., Dichotic ear preferences of stuttering children and adults. *Perceptual Motor Skills*, **41**, 931–38 (1975).

Starkweather, C. W., Hirschman, P., and Tannenbaum, R. S., Latency of vocalization onset: Stutterers versus non stutterers. *Journal of Speech and Hearing Research*, **19**, 481–92 (1976).

Stewart, J. L., The problem of stuttering in certain North American Indian societies. *Journal of Speech and Hearing Disorders Monograph Supplement*, **6** (1960).

St. Louis, K. O., Linguistic and motor aspects of stuttering. In N. J. Lass (Ed.), *Speech and Language: Advances in Basic Research*. New York: Academic Press (1979).

St. Louis, K. O., and Martin, R. R., Motor speech awareness in stutterers: Reorganization of distinctive features? *Asha*, **18**, 593, 1976 (Abstract).

Sutton, S., and Chase, R. A., White noise and stuttering. *Journal of Speech and Hearing Research*, **4**, 72 (1961).

Taylor, I. K., The properties of stuttered words. *Journal of Verbal Learning and Verbal Behavior*, **5**, 112–18 (1966).

Trotter, W. D., Relationship between severity of stuttering and word conspicuousness. *Journal of Speech and Hearing Disorders*, **21**, 198–201 (1951).

Trotter, W. D., and Silverman, F. H., Does the effect of pacing speech with a miniature metronome on stuttering wear off? *Perceptual Motor Skills*, **39**, 429–30 (1974).

Tuthill, C., A quantitative study of extensisual meaning with special reference to stuttering. *Journal of Speech Disorders*, **5**, 188–91 (1940).

Ushijima, T., Kamiyama, G., Hiydse, H., and Niimis, S., Articulatory movements of the larynx during stuttering, a film produced at the Research Institute of Logopedics and Phoniatrics, Faculty of Medicine, University of Tokyo (1965).

Van Riper, C., *Speech Correction: Principles and Methods*. (4th Ed.) Englewood Cliffs, N.H.: Prentice-Hall (1963).

Van Riper, C., Clinical use of intermittent masking noise in stuttering therapy. *Asha*, **7**, 381 (1965).

Van Riper, C., *The Nature of Stuttering*. Englewood Cliffs, N.J.: Prentice-Hall (1971).

Van Riper, C., *The Nature of Stuttering*. (Rev. ed.) Englewood Cliffs, N.J.: Prentice-Hall (1982).

Van Riper, C., *The Treatment of Stuttering*. Englewood Cliffs, N.J.: Prentice-Hall (1973).

Voelker, E. X., and Voelker, C. H., Spasmophemia in dyslalia copotica. *Annals of Otorhinolaryngology*, **46**, 740–743 (1937).

Webster, L. M., and Brutten, G., An audiovisual behavioral analysis of the stuttering moment. *Behavior Therapy*, **3**, 555–60 (1972).

Webster, L. M., and Brutten, G. J., The modification of stuttering and associated behaviors. In S. Dickson (Ed.), *Communicative Disorders*. Glenview, Ill.: Scott, Foresman and Company (1974).

Webster, R. L., A behavioral analysis of stuttering: Treatment and theory. In K. S. Calhoun, H. E. Adams, and K. M. Mitchell (Eds.), *Innovative Treatment Methods in Psychopathology*. New York: Wiley (1974).

Webster, R. L., Empirical considerations regarding stuttering therapy. In H. H. Gregory (Ed.), *Controversies in Stuttering Therapy*. Baltimore: University Park Press (1979).

Webster, R. L., Schumacher, S. J., and Lubker, B. B., Changes in stuttering frequency as a function of various intervals of delayed auditory feedback. *Journal of Abnormal Psychology*, **75**, 45–49 (1970).

Wepman, J. M., Familial incidence in stammering. *Journal of Speech Disorders*, **4**, 199–204 (1939).

West, R., An agnostic's speculations about stuttering. In J. Eisenson (Ed.), *Stuttering: A Symposium*. New York: Harper and Row (1958).

Williams, D. E., A point of view about "stuttering." *Journal of Speech and Hearing Disorders*, **22**, 390–97 (1957).

Williams, D. E., Stuttering therapy: An overview. In H. H. Gregory (Ed.), *Learning Theory and Stuttering Therapy*. Evanston, Ill.: Northwestern University Press (1968).

Williams, D. E., A perspectives on approaches to stuttering therapy. In H. H. Gregory (Ed.), *Controversies on Stuttering Therapy*. Baltimore: University Park Press (1979).

Williams, D. E., and Kent, L. R., Listener evaluations of speech interruptions. *Journal of Speech and Hearing Research*, **1**, 124–31 (1958).

Williams, D. E., Silverman, F. H., and Kools, J. A., Disfluency behavior of elementary-school stutterers and non stutterers: Loci of instances of disfluency. *Journal of Speech and Hearing Research*, **12**, 308–18 (1969).

Wingate, W. E., A standard definition of stuttering. *Journal of Speech and Hearing Disorders*, **29**, 484–89 (1964).

Wingate, M. E., Criteria for stuttering. *Journal of Speech and Hearing Research*, **20**, 596–607 (1977).

Wischner, G. J., Stuttering behavior and learning: A preliminary theoretical formulation. *Journal of Speech and Hearing Disorders*, **15**, 324–35 (1950).

Yates, A. J., Delayed auditory feedback. *Psychological Bulletin*, **60**, 213–32 (1963).

Young, M. A., Predicting ratings of severity of stuttering. *Journal of Speech and Hearing Disorders*, Monsgram Supplement, **7**, 31–54 (1961).

Zaliouk, D., and Zaliouk, A., Stuttering, a differential approach in diagnosis and therapy. *De Therapia Vocis et Loquelae*, Vol. 1, XIII Congress, International Society of Logopedics and Phoniatry (1965).

Zimmermann, G., Articulatory behaviors associated with stuttering: A cinefluorographic analysis. *Journal of Speech and Hearing Research*, **23**, 108–21 (1980a).

Zimmermann, G., Stuttering: A disorder of movement. *Journal of Speech and Hearing Research*, **23**, 122–36 (1980b).

5 Voice Remediation and the Teaching of Alaryngeal Speech

James C. Shanks
Marshall Duguay

Laryngeal voice disorders may be attributed to many factors. A structural anomaly of the laryngeal mechanism, an improper use of the laryngeal organs, or certain attitudes about speaking may all account for phonatory behaviors judged to be aberrant. It is thus essential that in studying a particular problem and determining steps to be taken for its alleviation, the traditional function of the voice clinician or pathologist be supplemented by the services of the laryngologist, the laryngeal physiologist, and the psychiatrist in a team approach. Their combined knowledge and skills afford a patient the best opportunity for successful remediation.

Depending on the particular problem, medical (surgical) treatment may be indicated, or learning to modify vocal behavior may be prescribed. It is the purpose of this chapter to acquaint the voice clinician who will be dealing primarily with the modification of vocal behavior with methods of analyzing disorders of phonation and techniques of vocal remediation. The first section deals with laryngeal phonation disorders and the second with alaryngeal phonation.

LARYNGEAL PHONATION DISORDERS

Despite the advantages of the team approach to laryngeal voice disorders, the notion has persisted that each of the factors influencing normal or abnormal laryngeal phonation is the primary province of a particular specialist, as follows:

1. the physical condition of the larynx—the laryngologist or laryngeal physiologist;
2. vocal habits in speaking—the voice clinician;
3. the feelings of the speaker—the psychiatrist.

Ideally, however, each discipline should contribute to the general fund of information and work together in the rehabilitation of laryngeal voice disorders, with the respective specialists understanding phonation in its entirety.

240

The Study of Phonation Disorders

It should be clear that the role of the voice clinician goes far beyond that of a technician, and that limiting the study of voice disorders to diagnostic and remedial techniques is shortsighted and dangerous. However, a thorough understanding of phonation is not easy to achieve. The phonatory process is a significant blend of science and art in which the terms "functional" and "organic" lose precise lines of demarcation. Voice is disordered if it sounds unpleasant, is inappropriate for comparable speakers, or results from deviant feelings or defective neuromuscular structures.

The terms "hypertonic" and "hypotonic," as applied to the force of glottal approximation, are indicative of excessive and insufficient force, respectively. The principle of voice therapy is deceptively simple: to strive for an optimal balance of muscular tensions, while avoiding extremes of hypertonic and hypotonic function (Brodnitz, 1959; Perkins, 1957; Von Leden, 1968). The clinician, in applying that principle, must decide whether to decrease or increase tension, and determine which techniques to use in trying to effect the desired change (Murphy, 1964). If therapy is effective, the clinician must appreciate the physiology of phonation in order to know how and why the voice is improved.

The present section, which is intended to foster that understanding, is based on certain premises: (1) the myoelastic-aerodynamic theory of Van den Berg (1958), which, stated simply, relates vocal fold activity to well-established principles of aerodynamics, gives the most reasonable theoretic model of phonation; and (2) a client's phonatory behavior can and should be analyzed if it is to be understood and if remediation efforts are to succeed. The present discussion focuses on phonation, although the processes of phonation, respiration, and resonation are interwoven. Respiration will be considered only to the extent that air, moving through the larynx, is needed to achieve phonation. (For a discussion of resonance problems associated with cleft-palate speech, see chapter 6.)

Analyzing Disorders of Phonation

For purposes of evaluation and diagnosis, a patient's phonatory behavior may be analyzed by various methods of study, each of which uses a particular sensory avenue and unique units of measurement or description:

1. physiological (including aerodynamic and neuromuscular) analysis;
2. psychological analysis;
3. auditory (including acoustic, perceptual, and clinical) analysis.

Although each method is considered separately in the following discussion, it should be noted that added insights into a patient's condition are gained by correlating the findings of two or more methods. (See case study of T. R., p. 245.)

Physiological Analysis. The physiological function of the larynx during phonation may be discerned through the aerodynamics of measured pressure and flow of air through the larynx, through visible evidence of physical activity, and through neuromuscular activity within the larynx.

Aerodynamic analysis. The purpose of aerodynamic analysis is to measure air flow and pressure below, at, and above the glottis. The movement of air across the vocal folds sets them into vibration. We refer to this phenomenon as phonation. Clearly, if subglottic air pressure were neutralized by equivalent pressure of air downward from above the larynx, phonation would not occur. The flow of air can be upward or downward, as indicated by the fact that one can phonate on inhalation. It can occur without vibrating the vocal folds. It can be audible (breathing), produce speech sounds (voiceless consonants), be intelligible (whispered speech), and yet not produce phonation.

To maintain phonation at low intensity, there must be an air flow of at least 33–50 cc/sec (cubic centimeters per second) (Cavagna and Margaria, 1968). The rate can range up to 220 cc/sec at high intensity (Van den Berg, 1964). The following flow rates have been reported for various activities.

1. Phonating: 100–110 cc/sec reported by Yanagihara (1967), and 130 cc/sec by Von Leden (1968).
2. Singing: 110–200 cc/sec reported by Proctor (1968).

Understandably, flow rates increase in whispering and are as much as 100 cc/sec higher in the presence of laryngeal pathology. They also become greater with increases in pitch (Van den Berg, 1968) and with increases in intensity (Yanagihara, 1967), varying up to sevenfold for tones of constant frequency at low-middle intensity levels (Cavagna and Margaria, 1968).

Subglottic air pressures often average 7 mm Hg (millimeters of mercury), but may range up to 37 mm Hg. A given subglottic pressure may be achieved by the release of the stretched respiratory tree, which varies with lung volume, as well as by the action of the respiratory muscles (Bouhuys et al., 1968). As pressure increases, so does the intensity of phonation.

The efficiency of the vocal instrument may be measured by relating the input of aerodynamic power (in watts) to the output of sound, as has been done by Cavagna and Margaria (1968) and Van den Berg (1964). In the latter study, Van den Berg reported values ranging from .0005 to .05 percent, with efficiency increasing by a factor of 100 with increased voice fundamental frequency. Clearly, efficiency is a function of increased subglottic air pressure and flow rate (Bouhuys et al., 1968), while dysphonia is characterized by turbulence and air waste. Differences in air volume and flow rate for hypertensive and hypotensive disorders have been noted by Von Leden (1968), with both having been found to be greater in hypotensive cases by Rubin and Hirt (1960). Gould (1975) indicated that maximum phonation time provides a measure of the overall status of laryngeal function, laryngeal tension and neuromuscular disability. A short phonation time, accompanied by a significant escape of air, suggests a neurological deficit such as a laryngeal nerve paralysis. Iwata, Von Leden and Williams (1972) stated that the presence of higher mean air flow rates reflect laryngeal hypotension, whereas lower mean air flow rates suggest hypertension of the cords. Boone (1977) writes, "Another respiration-phonation task is to ask the patient to take a breath and sustain a hissing, non-vocalized 's.s.s.' as long as he can. The typical prepubertal child can sustain the voiceless exhalation for about ten seconds; the average adult in the voice clinic can do so for about twenty seconds"

(p. 86). These duration times appear somewhat short since Tait, Michel, and Carpenter (1980), testing a group of nine-year-olds report nonvocalized exhalation times for /s/ of almost sixteen seconds. It seems then that typical prepubescent children and adults should produce the /s/ sound longer than Boone suggested.

Physical Analysis. The fundamental frequency of the voice is changed by tensing or relaxing the vocal cords. This physical change is accompanied by alterations in the stiffness, length, elasticity, and size of the vocal cords (Hollien and Coleman, 1970; Moore, 1957). They may be studied directly and indirectly by means of laryngoscopy, photography, stroboscopy, and radiography, including laminography (Hollien and Coleman, 1970; Sedlackova, 1965; Von Leden and Koike, 1970). The physical property of mass, a factor which also affects the function of the vocal cords and the frequency of the sounds produced by their vibrations, is altered by pathological changes such as neoplasms, and procedures such as therapeutic intra-cordal injections, and surgical intervention. Increases in mass will lower the frequency of the voice, while decreases will raise it.

Vocal fold length is reduced in falsetto, where maximal voice fundamental frequency is achieved by shortening the vibrating segments of the cords through progressive damping or stoppage of the posterior section of the folds (Briess, 1964; Moore, 1957; Rubin and Hirt, 1960). The length of the folds is also reduced during vocal fry, an atypical vibratory pattern involving a rapid double opening of the vocal folds with a long closure (Moore and Von Leden, 1958; Wendahl, Moore, and Hollien, 1963).

Other factors studied in the physical analysis of phonation include the symmetry and contour of the vocal folds during the vibratory cycle, as well as the synchrony and pattern of motion (Von Leden, Moore, and Timcke, 1960). A bulge on one or both folds, or a notching or bowing of one or both, will be revealed by disturbances in the glottic wave. (See figure 5–1.) In bulging, the problem may be a consequence of a vocal nodule (a small protuberance or aggregation of cells on vocal folds), a polyp (a small mass composed of new tissue, primarily vascular in origin), a papilloma (a benign new growth, wart-like in nature, occurring primarily in children), or edema.

Irregularities in the contour of the folds, with consequent wastage of air, alter both respiration and phonation. Post-surgical analysis may show that the removal of papillomata facilitates respiration more than phonation. Although the surgeon's removal of a polyp or nodule may be necessary, the removal of too much or too little tissue may disturb the contour of the fold (Brewer, Briess, and Faaborg-Anderson, 1960). After a cordectomy or hemilaryngectomy, the remaining tissue, even if cicatrical, can become a vibrating mass. A skin flap over the operated fold results in a faster recovery of voice, albeit low pitched, than is obtained with an irregular scar (Brodnitz, 1965).

If one or both of the vocal folds fail to move, their synchronous motion is disturbed. Bilateral paralysis of the folds does not preclude phonation; indeed, such phonation may sound less hoarse than if only one fold were paralyzed, or may not be perceived as hoarse at all (Arnold, 1959a). Although voice is dysphonic and inefficient with one paralyzed fold in the paramedian position, the other fold can be abducted for breathing. Phonation can be facilitated in such cases by injecting the paralyzing fold with a substance such as Teflon, which effectively shifts it from the paramedian to a

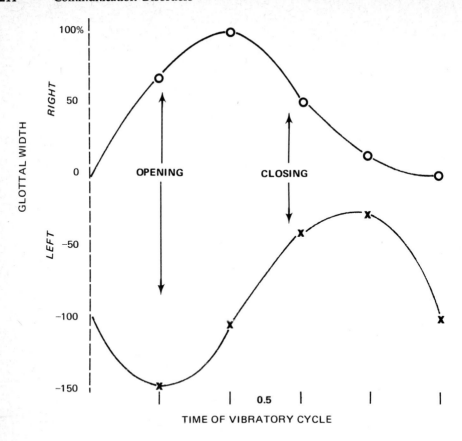

GLOTTAL WIDTH

RIGHT

LEFT

100%

50

0

−50

−100

−150

OPENING

CLOSING

0.5

TIME OF VIBRATORY CYCLE

Figure 5–1. Illustration of Asymmetric Vocal Fold Motions.

phonatory position. However, this procedure reduces the maximal exchange of air for breathing and must be carefully evaluated (Arnold, 1963a; see also the case study of Mrs. N. D., p. 256).

Altered duration of fold approximation during a vibratory cycle affords the examiner a useful index of irregularities of the folds' contour and motion. Two values allow comparison between normal cord function: open quotient (OQ- the ratio of the fraction of the cycle during which the glottis is open to the duration of the entire cycle) and speed quotient (SQ- the ratio of the time of abduction, or lateral excursion, to the time of abduction, or medial excursion) (Timcke, Von Leden, and Moore, 1958; Von Leden et al., 1960). Such measurements may be used in evaluating progress in therapy for vocal nodules (Fisher and Logemann, 1970).

Neuromuscular Analysis. An understanding of neuromuscular activity may proceed from electromyographic (EMG) analysis (Faaborg-Anderson, 1964; Hirano, Ohala, and Vennard, 1969; Snidecor, 1940) or from the laryngologist's observation of the extent to which individual muscles function excessively or insufficiently (Brewer, 1964). The laryngologist is assisted in his observations by a series of vocal tests developed by Briess (1957). These divergence and endurance tests for specific muscles have been based on the premises that the thyroarytenoid muscle and cricothyroid muscle normally work antagonistically. As voice fundamental frequency is increased, the ratio of thyroarytenoid to cricothyroid function is decreased, even for voices of differing type and character (Briess, 1959; Van den Berg, 1968). Thus, the cricothyroids have been termed the "pitch muscles" (Moore, 1971). Hirano and his associates (1969) found the lateral cricoarytenoids to aid in controlling intensity at low voice fundamental frequency, while Briess (1964) reported that shifting from full to breathy phonation involves the interplay of lateral and posterior cricoarytenoid muscles. Briess' clinical assessment of muscle function was confirmed by EMG in 99 percent of 200 patients examined by Faaborg-Anderson (1964).

Most voice clinicians do not try to determine the tension of individual muscles because they have no practical reason for doing so. Rather, they assume that hyperfunction (excessive tension) in some form (Briess, 1959; Flower, 1959; Froeschels, 1943) will make itself known. Thus, disturbance in the balance of respiratory and phonatory activity will impair voice quality.

Psychological Analysis. The voice is commonly regarded as a barometer of personality. Many writers (Barton, 1960; Briess, 1959; Perkins, 1957; Van Riper and Irwin, 1958; Cooper and Cooper, 1977; Boone, 1977) have noted the association between vocal pathology and disturbed attitudes and personality. For a detailed analysis of the ways in which voice deviations are symbolically interpreted, the reader is referred to *The Voice of Neurosis* (Moses, 1954). In the present discussion, factors of personality and attitudes are considered only with respect to their role in creating excessive or insufficient muscular tension between respiratory and phonatory forces.

Excessive tension appears to be closely related to the occurrence of vocal nodules. Consistent with the concept that emotional tension leads to physical tension, it is valuable to ascertain if the person with vocal abuse is "uptight." As Moore (1971) has noted, a vocal disorder associated with nodules may be "caused" by other factors. A case in point is that of T. R.:

> T. R., twenty-five, earned his living by singing country and western music. When small bilateral vocal nodules were discovered, he worried about what they would mean to his career. His ear, attuned to music, failed to note a recently acquired habit of clearing his throat frequently or of dropping into a dicrotic (quavering) voice at the ends of sentences. During his third clinical visit, he wondered aloud as to the possible effect on his voice of worries connected with his recent divorce and the impending dissolution of his musical group.

The diagnosis of T. R.'s voice problems required an understanding of his physical condition, his feelings, and his vocal habits.

Insufficient tension is reflected in hypotonia, in one form or another. The behavior labeled as hysterical aphonia may be viewed as an extreme form of hypotonia. The speaker continues to breathe for pulmonary purposes, as well as for vital functions, such as coughing. Indeed, coughing and clearing the throat indicate that he can achieve glottal function, but he fails to use this function in speaking for fear of what he might say (Barton, 1960). This behavior is illustrated by the case of Mrs. L., 60, respected for her family, civic and church work, who incurred a sudden loss of phonation upon learning that her son had been jailed for a felony.

Elective mutism is a smaller form of hypotonia, in which the person can, but sometimes elects not to, phonate. A less severe form is associated with a dicrotic quality suggestive of fatigue or old age. Some persons, with reduced breath support, manifest hypotonia at the ends of words or sentences (Moore, 1971).

Auditory Analysis. The sound produced in phonation has properties which may be assessed in three dimensions: how high, how much, and how long. Each dimension of sound may be "heard" in three ways:

1. acoustically, with instruments;
2. perceptually, with the human ear;
3. clinically, with indices of vocal use.

Although quality of sound usually is considered a subjective criterion, the quality of phonation has correlates in each method of hearing.

Acoustic Analysis. In acoustic analysis, phonation is measured in terms of frequency (F), intensity (I), and time (T). The voice of good quality has these characteristics in appropriate degrees; it is acoustically *FIT*.

Voice fundamental frequency and relative intensities of overtones are measured by the visecorder or spectograph, while a less precise measure of fundamental frequency is provided by the pitchmeter (developed at Purdue University and available from PAD Laboratories, Cleveland, Ohio).

Intensity of phonation may be measured with a graphic level meter, making it possible to determine the periodicity and mathematical relationship of harmonics associated with voices of varying quality (Curry, 1953; Sansone and Emanuel, 1970; Von Leden, 1968). In such tests, for example, hoarseness has been related to aperiodicity, especially in the frequency regions approximating the second and third formants of vowels (Yanagihara, 1967).

Findings expressed as a function of time include rate of air usage, frequency change in vibrato, and rate of breathing. Precise time measurements may be made of the speed of onset of phonation, percent time phonation, and speed quotient, as well as the more customary duration of phonation.

Abnormal voice production has been related to laryngeal vibratory patterns that deviate from "normal" periodicity. "Vocal jitter" refers to cycle-to-cycle variations in period that occur when a person tries to sustain a constant frequency at a constant intensity. When such variations become excessive, as they do in pathological cases, the voice is perceived as abnormal. "Vocal shimmer" refers to cycle-to-cycle variations in amplitude that occur when a person tries to sustain a constant frequency at a constant intensity. Wide and random variations in shimmer, just as in jitter, will result in the auditory impression of abnormal voice. Glottograms can be plotted and used to measure the amount of jitter and shimmer present in a speaker's voice. They provide objective measures of the initial status as well as improvement in therapy. The terms "pitch perturbation" and "amplitude perturbation" also are used in the literature to refer to jitter and shimmer. Measures of perturbation can be made by transcribing on an oscilloscope an audiosignal of a sustained vowel at constant pitch and constant intensity. The period and amplitude of successive waves can be measured and mathematically computed as changes in perturbations (Iwata and Von Leden, 1970).

Figure 5–2. Voice Profile by Frank B. Wilson

VOICE PROFILE

NAME: _____ AGE: _____ SEX: _____

(circle one)

VOICE RATING: 1 2 3 4 5 6 7

LARYNGEAL CAVITY	RESONATING CAVITY	INTENSITY		
PITCH	NASALITY	−2	1	+2
high	hypernasal	soft		loud
B	C			
+3	+4			
+2	+3			
	+2			
A open −4 −3 −2 1 +2 +3 closed	−2 1 +2	VOCAL RANGE		
−2	−2	−2	1	+2
−3	hyponasal	monotone		variable
low				pitch

		YES	NO
INTERMITTENT DIPLOPHONIA	*Indicate presence or absence of acoustic feature by (✓)*	____	____
DIPLOPHONIA		____	____
AUDIBLE INHALATION		____	____
PITCH BREAKS		____	____
ERRATIC PHRASING		____	____
IMMATURE RESONANCE		____	____

MARKING SYSTEM

Primary Feature   *x*   Secondary Feature
Intermittent Feature (*int*)   Noted Feature

Perceptual analysis. Sound which is heard by the ear and has meaning attributed to it by the mind is said to be perceived. The phonatory attributes thus perceived are described in terms of pitch, loudness, and quality (Perkins, 1957; Van Riper and Irwin, 1958).

Pitch and loudness may be scaled in degrees and correlated with data derived from other methods of study (Aronson, 1969; Briess, 1959; Faaborg-Anderson, 1964; Hirano et al., 1969; Isshiki, 1965; Perkins and Yanagihara, 1968).

Impaired voice quality, or dysphonia, is most frequently perceived as hoarse. Although other terms, such as harsh, strident, thin, and metallic have been used to describe impaired voice quality (Van Riper and Irwin, 1958), they appear to have less universal meaning and acceptance. Hoarseness is aesthetically unpleasant and suggests some degree of air loss and/or noise (Moore, 1971). Although hoarseness can be perceived auditorily, there is no current method by which degrees of perceived hoarseness can be scaled and related unequivocally to acoustic or physiological parameters (Von Leden, 1968).

There has been some attempt to devise rating scales to quantify the perceptual attributes of abnormal voice. Wilson's Voice Profile (1970): assigns a number from 1 to 7 whereby 1 represents a barely perceptible problem and 7 a very significant problem (top right of fig. 5–2). A measure of the patient's ability to sustain an /a/ is made to get an impression of laryngeal ease, efficiency, and amount of air escape. The parameters of pitch, laryngeal fold opening, and resonation are rated. Pitch is judged along a continuum in which +3 represents the abnormal high point, −3 the abnormal low point, and 1 the normal pitch for the person's age, sex, and size. Laryngeal opening also is viewed along a continuum, from completely open, represented by a − 4, to extreme tension and hyperadduction which would be rated as a + 3. Normal is rated as a 1. It is possible along this laryngeal opening dimension to have a voice rated as a + 2 − 2. This would indicate a breathy voice (− 2) and a voice exhibiting a serious amount of tension (+ 2). Clinically, this could be the voice of one with vocal nodules. Although not central to the present discussion of voice, Wilson also scaled the resonance feature of nasal balance, i.e., resonating cavity ratings range from + 4 (extreme nasality and nasal distortion) to a − 2 where the perception is one of hyponasality. The bottom part of the scale (see fig. 5–2) provides the opportunity to judge and score rate, intensity, and vocal range.

The Buffalo Voice Profile (Wilson, 1979) (fig. 5–3) utilizes seven equal-appearing intervals in which 1 represents a slight deviation and 7 a severe deviation. The vocal dimensions of laryngeal tone, laryngeal tension, vocal abuse, loudness, pitch, vocal inflections, pitch breaks, diplophonia, resonance, nasal emission, rate, and overall voice efficiency are the parameters considered.

These two scales are especially useful for the beginning clinician and for the exchange of information. They not only specify vocal attributes to be evaluated, but also require numbers for greater quantification.

Quality of phonation may be perceived on another scale related to, but not synonymous with, pitch and not suggestive of impairment. Although it has been primarily used to describe singing voices, this specialized scale of perception, termed register, has value for scientists and clinicians dealing with spoken voice (Van den Berg, 1968).

Garcia, credited with developing the mirror for indirect laryngoscopy, advanced the theory of a register as "a series of consecutive homogenous sounds produced by one mechanism" (see Appleman, 1967, p. 88). Every voice has three distinct registers (Appleman, 1967) separated by breaks, shifts, or modes (McGlone and Brown, 1969; Moses, 1954). Each register has a distinctive quality or timbre (Luschinger and Arnold, 1965), as well as a distinctive mechanism. Voices have been classified as exhibiting head, chest, and falsetto register, as well as vocal fry, best considered a register as opposed to a pathology.

Singing with head register has been equated with lyric quality while chest register conveys dramatic quality (Moses, 1954). In an effort to reduce the impression that the physiological activity of head register occurs primarily in the head, it has been labelled falsetto (Van den Berg, 1968). Similarly, chest register, commonly employed while speaking, has been described as fundamental (Rubin and Hirt, 1960) or modal (McGlone and Brown, 1969).

Hollien (in Cooper and Cooper, 1977) uses the classification of pulse, modal, and loft to refer to registers, attempting to avoid those terms that might be contaminated by concepts "lingering in the minds of the phoneticians, voice pathologists, laryngologists, voice teachers, or, 'for that matter, any class of professionals who must deal with the human voice (p. 79)." The pulse register represents the lowest range of phonation, pulse-like in nature and synonymous with glottal fry. Modal register is the register customarily employed in speaking and singing. The loft register is the one commonly thought of as falsetto. Table 5–1 summarizes the differences between chest and falsetto registers in terms of specific physical differences.

Figure 5–3. The Buffalo Voice Profile

Name _____ Birth Date _____ Age ___ Sex ___

Rater _____ Date _____ Time of Day _____ Place _____

1. *Laryngeal Tone*
   Normal
   Breathy
   Harsh
   Hoarse   1   2   3   4   5   6   7

2. *Laryngeal Tension*
   Normal
   Hypertense
   Hypotense   1   2   3   4   5   6   7

3. *Vocal Abuse*
   No
   Yes   1   2   3   4   5   6   7

4. *Loudness*
   Normal
   Too loud
   Too soft   1   2   3   4   5   6   7

5. *Pitch*
   Normal
   High
   Low   1   2   3   4   5   6   7

6. *Vocal Inflections*
   Normal
   Monotone
   Excessive   1   2   3   4   5   6   7

7. *Pitch Breaks*
   None
   Amount   1   2   3   4   5   6   7

8. *Diplophonia*
   None
   Amount   1   2   3   4   5   6   7

9. *Resonance*
   Normal
   Hypernasal
   Hyponasal   1   2   3   4   5   6   7

10. *Nasal Emission*
    No
    Yes   1   2   3   4   5   6   7

11. *Rate*
    Normal
    Fast
    Slow   1   2   3   4   5   6   7

12. *Overall Voice Efficiency*
    Adequate
    Inadequate   1   2   3   4   5   6   7

Circle the appropriate descriptive term under *each* item. For each item *not* normal or adequate, circle a number on the scale for that item. Do *not* mark between numbers.

Key: 1 = slight deviation   4 = moderate deviation   7 = severe deviation

COMMENTS:

Table 5–1. Differences Between Chest and Falsetto Registers

Parameter	Chest	Falsetto
Vocal fold		
Appearance		
Frontal	Thick, rounded	Thin, sharp
Coronal		Elongated
Mass	Increased	Decreased
Longitudinal tension		
Ligament (medial)	Small, slack	Increased
Vocalis (lateral)	Variable, greater	Small
Amplitude of movement		
Lateral	Increased	Decreased
Vertical phase difference	Marked	Negligible
Mechanics of movement		
Abduction		
Subglottal air pressure		Increased
Ligament tension		Increased
Adduction		
Bernoulli force	Increased	Decreased
Ligament tension		Increased
Mechanics of air release		
Pattern	Discrete puffs	Like sine wave
Open Quotient		Increased
With increased subglottal pressure		
Flow rate		Increased
Open Quotient	Decreased	
Glottal		
Closure	Firm	Light, absent
Resistance		Increased
Tone		
Voice fundamental frequency	Up to 300 Hz	Down to 150 Hz
Harmonic partials	Many	Few

Pitch placement during pubertal voice change is related to the concept of register. Brodnitz (1959) has described three types of post-mutational disturbances in the male basso, incomplete falsetto, and persistent falsetto.

By itself, a perceptual analysis of vocal attributes is limited to the use of subjective terms whose reliability depends on matching an acoustic signal with a verbal label. Such matching is refined by experience. Describing a vocal attribute in words is not the same as hearing it demonstrated. Clearly, a recorded or face-to-face demonstration of different registers, mutational changes, or degrees of hoarseness is of much value to voice clinicians. In a similar way, even when spastic dysphonia—a spastic condition resulting in vocal irregularity—is described as a "stuttering of the vocal cords" (Arnold, 1959b; Aronson et al., 1968), the meaning is incomplete until one has heard a voice that manifests that condition.

Clinical Analysis. A thorough history of a patient frequently reveals such physical symptoms as dryness, tickle, choking, scratchiness, lump, ache, or burn. These symptoms may be related to vocal abuse. As indicated by the following summary of research studies, vocal abuses which have been identified can be classified in terms of pitch, loudness, and time, and in terms of the imbalance between respiratory and phonatory forces:

- Pushing limits of pitch range: Perkins (1957), Proctor (1968)
- Pushing limits of loudness: Rubin and Lehrhoff (1962)
- Throat-clearing: Brewer et al. (1960), Gardner (1958), Peacher (1966)
- Glottal attack: Briess (1959), Brodnitz (1959)
- Using undue subglottal pressure for intensity: Proctor (1968)
- Using voice unduly during laryngitis: Proctor (1968)
- Stage whisper: Briess (1959)
- Breathing with vocal folds partly closed: Briess (1959)
- Vocal fatigue: Gardner (1958)
- Voice deterioration late in the day: Gardner (1958)

Excesses of pitch are revealed by vocal nodules among persons who are more apt to attempt to sing above their natural range, such as a baritone attempting to sing as a tenor (Brodnitz, 1959). Excesses of loudness imputed to juveniles by the use of the descriptive term "screamers' nodes" are confirmed by the high incidence of nodules among cheerleaders. Excesses in the amount of talking are revealed by the higher incidence of voice disorders among persons in the "vocal" professions—such as singers, ministers, and teachers—even though they have greater vocal competence.

Indices of vocal abuse may be elicited by specific tests of phonatory habits, the effect of masking noise on vocal production, and the effect of physical manipulations of the larynx or tongue.

The range of voice fundamental frequencies, on which habitual pitch may be located, reveals register divergence as well as tension (Briess, 1964). In assessing intensity, the clinician may note the quality and muscular effort associated with the extremes of loud and of quiet (non-whispered) phonation. Having the speaker, on signal and without delay, initiate phonation at a comfortable pitch may reveal symptoms of glottal attack or undue muscular effort. Such effort may be manifested in an elevation of the larynx, a bulge of the sternal notch, a protrusion of the sterno-cleidomastoids, or an extraneous mandibular drop. Reduced prolongation (phonation time) suggests excessive air loss.

Using the Lombard test to determine the effect of loud masking noise on phonation may evoke significant changes in vocal behavior (Freud, 1962; Weiss, 1965). For example, there may be an increase in loudness or a rise in pitch.

In tests involving manipulations of the larynx, the voice clinician may defer to the physician. Application of digital pressure against the notch of the thyroid, either in a posterior (Brodnitz, 1959) or inferior (Aronson, 1969) direction, combats the excessive tension produced by the cricothyroid muscle, as in persistent falsetto. The modal register thus achieved may also be accomplished through marked extension of the head before phonating. These tests are more valuable when the patient begins with an ample supply of air and employs a forceful method of expiration during phonation.

Medial pressure against one thyroid cartilage may also enhance voice quality, as in cases involving unilateral paralysis (Arnold, 1962); or it may evoke voice, as in cases involving psychogenic aphonia (Aronson, 1969; Barton, 1960). One also should assess the patient's laryngeal abilities in non-speech activities such as coughing, clearing the throat, grunting, groaning, humming, laughing, crying, or producing glottal fry. The patient presenting with a psychogenic dysphonia may be expected to perform these laryngeal maneuvers in a normal manner.

The effect of varying pitch and intensity (high pitch-low intensity, low pitch-high intensity, etc.) may provide clinical clues for locating a starting point for voice remediation.

Remediation of Phonation Disorders

At the start of this chapter, it was noted that laryngeal voice disorders judged to be aberrant can be caused by a variety of factors, organic as well as functional. Whatever the problem, remediation calls for a team approach by a laryngologist or laryngeal physiologist, a voice clinician, and a person qualified to deal with the speaker's psychic need, in other words, psychiatrists, psychologist, social worker. Concern here is only with the remediation of hypertonic and hyptonic voice disorders and not problems associated with removal of the laryngeal mechanism. The techniques to accomplish alaryngeal phonation are varied, different, and the subject of the section on alaryngeal phonation.

Principles of Remediation. The following general principles, elaborated in the subsequent discussion, should serve as a guide to effective voice remediation:

1. A laryngeal examination should precede voice therapy (Moore, 1957) because disturbances of laryngeal structure and function are, primarily, laryngeal diseases (Rubin and Hirt, 1960; Von Leden, 1968; Von Leden and Koike, 1970). In harmony with this concept is the fact that the laryngologist frequently determines not only which persons need to correct vocal habits or to acquire compensating vocal patterns, but also which ones should receive psychiatric help. Speech (voice) clinicians should also consider psychiatric referrals when appropriate.

2. If surgery for vocal nodules appears to be indicated, three factors to be considered are the age of the patient, the vocation of the patient, and the condition of the nodule.

3. Voice therapy is particularly appropriate for persons whose conditions are presumed to be associated with significant elements of vocal abuse, that is, those with vocal nodules, vocal polyps, contact ulcers, and other functional disorders (Arnold, 1962; Aronson, 1980; Boone, 1977; Brewer, 1964; Gardner, 1958; Moore, 1957; Wilson, 1979).

4. Although the reduction of abuses associated with hypertonic voice disorders may be the chief concern of the voice therapist, stronger efforts may be needed to combat hypofunction or to establish voice habits that will compensate for cord asymmetry or the limited motion that interferes with cord approximation.

Vocal Nodules—Determining the Need for Surgery. Medical management of vocal nodules may include surgical removal, depending, in each case, on the age and vocation of the patient and the condition of the nodule. Prepubertal nodules do not need surgery, and neither do small, soft, incipient ones; but surgery is needed for those which are firm and fibrotic. For the adult whose healthy vocal folds are necessary for income, such as a professional singer, surgical removal of nodules represents a considerable financial risk.

The case of Mrs. P. S. demonstrates that surgery is not always needed nor are the results permanent. Mrs. P. S., 38, was a singing teacher who had taught full-time for seven years, part-time for five. For many years she was apt to develop laryngitis after getting a head cold. When the hoarseness eventually persisted unduly, a laryngeal examination was performed and proved negative. In the ensuing two years, the laryngologist twice noted a nodule evolve, only to disappear for months with no special treatment. The third time a nodule developed, however, surgical removal was elected. Seven months after surgery, an incipient nodule was noted, and a voice evaluation was initiated. During the evaluation, tension was noted, as phonation was initiated, by a marked bulge of the abdomen and sternal notch. Mrs. P. S. accepted the clinician's suggestion to use a mirror to discern degrees of effort in progressing from quiet respiration to sighed /a/, /h/ words and phrases. In addition, she began to use a portable amplifier while teaching. The nodule was not evident two months later, but Mrs. P. S.'s voice quality was deemed unsatisfactory, a judgment that persisted until two more months had passed. At that point, she reported that a slight restriction of her vocal range for high tones was her only concern.

Correcting Vocal Abuse. While therapy is designed to correct specific misuses, it must also be directed at the elimination or modification of vocal abuse. Thus, the clinician may set forth guidelines in the form of "don'ts:" *don't* clear the throat, shout, sing, lead cheers, or tax the pitch limits of the voice; *don't* talk too much when tired, tense, or suffering from laryngeal infection (Moore, 1957); and *don't* expend undue physical energy while talking (Burkowsky, 1968).

Mrs. A. L., thirty-nine years old, was married and the mother of two teenage children. Hoarseness had persisted for six weeks, when indirect laryngoscopy revealed the presence of vocal nodules. Although during an initial clinical visit, the evaluation of her phonation suggested no significant vocal abuse, her history indicated that there were two potential sources of abuse of vocal intensity—frequently calling her children in from outside and trying to make herself heard in large groups. She helped evolve a plan for summoning her children with a whistle instead of shouting, and for intentionally speaking with less than average intensity in noisy social situations. At a progress check six months later, she reported that at first people responded to her lowered voice with "what?," but then they really began to listen to her through the competing noise. The laryngologist reported that the nodules had disappeared.

Cutting down on the amount of talking should reduce the amount of vocal abuse. Restrictions may take many forms, such as imposing a period of silence on the speaker, limiting the amount of talking time, or avoiding specific vocal situations. A forceful, or stage whisper, does not afford voice rest. On the contrary, it is harmful since this respiratory attack increases laryngeal tension and thus contributes to vocal misuse.

Some clinicians have patients work for ease of phonation by concentrating on muscle balances which are free of hypertonic function, as in chewing. Others emphasize treatment of the whole person, rather than limiting the treatment to control of pitch (Boone, 1977; Brodnitz, 1959; Flower, 1959; Moore, 1957; Perkins, 1957). On the assumption that anxiety and tension may have become generalized in the person with vocal nodules, reciprocal inhibition—in which the speaker learns to become aware of and to inhibit tensions, especially laryngeal tensions, while imagining anxiety-evoking stimuli—has been suggested as a means of facilitating muscle relaxation (Gray, England, and Mohoney, 1956).

A study of the vocal nodule psyche may be conducted. It might be hypothesized that some people actually prefer a hoarse vocal quality. Consider for example, the case of D. W.

D. W., nine years old, was found to have small bilateral vocal nodules. He participated extensively in athletics with much enthusiasm and shouting. His phonation was initiated in a glottal manner and was sustained with bulging of the abdomen and sternal notch. He habitually spoke two semitones above his lowest tone, with frequent throat-clearing. His parents were asked to note, but not to correct, his vocal usage at home. On the basis of their reports, the clinician asked the boy to restrict his throat-clearing and shouting and to raise his pitch slightly, so as to phonate more easily. D. W. recorded daily a letter grade on his efforts to restrict vocal abuse.

There was no apparent carry-over from practice in the clinic to outside situations. When simulating in the clinic loud speech at an imaginary athletic contest, D. W. found phonation easier, yet he continued to shout abusively at actual ball games. He intimated that he rather liked his husky voice, that it made him sound "strong."

After six months of biweekly visits with no observable improvement, D. W.'s clinic visits were reduced to one every other month. A year later, the sessions were dropped, although the voice was still hoarse.

In addition to using negative suggestions, the clinician may use positive admonitions aimed at using the least air pressure and glottal resistance. These are offered in the form of do's, such as *do* try to phonate with as much ease as possible, that is, quietly, with inflection in a restricted pitch range (Moore, 1957). Such an approach does not involve getting an optimal pitch, which is a difficult task at best (House, 1959; Perkins, 1957). Inflection in a restricted pitch range, however, implies avoiding extremes in pitch (Arnold, 1963b), as well as avoiding laryngeal tension by adjusting muscles to alter pitch, especially in a downward inflection (Curry, 1953). The controversy over raising or lowering pitch has not been adequately resolved. (Connelly et al., 1970; Cooper, 1974; Fisher and Logeman, 1970; Laguaite and Waldrop, 1964; Mueller, 1975; Perkins, 1971).

Generally most people with vocal nodules and polyps (certainly contact ulcer cases) are phonating at a pitch too close to the bottom of their range and need to raise pitch (actually avoid the basal pitch) in order to improve phonation.

Wilson (1979) expressed a major remedial consideration in recommending "normalizing pitch when it is inappropriate to a child's size, age and sex and is thought to have a relationship to voice misuse or vocal pathology" (p. 140). This holds true for adults as well.

Paradoxical as it may seem, therapy for hypertonic function often aims at a breathy attack and quality (Moore, 1971). Even though hypertonic function frequently is associated with hoarseness, which presumes air loss, a breathy voice reduces the likelihood of undue firmness in vocal fold contact, such as that characterizing a glottal attack. Thus, as suggested by Fox (1969), working for a markedly breathy voice is a valid therapy procedure for cases involving spastic dysphonia. This is demonstrated in the case of E. S.:

> E. S., 49 years old, taught at a seminary. Within a period of two months he noted an inconsistent interruption of phonation, first when lecturing, and then in conversation. Generally physical, laryngeal, and neurologic examinations were suggestive of no pathology.
>
> A voice examination revealed appropriate pitch level and range, and absence of dysphonic quality. Phonation was initiated quickly and was sustained for more than twelve seconds. However, when some words were attempted during conversation, there appeared to be cessation of exhalation and an abrupt emergence of phonation. During production of the first phoneme, his pitch rose rapidly, then dropped to his habitual level as he spoke fluently. The loci of spasms were not limited to specified sounds or words. Consistent with an impression of spastic dysphonia, indirect laryngoscopy was requested with the medical diagnosis. The laryngologist observed one laryngeal spasm. During the next four months, a psychiatrist noted marked feelings of anger in E. S. Voice therapy was begun, aimed at establishing a breathy attack of phonation. At times, phonation was so weak that E. S. appeared to whisper, an activity that was asymptomatic. He secured a change in his duties from teaching to counseling, but otherwise he engaged in his usual situations, including telephoning. Spasms continued to exist in E. S.'s speech during conversation, but were considerably less noticeable. In fact, his listeners reported less awareness of his breathy voice. Therapy was terminated on the assumption that E. S. was aware of the ongoing need to compensate for his hypertonic laryngeal function with minimal vocal fold adduction. At a follow-up evaluation a year later, he handled about half of his spasms in ways that would not be noticed by most listeners.

With the current interest in techniques for behavior modification, several approaches to programmed instruction in voice therapy have been devised and reported. For a better understanding of these approaches the reader should examine Cook et al. (1979), Deal et al. (1976), Drudge and Philips (1976), Johnson (1976), and Wilson and Rice (1977). In general, a programmed approach first isolates an improper response, determines its baseline or frequency of occurrence, and then proceeds via an operant shaping-training program to phase out the original aberrant behavior, usually in small increments, until the desired goal is achieved.

Consistent with these views is the concept that for the large majority of patients with hypertonic vocal disorders (whose disorders do *not* serve some emotional need), a symptomatic approach to therapy as described by Boone (1977) is very effective. This approach seeks to identify and then to eliminate the "possible misuses of respiration, phonation, or resonance which contribute to the patient's vocal impairment" (page 12). The individual who has a voice disorder often misuses and abuses his voice because he does not know healthier ways to use it. He must be helped to find the cause(s) of his abuse or misuse, to systematically discard these and then to employ only correct vocalization throughout his speaking day. This symptom-oriented approach has been extremely successful with a variety of voice disorders.

Correcting Hypotonic Problems. Except as noted, the remedial goal in hypotonic problems is to deliberately seek glottal tension. Thus, an intentional glottal attack, even accompanied by increased tension in the arms and trunk by means of pushing forcefully, facilitates the approximation of the vocal folds (Froeschels, 1943; Van Riper and Irwin, 1958). An approach to "tension increase therapy" for children (Wilson and Rice, 1977) can be adapted for use with adults since the goals are the same.

Some apparent cases of hypotonic function are not aided by increased tension, however. For example, although phonating with bowed vocal folds might appear to be the result of hypotonic function and warrant greater muscular effort, bowed cords, like vocal nodules, may be *caused* by excessive tension. And, myasthenia laryngia, exemplified by a fifty-five-year-old man who, thirty years earlier, had taken pride in "calling hogs all day and square dances at night," is another apparent hypotonic function that is not aided by increased tension (Moore, 1957).

The voice clinician need not become an amateur psychiatrist in order to discuss the relationship between emotional and voice disorders. In the case of hypofunction known as hysterical aphonia, the clinician can provide symptom therapy through the use of hypertonic techniques, including coughing and throat clearing.

There are forms of dysphonia whose management must rely on medical as well as voice therapy (Damsté, 1967; Moore, 1971). For example, the efficiency of breathing is a primary factor when considering remedial techniques for unilateral vocal fold paralysis of the kind described on p. 243. The case of Mrs. N. D. serves as an illustration.

Mrs. N. D., sixty-one years old, had a unilateral vocal paralysis after thyroid surgery. Hoarseness diminished dramatically when slight medial pressure was exerted against the thyroid lamina on the side of the paralyzed cord in the Gutsmann test. The laryngologist, however, decided against injecting the affected cord with Teflon, as it would further compromise the respiratory stridor attendant upon the reduced glottal airway. Under the circumstances, it was best to settle for the limited voice improvement that could be achieved from efforts to phonate with increased muscular effort and glottal attack.

Other examples of medical or voice therapy management are patients with myasthenia gravis and parkinsonism. The former can sometimes be helped vocally by ". . . the administration of anticholinesterase drugs or thymectomy . . ." and even by the use of a palatal lift prosthesis (Aronson, 1980). Patients with parkinsonism, who have breathiness, monopitch and inadequate intensity, sometimes show improved vocal ability when undergoing drug therapy with L-dopa and by using electronic devices to amplify speech (Aronson, 1980). For an excellent coverage of the complex area of organic voice disorders and neurologic disease, the reader is encouraged to read *Clinical Voice Disorders by Aronson (1980)*.

ALARYNGEAL PHONATION

The rehabilitation of the laryngectomee presents the team of specialists engaged in the effort with a significant challenge. To be effective, their approach requires a consideration of the physiological and psychological changes that accompany the surgical removal of the vocal folds, together with a thorough understanding of the given case so that enough information can be communicated to the patient to enable him to understand and cope with those changes. Obviously, then, more is involved than instructing a patient in methods of charging the esophagus with air in order to achieve phonation and assessing and helping to refine speech efforts, although these are important goals of rehabilitation.

Since the entire story of alaryngeal voice rehabilitation cannot be covered in these pages, we shall focus our discussion on the following topics that are of interest to the speech clinician: factors affecting the learning of alaryngeal speech; the physiology of alaryngeal phonation; and the principles of techniques of alaryngeal phonation.

There are many reasons why the speech clinician must be concerned with vocal rehabilitation after laryngectomy. One of the main ones is the continued increase in the incidence of larynx cancer. It has been estimated that approximately 11,000 new cases of laryngeal cancer occur each year in this country (American Cancer Society, 1976). Moreover, in the past, the voice and speech therapy for this particular condition has been handled by persons other than speech pathologists to a degree greater than has been shown for any other speech disorder (Duguay, 1980; Horn, 1962; Lauder, 1965). The rehabilitation of laryngectomees is by no means new, but as recently as twenty years ago, the development of a new postoperative voice was left largely to chance or to well-meaning but poorly trained laymen. This unfortunate situation is rapidly changing mainly because of the efforts of the International Association of Laryngectomees (IAL) and the American Speech, Language and Hearing Association (ASHA).

Factors Affecting the Learning of Alaryngeal Speech

Like beauty, alaryngeal phonation is perceived uniquely by each beholder. To some laryngectomees, for example, it simply means talking differently by getting air into and sound out of the esophagus, while to others, it means using a voice whose hoarseness resembles that of a person with a cold. To surgeons, it represents a desirable by-product of a procedure in which they attempt to remove enough tissue to preserve health but leave enough to preserve normal physiology. To counselors, the effort to achieve alaryngeal speech is part of a total adjustment in which the patient's self-acceptance and interpersonal relationships are important factors. To employers, the rehabilitation effort may be viewed in terms of the dollar cost of renewing the employee's capacity to perform a job. The speech clinician needs to appreciate all of these views as they may affect the aphonic person's ability to acquire and use a compensatory substitute voice.

As therapy begins, two questions confront the speech clinician: What kind of person was the laryngectomee before his operation? In what ways has he changed since the operation? Increasingly, there has been systematic investigation of the physiology of alaryngeal voice (Damsté, 1957, 1959; Damsté, Van den Berg, and Moolenaar-Bijl, 1956; Diedrich and Youngstrom, 1966; Murry and Brown, 1975;

Snidecor, 1969; Winans and Waldrop, 1974; Weinberg, 1980), as well as the psycho-logical aspects of laryngectomy (Amster et al., 1972; Gardner, 1966; Greene, 1947; Locke, 1966; Pitkin, 1953; Sanchez-Salazar and Stark, 1972; Schall, 1938; Stoll, 1958; Weinberg, 1980). Besides knowing what these changes are, it is important for the clinician to know how the laryngectomee views these changes, and the implications for his learning alaryngeal speech.

Background Information Needed by the Clinician. To get acquainted with a given case, the speech clinician should obtain a thorough case history, either directly from a referring physician or counselor, or abstracted from a medical record or other types of reports. The essential data pertain to the patient's health, social, vocational, family, and educational history, as well as to his receptive and expressive communica-tion skills (Shipp, 1968). Communication items which assume special significance relate to hearing loss, inability to read (as in illiteracy or blindness), inability to write English (as in illiteracy or reliance on another language), amount of and enjoyment in talking, and difficulty with teeth, palate, or tongue in talking. Information about the patient's health has a bearing not only on his acquisition of alaryngeal speech, but also on his chances of staying alive, for laryngectomy, after all, is performed to save the patient's life.

The Patient's Understanding of His Condition. For an understanding of his condition and the nature of his operation and its consequences, the patient must rely on information given to him. The physician is in the best position to provide that information, because he not only knows the patient's health better than anyone else, but he also is the one who must tell the patient of the need for surgery and explain something of its consequences. Unfortunately, however, the information the surgeon provides is often extremely meager and does not fully prepare the patient for what will happen.

Kalfuss (1969) studied the questionnaire responses of forty-one surgeons perform-ing laryngectomies in a metropolitan area and tabulated the responses in terms of preoperative counseling about surgery and its consequences, including tracheostomy and postoperative speech. The results of her study are cited below, not as indictments of these specific surgeons, but rather as indications of the nature of counseling attempts presumed to prevail throughout the country.

Some 8 percent of the surgeons responding to the questionnaire reported that they do not tell their patients that "the hole in their neck will be permanent"; 5 percent do not tell them that "they will cough through the tracheostomy"; and 24 percent do not tell them that "mucous secretions will have to be coughed up and wiped from the stoma." Some of these surgeons added that reporting such information is distasteful to them and that, in many cases, they leave the task to the nurses.

Information about speech after laryngectomy is not given preoperatively by 9 percent of the surgeons. Some 16 percent do not tell patients about a specific agency where they can get speech training, while 26 percent give no information as to where speech training is available.

The information that is given to patients includes statements that "they will swallow air to talk" (71 percent); that "they will talk with their stomachs" (16 percent); and that "tracheostomy air will be used for speech" (11 percent).

The finding that 63 percent of the surgeons do not tell patients "that it will be difficult to talk again," while 89 percent do not tell them that it will be "easy" indicates that the topic is seldom discussed in preoperative counseling. Similarly, information is not given by surgeons to enable patients to expect a postoperative lessening of the sense of smell (84 percent failing to do so) or taste (17 percent). More than half of the surgeons replied negatively to questions dealing with the provision of preoperative explanations to patients through such means as discussing or drawing the anatomy of the larynx, drawing the surgical procedure, explaining the physiology of the larynx, and explaining the mechanism of esophageal speech. Indeed, 18 percent of the surgeons reported that they do not know how esophageal speech is produced, and 93 percent that they are not able to speak esophageally. The attitudes of the surgeons sampled indicated that 26 percent do not feel that their p operative counseling is adequate.

Five surgeons in eight (63 percent) do not like the sound of esophageal speech, while seven out of eight (87 percent) do not like the sound of an artificial larynx. Half of the surgeons responding felt that esophageal speakers do not look like normal speakers, and 60 percent thought that esophageal speakers are very conspicuous.

Some common misconceptions among laryngectomy candidates are often noted by clinicians. As indicated previously, the patient's understanding of his health status, and of the operation and its consequences, depends not only on what his physician knows and reports, but also on how he himself interprets those reports in the light of his prior knowledge and attitude. Thus, different patients react differently to similar information. One patient may fixate upon the word cancer in the diagnosis. Another may focus on the report that he will die unless he has the operation. Another may dwell on the financial consequences—either the cost of the operation, or a reduced income. And still another may despair at the prospect of losing friends or the ability to use laryngeal speech.

Duguay (1966) had occasion to record more than fifty different preoperative interviews with laryngectomy candidates who had been counseled by their surgeons regarding their impending surgery. In each interview, the individual was encouraged to verbalize his ideas about how he would be able to talk without his "voice box." The following verbatim comments represent a cross section of the ideas expressed.

Case 1, a forty-three-year-old furniture salesman: "I know it's going to be quite a struggle to learn to speak all over again. It would be, I assume, much harder than teaching a child how to talk, because the air is then shut off somewhere at the nose and mouth. There is no intake there, only through the aperture, which I must use for speech and for breathing, I imagine I'll have to take a deep breath, and when I let it out, that's when I form the speech—talk through the opening in my neck."

Case 2, a sixty-two-year-old housewife: "When they operate, they put in a switch. I don't know—like a little box. I never saw it."

Case 3, a forty-two-year-old male postal worker: "I'll use the diaphragm method to talk. I saw a man talk like that. He was breathing heavy and talking out of the hole in his neck. I'll breathe air in. The sound's made there by cartilage moving on cartilage or flesh. Something must already be there. I don't think they'll put anything in."

Case 4, a sixty-three-year-old retired steel plant foreman: "They put something in there, don't they? You draw breath in some way into your lungs—develop some kind of pressure. The sound comes from your lungs. The words are formed down there too."

Case 5, a sixty-two-year-old millwright: "I haven't the least idea of how I can talk with no voice box."

Case 6, a fifty-nine-year-old automobile factory foreman: "You can talk from the stomach. It comes all the way up—take a deep breath."

Case 7, a fifty-six-year-old farmer: "They claim that after a while you can get to whisper a bit. They have some of these other things you put up there and throw your voice some way. There's a fellow back home who had it. He talks just the same as I do now, only it's all messed up—hoarse and sounds as if his mouth were full of water. He gets by with it."

Case 8, a sixty-one-year-old carpenter: "I don't know how it's gonna be. Air will come up from my stomach. It will get into my stomach, I guess, through the hole in my neck."

Case 9, a fifty-eight-year-old club steward: "I have no idea. There was one man at home—he had a little tube that fit in his mouth and in the hole there. He spoke well. Of course, he died in Florida a few years later. He carried this tube in his pocket and you could understand him. I don't know—that's what worries me. What in the hell will I do?"

Case 10, a fifty-nine-year-old chef: "My sister in-law has no voice box. It was an accident. They cut her vocal cords out when they took her tonsils out. She talks from her stomach. They wanted her to go to a clinic in Cleveland and explain how she does it. She learned by herself. That's just one idea of mine. I suppose they have electronic devices now, too. I was never in a hospital before, so I don't know too much about it."

The interviews thus were indicative of unrealistic, often inaccurate, ideas among laryngectomy candidates about postoperative speech. Certain misconceptions were very common, including the beliefs that they would have to do the following:

1. swallow air all the way down into the stomach in order to talk;
2. talk from the stomach;
3. talk from the diaphragm;
4. talk from the lungs;
5. talk through the hole in the neck (that is, the tracheostoma);
6. have to cover the hole in the neck in order to talk; or
7. talk from some kind of voice box "put in" by the surgeons.

It is difficult to determine whether these misconceptions were due to inadequate preoperative counseling, to the patients' mistaken assumptions or interpretations stemming from their concern with death or cancer, or to their general anxiety. The voice clinician may feel that the statements of these patients are naive as well as inaccurate, but most of the patients expressed one or more of these seven common misconceptions.

Accurate Information About Physiologic Changes. Giving a patient accurate information about anatomical and physiologic changes stemming from laryngectomy

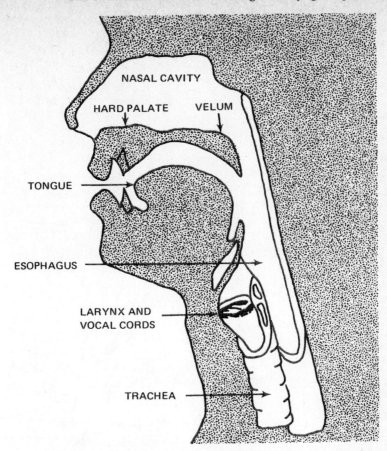

Figure 5–4. Sagittal View of the Phonatory Mechanism Before Laryngectomy

may reduce the likelihood of misconceptions. In addition, it may reassure him concerning changes that will take place in his daily activities.

Major features of the operation include total removal of the larynx (thyroid cartilage) and the creation of a permanent opening into the trachea (tracheostoma) through which the person will breathe for the remainder of his life. Figures 5–4 and 5–5 illustrate the changes effected by surgery.

Who should present the information? It would appear to be the physician's perogative, but one that is not always exercised. It may be given by an informed speech clinician. It may be given orally or as published statements (American Cancer Society, 1964a; International Association of Laryngectomees, 1964; Keith et al., 1977; Lauder, 1979).

It does not appear desirable to have such information presented by a previously operated laryngectomee in personalized anecdotal form, although the question of whether to have the laryngectomy candidate visited preoperatively by a well-rehabilitated and well-spoken laryngectomized person has not been satisfactorily resolved. Those advocating such visits suggest that they can provide a favorable psychological

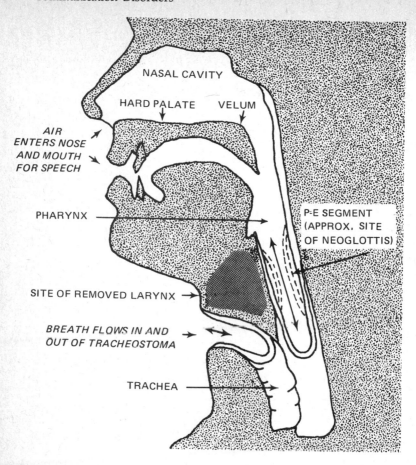

Figure 5-5. Changes Effected by Laryngectomy. Separate air supplies are needed for breathing and esophageal speech.

experience in terms of motivation and of reducing anxiety regarding living, speaking, and general adjustment. Others suggest that they may have deleterious effects on the candidate's well-being.

To one who still has a larynx, the sound of esophageal voice can be most discouraging, and the efficacy of the preoperative visit is speculative at best. Although the overwhelming majority of a large group of well-rehabilitated laryngectomees indicated approval of a preoperative visit by another laryngectomee (Horn, 1962), 3 percent of the group disapproved. If only one prospective laryngectomee refused surgery on the basis of a preoperative visit by a laryngectomee, few speech clinicians would want the responsibility for having influenced that decision. Both authors of this chapter have experienced situations in which a patient has refused surgery, knowing that death was inevitable, rather than "end up like that." On the other hand, the authors have seen instances where surgery was agreed to primarily because of the positive effect of talking with a laryngectomee. The question of whether such a visit will be beneficial or not in a given case may be resolved by the attending physician.

Regardless of who informs the patient about post-laryngectomy changes, someone should do it—enumerating specific changes in bodily function and relating them to normal respiratory physiology. Special consideration should be given to the role of the larynx in the categories of pulmonary inhalation, pulmonary exhalation, laryngeal valving, and changes necessitated by total laryngectomy (Walsh, 1972).

Changes in Inhalation. Pulmonary inhalation normally involves moving atmospheric air (via the nasal and oral cavities) through the pharynx into the respiratory tree (trachea, bronchi, and bronchioles of the lung). Stretching this tree by contracting the diaphragm and rib-moving muscles of inspiration lowers air pressure in the trachea and in the esophagus behind it. With the laryngeal valve open, tracheal air pressure equals pharyngeal air pressure which, in turn, equals atmospheric air pressure. As tracheal air is drawn deeper into the expanding lungs, a tendency for air pressure in the trachea to drop below atmospheric pressure is offset by air moving into the trachea through the nose (if not blocked by velopharyngeal closure) or the mouth (if not blocked by lip/tongue seal). Concomitantly, esophageal pressure, which is 4–7 mm Hg below atmosphere at rest, drops to -15 mm Hg during inhalation. Atmospheric air would move from the pharynx into the esophagus if the pressure differential were great enough to break the resistive seal of the pharyngoesophageal juncture, which is 10 mm Hg at rest (Dey and Kirchner, 1961).

Inhaling air through the nose and mouth is involved in such activities as smelling, sniffing, tasting, sipping, snoring, and yawning—all of which are altered by laryngectomy, since it precludes the movement of air into the lungs through the throat and mouth or nose. (The same statement applies to smoking, assuming that the object being smoked is held between the lips. It is possible to smoke an object held at the tracheostoma where pulmonary respiration will allow smoke to get in and out of the lungs.)

Changes in Exhalation. Pulmonary exhalation normally involves moving air from the respiratory tree through the pharynx and into the nose and mouth enroute to atmospheric air outside the body. Compressing the respiratory tree (by contracting the abdominal and rib-moving muscles of exhalation) raises air pressure in the trachea and in the esophagus behind it. With the laryngeal valve open, tracheal air of increased pressure is forced up.

Exhaling air through the nose and mouth is involved in activities such as speaking, whistling, smoking, sneezing, blowing the nose, gargling, snoring, spitting, puffing out of the cheeks, emitting a Bronx cheer ("raspberries"), snorting, and sighing. All of these activities are, of necessity, altered by laryngectomy, since it precludes the movement of air from the lungs out through the throat and mouth or nose.

Changes in Laryngeal Valving. Laryngeal valving—that is, complete vocal-fold adduction, normally is used to (1) prevent inappropriate aspiration, or (2) effect changes in air pressure in the respiratory tree without movement of air between the tree and the atmosphere.

Valving (which serves the first purpose listed above) occurs during the second stage of swallowing—effectively preventing objects such as water, food, insects, and noxious particles suspended in the air (such as dust and fumes) from entering and injuring the respiratory tree.

An increase in air pressure in the respiratory tree is effected in activities such as coughing, clearing the throat, lifting, defecation, and parturition, where laryngeal valving resists egress of air placed under increased pressure by abdominal contractions to exhale.

Although not done frequently by a laryngeal person, it is possible to decrease air pressure in the respiratory tree with the laryngeal valve closed. This is done by some laryngeal persons who inhale air for esophageal phonation. In addition, it is possible to increase air pressure above the closed laryngeal valve. Activities such as whistling, saying voiceless consonants, whispering, emitting a "Bronx cheer," and puffing out the cheeks may be performed while holding the breath or while maintaining complete vocal-fold adduction.

Decreased air pressure in the oral-pharyngeal cavities with laryngeal valve closure is exemplified in sipping, kissing, tongue-clicking, and sucking in the cheeks. All of these activities are of necessity altered by laryngectomy, since the laryngeal valve is removed.

Changes Necessitated by Total Laryngectomy. The risk of aspirating food is obviated by the surgical tie-off between the pharynx and the trachea, but there is an increased risk of aspirating water at the tracheostoma during activities such as showering and swimming, for which the laryngectomee must take precautions. Similarly, he will have to guard against the entry of insects, dust, and fumes via the tracheal stoma into the respiratory tree.

The fact that changes will occur in his daily activities should not surprise the laryngectomee—they are to be expected. To regain any of the aforementioned activities, even partially, he must learn to change air pressure in the pharyngeal, nasal, and/or oral cavities. It would appear that such pressure changes can be accomplished only by expanding and/or contracting the size of the oropharyngeal tube, for which the necessary muscular action may involve moving the tongue, cheeks, velum, and walls of the pharynx. To assess the patient's capacity to alter air pressure in the oropharyngeal tube, an oral manometer can be used. If he fails to demonstrate increased pressure, positive or negative, it may mean that he has not yet learned to expand and/or contract his oropharyngeal tube. By attempting to blow strips of paper, small whistles, matches, etc., he can become more aware of and learn to change pressures in the mouth or throat.

The Physiology of Alaryngeal Phonation

A description of how the laryngectomee achieves increased air pressure in the hypopharynx and decreased negative pressure in the esophagus requires a review of the elements of alaryngeal phonation: the *vibrata*, the *power source*, and the dynamics of *air intake* and *air expulsion*.

The Vibrata. The esophagus becomes the reservoir of air for speech production in the esophageal speaker. The muscular structure at the mouth of the esophagus, which at rest is adducted and resembles a slit, becomes the neoglottis. Most authorities agree that the cervical level of the neoglottis in the majority of patients is between cervical vertebrae four and six. Thus, the vibrating agents that substitute for the removed vocal folds would include the cricopharyngeal muscle, perhaps strands of the inferior pharyngeal constrictor, and the superior esophageal sphincter. However, it is necessary only to examine the radiographic studies of Damsté (1958), Diedrich and Youngstrom (1966), Hodson and Oswald (1958), and Vrtica and Svaboda (1961) to appreciate the striking variability from case to case in the site and configuration of the neoglottis. Diedrich and Youngstrom (1966) employ the term pharyngoesophageal segment (or PE segment) to designate the area of the neoglottis. Its tonicity of 5–10 mm Hg (Dey and Kirchner, 1961) is essential to retain air in the esophagus. Unlike the glottis, the neoglottis cannot maintain partial abduction or a paramedian position, such as is needed for /h/ and other voiceless consonants.

Power Source. Air, the power source that drives the glottis in the laryngeal speaker, drives the neoglottis in the esophageal speaker. Air must pass down through the closed PE segment and into the esophagus. The normal physiological contraction of the pharyngoesophageal fibers prevents air from entering the esophagus. Once in, the air must be forced back out to create sound, since rapid, voluntary charging and expelling of air is critical to fluent esophageal speech.

The air reservoir, the esophagus, may be compared to a long balloon. Collapsed at rest, it stretches in diameter when filled with food or air. Swallowing a bolus of food, for example, results in a peristaltic bulge which ripples toward the stomach in approximately one second (Best and Taylor, 1950). Accompanying this esophageal bulge are peaks of esophageal pressure which progress downward (McNally, 1969).

Air Intake. An understanding of air intake for esophageal speech demands an appreciation of the pressure at the PE segment in relation to the positive pressure above it (in the hypopharynx) and to the negative pressure below it (in the esophagus). To permit air to enter the esophagus, a significant pressure differential must exist.

The esophagus can be charged with air by two methods, inhalation and injection (Damsté, 1958; Diedrich and Youngstrom, 1966; Snidecor, 1969). Inhalation involves further lowering of the negative pressure below the PE segment, while injection raises the positive pressure above the PE segment to above atmospheric level. Techniques for using each method will be explained in a subsequent section.

Air Expulsion. The dynamics of expelling air from the esophagus and achieving phonation are complex and interrelated. Accounting for air expulsion are such factors as increased pressure of air in the esophagus, the recoil and elastic properties of the esophagus, and external pressures stemming from intrapulmonary pressure changes, diaphragmatic tension, and abdominal muscle contractions. Positive pressure of air retained in the esophagus reaches 15–25 mm Hg (Dey and Kirchner, 1961), and may go as high as 74 mm Hg (Van den Berg and Moolenaar-Bijl, 1959).

The upper third of the esophagus is surrounded by striated muscle, in contrast to the lower esophagus, which is surrounded by smooth muscles. This fact has led to the assumption that air is subject to voluntary control by expulsion in an antiperistaltic bulge moving upward only if it is retained in the upper esophagus (Diedrich and Youngstrom, 1966). However, radiographic studies of esophageal speech—frames which are depicted in figure 5–6—indicate that air is distributed along the entire length of the esophagus. Moreover, there is little evidence that air expulsion creates upward ripples, like the regurgitation of food. On the contrary, expulsion of esophageal air may be viewed as effecting a reduction of esophageal diameter throughout its length, with complete collapse effected first near the cardiac sphincter, then moving upward to the PE segment.

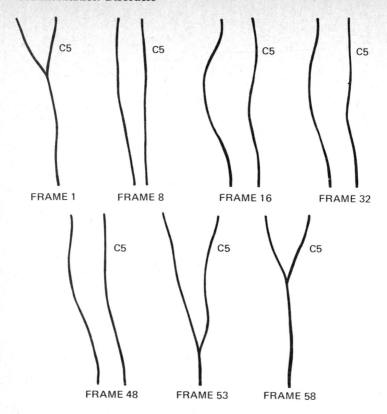

Figure 5–6. Radiographic Studies of Air Expulsion During Esophageal Speech

Principles and Techniques of Alaryngeal Phonation

The techniques used in instructing the laryngectomee to accomplish alaryngeal speech are described below, following a discussion of the principles of inhalation and injection on which they are based.

The Principle of Inhalation. As mentioned earlier, the inhalation process may be described as an inspiring or drawing of air quickly into the esophagus; by means of that activity there is a decrease in sub-neoglottic pressure. When a patient inhales pulmonary air via the tracheal opening, there is a pressure drop, or an increase in the negative pressure that normally exists in the esophagus at rest. In other words, it goes from − 4 to − 8 mm Hg (Atkinson et al., 1957) to as low as − 10, − 15, or − 20 mm Hg (Dey and Kirchner, 1961), or − 26 mm Hg (Damsté, 1958).

Since this air pressure is substantially less than that in the hypopharynx, which is essentially atmospheric (Damsté, 1958), a significant pressure differential is created. Air is pulled from the hypopharynx into the esophagus through the closed PE segment, if the tonic closure of the PE segment is not increased unduly. Similarly, air for speech may be inhaled into the esophagus in the absence of a significant PE sphincter or resistance (Dey and Kirchner, 1961).

The Principle of Injection. In injection, which may be described as a method of charging the esophagus with air by compressing and forcing the air into it, there is an increase in supra-neoglottic (hypopharyngeal) pressure. Injection is more than merely swallowing air, although the terms have been used synonymously (Doehler, 1953) and some confusion has resulted from the practices. Thus, it may be well to clarify the relationship between the two activities before detailing what happens in injection.

Research findings differentiate between injection and swallowing on the basis of—

1. muscle activity (Shipp, Deatsch, and Ross, 1967);
2. sequence of esophageal pressures (McNally, 1969);
3. minimal time requirements (Berlin, 1965).

The authors are of the opinion that true swallowing of air into the esophagus—that is, using all of the movement patterns observed in the oral cavity (with the tongue and palate), pharynx, and esophagus during swallowing—can be considered under the heading of air injection. Indeed, a beginning esophageal speaker may seem to swallow air. The inefficiency of such true swallow injection, however, imposes unnecessary demands on the speaker's time and effort. To achieve rapid, fluent, and effortless esophageal speech, the esophageal speaker must progress to a method other than the true swallow type of air injection. This is not to say that the word swallow, with all of its semantic information, cannot be used in instructing the laryngectomee. On the contrary, a selective use of its connotations is often of value in helping "program" the laryngectomee to load air into the esophagus. By using some descriptive term, such as *partial, modified,* or *beginning,* before *swallow,* the clinician may facilitate the patient's approach to unfamiliar behavior via the familiar motor act, and still keep the patient from succumbing to the total physiological performance of a true swallow. Therefore the clinician may exercise a "teaching license" concerning the use of the word *swallow* when instructing laryngectomees. Because it is such a cumbersome and uneconomical way of loading air, true swallowing should not be reinforced.

The injection method results in an elevation of hypopharyngeal air pressure by 7–22 mm Hg or up to 48 mm Hg (Damsté, 1958). The compression can be achieved in several different ways (described in the section on techniques for air injection). Such an increase in pressure presumes that air cannot be dissipated through an opening or port, such as the mouth and/or the velopharyngeal isthmus. A lip and/or tongue seal prevents air in the hypopharynx from escaping through the mouth, while a velopharyngeal closure prevents it from escaping through the nose. Pressure in the hypopharynx can be influenced by tongue action and/or expansion and contraction of the oral-pharyngeal tube.

Two kinds of tongue action can occur (Diedrich and Youngstrom, 1966), both of which result in a reduction in the size of the pharyngeal cavity and an increase in hypopharyngeal air pressure.

1. There can be a glossopalatal press in which the tongue tip contacts the teeth or alveolar process, while the middle of the tongue makes a backward excursion. Here, the linguapalatal seal precludes the need for a lip seal because it requires a velopharyngeal closure.
2. There can be glossopharyngeal press which differs from the preceding one in that the posterior portion of the tongue makes a dorsal movement, contacting the

posterior pharyngeal wall. Theoretically, velopharyngeal closure is not essential, although it may exist (Diedrich and Youngstrom, 1966).

Clinically, it seems that most patients using an injection method of air intake do employ velopharyngeal closure. Failure to close this port will be heard as a snort with nasal escape of air, rather than the sound of a "klunk" (Diedrich and Youngstrom, 1966) when air is injected into the esophagus.

A third way of injecting air is by contracting the oral-pharyngeal tube. This contraction reduces cavity size and hence increases air pressure. (A given amount of air is forced into a smaller space, thus increasing its pressure.) This increased pressure is usually sufficient to override the closed PE segment. One might conceptualize this maneuver as reversing the process of puffing up the cheeks and throat with air and then pushing on them with the fingers. In other words, the pushing occurs because of buccal and pharyngeal contraction and it results in air being "squirted" down into the esophagus.

The Use of Loading Phonemes (Consonant Injection). Injection is facilitated through the use of voiceless consonants; that is, the taking in of air during the forceful articulation of the consonants permits esophageal phonation on the ensuing vowel. Without conscious attention to taking in air before talking, the patient can utter a syllable (puh, tuh, skuh) or a word (pie, tow, car, star, sky). The value of the plosive sounds /p/, /t/, and /k/ to aid injection has been described by Damsté (1959), McClear (1960), Moolenaar-Bijl (1953a, 1953b), and Stetson (1937). Nonplosive consonants, such as /s/ and /f/, also have been shown to help patients load air, according to clinical research done by Berlin (1963b) and Diedrich and Youngstrom (1966). Accounting for the use of voiceless consonants in aiding injection is the greater oral air pressure used in their articulation, as compared with the articulation of voiced consonants.

Consonant injections utilize both aspects of injection—tongue action and oral pharyngeal contraction. Phonemes that call for tongue action, such as /t/ and /k/, utilize a glossal press (strictly speaking, a glossopalatal and a glossopalatal/glossopharyngeal press respectively). Others, such as /s/ and /p/, call for contractions of the oral-pharyngeal tube. (See the section on techniques for air injection.)

The ability of some patients to load air easily and to phonate using a voiceless consonant as a "starter" has extremely important implications for therapy. If the patient can inject air naturally, easily, and unconsciously, using selected initial or releasing phonemes, the clinician can bring this ability from an unconscious to a conscious, controlled level.

Techniques for Air Inhalation. The following techniques can be used to accomplish air inhalation as a method of charging the esophagus:

1. expanding the pharyngoesophageal tube
2. feigning oral inhalation
3. resisting pulmonary inhalation

1. *Expanding the pharyngoesophageal tube.* To cause an expansion of the pharyngoesophageal tube, the patient should be instructed to relax and yawn as real-

istically as possible. At the height of the yawn, the clinician should listen very carefully for the clicking sound of air entering the esophagus. If it occurs, he should identify and reinforce it. Help may be needed at this point to get a quick return of the inhaled air, for the patient should try to bring air back out quickly, thereby phonating as soon as the air is felt or heard entering the upper esophagus. He can try to suck his cheeks in, to kiss audibly, or to draw air in via an oral manometer.

Frequently, the head is extended during the yawning exercise. The head may be raised even more consciously by simulating an activity such as tossing a food particle (peanut or popcorn) into the air and catching it with the mouth. Similarly, the patient may open the pharyngo-esophageal tube by pretending to swallow a sword, to reach for a kernel of corn like a chicken, or to drink a glass of beverage in chugalug fashion without taking a breath.

2. *Feigning oral inhalation.* To practice this technique, the patient may be told to hold a mirror for the purpose of visualizing and identifying his uvula, then to hold his breath and quickly try to suck in his uvula. As he does, the clinician should listen for air passing through the PE segment. In an attempt to provide a "semantic" feel of air entering the esophagus, the patient can pretend that he is inhaling cigarette smoke or gasping for air after prolonged swimming under water, with the clinician then working to get him to return the air quickly. Sometimes phonation will occur upon inspiration. After identifying the target sound present in the inspiratory behavior, the clinician needs to help the patient reverse the pattern so that phonation will occur on exhalation.

3. *Resisting pulmonary inhalation.* This technique involves showing the patient that he can "hold his breath" for a few seconds by occluding his stoma. He can do this simply by placing a finger over the stoma, the cannula, or the tracheotomy tube. To show that there is no danger, the clinician should hold his own breath for a few seconds by covering his nose and mouth with his hand, then uncovering his nose and mouth and breathing, then covering them again and holding his breath. When the patient has held his breath a few times, by occluding his stoma and realizes that he will not suffocate, the following technique might be tried: after exhaling pulmonary air through the stoma, the patient opens his mouth, occludes his stoma, and quickly sucks air into his mouth while attempting pulmonary inhalation. The stoma should then be uncovered for him to breathe before further attempts are made to phonate or inhale air. Once again, the clinician listens carefully for the sound of air entering the esophagus, identifying and reinforcing the behavior if it occurs.

When instructing a patient in an inhalation method of air intake, the clinician needs to be aware of several important factors. One is that rapid and deep inhalation can easily result in hyperventilation, with the patient becoming dizzy. Consequently, it is advisable to use short practice sessions together with periods of normal pulmonary respiration between therapy activities. Sometimes as indicated previously, a patient learning to load air may phonate and even articulate on the phonation that occurs during inhalation. Since this is out of phase with desired speech production, and since it is difficult to prolong the "inhaled sound" for any length of time, the practice should be discouraged and the pattern reversed so that phonation occurs upon expiration of the inhaled air. Finally, the clinician may find that when using an inhalation method with a patient who has emphysema, bronchitis, or residual effects upon his lungs from some other disease, the "tracheal noise" created during inspiration and expiration may be so disturbing that it affects esophageal intelligibility or even masks the esophageal phonation. When this occurs, the clinician will need to consider an alternate method of air intake.

Techniques for Air Injection. There are a number of techniques to obtain satisfactory air intake for esophageal phonation. The following ones are used to accomplish air injection as a method of charging the esophagus:

1. expanding and contracting the oral-pharyngeal tube
2. using a glossal press
3. using a glossopharyngeal press
4. using a modified swallow
5. using a glossopalatal/glossopharyngeal press

1. *Expanding and contracting the oral-pharyngeal tube.* When this is the goal, the patient should try to blow out a match or blow strips of paper, a whistle, or a manometric tube held at the lips. In addition, he should try to puff out his cheeks, pushing the air from one cheek into the other. He should move the air up to the roof of his mouth, then back into his throat. Sometimes, the air will escape through the nasopharynx, and he must raise the velum when he pushes. He may attempt to "gargle" the air that he has in his mouth.

2. *Using a glossal press.* To perform a glossal press, the patient should place the tongue tip on the upper alveolar ridge and push hard while he "squeezes" the muscles of the pharynx and neck. An alternative is to produce a lingual click by rapidly pulling the sides of the tongue from the inner border of the alveolus—as in urging a horse to "giddap." Then he may try to make a similar sound with the back of the tongue against the posterior pharyngeal wall.

3. *Using a glossopharyngeal press.* To perform a glossopharyngeal press, the patient should place his tongue tip on the lower alveolar ridge and push air while he squeezes the muscles of his neck and pharynx.

If the patient wears an upper denture, he should perform the exercises for achieving sounds with a glossal and a glossopharyngeal press with the denture out as well as with it in. Some patients are helped by the use of dentures, while others, especially those with poorly fitting plates, will tense muscles in order to retain the plate, and thus interfere with tongue motions needed to inject air. The use of a good dental plate cement may prove helpful in such cases.

4. *Using a modified swallow.* To help the patient use a modified swallow injection, the direction to "start a swallow," "begin to swallow," or "try to swallow" can sometimes achieve the desired result. Care should be taken that he does not attempt to swallow too forcefully, which would be indicated by head flexion, lip closure, eye closure, or prolonged duration. It may help to have the patient "sip" air from a spoon, small glass, or straw.

5. *Using a glossopalatal/glossopharyngeal press.* To perform a glossopalatal or glossopharyngeal press, the patient can be requested to "use the tongue like a piston to force the air into your throat," or to "use your tongue like a scoop or shovel to put the air

into your throat." It may be helpful to encourage movement of the middle of the tongue upward toward the hard and soft palate while the posterior portion makes an accompanying backward motion. The additional cue of squeezing or contracting pharyngeal musculature along with the tongue movement may provide an assist to air intake.

Eliciting Alaryngeal Phonation. The previous section described ways of teaching the skills needed for taking air into the esophagus and expelling it as sound. Before becoming directive and trying to teach these new motor skills, however, the clinician should determine where the patient is in terms of his ability, that is, what he can already do. A great deal of time and effort may be saved if the patient can already phonate.

Chance Recreation of Sound. One way of determining a patient's ability to phonate esophageally is by taking a modified case history from the patient, not from a relative or anyone with him. He may need encouragement to respond verbally. The clinician can observe not only what is said, but especially, how it is said. The patient who is mouthing words with minimal force should be asked to speak louder. If whispered speech is audible but has a "Donald Duck" quality, the clinician should realize that this pharyngeal voice is not true esophageal phonation.

The clinician may see or hear attempts to put air into the esophagus. He may even hear phonation. Whenever he hears air enter the esophagus or sound produced by the neoglottis, he should ask the patient to reproduce the activity. Careful note should be made of what is heard, as well as when and how the sound is created. If there is success in producing the sound, the laryngectomee should tell, in his own words, how he accomplished it. Later, that description can be used in instructing him to recreate the sound. A significant number of laryngectomees arrive at the initial therapy session able to create esophageal sound, and many times they are not even aware of their ability. For such patients, therapy consists of refining this phonation. However, if air is not heard entering the esophagus or sound is not excited in attempts to talk, another step is needed.

Recall of Successful Phonation. The patient may be asked if, since his operation, a word has "just popped out" with sound, not merely a whisper. If so, he should recall and repeat the word. In addition, he should try to count, to name the days of the week, or to name the months of the year. The clinician should listen dynamically to such serial speech of low propositionality, being especially aware of any sound occurring because of the use of a "loading" phoneme. Behavioral clues may indicate the method of air intake which the patient is employing.

Loud Whispering. The patient may seek consonant injection by rapidly, successively, and loudly repeating the syllables, puh, tuh, kuh, stuh, or skuh. He should be asked to utter ten times, quickly and loudly, such words as pop or pep, taste or test, cake or kick, pick or pet, tap or take, cap or Kate, step or stop, scotch or scratch. If phonation occurs, he should seek to make this phonation more conscious and consistent.

Concerning the suggestion to say a word louder, it may be recalled that external pressures, using abdominal muscles, provide some of the force needed to expel the insufflated or injected air. Consequently, rather than going into a lengthy discourse with the patient as to what he needs to do to increase such abdominal pressure, simply asking him to "say it louder" may cause him to exert more effort automatically, thereby increasing abdominal pressure. At some later time, when he has habituated the action, he can attempt to reduce pulmonary exhalation without sacrificing articulatory force. Then he can discover that "it's the tongue, not the lung" which injects air.

It may be noted that the first three ways of initiating esophageal phonation—chance, recall, and loud whisper—are nondirective and do not solicit imitative responses. In contrast, the clinician may demonstrate the specific stimulus he wants the patient to copy.

Imitation of Demonstrated Speech. In exhibiting the motoric, visual, and acoustic stimuli present in esophageal speech for the patient to copy, the rationale is to combine the three air-intake principles of inhalation, injection, and the use of loading phonemes (Diedrich and Youngstrom, 1966). It is hoped that one or a combination of the methods will succeed in charging the esophagus with the necessary air.

One model that the clinician may present to the patient involves sniffling, as if inhaling air, and lifting the head and mandible forward and up. Then air is injected, using a visible but not exaggerated squeezing together of the lips (as might occur in a "swallow"), following which one of the /p/, /t/, or /k/ syllables or words is uttered. The clinician may offer this model to the patient several times so that he may observe carefully.

The clinician may feel inadequate if he is unable to produce esophageal tone. However, it is not essential to be able to phonate esophageally in order to successfully teach laryngectomized patients. Some very successful esophageal speech instructors have never been able, and may never be able to produce esophageal eructation. They may "fake it" with a glottal fry, a low gutteral sound, or a word that is laryngeally phonated. If a clinician is still reluctant to serve as a model, he can use a well-rehabilitated laryngectomee for that purpose. The latter, in fact, may help motivate the beginning patient to make speech attempts.

Whether the demonstration is given by the clinician or a rehabilitated laryngectomee, the goal is to get the patient to imitate. Then, if it occurs, it should be determined what method the patient used for loading air. That seemingly successful method should be reinforced. If the patient does not succeed in creating an esophageal eructation, however, the clinician must become more directive and furnish more precise stimuli.

Assessing and Refining Alaryngeal Speech. Assessing the proficiency of alaryngeal speech and refining that speech are two sides of the same coin. The assessment criteria developed by Berlin (1963a) focused on the time aspects of phonation skills, whereas the seven-point rating scales of Wepman et al. (1953) and Barton and Hejna (1963) focused on the fluency of speech in polysyllabic phrases. Snidecor (1969) suggested that assessment be based on the factors of rate, stress, pitch, loudness, and quality, while Diedrich and Youngstrom (1966) listed ten criteria, with special emphasis on articulation. On the basis of such studies, it would seem that proficiency in alaryngeal speech may be assessed and improved in terms of the following skills:

1. consistency of phonation
2. ability to (a) take air in and get sound out quickly and/or (b) prolong sound output

3. satisfactory rate, loudness, pitch, and quality of voice
4. articulatory accuracy
5. intelligibility and acceptability.

The following discussion reflects the conviction that such skills can be expected to be influenced by the method of air intake which the laryngectomee uses.

Consistency of Phonation. It would appear that phonation, either on demand or in connected speech, may be expected on virtually 100 percent of the attempts of those who use inhalation or injection before speaking. If the patient relies on consonant injection, he may be expected to phonate consistently on words starting with voiceless consonants. To initiate vowel phonation of equal consistency, he must intrude a releasing voiceless consonant (or the motor movement for one), or shift to another form of air intake.

Rapid Air Intake and Prolonged Phonation. Ideally, an alaryngeal speaker should be able to get air in and sound out quickly and to produce prolonged phonation. However, clinical experience has indicated that good speakers may develop one ability more than the other, depending, in part, on their manner of air intake. The consonant injector, for example, may be expected to get "air in, sound out" rapidly (up to .2 second), yet have difficulty in prolonging tone for as long as 2 seconds. Inhalers, as well as injectors who do not use consonant injection, may take slightly longer in getting air in and sound out, at best in 15 seconds, yet prolong phonation for 2 or more seconds. Those whose behavior during air injection seems to resemble swallowing use even greater effort and time, that is, more than 1 second. This longer, less efficient injection, however, does not preclude the ability to prolong phonation for as much as 2–4 seconds.

Rate of Speech. Rate of connected speech is usually recorded in terms of words per minute. It includes such factors as (a) time to get air in and sound out, (b) words per air charge, and (c) duration of each phrase, including pauses not involving air-charging. Snidecor (1969) has reported rates of 120 words per minute (wpm) for excellent alaryngeal speakers. On the average, there were 5 words per charge. Similar wpm rates may represent differing proportions of component times, when for example a longer prolongation may be offset by a longer loading time. On the other hand, the quick air-charge from plosive injection may result in fewer words per charge, but with no sacrifice in words per minute. Pitch, loudness, and voice quality do not appear to vary significantly by type of air intake.

Articulation. It is hypothesized that variations in articulatory accuracy depend in part on the manner of air intake employed by a speaker. However this distinction implies that a confusion matrix of alaryngeal speech (Sacco, Mann, and Schultz, 1967) must take into account the type of air intake. Otherwise, pooling subjects cancels out differences between them in articulation errors stemming from their different kinds of air intake. On the surface, it would appear that alaryngeal phonation is an on-off phenomenon in which voiced phonemes, vowels and voiced consonants, are favored. The person who takes in air without benefit of initial voiceless consonants may err in articulating a voiceless consonant so that it resembles its voiced cognate, as when *pie* sounds like *by*. (Gargan, 1969, p. 251, reported particular difficulty in saying /p/.)

Such a tendency may be combated by increasing intraoral air pressure when articulating voiceless consonants at the beginning of words.

Articulating a voiceless consonant which arrests a phrase may be improved by stopping esophageal phonation and relying on compression of the oropharyngeal tube for the necessary air pressure. Thus, *up, out, ache, off, ice, each,* and so on, may be spoken by terminating phonation at the end of the vowel, then articulating the remaining consonant, using only compressed oral air.

Some laryngectomees are able to take advantage of increased oral air pressure inherent in articulating voiceless consonants. A simple test will demonstrate that capacity. The clinician should count the number of /a/ sounds the speaker can utter at the rate of 1–2 per second, with the mouth open after one air-charge. He should repeat the test using /ta/, seemingly with one air-charge. The speaker who can say considerable more /ta/ than /a/ syllables probably does so because he has recharged the esophagus while saying the /t/. In order to recharge before each /a/ in a series, the speaker will display audible and visible evidence of such recharging. That is, he will be seen to move the tongue back and forth, pulse the chest cage, and breathe pulmonary air in and out with each intake. The injector who has his mouth open will also reveal any tongue action that is not part of articulating the /a/.

The laryngectomee who takes advantage of pressure-laden voiceless consonants may be expected to unvoice a voiced consonant so that it resembles its voiceless cognate, as when *by* sounds like *pie*. He also may intrude a releasing voiceless stop-plosive (usually /t/ or /k/) when saying a vowel-initiated word. Thus, he may make the word *apple* sound like *tapple* or *kapple.*

Nasal consonants have been found to be impaired, either mildly (Hyman, 1955) or severely (Di Carlo, Amster, and Herer, 1956). In a study of lateral X-rays, Diedrich and Youngstrom (1966) found that velopharyngeal closure is present during articulation of nasal consonants and may be related to the injector's need to achieve a velopharyngeal seal sufficient to resist high pressures generated in the pharynx. The tendency for a nasal consonant to sound muffled may be combated by exercises whereby the laryngectomee attempts to hum or to prolong a nasal consonant.

Difficulty in saying the glottal aspirate /h/ is both predictable and rather difficult to overcome. Auditory perception of /h/ may be enhanced by at least five factors:

1. prolonged duration of the vowel following /h/
2. increased force or loudness
3. intrusion of a /k/
4. added release of stomal air
5. expulsion of air from the pharynx by posterior tongue movement.

Whether or not the laryngectomee has succeeded in producing alaryngeal phonation, the clinician should bear in mind that phonation can be achieved through the use of an artificial larynx, a device designed to transmit sound into the oral cavity for production of speech by the articulators.

The Use of an Artificial Larynx

It is not the purpose of this chapter to compare the characteristics and acceptability of alaryngeal speech as discussed above with those of speech resulting from the use of an artificial larynx. Nor is it the purpose to suggest when and where artificial devices are best used. How the artificial larynx is used is the primary concern. The reader who is interested in investigating other variables may want to examine the reports of Diedrich and Youngstrom (1966), Hyman (1955), Lauder (1970), Martin (1963), McCroskey and Mulligan (1963), Nichols (in Snidecor, 1969), Salmon and Goldstein (1978), Shames, Font, and Matthews (1963), and Shanks (1966). The reader should find the Salmon and Goldstein (1978) reference particularly interesting since an audiotape demonstrating the various artificial larynxes accompanies the text.

The following discussion is predicated on the belief that the artificial larynx is a suitable alternative or even a "partner" to esophageal voice. In fact, it is a more desirable method of post-laryngectomy communication than poor esophageal speech.

Since many laryngectomy patients cannot, or will not, learn to use alaryngeal speech (Diedrich and Youngstrom, 1966; Gardner and Harris, 1961; Martin, 1963; Putney, 1958), the clinician should have some familiarity with the artificial larynxes. (Some are pictured in figure 5–7.) As Miller (1959) has stated, "We dare not be committed to one method of speech production alone" (p. 215). Moreover, an artificial larynx may be recommended in place of esophageal speech, prior to the initiation of esophageal speech, or in addition to esophageal speech. Since there are a number of artificial devices commercially available (Salmon and Goldstein, 1978), a clinician may find it very difficult to have all the artificial larynxes at his disposal. Therefore, the question is, *which instruments should be available for demonstration?*

Suiting a Model to the Patient. No formula can be applied for selecting a particular device; the suitability of a model for a patient must be determined on an individual basis. In order to meet the varied needs of most laryngectomees, the clinician should have available *at least* three different commercial models of electrolarynxes—the Western Electric (Bell Telephone, 5A for males, 5B for females), the Aurex, and the CooperRand (shown in fig. 5–7). Electrolarynxes that are held to the neck, such as the Western Electric and the Aurex, differ in the size of their vibrating heads. Patients also differ with respect to a suitable neck area. A thick, fleshy neck tends to absorb the sound delivered by the device, thus taxing its ability to transmit the sound into the oral cavity for articulation. A small, thin neck may not provide an area of sufficient size to accommodate the device. In some cases, the post-surgical anatomical configuration and/or submental firmness (edema or scar tissue) may interfere with transmission of sound through the neck wall.

The diameter of the vibrating head of the Aurex electrolarynx is smaller than that of the Western Electric. The clinician should try them both. If the available flat area of the neck is too limited in size for either instrument, the Cooper-Rand electrolarynx may be preferred. It differs from the other two devices both in design and operation. It consists of two parts, an electronic pulse generator and a tone generator allowing sound to be piped into the oral cavity via a plastic tube affixed to the tone generator.

Training the Patient to Use the Device. A patient should not just be given an electrolarynx; he should be instructed in its use. This instruction requires the clinician to consider several factors. With models held to the neck, the first determination to be made is the best site for the instrument head.

The electrolarynx should be tried on each side of the neck below the mandible and should be held so that the generated sound can enter the oropharyngeal area in the most direct manner. Care should be taken to avoid direct application of the instrument to the mandible, as this will serve only to dampen the sounds. Shifting it along

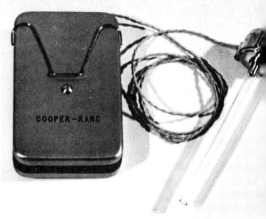

Figure 5–7. Three Models of Electro-larynxes. From left, the Cooper-Rand Electronic Speech Aid (Luminaud, 8688 Tyler Blvd., Mentor, Ohio 44060); the Aurex Neovox (Aurex Corp., Chicago, Illinois); and the Western Electric #5C Electrolarynx (available from local Bell Telephone Company).

the neck toward and away from the midline while mouthing words should help in determining the best sounding site. In some patients, this is just above the point where the notch of the thyroid cartilage had been located prior to surgery.

When holding the instrument to the preferred neck site, it is important that the vibrating head be in firm and even contact with the tissues. Otherwise, sound will escape, creating an annoying masking buzz and reducing the phonation available for articulation. The same thing will happen if part of the vibrating head is in contact with an irregular skin surface, such as a line of surgical incision.

In addition, the clinician should pay attention to the handedness of the patient and to the most effective way for him to control the on-off switch. Generally, patients prefer to use the thumb to depress the "button" to turn sound on and, in the case of the Western Electric device, to further depress it to raise pitch. Using the instrument with the non-dominant hand allows patients to continue with other functions, such as writing or telephoning.

When the best site has been located and the patient can maintain a flush contact of the instrument with the neck, he may be able to monitor his speech production. But if he does not appear to have good auditory feedback, the clinician may need to train him to use a different feedback system for locating the best placement. With a grease or felt-tip pen, the clinician can mark the desired target site on the neck. Then the patient can monitor visually, by practicing in front of a mirror until he develops a motor pattern and kinesthetic feedback that will ensure satisfactory placement of the electrolarynx.

The patient should be advised to exaggerate his articulation movements, especially in opening his mouth and moving his tongue. Skill in articulating consonants is vital to the intelligibility of speech when an artificial larynx is used, even if the user is a laryngeal speaker (e.g., a person who stutters, or one who requires vocal rest and is using an artificial larynx). Moreover, the patient must learn to coordinate the instrument with the articulation movements of running speech. Phrasing assumes added importance as a means of avoiding choppy, single-word utterances or unduly prolonged, droning speech patterns.

Since pitch variation may affect listener reaction and the acceptability of alaryngeal speech, a patient who uses the Western Electric larynx can seek varying pitch levels, as well as inflection. In this respect, the exercises for developing laryngeal inflection

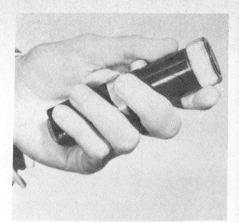
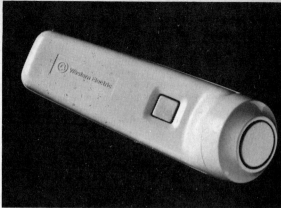

and pitch from Fairbank's *Voice and Articulation Drillbook* (1960) or some other conventional text dealing with speech improvement can be used.

Occasionally, a laryngectomee seems to hold his tongue in a humped and somewhat retracted position, with the result that the sound created by the electrolarynx can enter the pharynx but cannot progress into the oral cavity for articulation. When working with such a patient, the clinician may find it effective to have him try to talk on the inspiratory phase of the respiratory cycle. This seems to encourage a lower tongue carriage, allowing sound to get into the oral cavity. A lower tongue position is also achieved by speaking with the tongue protruded out of the mouth. After perceiving the benefits from talking in this manner, the patient can work toward a more synchronous and normal pattern of speaking.

In order to reduce its mechanical quality which might attract undue attention, the patient should be taught to vary the intensity level of the device so that it can be softened for situations that require a softer voice (theatre, restaurant, telephone, etc.)

Using the Cooper-Rand larynx may present special problems. The plastic conducting tube must be kept away from the teeth and the tongue tip, because biting or occluding the tube with the tongue interrupts the sound. Although some distortion may occur on velar consonants, the tube may be placed well into the mouth, with the tip toward the palatal vault. A patient who has difficulty swallowing saliva may not be a favorable candidate for the appliance, since the tube may become occluded with muscles, thereby preventing sound transmission. Sometimes the use of a firm dental saliva ejection tube may reduce the problem. Inflectional patterns and pitch variations are less feasible therapy goals with the Cooper-Rand than with the Western Electric models. It is valuable, however, to have the patient talk at different pitch levels by changing settings on the pitch dial. Factors which may influence choice of a particular pitch level include the patient's size, sex, and individual resonance characteristics.

Surgical and Surgical Prosthetic Voice Restoration

The large amount of work currently going on in this surgical area will certainly make much of the information to be reported here outdated by the time this chapter goes to print. Nevertheless, it would be remiss to omit an overview of these procedures in a

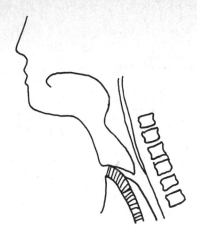

Figure 5–8. Calcaterra and Jafek's Tracheo-Esophageal Shunt Method

chapter of this nature. Consequently, rather than focusing on a specific surgical procedure we will generalize "directions" receiving current attention.

The work by Conley et al. (1958) to construct a shunt for tracheal air into the esophagus has been adapted, modified, and redesigned by a number of surgeons since that time (Conley, 1959; Calcaterra and Jafek, 1971; Zwitman and Calcaterra, 1973; Korman et al., 1973; Korman, 1974). Figure 5–8 shows one example of this technique. Since the air enters the esophagus inferior to the PE segment, the resultant voice is an esophageal voice in terms of sound source, quality and pitch. However, this type of voice, and in fact all surgically restored voices that "hook up" to a pulmonary air supply, have some distinct advantages. Dworkin and Sparker (1980) write that

> individuals using the shunt method are able to (a) initiate voice and speech more easily, (b) produce more words per breath, with a greater supply of continuous air from the lungs, (c) achieve more intensity of voice, (d) establish more appropriate stress patterns, (e) prolong phonation for longer durations, (f) eliminate clunking and stoma noises, and (g) speak as intelligibly as superior esophageal speakers, thereby more closely approximating the parameters of normal speech. (p. 340)

Other surgeons (Miller, 1967, 1968, 1971; Montgomery and Toohill, 1968; McGrail and Oldfield, 1971), and most notably Asai (1965, 1972), have chosen to shunt the tracheal air into the pharyngeal area. As with the previous procedure, voice is achieved by occluding the tracheal stoma, thus forcing air into the surgically created shunt and into the pharynx to create phonation. (See fig. 5–9 for an example of this method.)

Another group of surgeons (Arslan and Serafini, 1972; Arslan, 1975; and Vega, 1975) attempt, with variations, to retain the epiglottis and/or hyoid bone at the time of laryngectomy. The trachea is raised and sutured to the hypopharynx just below the supra-hyoid stump of the epiglottis or hyoid bone. A "temporary" tracheostoma is constructed with the hope of subsequent decannulation (removal of cannula—tube in neck). In effect, the patient has a tracheo-pharyngeal shunt using tracheal cartilage.

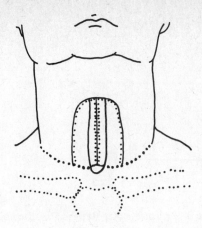

Figure 5–9. Asai's Tracheo-Pharyngeal Dermal Tube Shunt Method

These air shunting procedures are not without their drawbacks. A connection from trachea to esophagus/pharynx for air, also provides a hazardous connection from esophagus/pharynx into trachea for the aspiration of liquid and food.

In an attempt to avoid the problems inherent in internal air shunts, others (Taub and Spiro, 1972, 1973; Taub, 1975; Shedd, 1972, 1976; Edwards, 1974, 1975, 1976; and Sisson et al., 1975), surgically create a fistula in the neck or pharynx. An external prosthetic air shunt is then attached from the tracheal opening to the pharyngeal fistula. Pulmonary air can then be forced through the prosthetic connection to set structures into vibration. A pressure sensitive valve is used in some of the devices so that low pulmonary pressure, as in normal breathing, does not activate the valve. Increased pulmonary pressure closes the valve, shunting the air through the prosthesis and into the fistula for speech. At the present time, only the Shedd prosthesis houses a musical rubber-reed that functions as a sound source. The others depend upon pulmonary air to excite surrounding soft tissue. External air shunt speech has the same speech advantages attributed to internal air shunt speech (Dworkin and Sparker, 1980). For examples see figures 5–10, 5–11, and 5–12.

In 1979, Blom and Singer altered a procedure devised by Amatsu et al. (1977) to create a simple tracheo-esophageal puncture (Singer et al., 1981). An inexpensive valved tube is placed into the tracheo-esophageal puncture. This "duckbill" speech tube (see figure 5–13) has a thin slit at its proximal end which permits air to flow in only one direction, thus eliminating the possibility of the reflux of food or liquid from the esophagus. The procedure can be accomplished in a matter of minutes. If the duckbill prosthesis is removed for several hours, the T-E puncture will spontaneously close to restore the patient to preoperative anatomical status. A "paste on" or fitted pressure-sensitive valve promises to eliminate the need for digital occlusion of the stoma.

The work of Blom and Singer (1979) has encouraged exploration and changes by others of their basic T-E puncture utilizing a tube (Panje, 1981), and variations are being reported even as this chapter goes to print.

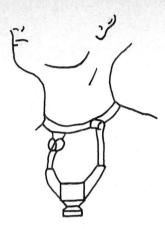

Figure 5-10. Taub's Air-Bypass Prosthesis Method

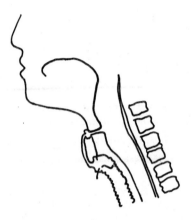

Figure 5-11. Sisson and McConnel's Prosthesis Method

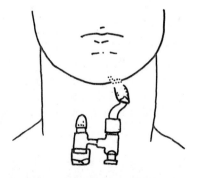

Figure 5-12. Shedd's Reed Fistula Prosthesis Method

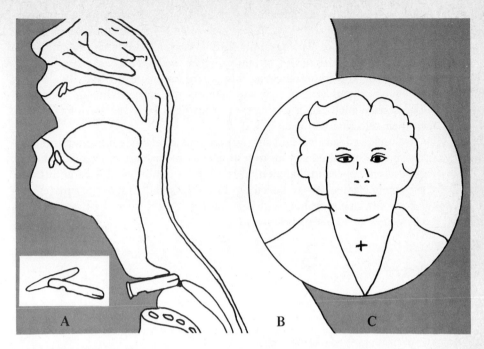

Figure 5–13. Blom and Singer's Tracheo-Esophageal Puncture Method: A. duckbill speech tube in isolation; B. duckbill speech tube in place; C. duckbill speech tube taped in place at top of stoma

The reader will find the book by Shedd and Weinberg (1980) an excellent source for readings in the area of surgical and surgical-prosthetic speech restoration.

The surgical and surgical prosthetic procedures noted are both innovative and promising. Advances are dramatic, exciting, and provide more options for the individual who is faced with the loss of his larynx.

SUMMARY

This chapter has had two main emphases: the remediation of laryngeal phonation disorders and the teaching of alaryngeal speech. In the first section, an understanding of laryngeal voice disorders was enlarged by synthesizing data from many methods of study, variously employing physiological, psychological, and auditory methods of measurement. Voice remediation employs techniques to correct hypertonic and hypotonic muscle function and to achieve a balance of respiratory and phonatory forces, with attention being directed primarily toward abuses of pitch, loudness, and duration.

The patient whose voice disorder requires surgical removal of the larynx has varied and present different remedial problems. The changes, both physiological and psychological, that confront the laryngectomee underscore the significance of preoperative counseling. A patient will be more likely to adjust satisfactorily to his condition and to learn alaryngeal speech if he understands what is involved in the surgical procedure as well as how it will affect his breathing and speech.

The physiology of alaryngeal phonation was discussed in terms of vibrata, power source, air intake, and air expulsion, all of which provided a basis for delineating the principles and techniques of alaryngeal phonation. Ways of instructing the patient in the methods of air inhalation and air injection, as well as in the use of loading phonemes, were of key importance in this regard, as were methods of eliciting alaryngeal phonation and of assessing and refining the laryngectomee's speech attempts. The section included a description of artificial larynxes and of factors to consider in their selection and use.

Finally, we reviewed surgical and surgical prosthetic methods using both internal and external shunts for pulmonary air to restore voice to laryngectomized individuals.

Post-laryngectomy speech rehabilitation is, without doubt, complex and difficult. It is also extremely challenging and exciting. From the standpoint of the authors, it is an area that professionals dealing with communication disorders have avoided too long. We have no choice but to become involved.

BIBLIOGRAPHY

American Cancer Society, ACS Florida Division, *Your Latest Challenge, That New Voice* (1964).

American Cancer Society, *NCI Third National Cancer Survey*, American Cancer Society (1976).

Amatsu, M., Matsui, T., and Maki, T., Vocal rehabilitation after total laryngectomy: A new stage surgical technique. *Jr. Otolaryngol.*, Jpn. **80**, 779–785 (1977).

Amster, W. W., Love, R. J., Menzel, O. J., Sandler, J., Sculthorpe, W. B., and Gross, F. M., Psychosocial factors and speech after laryngectomy. *J. Commun. Dis.*, **5**, 1–18 (1972).

Appleman, D. R., *The Science of Vocal Pedagogy*. Bloomington: Indiana University Press (1967).

Arnold, G. E., Vocal rehabilitation of paralytic dysphonia: V. Vocal symptomatology after bilateral loss of abduction. *Arch. Otolaryngol.*, **70**, 444–453 (1959a).

Arnold, G. E., Spastic dysphonia. *Logos*, **2**, 3–14 (1959b).

Arnold, G. E., Phoniatric methods of vocal compensation: VIII. *Arch. Otolaryngol.*, **75**, 76–83 (1962).

Arnold, G. E., Alleviation of aphonia or dysphonia through intrachordal injection of teflon paste. *Ann. Otolaryngol. Rhinol. Laryngol.*, **72**, 384–395 (1963a).

Arnold, G. E., Vocal nodules. *N.Y. State J. Med.*, **63**, 3096–3098 (1963b).

Aronson, A. E., Speech pathology and symptom therapy in the interdisciplinary treatment of psychogenic aphonia. *J. Speech Hearing Dis.*, **34**, 321–341 (1969).

Aronson, A., *Clinical Voice Disorders*. New York: Brian C. Decker, a division of Thieme-Stratton, Inc. (1980).

Aronson, A., Brown, J. R., Litin, E. M., and Pearson, J. S., Spastic dysphonia: I Voice, neurologic, and psychiatric aspects. *J. Speech Hearing Dis.*, **33**, 203–218 (1968).

Arslan, M., Technique of laryngeal reconstruction. *Laryngoscope*, **85**, 862–865 (1975).

Arslan, M., and Serafini, I., Restoration of laryngeal function after total laryngectomy: Report of the first 25 cases. *Laryngoscope*, **82**, 1349–1360 (1972).

Asai, R., A new voice production method: A substitution for human speech. Paper presented at the Eighth International Congress for Otolaryngology, Tokyo (1965).

Asai, R., Laryngoplasty after total laryngectomy. *Arch. Otolaryngol.*, **95**, 114–119 (1972).

Atkinson, M., Kramer, P., Wyman, S., and Ingelfinger, F. J., The dynamics of swallowing: I. Normal pharyngeal mechanisms. *J. Clin. Invest.*, **36**, 518–558 (1957).

Barton, R. T., The whispering syndrome of hysterical dysphonia. *Ann. Otolaryngol. Rhinol. Laryngol.*, **69**, 156–164 (1960).

Barton, J., and Hejna, R., Factors associated with success or non-success in acquisition of esophageal speech. *J. Speech Hearing Assoc.*, **4**, 19–20 (1963).

Berlin, C. I., Clinical measurement of esophageal speech: I. Methodology and curves of skill acquisition. *J. Speech Hearing Dis.*, **28**, 42–51 (1963a).

Berlin, C. I., On the use of /s/ in esophageal inflation, letter. *J. Speech Hearing Dis.*, **28**, 208 (1963b).

Berlin, C. I., Clinical measurement of esophageal speech: III. Performance of non-biased groups. *J. Speech Hearing Dis.*, **30,** 174–183 (1965).

Best, C. H., and Taylor, N. B., *The Physiological Basis of Medical Practice.* (5th ed.) Baltimore: The Williams & Wilkins Co. (1950).

Blom, E. D., and Singer, M., Surgical prosthetic approaches for post-laryngectomee voice restoration. In R. I. Keith and F. L. Darley (Eds.), *Laryngectomee Rehabilitation.* Houston: College Hill Press (1979).

Boone, D. R., *The Voice and Voice Therapy.* Englewood Cliffs, N.J.: Prentice Hall, Inc. (1977).

Bouhuys, A., Mead, J., Proctor, D. F., and Stevens, K. N., Pressure-flow events during singing. In A. Bouhuys (Ed.), *Sound Production in Man. Ann. N.Y. Acad. Sci.*, **155,** 164–176 (1968).

Brewer, D. W., Medical and surgical aspects. In D. W. Brewer (Ed.), *Research Potentials in Voice Physiology.* Syracuse: State University of New York (1964).

Brewer, D. W., Briess, F. B., and Faaborg-Anderson, K., Phonation-clinical testing versus electromyography. *Ann. Otolaryngol. Rhinol. Laryngol.*, **69,** 781–804 (1960).

Briess, F. B., Voice therapy: I. Identification of specific laryngeal muscle dysfunction by voice testing. *Arch. Otolaryngol.*, **66,** 375–382 (1957).

Briess, F. B., Voice therapy: II. Essential treatment phases of specific laryngeal muscle dysfunction. *Arch. Otolaryngol.*, **69,** 61–69 (1959).

Briess, F. B., Voice diagnosis and therapy. In D. W. Brewer (Ed.), *Research Potentials in Voice Physiology,* pp. 259–295. Syracuse: State University of New York (1964).

Brodnitz, F. S., *Vocal Rehabilitation.* Rochester, Minn.: American Academy of Ophthalmology and Otolaryngology and Whiting Press (1959).

Brodnitz, F. S., Vocal rehabilitation after reconstructive surgery for laryngeal cancer. Vienna: *De Therapia Vocis et Loquelae,* III Congress, **2,** 151–154 (1965).

Burkowsky, M. R., Vocal ulcers in a seventy-one year old male. *J. Speech Hearing Dis.*, **33,** 268–269 (1968).

Calcaterra, T. C., and Jafek, B. W., Tracheo-esophageal shunt for speech rehabilitation after total laryngectomy. *Arch. Otolaryngol.*, **94,** 124–128 (1971).

Cavagna, G. A., and Margaria, R., Airflow rates and efficiency changes during phonation. In A. Bouhuys (Ed.), *Sound Production in Man,* pp. 152–163. *Ann. N.Y. Acad. Sci.*, **155,** 152–163 (1968).

Conley, J. J., Vocal rehabilitation by autogenous vein graft. *Ann. Otol. Rhinol. Laryngol.*, **68,** 990–995 (1959).

Conley, J. J., DeAmesti, F., and Pierce, J. K., A new surgical technique for the vocal rehabilitation of the laryngectomized patient. *Ann. Otol. Rhinol. Laryngol.*, **67,** 655–664 (1958).

Connelly, M. K., Wilson, F. B., and Leeper, H. A., A group voice therapy technique for decreasing vocal abuse in children with vocal nodules. *J. Mo. Speech Hearing Assoc.*, **3,** 7–18 (1970).

Cook, J. V., Palaski, D. J., and Hanson, W. R., A vocal hygiene program for school age children. *Language Speech and Hear. Ser. in Schools*, **1,** 21–26 (1979).

Cooper, M., Spectographic analysis of fundamental frequency and hoarseness before and after vocal rehabilitation. *J. Speech Hearing Dis.*, **39,** 286–299 (1974).

Cooper, M., and Cooper, M. M., (Eds.), *Approaches to Vocal Rehabilitation.* Springfield, Ill.: Charles C. Thomas (1977).

Curry, E. T., A vocal frequency analysis in voice dysfunction. *EENT Monthly,* **32,** 518–520 (1953).

Damsté, P. H., Improvement of the voice after total laryngectomy by changing the site of the pseudoglottis. *Pract. Otorhinol.*, **19,** 309–312 (1957).

Damsté, P. H., *Oesophageal Speech after Laryngectomy.* Groningen, the Netherlands: Hoitsema (1958).

Damsté, P. H., The glosso-pharyngeal press. *Speech Pathol. Ther.*, **2,** 70–76 (1959).

Damsté, P. H., Voice change in adult women caused by virilizing agents. *J. Speech Hearing Dis.*, **32,** 126–132 (1967).

Damsté, P. H., Van den Berg, J., and Moolenaar-Bijl, A. J., Why are some patients unable to learn esophageal speech? *Ann. Otolaryngol. Rhinol. Laryngol.*, **65,** 998–1005 (1956).

Deal, R. E., McClain, B., and Sudderth, J. F., Identification, evaluation, therapy, and follow-up for children with vocal nodules in a public school setting. *J. Speech Hearing Dis.*, **41,** 390–397 (1976).

Dey, F. L., and Kirchner, J. A., The upper esophageal sphincter after laryngectomy. *Laryngoscope,* **71,** 99–115 (1961).

Di Carlo, L., Amster, W., and Herer, G., *Speech after Laryngectomy.* Syracuse: Syracuse University Press (1956).

Diedrich, W., and Youngstrom, K., *Alaryngeal Speech.* Springfield, Ill.: Charles C. Thomas (1966).

Doehler, M., *Esophageal Speech.* Boston: American Cancer Society (1953).

Drudge, M. K. M., and Philips, B. J., Shaping behavior in voice therapy. *J. Speech Hearing Dis.*, **41**, 398–411 (1976).

Duguay, M. J., Preoperative ideas of speech after laryngectomy. *Arch. Otolaryngol.*, **83**, 69–72 (1966).

Duguay, M. J., The speech-language pathologist and the laryngectomized lay teacher in alaryngeal speech rehabilitation. *ASHA*, **22**, 965–966 (1980).

Dworkin, J. P., and Sparker, A., Surgical vocal rehabilitation following total laryngectomy: A state-of-the-art report. *Clin. Otolaryngol.*, **5**, 339–350 (1980).

Edwards, N., Post-laryngectomy vocal rehabilitation: Preliminary report of a one stage method using air and a valved prosthesis. *J. Laryngol. Otol.*, **88**, 905–918 (1974).

Edwards, N., Post-laryngectomy rehabilitation by the external fistula method: Further experiences. *Laryngoscope*, **85**, 690–699 (1974).

Edwards, N., New voices for old: Restoration of effective speech after laryngectomy by the pulmonary air-shunt vocal fistula principle, *Bristol Med. Chir. J.*, **90**, 11–17 (1976).

Faaborg-Anderson, K., Electromyography of the laryngeal muscles in man. In D. W. Brewer (Ed.), *Research Potentials in Voice Physiology*, pp. 105–123. Syracuse: State University of New York (1964).

Fairbanks, G., *Voice and Articulation Drillbook.* (2nd ed.) New York: Harper & Row (1960).

Fisher, H. B., and Logemann, J. A., Objective evaluation of therapy for vocal nodules: A case report. *J. Speech Hearing Dis.*, **35**, 277–285 (1970).

Flower, R. M., Voice training in the management of dysphonia. *Laryngoscope*, **69**, 940–946 (1959).

Fox, D. R., Spastic dysphonia: A case presentation. *J. Speech Hearing Dis.*, **34**, 275–279 (1969).

Freud, E. D., Functions and dysfunctions of the ventricular folds. *J. Speech Hearing Dis.*, **27**, 334–340 (1962).

Froeschels, E., Hygiene of the voice. *Arch. Otolaryngol.*, **38**, 122–130 (1943).

Gardner, W., Executives' dysphonia. *Cleveland Clin. Quart.*, **25**, 177–186 (1958).

Gardner, W., Adjustment problems of laryngectomized women. *Arch. Otolaryngol.*, **83**, 57–68 (1966).

Gardner, W., and Harris, H., Aids and devices for laryngectomees. *Arch. Otolaryngol.*, **73**, 145–152 (1961).

Gargan, W., *Why Me?* Garden City, N.Y.: Doubleday & Company, Inc. (1969).

Gould, W. J., Quantitative assessment of voice function in microlaryngology. *Folia Phonation.*, **27**, 190–200 (1945).

Gray, B. B., England, G., and Mohoney, J. L., Treatment of benign vocal nodules by reciprocal inhibition. *Behav. Res. Ther.*, **3**, 187–193 (1956).

Greene, J. S., Laryngectomy and its psychologic implications. *N.Y. State J. Med.*, **17**, 53–56 (1947).

Hirano, M., Ohala, J., and Vennard, W., The function of laryngeal muscles in regulating fundamental frequency and intensity of phonation. *J. Speech Hearing Res.*, **12**, 616–628 (1969).

Hodson, C. J., and Oswald, M. V., *Speech Recovery after Total Laryngectomy.* Baltimore: The Williams & Wilkins Co. (1958).

Hollien, H., and Coleman, R. R., Laryngeal correlates of frequency change: A STROL study. *J. Speech Hearing Res.*, **13**, 271–278 (1970).

Horn, D., Laryngectomee survey report summary presented at the 11th Annual Meeting of the I.A.L., Memphis, Tenn. (August 21, 1962).

House, A. S., A note on optimal vocal frequency. *J. Speech Hearing Res.*, **2**, 55–60 (1959).

Hyman, M., An experimental study of artificial larynx and esophageal speech. *J. Speech Hearing Dis.*, **20**, 291–299 (1955).

International Association of Laryngectomees. *Helping Words for the Laryngectomee.* 219 East 42 Street, New York, N.Y.: I.A.L. (1964).

Isshiki, N., Vocal intensity and air flow rate. *Folia Phoniat.*, **17**, 92–104 (1965).

Iwata, S., and Von Leden, H., Pitch perturbations in normal and pathologic voices. *Folia Phoniats.*, **22**, 413–424 (1970).

Iwata, S., Von Leden, H., and Williams, D., Air flow measurement during phonation. *J. Commun. Dis.*, **5**, 67–69 (1972).

Johnson, T. S., *Vocal Abuse Reduction Program.* Department of Communicative Disorders, Utah State University (1976).

Kalfuss, H. A., Counselling the laryngectomee: A study of the surgeon's approach. Paper presented by H. R. Hoops at the ninth I.A.L. Voice Institute, University of Pittsburgh (July 17, 1969).

Keith, R., Shane, H., Coates, H., and Devine, K., *Looking forward . . . A Guidebook for the Laryngectomee.* Rochester Memorial.: Mayo Foundation (1977).

Korman, R. M., Vocal rehabilitation in the laryngectomized patient with a tracheo-esophageal shunt. *Ann. Otol. Rhinol. Laryngol.*, **83**, 445–451 (1974).

Korman, R. M., Weyger, J. S., Sessions, R. B., and Malone, P. E., Vocal rehabilitation with a tracheo-esophageal shunt. *Arch. Otolaryngol.*, **97**, 303–335 (1973).

Laguaite, J., and Waldrop, W., Acoustic analysis of fundamental frequency of voice before and after therapy. *Folia Phoniats.*, **16**, 183–192 (1964).

Lauder, E., The role of the laryngectomee in post-laryngectomy voice instruction. *J. Speech Hearing Dis.*, **30**, 145–158 (1965).

Lauder, E., The laryngectomee and the artificial larynx—a second look. *J. Speech Hearing Dis.*, **35**, 62–65 (1970).

Lauder, E., *Self-Help for the Laryngectomee*. San Antonio, Texas: E. Lauder (1979).

Lieberman, P., Vocal cord motion in man. In A. Bouhuys (Ed.), *Sound Production in Man*, Ann. N.Y. Acad. Sci., **155**, 28–38 (1968).

Locke, B., Psychology of the laryngectomee. *Milit. Med.*, **131**, 593–599 (1966).

Luschinger, R., and Arnold, G. E., *Voice-Speech-Language, Clinical Communicology*. Belmont, Calif.: Wadsworth Publishing Co., Inc. (1965).

McClear, J., *Esophageal Voice Production: An Instruction Manual*. New York: National Hospital for Speech Disorders (1960).

McCroskey, R., and Mulligan, M., The relative intelligibility of esophageal speech and artificial larynx speech. *J. Speech Hearing Dis.*, **28**, 37–41 (1963).

McGlone, R. E., and Brown, W. S., Identification of the "shift" between registers. *J. Acous. Soc. Am.*, **46**, 1033–1036 (1969).

McGrail, J. S., and Oldfield, D. L., One-stage operation for vocal rehabilitation at laryngectomy. *Trans. Am. Acad. Opthalmol. Otolaryngol.*, **75**, 510–512 (1971).

McNally, E. F., Use of intraluminal pressure measurements in esophageal speech. Paper presented at the 18th Annual Meeting of the I.A.L., Pittsburgh, Pa. (July 13, 1969).

Martin, H., Rehabilitation of the laryngectomee. *Cancer*, **16**, 823–841 (1963).

Miller, A. H., First experiences with the Asai technique for vocal rehabilitation after total laryngectomy. *Ann. Rhinol. Laryngol.*, **76**, 820–833 (1967).

Miller, A. H., Further experiences with the Asai technique for vocal rehabilitation after laryngectomy. *Trans. Am. Acad. Opthalmol. Otolaryngol.*, **72**, 779–781 (1968).

Miller, A. H., Four years experience with the Asai technique for focal rehabilitation for the laryngectomized patient. *J. Laryngol. Otol.*, **85**, 567–576 (1971).

Miller, M., The responsibility of the speech therapist to the laryngectomized patient. *Arch. Otolaryngol.*, **70**, 211–216 (1959).

Montgomery, W. W., and Toohill, R. J., Voice rehabilitation after laryngectomy. *Arch. Otolaryngol.*, **88**, 499–506 (1968).

Moolenaar-Bijl, A., Connection between consonant articulation and the intake of air in esophageal speech. *Folia Phoniat.*, **5**, 212–215 (1953a).

Moolenaar-Bijl, A., The importance of certain consonants in esophageal voice after laryngectomy. *Ann. Otolarygol. Rhinol. Laryngol.*, **62**, 979–989 (1953b).

Moore, G. P., Voice disorders associated with organic abnormalities. In L. E. Travis (Ed.), *Handbook of Speech Pathology*, pp. 653–703. New York: Appleton-Century-Crofts, Inc. (1957).

Moore, G. P., *Organic Voice Disorders*. Englewood Cliffs, N.J.: Prentice-Hall, Inc. (1971).

Moore, G. P., and Von Leden, H., Dynamic variations of the vibratory pattern in the normal larynx. *Folia Phoniat.*, **10**, 205–238 (1958).

Moses, P. J., *The Voice of Neurosis*. New York: Grune & Stratton, Inc. (1954).

Mueller, P. B., Vocal nodules in children. *J. Wisc. Speech Hearing Assoc.*, **9**, 5–15 (1975).

Murphy, A. T., *Functional Voice Disorders*. Englewood Cliffs, N.J.: Prentice-Hall, Inc. (1964).

Murry, T., and Brown, W. S. J., Intraoral air pressure variability in esophageal speakers. *Folia Phoniat.*, **27**, 227–249 (1975).

Panje, W. R., Prosthetic vocal rehabilitation following laryngectomy; A voice button. *Ann. Otol. Rhin. Laryng.*, **90**, 116–120 (1981).

Peacher, G., *How To Improve Your Speaking Voice*. New York: Frederick Fell, Inc. (1966).

Perkins, W. H., The challenge of functional disorders of voice. In L. E. Travis (Ed.), *Handbook of Speech Pathology*, pp. 832–877. New York: Appleton-Century-Crofts, Inc. (1957).

Perkins, W. H., Vocal function: Assessment and therapy. In L. E. Travis (Ed.), *Handbook of Speech Pathology and Audiology*, pp. 505–534. New York: Appleton-Century-Crofts, Inc. (1971).

Perkins, W. H., and Yanagihara, N., Parameters of voice production: I. Some mechanisms for the regulation of pitch. *J. Speech Hearing Res.*, **2**, 246–267 (1968).

Pitkin, Y. N., Factors affecting psychologic adjustment in the laryngectomized patient. *Arch. Otolaryngol.*, **58**, 38–49 (1953).

Proctor, D. F., The physiologic basis of voice training. In A. Bouhuys (Ed.), *Sound Production in Man*, Ann. N.Y. Acad. Sci., **155**, 208–228 (1967).

Putney, F., Rehabilitation of the post-laryngectomized patient. *Ann. Otolaryngol. Rhinol. Laryngol.*, **67**, 544–549 (1958).

Rubin, H. J., and Hirt, C. C., The falsetto. A high speed cinematographic study. *Laryngoscope*, **70**, 1305–1324 (1960).

Rubin, H. J., and Lehroff, I., Pathogenesis and treatment of vocal nodules. *J. Speech Hearing Dis.*, **27**, 150–161 (1962).

Sacco, P. R., Mann, M. B., and Schultz, M. C., Perceptual confusions among selected phonemes in esophageal speech. *ISHA*, **26**, 19–33 (1967).

Salmon, S., and Goldstein, L., *The Artificial Larynx Handbook*. New York: Grune Stratton (1978).

Sanchez-Salazar, V., and Stark, A., The use of crisis intervention in the rehabilitation of laryngectomees. *J. Speech Hearing Dis.*, **37**, 323–328 (1972).

Sansone, F. E., and Emanuel, F. W., Spectral noise levels and roughness severity ratings for normal and simulated rough vowels produced by adult males. *J. Speech Hearing Res.*, **13**, 489–502 (1970).

Schall, L. A., Psychology of laryngectomized patients. *Arch. Otolaryngol.*, **28**, 581–584 (1938).

Sedlackova, E., Laryngostroboskopische und electroakustiche befunde bei spastischer dysphonie. Vienna: *De Therapia Vocis et Loquelae*, III Congress, **2**, 1–3 (1965).

Shames, G., Font, J., and Matthews, J. Factors related to speech proficiency of the laryngectomized. *J. Speech Hearing Dis.*, **28**, 273–287 (1963).

Shanks, J., Advantages in the use of esophageal speech by a laryngectomee. *Laryngoscope*, **76**, 239–243 (1966).

Shedd, D., Bakamijian, V., Sako, K., Mann, M., Barba, S., and Schaaf, N., Reed fistula method of speech rehabilitation after laryngectomy. *Am. J. Surg.*, **124**, 510–514 (1972).

Shedd, D., Schaaf, N., and Weinberg, B., Technical aspects of reed fistula speech following pjaryngolarynectomy. *J. Surg. Oncol.*, **8**, 305–310 (1976).

Shedd, D., and Weinberg, B., *Surgical and Surgical Prosthetic Approaches to Speech Rehabilitation*. Boston, Mass.: G. K. Hall (1980).

Shipp, T., Frequency, duration, and perceptual measures in relation to judgments of alaryngeal speech acceptability. *J. Speech Hearing Res.*, **10 (3)**, 417–422 (1967).

Shipp, T., Procedures with laryngectomy patients prior to speech training. Paper presented at a seminar directed by E. Hendrichson and supported by VRA grant 67–71. University of Minnesota (June 10–14, 1968).

Shipp, T., Deatsch, W. W., and Ross, J. A. T., Pharyngoesophageal activity in laryngectomees. Progress report submitted to the National Institute of Neurological Disease and Blindness (March 10, 1967).

Singer, M. I., Blom, E. D., and Hamaker, R. C., Further experience with voice restoration after total laryngectomy. *Ann. Otol. Rhin. Laryng.*, **90 (5)**, 498–502 (1981).

Sisson, G. A., McConnel, F. M., Logemann, J. A., and Yeh, S., Voice rehabilitation after laryngectomy. *Arch. Otolaryngol.*, **101**, 178–181 (1975).

Snidecor, J. C., Experimental studies of the pitch and duration characteristics of superior speech. Unpublished doctoral dissertation, State University of Iowa (1940).

Snidecor, J. (Ed.), *Speech Rehabilitation of the Laryngectomized*. (2nd ed.) Springfield, Ill.: Charles G. Thomas (1969).

Stetson, R. H., Esophageal speech for any laryngectomized patient. *Arch. Otolaryngol.*, **26**, 132–142 (1937).

Stoll, B., Psychological factors determining the success or failure of the rehabilitation program of laryngectomized patients. *Ann. Otolaryngol. Rhinol. Laryngol.*, **67**, 550–557 (1958).

Tait, N. A., Michel, J. F., and Carpenter, M. A., Maximum duration of sustained /s/ and /z/ in children. *J. Speech Hearing Dis.*, **45**, 239–246 (1980).

Taub, S., Air bypass voice prosthesis for vocal rehabilitation of laryngectomies. *Ann. Otol. Rhinol. Laryngol.*, **84**, 45–48 (1975).

Taub, S., and Bergner, L. H., Air bypass voice prosthesis for vocal rehabilitation of laryngectomees. *Am. J. Surg.*, **125**, 748–756 (1973).

Taub, S., and Spiro, R. H., Vocal rehabilitation of laryngectomees: Preliminary report of a new technic. *Am. J. Surg.*, **124**, 87–90 (1972).

Timcke, R., Von Leden, H., and Moore, P., Laryngeal vibrations: Measurements of the glottic wave: I. The normal vibrating cycle. *Arch. Otolaryngol.*, **68**, 1–19 (1958).

Van den Berg, J. W., Myoelastic-aerodynamic theory of voice production. *J. Speech Hearing Res.*, **1**, 227–244 (1958).

Van den Berg, J. W., Register problems. In A. Bouhuys (Ed.), *Sound Production in Man*, pp. 129–134. Ann N.Y. Acad. Sci., 1955 (1968).

Van den Berg, J. W., Some physical aspects of voice production. In D. W. Brewer (Ed.), *Research Potentials in Voice Physiology*, pp. 63–101. Syracuse: State University of New York (1964).

Van den Berg, J. W., and Moolenaar-Bijl, A., Cricopharyngeal sphincter, pitch, intensity, and fluency in esophageal speech. *Pract. Otorhinolaryngol.*, **21**, 298–315 (1959).

Van Riper, C., and Irwin, J., *Voice and Articulation*. Englewood Cliffs, N.J.: Prentice Hall, Inc. (1958).

Vega, M. F., Larynx reconstructive surgery—a study of three year findings—a modified surgical technique. *Laryngoscope*, **85**, 866–881 (1975).

Von Leden, H., Objective measures of laryngeal function and phonation. In A. Bouhuys (Ed.), *Sound Production in Man*, Ann N.Y. Acad. Sci., **155**, 55–56 (1968).

Von Leden, H., and Koike, Y., Detection of laryngeal disease by computer technique. *Arch. Otolaryngol.*, **91**, 3–10 (1970).

Von Leden, H. P., and Timcke, R., Laryngeal vibrations: Measurements of the glottic wave: III. The pathologic larynx. *Arch. Otolaryngol.*, **71**, 16–35 (1960).

Vrticka, K., and Svoboda, M., A clinical and X-ray study of 100 laryngectomized speakers. *Folia Phoniat.*, **13**, 174–186 (1961).

Walsh, T. F., Rehabilitation: Sound the way for laryngectomees. *Patient Care*, **6**, No. 14, 58–89 (1972).

Weinberg, B., *Readings in Speech Following Total Laryngectomy*, Baltimore, Md.: University Park Press (1980).

Weiss, D. A., Spastic dysphonia and stammering. Vienna: *De Therapia Vocis et Loquelae*, III Congress, **2**, 251–255 (1965).

Wendahl, R. W., Moore, G. P., and Hollien, H., Comments on vocal fry. *Folia Phoniat.*, **15**, 251–255 (1963).

Wepman, J., MacGahan, J., Richard, J., and Skelton, N., The objective measurement of progressive esophageal speech development. *J. Speech Hearing Dis.*, **18**, 247–251 (1953).

Wilson, D. K., *Voice Problems of Children*. (2nd. ed.) Baltimore: The Williams and Wilkins Co. (1979).

Wilson, F. B., The voice disordered child: A descriptive approach. *Lang. Speech. Hearing Ser. in Schools.*, **4**, 14–22 (1970).

Wilson, F. B., and Rice, M., *A Programmed Approach to Voice Therapy*. Austin: Learning Concepts Inc. (1977).

Winans, C. S., and Waldrop, W. F., Esophageal determinants of alaryngeal speech. *Arch. Otolaryngol.*, **99**, 10–14 (1974).

Yanagihara, N., Significance of harmonic changes and noise components in hoarseness. *J. Speech Hearing Res.*, **10**, 531–541 (1967).

Zwitman, D., and Calcaterra, T., Phonation using the tracheosophageal shunt. *J. Speech Hear. Disord.*, **38**, 369–373 (1973).

6 Communication Therapy for Problems Associated with Cleft Palate

Rolland J. Van Hattum

The extreme importance of communication ability to each individual has frequently been described in the literature (Van Hattum, 1980). Social, emotional, educational, and occupational success are intimately related to the individual's ability to communicate to the limit of his or her ability. Thus, any interference with this ability will likely have far-reaching effects on the individual. Craniofacial anomalies which affect the speech and hearing mechanisms are major contributors to communication disorders. Absent, misplaced, malformed, or malfunctioning parts of the system are likely to lead to varying degrees of abnormal speech production. The fact that these aberrations are most often congenital adds to the complexity of the problems presented.

Craniofacial anomalies in which the palatal partition between the oral and nasal cavities is missing to some degree has been labeled "cleft palate" and usually has serious ramifications for the acceptable production of voice and articulation, as well as frequent interference with language acquisition. Cleft palate and cleft lip, the lack of fusion of lip structures, may occur singly or together. In addition, the palate may be too short for adequate function (foreshortened velum) or submucous clefts (clefts involving absence of bony structures but with mucousal tissues intact) may exist. Cleft palates are also often associated with specific syndromes (McWilliams, 1980). All of these factors suggest that there is virtually an infinite variety of types, combinations, and severities of clefts among the approximately 1 in 700 persons who bear this label. Additionally, each of these individuals varies in social, emotional, and intellectual resources and has been subjected to a wide variety of medical and dental management techniques. It is not surprising that persons with clefts of the lip and/or palate range over the entire spectrum of communication ability, from normal to severe defectiveness.

ORAL-FACIAL CLEFTS

Throughout history, physical malformations have been mired in views of divine providence and superstition, reflecting society's dependence on the supernatural for explanations of the unknown. Such beliefs continue even today in the minds of some parents and grandparents. These beliefs would be more easily eradicated if scientific fact could produce substantiated explanations. However, that is not currently possible. We do not know why a child is born with a cleft condition or how the cleft occurs during the prenatal period.

Causes of Clefts

More recent scientific exploration has focused on two major views regarding causation. The first view considers congenital clefts of the palate as the result of genetic factors, while the second view suggests that these clefts are the result of influences in the uterine environment. A rapidly growing belief in the scientific community combines interactions between these two factors as the most likely causation. Fraser (1955) summarized it well in noting his belief that clefts are caused by a genetic predisposition, probably multifactorial, interacting with undefined environmental circumstances. Some of these teratogenic (agents capable of causing a physical defect in a developing embryo) include rubella virus, thalidomide, valium, radiation, and some other yet unidentified medications (McWilliams, 1980).

Palatal Formation

The second part of the two questions, "how" the cleft occurs, is similarly unanswerable at this time. Congenital clefts of the lip and palate are related to either the failure of fusion of palatal structures or the failure of the fusion of these structures to hold together rather than to separate after fusion occurs. A brief overview of embryological development suggests where a cleft of oral structures is more likely to occur.

The three primordial cell layers that ultimately become all the organs and structures of the body are the ectoderm, or outer layer, the endoderm, or inner layer, and the mesoderm, or middle layer. Toward the end of the third week following conception the embryo produces a groove known as the stomodeum or primitive mouth. The stomodeum deepens and leads to an ectodermal-endodermal cell layer which begins to rupture during the fourth month establishing the mouth opening. The face develops around the mouth and involves the merging of five processes: the frontal prominence, two maxillary prominences, and two mandibular prominences. The frontal prominence becomes the frontonasal process and divides into the median nasal and two lateral processes. These processes develop into the nose, middle part of the upper lip, and primary palate (the part of the palate anterior to the incisive foramen). The upper lip is formed by the merging of the median nasal process with the two maxillary processes. Failure of the structures to join by the end of the eighth week will result in a cleft of the lip. The maxillary processes lead to the posterior two thirds of the hard palate, the soft palate and part of the alveolar ridge.

The hard palate is comprised of two palatal shelves that emerge out of the maxillary processes in the eighth week. The palatal shelves have the tongue positioned between them. During the ninth week there is a sudden growth spurt which allows the tongue to drop down and the two shelves to begin to merge, also joining with the primary palate. The velum, or soft palate, also evolves from the palatal processes and merges at the midline. Fusion of the palatal structures, which takes place in an anterior-to-posterior direction, is completed by the twelfth week. However, the crucial period appears to be between the sixth and ninth weeks.

The exact manner in which these facial structures join is not well understood, but, it is believed that ectodermal covering of the abutting surfaces breaks down and the mesodermal layers merge. Clefts of the lip and palate appear to be the result of the failure of the ectodermal layer to break down and/or the failure of the mesoderm to fuse together.

It is understandable that parents and other members of families of children with clefts of the lip and palate would want to know why and how the physical defect occurred. The problem of interpretation with our current level of understanding is obvious. The best course for the professional to pursue is to attempt to dispel superstition or myth and to be honest and forthright in advising parents on our current level of understanding. Figure 6–1 shows a child born with a unilateral cleft of the lip and palate before and after surgical closure of the lip.

Types of Clefts

It would be helpful, for the purposes of professional discussion, to have a systematic classification of clefts; unfortunately this does not currently exist (Berlin, 1971). Various systems of classification exist which recognize a progression of palatal involvement often beginning with a bifid or split uvula (associated with a foreshortened velum with some frequency), progressing to a cleft of the soft palate, or velum, and continuing on to clefts of the hard palate in varying types and degrees. The classification system of Veau (1931) was used for a number of years. Veau included four types of clefts:

Group I: Cleft of the soft palate only

Group II: Cleft of the hard and soft palate to the incisive foramen (i.e., the incisive foramen are openings in the hard palate approximately at the apex of the palatal vault through which the nasopalatine nerves pass).

Group III: Complete unilateral cleft of the soft and hard palate and of the lip and alveolar ridge on one side.

Group IV: Complete bilateral cleft of the soft and hard palate and of the lip and alveolar ridge on both sides.

Because Veau's system omitted the possibility of classifying many variations, many authors sought to improve on it. Kernahan and Stark (1958) suggested a system which was more complete and which was more closely related to embryological development. They differentiated between clefts of the primary palate (anterior to the incisive foramen) and the secondary palate (posterior to the incisive foramen). Mc-Williams (1980) points out that this system draws a clearer distinction between these two conditions which develop independently of one another. The Kernahan and Stark system is as follows:

Clefts of the Primary Palate—Right or left unilateral: Complete or incomplete

Median: Complete (premaxilla absent) or incomplete (premaxilla rudimentary)

Bilateral: Complete or incomplete

Clefts of the Secondary Palate—Complete, incomplete, or submucous

Figure 6–1. A Left Complete Unilateral Cleft of the Lip and Palate of the Same Child Before and After Initial Surgical Intervention.

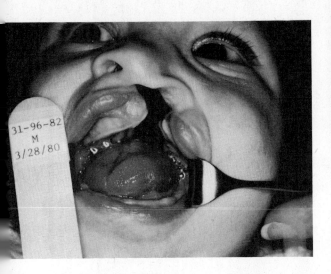
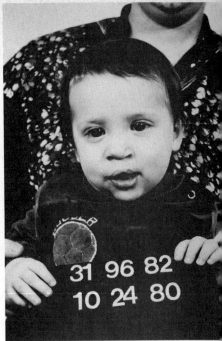

Clefts of the Primary and Secondary Palates—Right or left unilateral: Complete or incomplete

    Median: Complete or incomplete

    Bilateral: Complete or incomplete

    A similar classification system, presented by the 1968 Subcommittee on Cleft Lip and Palate Nomenclature of the International Confederation for Plastic and Reconstructive Surgery, attempted to improve on Kernahan and Stark. It has not received wide acceptance and the search continues for a system which is efficient and acceptable to all specialists interested in the problems associated with clefts. Figure 6–2 shows examples of different types of oral clefts.

COMMUNICATION PROBLEMS ASSOCIATED WITH PALATAL CLEFTS

The term *cleft-palate speech* has been a common one in the literature in the past. However, the communication abilities are far too complex and variable to be represented by a single label. The stereotype of the speech associated with cleft palate which includes misarticulation and inappropriate nasal resonance is present in some individuals. It is misleading to assume that this is characteristic of all speech of individuals with cleft palates. It is much more accurate to carefully describe the communication ability of each individual in the diagnostic process. Some of the problems of misdiagnosis and consequent mishandling of therapeutic efforts, as well as problems which have been associated with confusing research results, may be directly attributable to the fallacy of the concept of *cleft-palate speech*.

    Three possible types of deviation in communication abilities are associated with

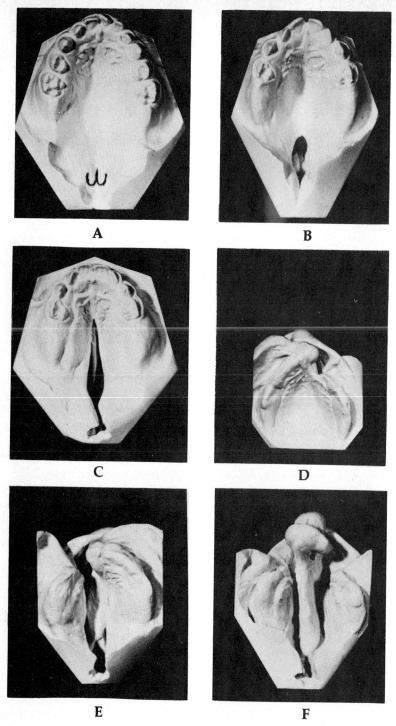

Figure 6–2. Examples of Palato-Facial Clefts. From upper left to right: A. bifid uvula; B. cleft of the soft palate; C. cleft of the palate extending to the incisive foramen; D. cleft of the lip only; E. unilateral cleft of the lip and palate; F. bilateral cleft of the lip and palate.

palatal clefts: (1) communication disorders presumed to be unrelated to the physical defect; (2) those disorders presumed to be indirectly related; and (3) those directly related.

Unrelated Problems

Problems of communication unrelated to the palatal cleft may include developmental disorders, for example, below average intellectual function, lack of motivation in an unstimulating environment, and other similar problems found throughout the entire population, with or without appropriate palatal structures.

In the normal process of developing communication, children initially make errors in articulation, display nonfluencies, or reveal immaturities in language performance. The child with a palatal cleft is not different in this respect and, further, a cleft palate does not provide immunity to articulatory problems, voice problems, or stuttering and language disorders presumably unrelated to this physical defect.

Indirectly and Directly Related Problems

Problems presumed to be indirectly related to the palatal cleft may result from early feeding difficulties, early conductive hearing loss or psychosocial influences. Infants with palatal clefts are difficult to nurse or to bottle feed in the usual manner due to the absence of palatal and lip structures and the difficulty in sucking associated with loss of oral pressure. Thus, even following reconstructive surgery, the child often has not experienced the "exercise" or use of the lips and mandible that other children have experienced. This lack of experience and other difficulties in sucking, chewing, and swallowing may lead to aberrant development of lingual and labial skills, adversely affecting adequate articulatory movements. Hearing disorders, which are now believed to occur in almost all children with palatal clefts (Paradise, Bluestone and Felder, 1969), may affect many aspects of communication development, particularly articulatory ability and language skills. Finally, the emotional reactions of parents to the birth of a child with a defective structure, the rejection the child may experience from persons in his or her environment during the developmental years, and the reactions of parents and child to the frequent special needs, such as medical or dental treatments, may lead to disturbance in the child's psychosocial development. Further, the child's first speech attempts may be so unintelligible that they are not recognized as such and the family may fail to provide the stimulation and reinforcement necessary to the development of adequate communication, particularly language. Persons with defective communication skills may be self-conscious and self-critical. Self-criticism, sometimes observed even among preschool children, may result in attempts to avoid or minimize communication and may lead to compensatory behaviors, such as inadequate volume aimed at minimizing nasal resonance (McWilliams, 1980). All of these factors may result in the delay or further complication of communication efforts.

The major problems in communication are directly related to the palatal cleft itself. The absence of the palatal partition between the oral and nasal cavities creates a problem of aberrant aerodynamics. Both pressure and flow activities are disrupted in varying degrees, leading to unnatural physiological relationships for speech production.

To produce acceptable speech patterns, an air stream originates in the lungs and proceeds through the trachea over the vocal folds. The air stream may continue on in a voiceless, non-vibrated fashion or it may be set in vibration, creating voicing. For all but the /m/, /n/, and /ŋ/ consonants the air stream is directed past a variably sealed velopharyngeal sphincter through the oral pharynx and oral cavity and out through the lips. For the three nasal consonants, the sounds are given articulatory postures in the oral cavity but resonated in the nasal cavity. In other words, the sound energy passes through the nasal cavity. The valves which control air pressure and the direction of the air flow function in three ways.

The first type of valve, illustrated by the vocal folds, alters the acoustical characteristics. The second type of valve, the velopharyngeal valve, for example, directs the air stream and acoustic energy. The third type of valve alters the air stream, either by damming it up to build pressure behind a relatively tight structure and then exploding it as in plosives, or by creating a constriction of the oral pathway so that the air stream is forced through varying degrees of narrowed orifices to create a friction type of sound, as in the fricatives. The acoustic nature of the air stream is also changed without valving per se when the resonance characteristics of the oral cavity are changed as the air stream is modified in the oral cavity by adjustments in the height, shape, and position of the tongue, as in the production of vowels.

The eight musculoskeletal valves which are responsible for the production of the consonants are illustrated in figure 6–3. They are (1) the teeth in the maxillary arch and the lower lip; (2) the lower and upper lips; (3) the tongue tip and the teeth; (4) the tongue tip and the alveolar ridge; (5) the tongue and the hard palate; (6) the posterior portion of the tongue and the velum; (7) the velum and the pharyngeal constrictors; and (8) the glottis.

Although it is not a valve, the patent egress from the nasal cavity at the nares is the terminal boundary of the speech production mechanism.

American speech production utilizes an oral, in contrast to a nasal, system of speech production. To accomplish this, the valving must function properly, particularly the velopharyngeal valve, and the pathway through the pharynx and oral cavity must be relatively unimpeded. At the very least, valving must create a coupling system that makes it more likely that the preponderance of the air stream and sound energy will traverse the path through the oral cavity for all but the three nasal consonants, rather than being diverted through the nasal cavity.

Absence of the palatal partition seriously threatens the integrity of this valving system. Parts of the system's structures may be missing, misplaced, altered, or not functioning adequately. Bzoch (1979) points out that congenital disorders, such as clefts of the palate, have broader and more serious effects on speech and language acquisition than do similar disorders acquired later in life. Thus, even if surgical or dental measures may prove successful later in the child's life, there may be problems which are the result of the early difficulties the aberrations of the structures created. Compensatory behaviors may have developed in response to the defective structures which, though well intentioned, add to rather than assist in the amelioration of the communication disorders. For example, the child may hear the speech of other persons filled with plosive or fricative sounds. The child attempts to imitate these sounds but defects in the valving system make it impossible to direct the air flow and build up pressure to produce what is heard. The closest the child can come to producing the heard sounds is by approximating, through substitution of other types of articulation, for the correct manner and place of production. The glottis may be used so that glottal stops replace plosive sounds. The velopharyngeal valving problem

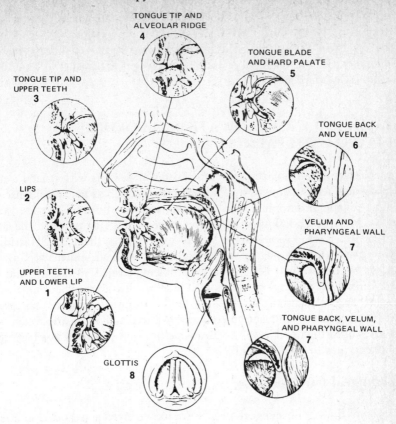

TONGUE TIP AND
ALVEOLAR RIDGE
4

TONGUE BLADE
AND HARD PALATE
5

TONGUE TIP AND
UPPER TEETH
3

TONGUE BACK
AND VELUM
6

LIPS
2

VELUM AND
PHARYNGEAL WALL
7

UPPER TEETH
AND LOWER LIP
1

TONGUE BACK, VELUM,
AND PHARYNGEAL WALL
7

GLOTTIS
8

Figure 6–3. The Eight Musculoskeletal Valves Produced by Oral and Pharyngeal Musculature During Articulation of Consonantal Sounds.

may be compensated for by approximating fricatives by retracting the tongue and producing a fricative with the back of the tongue and the posterior pharyngeal wall. Or, a fricative may be produced by attempting to elevate the velum with the posterior portion of the tongue, grooving the tongue and forcing some air through. This may result in a palatal fricative or nasal snort. Other types of undesirable compensation also may develop. If the child mismanages the air supply, he or she may try to compensate by using excessive amounts of air, giving the speech a characteristic of poorly phrased, short bursts of speaking efforts. The child may also attempt to avoid disordered production by using inadequate loudness, attempting to compensate for marginal adequacy of the mechanism by avoiding build up of any more than minimal pressure and flow. The child may also talk rapidly, attempting to complete the message before the supply of air is exhausted. This often results in a jerky, rapid, indistinct speech pattern, with any precision of which the child might be capable sacrificed.

The greater the inadequacies of the oral structure and the more time that elapses before restorative-remedial measures are begun, the more likely it is that compensatory measures will have become part of the child's speech production patterns. Inadequate compensations are also likely to become more severe and more deeply entrenched with time. Consequently, the major focus on communication should occur during the child's early years. Prevention should be the major goal for parents and professionals. Where early rehabilitation is not possible or not successful, remedial measures will be required and can yield varying degrees of success. However, this will almost certainly take longer and may well be less satisfactory than if early intervention was undertaken.

RESEARCH AND COMMUNICATION DISORDERS ASSOCIATED WITH PALATAL CLEFTS

The principal factors causing the speech problems of persons with palatal clefts are physiological and aerodynamic. Physiological factors, such as faulty velopharyngeal closure and tongue positioning, and the resultant aerodynamic factors, such as aberrant air pressure and flow, combine in various ways to produce the infinite variety of speech errors observed in individuals with clefts of the palate. Hearing loss, particularly during infancy, when speech and language development are in critical stages, plays an important role. Language problems related to hearing and other factors have received increasing attention. These are the areas where much of the research activity has focused. Examination of the literature suggests increased research activity in areas of language and reduced research activity in areas such as cleft palate. This is unfortunate. A review of available research will serve as a basis for the remedial techniques to be presented later.

Velopharyngeal Function

The function of the velopharyngeal mechanism has received a great deal of attention from specialists interested in the problems associated with cleft palates.

The four components of velopharyngeal function have been described by several authors, including Simpson and Colton (1980). The four functions are (1) velar movement in the superior-posterior direction, (2) mesial movement of lateral pharyngeal walls, (3) anterior movement of the posterior pharynx, and, (4) velar stretch. This latter factor, velar stretch, has only received significant attention since focused on by Graber et al. (1959). They called attention to the significant increase in the length of the soft palate from the rest position to an action position for function. Simpson and Colton point out that, as with other aspects of velopharyngeal function, this factor is variable with age. Normal function makes adjustments to achieve acoustically acceptable speech; the amount of adjustment is determined by structural characteristics of the mechanism and the specific sound or sound groups to be produced. The authors report on several studies which have shown the percent of elongation increasing with age. Although additional research is needed to quantify this phenomenon and to describe its role in the diagnostic and therapeutic processes, it is worthy of note and consideration in clinical planning.

The importance experts attach to this mechanism is summarized by McWilliams' view (1980) that velopharyngeal competency is necessary for adequate consonant articulation as well as for acceptable voice quality. Of all the factors in speech disorders associated with palatal clefts, none is more crucial than velopharyngeal function. Bzoch (1979) reports that the velum always makes firm seal or closure during syllable repetition for all but nasal syllables by normal speakers. This is not in agreement with a study of air flow in normal speakers reported by Van Hattum and

Worth (1967) which appeared to suggest continuous nasal air flow during connected speech in normal speakers. However, the preponderance of evidence suggests that velopharyngeal adequacy *is* necessary for acceptable speech production. Isshiki, Honjow and Morimoto (1968) created velopharyngeal incompetence in normal males by inserting tubes in the velopharynx. They found slight nasality when the size of the orifice was 5 mm in diameter, unquestionable nasality at 7 mm diameter, and extreme nasality at 9 mm and 12 mm. They concluded that the critical dimension of the opening is approximately 5 mm in diameter or 20 mm^2 in area. The researchers stated that there is no sudden point where velopharyngeal incompetence provides defective speech, since it is necessary to consider other factors, such as mouth opening and position of the tongue, along with the degree of velopharyngeal opening. In relating the size of velopharyngeal opening to age, they hypothesized that the degree of velopharyngeal competence is more critical before and during the acquisition of correct articulation. After articulation is learned, it can resist more velopharyngeal incompetence. This opinion is shared by other researchers (Shelton et al., 1969).

Subtelny, Koepp-Baker, and Subtelny (1961) reported that hypernasality results from inadequate velopharyngeal valving which permits excessive coupling of the nasal cavity with the remainder of the vocal tract, and consequently the transmission of air and sound energy through the nasal cavity. Non-nasal speech was found to be associated with good velopharyngeal function, and hypernasality with poor velopharyngeal function. It is interesting to note that their study included two hyper-nasal speakers, each with only a 1 mm opening, and two non-nasal speakers with 9–10 mm openings. Such findings continue to puzzle persons interested in this area and offer interesting opportunity for conjecture. It is an enigma that the two hypernasal speakers should have a very small velopharyngeal opening while the two non-nasal speakers should have such a large velopharyngeal opening.

Van Denmark (1964, 1966) examined factors associated with defectiveness of speech and found velopharyngeal closure to be the major factor. He found velopharyngeal closure the major factor in judged articulation defectiveness. Mazaheri, Millard and Erickson (1964) found no relationship between the degree of velopharyngeal adequacy and the severity of the speech defect, in contrast to the findings of Van Denmark. Loeb (1964) found no consistent correlation between hypernasality and the distance between the soft palate and posterior pharyngeal wall in children under ten years of age. With increasing age, the correlation increased, suggesting that velopharyngeal function becomes a more important variable in terms of hypernasality beyond childhood. These inconsistencies give rise to many speculative comments regarding the role of other variables in the understanding of hypernasality and defective articulation in cleft palate speech.

Research appears to support the importance of the adequacy of velopharyngeal integrity. It is critical but unstable among children becoming more stable with age. It appears to be more necessary for acceptable articulation than for acceptable voice quality, but this may be due in part to society's willingness to accept greater variability in voice quality than in articulation.

Tongue Positioning

Even if the velopharyngeal gap is small, speech may be affected by other factors, such as the size of the mouth opening, the rate of speech, the pitch level, and tongue positioning (Mazaheri et al., 1964). The latter factor has received considerable research scrutiny since McDonald and Koepp-Baker (1951) called attention to the possibility of "a high riding tongue." Hardy and Arkebauer (1966) stated that velopharyngeal closure may be less firm if the tongue position is relatively low in the oral cavity. Moll and Shriner (1967) reported that velar elevation is associated with tongue height, agreeing with Lubker (1968) that high vowels show greater velar elevation than low vowels. Lubker also stated that there seems to be considerable interdependence between tongue position and velar position; however, he found a low correlation between tongue movement and velar movement.

Buck (1960) reported that people with unrepaired clefts had markedly higher tongue position, and that the high point was more posterior than in people with normal palates or repaired clefts. On the other hand, Brooks, Shelton, and Youngstrom (1965) reported no significant difference between normal speakers and those with clefts for tongue retraction or for tongue mobility. Powers (1962) found the tongue retracted but not higher in subjects. In each study, the author noted that the retracted and elevated dorsum may occur, although it is probably not typical of the population with cleft palates. Brooks, Shelton and Youngstrom (1965) did note that the group with cleft palates tended to contact the soft palate or posterior pharyngeal wall during articulation, but that the control group did not.

The frequently conflicting views of authorities regarding the relationships between tongue and velar positions provides the clinician with grounds for confusion. It is likely that this is a variable factor, presenting problems in some persons but not in others. Thus, its influence is a necessary part of diagnostic evaluation.

Two other articles dealing with aspects of the tongue deserve mention. Fletcher (1966) reported the existence of a "blunt-ended" tongue in the cleft-palate population, which he felt should not be overlooked. He noted that Berry (1949) reported poor tongue tip and blade activity in cleft-palate subjects. Finally, Hochberg and Kabcenell (1967) found cleft-palate subjects to be significantly poorer than normals in oral stereognosis, or oral sensation ability. Since oral stereognosis may be related to velar and articulatory function, the deficiency is worthy of note, inasmuch as tongue function may thereby be deficient as well.

Speech and Language Differences

The speech and language differences of people with clefts have also been studied. Bzoch (1965) found two consonant types, the fricatives and the plosives, more difficult for cleft-palate than for normal subjects; and his preschool subjects were more proficient on voiced than unvoiced sounds. He found little difference between cleft-palate and normal subjects on the /w/, /m/, /n/, and /h/. Evaluating the types of errors, he found the cleft-palate subjects omitted sounds four times as frequently as the normals, and substituted and distorted sounds twice as often. Substitutions were most frequent in each group. Glottal stops, pharyngeal fricatives, and nasal snorts were frequent substitutions. Bzoch also pointed out the need for early therapy.

Spriestersbach, Darley, and Rouse (1956) studied cleft-palate children aged three to eight years. Most frequent misarticulations were the /z/, /θ/, /s/, /tʃ/, and /ʒ/, while /m/, /n/, /h/, /j/, and /ŋ/ were least defective. Inconsistency of articulation was reported, with omissions being most frequent, followed by substitutions and distortions.

Spriestersbach, Moll, and Morris (1961) studied a group whose ages ranged from 3 to 16 years. Affricates were most defective, followed by fricatives, plosives, glides, and nasals. Blends were more defective than nonblends, and voiceless sounds more defective than voiced ones, except that voiceless fricatives were less defective than voiced ones. Omissions and distortions were more common than substitutions. Errors on plosives consisted of glottal stops 40 percent of the time. They noted that the subjects with clefts of the lip only had essentially normal speech, and those with clefts of the palate only had poorer speech than those with clefts of both lip and palate. They concluded that the ability to impound intraoral breath pressure best accounts for variability in articulation.

McWilliams (1958), in a study of an adult population, found sibilants and plosives to be the most defective classes of sounds. Four sounds—/s/, /z/, dʒ/, and /tʃ/—were most often defective, but inconsistency of articulation was common, with most subjects producing error sounds correctly in some contexts. Distortions were the most common error (79.2 percent), followed by omissions (18.5 percent) and substitutions (2.4 percent). McWilliams stated that sibilants are most in need of attention, and although they may be harder to correct, the greatest improvement will be achieved by attacking them first. If the clinician is interested in early success, however, she noted that it may be better to start with other sounds.

Pitzner and Morris (1966) also found fricatives and plosives to be most often defective, and nasals and glides to be seldom defective. Dentition was found to have an effect on speech performance, and the group that had earlier surgical management had better articulatory skills. They also reported that people with inadequate intra-oral pressure ratios demonstrated errors on sounds that did not require great amounts of breath pressure.

In a study of oral breath pressure, Spriestersbach and Powers (1959a) found it to be greater during production of fricatives and plosives than during production of other consonants and vowels. More breath pressure was also required on voiceless than on voiced sounds. Hess and McDonald (1960) reported similar results, as did Van Hattum and Worth (1967) and Isshiki and Ringel (1964), when studying air flow. The correlation between air pressure, air flow requirements, and the most frequently defective sounds should be noted by speech clinicians for each case.

Less clinical research has been done on the voice quality characteristics of cleft-palate subjects. Hess (1959) stated that nasality may result either from deviations in the speech structures or from functional factors. He added that hoarseness may be due to inflamed and swollen tissue resulting from glottal articulation or ventricular voice; in addition, he related breathiness to faulty phonation, and harshness to lingual, pharyngeal, and laryngeal muscular imbalance. He found less nasality at higher pitches than at the habitual pitch, and also less nasality at more intense levels of pitch. Breathiness was not affected by pitch, but was less severe at more intense levels. Harshness was less severe for higher pitch and lower intensity, and hoarseness was less severe at higher pitch and higher intensity.

Van Hattum (1958) and McWilliams (1954) each found that articulation influences the perception of nasality. Poor articulation makes persons with cleft palates perceptually more nasal, and good articulation makes them perceptually less nasal.

Clinicians have long suggested that children with clefts of the palate were more likely to be delayed in speech and language development (Shames and Rubin, 1971). It has only been within recent years that increased interest in language behaviors of these children has been noted. However, research is still relatively sparse. Olson

(1965) studied children with unoperated cleft palate. The infants in the study used more back vowels and glottals at all levels and more pharyngeal fricatives with increasing age. Also, they displayed a more limited consonant repertoire. Spriesters-bach et al. (1958) noted that children with cleft palates were in general retarded in mean length of response and were retarded in vocabulary usage but not vocabulary recognition. Also, their structural complexity scores were not different from the normative group. Nation (1964), in contrast to the study just mentioned, found that the subjects in his study were also considerably behind in vocabulary comprehension at all age levels.

Smith and McWilliams (1968) found that when children with cleft palates were tested on the *Illinois Test of Psycholinguistic Ability* they tended to show depression in the areas measured by this testing instrument. The problem was more expressive than receptive.

Overall, the studies have shown some delays in the development of expressive language in children with cleft palates. Results are variable and not currently quan-tifiable. Again, each child's communication behavior must be evaluated individually, not assuming defects in a specific area but being alert to possible defects in any area.

Although we have insufficient information on the effects of early mild hearing losses on language acquisition, a study by Holm and Kunze (1969) on children without clefts found them significantly behind those without losses in vocabulary, articulation, receptive and expressive language, grammar, syntax and auditory mem-ory. McWilliams (1980) points out that these may be factors in children with clefts of the palate whom we know to experience early hearing difficulty. Thus, it may not be the cleft per se, but other aspects such as hearing or psychosocial factors, which result in slower maturation of language in some children with clefts of the palate who do reveal such delays.

To summarize, the research findings suggest that there is a critical size of opening of the velopharyngeal port where hypernasality will result, that tongue position is also related to cleft palate speech, and that defective valving alters the aerodynamic relationships necessary for satisfactory speech production. Consequently, cleft palate speech consists of defective voiceless fricatives, affricates, and plosives more than of other sounds. Errors of omission and distortion are more frequent than other articula-tory errors; and glottal stops, pharyngeal fricatives, and nasal snorts are frequent substitutions. Investigations support the observation that articulation errors influence the perception of nasality—the poorer the articulation, the more nasal the cleft palate speech may seem. Other voice problems may also be present. Finally, cleft-palate speakers generally show less verbal output and less vocabulary usage than normal subjects. The effects on language of cleft palate and its associated problems need further investigation.

Hearing

Since Alt (1878) commented on the link between palatal clefts and hearing loss, there has been a steadily increasing estimate of the extent of the relationship. At the present time there is general agreement that probably all children with palatal clefts have bilateral otitis media and conductive hearing losses (Paradise, Bluestone and Felder, 1969). It has been reported that these losses, usually in the 30 to 40 dB range, are related to malfunctioning of the eustachian tube. The losses tend to decrease with age with only a few children revealing permanent losses.

Heller (1979) notes that chronic otitis media develops prenatally or during the first weeks of life. Without treatment serious complications may result. Thus, prompt otological treatment is indicated. Further, the fluctuating nature of otitis media makes periodic follow-up essential.

The obstruction of the orifice of the eustachian tube by adenoidal tissue also may prove a problem for cleft-palate children. This poses a particular problem in the management of speech. The adenoidal tissue may provide a pad in assisting velopharyngeal closure, and its removal may lead to increased hypernasality. Careful team evaluation is necessary in arriving at a decision, often not totally satisfactory, before surgical measures are undertaken. The importance of maintaining the integrity of the hearing mechanism cannot be minimized. Measures aimed at improving speech production are also important, but those aimed at preserving the hearing mechanism, if its integrity is in jeopardy, are a major consideration and may take precedence.

Intelligence

Reports of the intelligence of individuals with palatal clefts have yielded varying results. Whereas earlier studies have reported a lower mean IQ for the cleft palate groups, more recent studies have disputed this. Clifford (1979) states that these individuals obtain IQ scores within the test norms for the normal range of intelligence. He adds that ranges for cleft palate children are slightly lower than for the normal subjects, but he does not feel that the differences are significant of and by themselves. He does feel that verbal scores tend to be lower than performance scores, a conclusion refuted by McWilliams and Musgrave (1972).

Persons with palatal clefts occupy the same range of intellectual skills as the normal population, from mentally retarded to gifted. The mean IQ of the group is likely slightly lower than that of the nonhandicapped population. However, when one considers the communication problems, both speech and language, and the heavy language weighting of intelligence tests, it is surprising that the discrepancy is not greater and adds further support for the importance of remedial measures.

DIAGNOSIS OF INDIVIDUALS WITH OROFACIAL ANOMALIES

The information derived from research is useful in revealing certain general characteristics of the cleft-palate population, but the fact that much of the information is conflicting makes it difficult for the clinician to determine principles of habilitation. Spriestersbach, Moll, and Morris (1964) emphasized this fact in their report on the variability of the cleft-palate population; in every study, there have been individuals who did not follow group performance. What this means is that each person with a cleft palate must be studied for his or her particular problems and needs. Each individual requires a carefully tailored therapy plan.

The speech-language pathologist's evaluation of a person's communication ability is not a medical or dental diagnosis. If there is a communication deficit, it is purely a symptom, a result, of the cleft. The communication deficit is not the basic defect; it is a result of the basic defect. The speech-language clinician deals only with the symptom, although he or she can deal with the basic defect by recommendation. The purpose of the evaluation, therefore, is to determine the adequacy of communication, the need for remediation, the type of remediation needed, the prognosis, and the barriers to success. Other specialists will have to advise the speech-language specialist as to whether the barriers to successful communication can be removed. This is the purpose of the team approach.

A Team Approach

In discussing diagnosis, it is necessary to describe the professional people involved in cleft-palate habilitation and their relationships with each other. Establishing the best possible communication for the individual and meeting her or his total habilitation needs requires many specialists, and the extent to which they can work cooperatively, share information, and complement one another's efforts determines the ultimate success. This suggests the use of a team approach—a term frequently used in the literature, although not always correctly. The team approach does not mean merely that a number of different specialists examine an individual, or that all of these examinations take place in one location. It means that significant dialogue occurs among the specialists regarding diagnosis and treatment. It means that planning is cooperative. It means that there is an ongoing program of mutual consultation throughout the habilitation program.

The team approach allows for the accumulation of objective data about the success or failure of various treatment methods, and it is a valuable means of training professionals from all fields of endeavor.

Figure 6–4 shows the specialists who serve as members of the team and the activities they engage in. The composition of teams varies, but the smallest possible team would have a communications expert, medical specialist, and dental specialist. The largest team known to the author consisted of a maxillofacial surgeon, pediatrician, otologist, general dentist, orthodontist, prosthodontist, speech-language pathologist, audiologist, psychologist, educational counselor, social worker, and nurse. The availability of personnel, the number of patients to be served, and the particular interests and skills of the team members help determine the exact composition. Two key people are necessary. The first is the team coordinator, usually the maxillofacial surgeon, dental specialist, or communications specialist. The second is the one responsible for scheduling, record keeping, and follow-up, usually either a social worker or nurse.

The diagnostic role of the communications specialist depends on the age of the patient. There are approximately four stages in the total diagnostic-habilitative process. The first occurs from birth to eighteen months; the second from eighteen months to three years; the third from three to five years; and the fourth from five years on. The first two stages require different evaluation procedures than the latter two.

Evaluating Children Under Three Years of Age

Evaluation of the child under 3 years of age is somewhat difficult. Obtaining the history of the child and family presents no unusual difficulty, but many standard test procedures cannot be used with a child so young, and the speech-language pathologist must rely on informal observation. The child may not be talking yet, or, if speech has developed, may be too shy to use it in a strange environment. In lieu of formal test procedures, the clinician may observe the child at play with one or both parents.

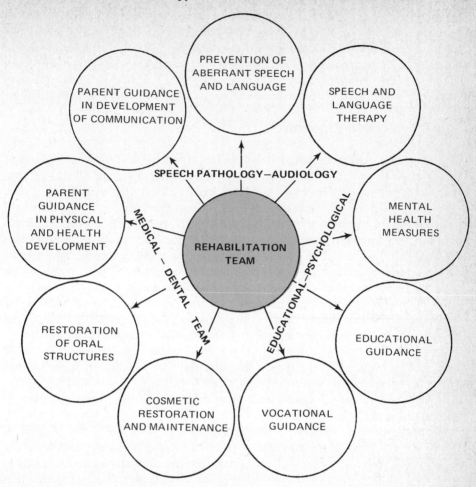

Figure 6–4. A Model for Diagnosis and Remediation of the Individual with a Cleft Palate.

Whether the observation is structured or unstructured, the clinician will want answers to the following questions: (1) does the child understand speech?, (2) does he or she use gestures rather than words for expression?, (3) is expressive oral language (words, phrases, and sentences) used?, (4) are correct articulation patterns emerging?, (5) does the child become frustrated when verbal communication is unsuccessful?, (6) is his or her use of the oral mechanism adequate for speech?, (7) are compensatory patterns (velar and glottal productions) beginning to appear?, (8) is nasal emission present?, (9) will the child try to imitate such oral activities as smacking the lips, clicking the tongue, or babbling?, (10) are the resonance characteristics of voice normal, or is hypernasality present?, (11) are the phonatory characteristics of voice normal?, (12) are the child's attempts at oral communication accepted, recognized, rejected, or reinforced by family members?, (13) are facial grimaces observable?, (14) is the child's hearing adequate?

As the child grows older, more sophisticated and objective measures can be used, and the different aspects of communication can be evaluated in more detail. Van Denmark and Swickard (1980) describe a promising procedure for assessing velopharyngeal competence in young children in this age group. They describe Morris' (1961) *Iowa Pressure Articulation Test* (Morris, Spriestersbach, and Darley, 1961) and used the *Peabody Articulation Deck* (1975) to develop their test, now in the developmental process. The following section is devoted to an overview of evaluation procedures.

Formal Evaluation Procedures

To achieve the purpose of evaluation that was expressed in the section on diagnosis of individuals with orofacial anomalies, the communication specialist should be concerned with getting answers to the following questions: (1) what defects exist in the patient's articulation, voice quality, rhythm, or language?, (2) does the patient have the physiological equipment necessary for adequate speech?, (3) are the oral structures and their functions adequate for speech?, (4) does the valving system function adequately?, (5) what is the relationship between the person's speech and language problems and the deficiencies in the speech mechanism?, (6) which defects are indirectly related or unrelated to the cleft? why are they present?, (7) what is the contribution of auditory acuity and discrimination?, (8) what effect do social, emotional, and intellectual factors have on the prognosis?, (9) what changes are indicated that would help the client develop communication skills to a greater degree?

The development of topics in this section follows the order suggested by the above questions. To begin with, the speech structure and function and the speech symptoms must be thoroughly described (questions 1–4); the factors to which they are related must be measured (questions 5–6); and finally, related factors must be explored (questions 7–9).

Whenever possible, objective measurement, rather than subjective judgment, should be used. Many of the problems in research and much of the confusion in our knowledge of communication problems accompanying cleft palate may be traced to the assumption that people with cleft palates make up a homogeneous population, but subjective judgments have also contributed to the misinformation. In examining subjective articulatory analyses, Philips and Bzoch (1969) found considerable disagreement not only among expert judges, but also in individuals, when rejudging the same material. The difficulties the experts have had in making subjective judgments should serve as a caution for all clinicians with respect to using subjective data in diagnoses.

To achieve objective measurement, certain instrumentation is essential. The complete diagnosis of a client with a cleft palate cannot take place in the usual clinical setting. Perhaps more than for any other communication problem, a laboratory setting is needed. When sufficient instrumentation is unavailable, the clinician will have to rely on his or her best judgment, realizing that considerable error is possible in diagnosis, therapy planning, and recommendations.

Speech and Language Evaluation. The clinician is concerned with discovering the defects that may exist in the subject's articulation, voice quality, rhythm, and/or language ability.

Articulation. A number of procedures can be used to evaluate articulation skills. They are familiar to all clinicians. However, in order to make an accurate assessment of articulation in someone with a cleft palate, the clinician must be thoroughly familiar with the particular types of misarticulations the client is likely to have.

In evaluating articulation, Bzoch's recommended procedure, in which the examiner asks the client to repeat the test word three times, is useful (Philips and Bzoch, 1969). Consistently produced errors suggest that articulatory patterns are firmly established, while inconsistent errors suggest that the variation is related to the phonetic context of the sound, or that a sound is in the process of correction.

Speakers with cleft palates, like all speakers, have better articulation ability on isolated words than in connected speech (Van Hattum, 1958), so the results of the phonetic analysis should be compared with the patient's performance in conversational speech. There is no standard scale for rating articulation in connected speech, but the clinician can devise one, such as by using the number *1* to denote mild articulation errors, *2* for moderate ones, and *3* for severe ones.

The intelligibility of speech can be similarly rated. Again, no standard scale is available, but a sample of connected speech or reading of a standard passage can be judged on a rating scale such as—

1. normal intelligibility;
2. slight unintelligibility—occasional words or phrases difficult to understand;
3. moderate unintelligibility—consistent errors cause listener confusion;
4. severe unintelligibility—meaning of speech almost lost; and
5. complete unintelligibility—speech cannot be understood.

A test of stimulability provides additional diagnostic information concerning articulation skills. Vowel-consonant syllables for each phoneme are produced by the examiner while the patient is directed to watch, to listen, and then to imitate. It is important to note not only whether the sound is imitated correctly in the acoustic sense, but also whether the articulatory placement for the phoneme is correct.

Finally, it is advisable to make a rough evaluation of the effect on articulation of differences in rate. The clinician can coach the person to read or converse at two or three speeds. One speed should be the habitual rate of speaking, one should be faster, and one should be slower. Speeding up or slowing down the rate of speech gives information about how well the articulators can function. Many people with cleft palates can produce isolated sounds, or even words, adequately, but they suffer a breakdown in performance when coarticulation and the rapid changes necessary for conversational speech are present.

The Iowa Pressure Articulation Test or IPAT (Morris, Spriestersbach, and Darley, 1961), helps assess articulation errors and permits inferences of intraoral pressure and velopharyngeal difficulty with specific types of articulation errors. Shelton, Brooks, and Youngstrom (1965) agree that this is a better method of evaluating velopharyngeal closure than measuring nasal air escape or oral breath pressure.

Voice Quality. Voice quality is a subjective characteristic encompassing aspects of phonation and resonance. The quality of voice provides the distinctiveness which allows us to distinguish one voice from another. Judgment of voice quality, even by expert examiners, is largely a subjective matter, and much disagreement exists over the use of terminology. For the study of speech associated with cleft palate, the specialist should determine whether the quality difference is related to a phonatory difference or a resonance difference. If the problem is phonatory, traditional descriptions of hoarse, harsh, or breathy and judgment of severity as mild, moderate, or severe are sufficient. The adequacy of pitch and loudness should also be noted. Shanks and Duguay, in chapter 5, discuss evaluation of voice quality disorders.

For nasal quality, a more refined measurement is indicated. Although there are instruments for measuring nasality, such as the accelerometer (Lipmann, 1981), these are more commonly used in the research laboratory than in the clinic. Measures of nasality can be made on vowels in isolation or in connected speech, but the degree of nasality in one cannot be inferred from the other (Van Hattum, 1958; Dickson, Barron, and McGlone, 1978). The clinician must learn to distinguish hypernasality (excessive nasality), hyponasality (lack of nasal resonance), and cul-de-sac ("blind alley") resonance. In addition, the speech-language pathologist must concentrate on voice quality and not be distracted by the influence of defective articulation on perceived voice quality (Van Hattum, 1958). Nasal emission should also be ignored in making this specific judgment. Again, a description of the nasality and a classification of mild, moderate, or severe should be presented.

Rhythm. The clinician should note if stuttering or cluttering is present and if speech is too fast or too slow, and the phrasing characteristic during conversational speech should be noted.

Language. Problems with expressive language are not uncommon among children with cleft palates. Both this and receptive language should be evaluated to see if there is a problem that warrants clinical attention. There are a number of tests available for this purpose. The Peabody Picture Vocabulary Test (PPVT) (Dunn, 1980) provides a measure of receptive vocabulary ability. The Northwestern Syntax Screening Test (NSST) (Lee, 1969) measures the client's use of syntax, being intended to identify children from three to eight years of age in need of remedial intervention.

Other tests of possible interest to the clinician are the Michigan Picture Language Inventory (MPLI) (Lerea, 1958) and the Verbal Language Development Scale (VLDS) (Mecham, 1958). In addition, measures such as the mean length of response (MLR) are described by Johnson, Darley, and Spriestersbach (1963). Some of these tests and others are described in chapter 2.

Evaluation of Physiological Concomitants Assessment to determine whether the individual possesses the needed physiological requirements for speech includes evaluation of the integrity of the velopharyngeal mechanism and the ability to impound sufficient air pressure and to direct the air stream adequately.

The Velopharyngeal Mechanism. The precise role of the velopharyngeal mechanism in the speech of people with cleft palates is still under investigation (see previous section on velopharyngeal function). While there is agreement that adequate velopharyngeal closure is related to good speech, and inadequate velopharyngeal closure to poor speech, exceptions cannot be currently explained.

Velopharyngeal closure can be evaluated in several ways. The IPAT (Morris, Spriestersbach, and Darley, 1961) has already been described. Physiological functions, such as blowing, sucking, and swallowing, have been used extensively but have given rise to considerable discussion. Hanson (1964), who obtained suction and positive pressure scores and judgments of nasality, reported that suction correlated higher with nasality judgments than did blowing, although neither correlation was significant. Moll (1965) found that all of his subjects exhibited closure during swallowing, gagging, and blowing. But sucking and puffing the cheeks seemed to involve a different mechanism, and Moll questioned their use, and that of blowing, in evaluating closure. McWilliams and Bradley (1965) also questioned the use of blowing on the basis that speech demands different velopharyngeal behavior than blowing does; and they also noted different activity when the nostrils were open and when they were occluded. Hardy and Arkebauer (1966) also felt that the velopharyngeal mechanism may perform differently during speech and blowing.

Hess (1970) described a procedure suggested by Robert J. Gorlin of the Divison of Oral Pathology, University of Minnesota, which Hess has called the TOM (tongue tip outside mouth) Puffed Cheeks test. Hess noted that the elimination of sucking and puffed cheeks tests left the clinician with few alternatives for assessing velopharyngeal competence, and suggested the TOM test as a useful alternative, particularly in combination with manometric testing. In the test, the subject is instructed to protrude the tongue, lock the tongue tip between the teeth (the lips may also surround the protruded tongue tip) and attempt to puff out the cheeks. The tongue tip must be clearly visible. Hess feels that when the cheeks are puffed out in this manner, without air escaping through the nose, adequate velopharyngeal closure can be inferred. He noted, however, that cinefluorographic study is necessary to confirm or not confirm the possibility that the test involves lingual-palatal valving.

As indicated by the published studies, there is general agreement that blowing, sucking, swallowing, gagging, and puffing do not parallel speech production sufficiently to offer useful diagnostic information. One possible exception is the TOM test.

Van Denmark and Van Denmark (1967) suggested that manometric ratios yield useful diagnostic measurements. Spriestersbach and Powers (1959b) suggested that a pressure of 8 ounces per square inch is minimal for the production of consonant sounds; if the client is able to demonstrate this amount of pressure on the manometer, velopharyngeal function is assumed to be adequate for speech. The "bleed" feature, available on most manometers, should be used to ensure a continuous flow of air through the oral cavity during testing. To measure pressure escape through the nasal cavity, U-tube water manometers are used, with measurements being made in centimeters of water displacement (Spriestersbach and Sherman, 1968).

Hess (1976) describes assessment of velopharyngeal adequacy using nasal manometric bleed testing. He found that speakers with cleft palates tended to have higher nasal pressure readings than speakers without clefts, whether or not bleed conditions are employed, and that controlled incremental bleed, coupled with nasal manometric testing appeared to have possible diagnostic utility, although there was further need for study of reliability.

A number of X-ray techniques permit excellent objective measurement of velopharyngeal function. The data supplied by these techniques are invaluable in the important clinical decisions to be made. Lateral head plates (lateral X-rays of the head) permit the measurement of velopharyngeal dimensions in an anteroposterior plane. Cephalometric tracings and measurements can be made of the size of the velopharyngeal opening, at least on one plane, during rest, while phonating a vowel such as /u/ and producing a consonant such as /s/. Head plates may also reveal the role of adenoid tissue in effecting closure, and the point of maximum constriction. The potential for improving function may also be studied. The deficiency of this approach is that only one plane is observed, making it impossible to see the extent of lateral closure.

Cinefluorographic films enable the clinician to study velopharyngeal function in motion without precluding a look at individual frames. The patient can be filmed saying phrases as well as isolated sounds, and a sound track can be used to relate velopharyngeal function to phonetic context. There is still the problem of a single plane of view, however. Speech-language pathologists sometimes complain that cinefluorography is not available, but most hospital and dental clinics can provide it, and diagnosis is most efficient when it can be located.

The Taub Oral Panendoscope and/or an instrument using fiber optic viewing techniques offers another method of studying velopharyngeal competence, but only skilled specialists are able to use it. These techniques include a light source and a viewing apparatus that can be inserted into the oral cavity or nasal cavity for a direct view of velopharyngeal function. Camera attachments are available for recording what is observed.

In all of these techniques, the importance of head positioning must be stressed (McWilliams, Musgrave, and Crozier, 1968). Tilting the head changes the position of the musculoskeletal structures, and should be avoided.

The presence of nasality, nasal emission, or facial grimaces may also suggest velopharyngeal incompetence. In measuring nasal escape of air, a cold mirror may be placed under the nostrils during phonation; it will become clouded if air is escaping. Movement of a small piece of thread, held under the nostril during phonation, also will reveal air escape. However, air escape which does not destroy the integrity of the phoneme is not objectionable. Furthermore, the examiner must realize that tests of nasal emission evaluate the adequacy of the nasal cavity as much as that of the velopharyngeal mechanism. Passage of the air stream may be prevented by inflamed membranes due to colds or allergies, by adenoid tissue, or by a deviated septum. These factors may lead to cul-de-sac resonance, which gives speech an undesirable quality. Facial grimaces usually suggest that the client is compensating for inadequate closure. Finally, the ability to imitate correct production of a sound or habitually use correct placement for the production of a sound, while producing it defectively, offers some evidence concerning the adequacy of velopharyngeal closure.

Even though use of instrumentation offers the best method of objectively and thoroughly evaluating velopharyngeal competence, this is often not possible in many clinical settings. Additionally, as Schneider and Shprintzen (1980) found, even in settings where instrumentation is available, 90 percent of evaluation uses subjective measures. In such instances, use of a structured rating scale can minimize subjectivity and lead to a more accurate assessment. McWilliams and Philips (1979) have demonstrated this in their weighted value scale shown in figure 6–5. Evaluating problems which are often associated with velopharyngeal incompetence can provide inferential information, which can enhance the diagnostic study, or assist in making decisions regarding speech-language remediation, medicine, and/or dentistry.

Air Pressure and Air Flow. Pitzner and Morris (1966) cite the importance of breath pressure for articulation, and several studies, such as that of Warren and Mackler (1965), point out that poor speech due to velopharyngeal incompetence is

Figure 6–5. Assessing Velopharyngeal Competence Using a Weighted Value Scale.

	Weighted Value		
	1	2	3
Nasal Emission (From nostril showing greatest amount of air escape)			
Mild, moderate; inconsistent; visible	A^1		
Mild, moderate; consistent; visible		A^2	
Severe; consistent or inconsistent; visible			A^3
Audible nasal emission			A^4
Nasal turbulence			A^5
(Add one point to any value if hyponasality also present)			
Resonance			
Mild or moderate hypernasality		B^2	
Severe hypernasality			B^3
Facial Grimace		C^2	
Phonation			
Mild hoarseness	D^1		
Moderate, severe hoarseness		D^2	
Very severe hoarseness			D^3
Reduced loudness		D^4	
(Add one point to D1, 2 or 3 if consistent visible or audible nasal emission is present)			
Articulation Fricatives or Plosives			
Omission of fricatives or plosives	E^1		
Anterior sibilant distortion	E^2		
Reduced intraoral pressure on fricatives		E^3	
Lingual-palatal sibilants		E^4	
Other Factors			
Omission of fricatives plus hard glottal attack for vowels			F^1
Reduced intraoral pressure, pharyngeal fricatives			F^2
Inhalation or exhalation substitutions			F^3
Glottal Stops			F^4
(Add three additional points to F3 or 4 if Visible or Audible Nasal Emission is present. Add only one if both Pharyngeal Fricatives and Glottal Stops are heard)			
Total			

Directions: Place points in the appropriate A, B, C, D, E, and F positions plus those additional points described. Total and compare with the following:

    0   Velopharyngeal competence assumed

    1-2   Velopharyngeal competence to borderline competence assumed

    3-6   Borderline velopharyngeal incompetence to mild incompetence

    7 +   Moderate to severe velopharyngeal incompetence assumed

characterized by low breath pressure. Dickson, Barron and McGlone (1978) found that hypernasal speakers revealed lower oral air pressure during reading although not for blowing or production of the vowel /i/. Their findings suggest that administration of a phonetic analysis involving only isolated words may not lead to accurate assessment. Connected speech or manometry likely would present more accurate information.

There has been little discussion recently in the literature of excessive intraoral breath pressure, although at one time McDonald and Koepp-Baker (1951) questioned whether there might not be an overemphasis on the necessity for high intraoral pressure. Some individuals with cleft palates do appear to overcompensate by using too much pressure, and the clinician should be aware of the possibility of too much as well as too little pressure.

Air flow is difficult to evaluate and has received little attention other than through efforts to establish normative data and describe its relationship to air pressure (Subtelny, Worth, and Sakuda, 1966). Isshiki and Ringel (1964) found flow rates greater for voiceless than voiced consonants, and greater for stops and fricatives than for other types of sounds. They reported that consonants in the terminal position are more variable than those in other positions. Van Hattum and Worth (1967) also reported more flow on voiceless than voiced sounds, and found the rank order of air use—by manner of articulation—to be affricates, plosives, fricatives, and nasals. They also reported air flow to be more variable in the beginning and end of an utterance than in the middle portion. These factors correlate highly with the conditions in which persons with cleft palate have their greatest speaking difficulty.

Dickson, Barron, and McGlone (1978) found that, in addition to higher oral pressure, their non-nasal speakers had lower nasal flow rates. They note, however, that the best discriminator between nasal and non-nasal subjects was a combination of the flow and pressure aerodynamic measures. The flow-pressure ratio (FPR) offers a good basis for diagnosis. However, the instrumentation for measurement is usually not available to most clinicians. The clinician can observe the individual's ability to produce pressure sounds and nasal air flow on non-nasal sounds but, as Dickson, Barron, and McGlone point out, this is better done in connected speech, which is the ultimate aim of remedial efforts, than on isolated measures such as blowing or the production of isolated sounds.

Evaluation of Oral Structures. It is best to postpone the examination of the oral structures and their function until a patient's speech has been described so as to minimize a prejudicial viewpoint. There is often a tendency to hear what we think we should hear. After the speech-language evaluation, the speech-language pathologist should study the data obtained and then evaluate the oral cavity. At this time, questions in the following categories should be answered:

Dental Structures. How is the patient's general oral hygiene? Are caries present? Are teeth widely spaced or missing? Are the dental arches in alignment, or are they maloccluded? (See the chapters by Koepp-Baker and Bloomer in Travis, (1971), for helpful information on the identification of dental abnormalities, classification of occlusion, and deviation of palatal structures which occur in cleft palate.)

The Tongue and Adjacent Structures. Does the tongue structure and function appear adequate for speech? Can the tongue be elevated independently of the mandible? Is the tip flexible? Can the tongue be moved adequately from side to side? Can it be grooved? Can the midpoint be elevated? Can it be retracted? Is the usual position low , and forward? Does it retract during swallowing? Is there any evidence of a consistently retracted tongue or a high riding tongue?

Next, does the oral cavity allow for free movement of the tongue? Is the palatal vault excessively low or high? Do enlarged tonsils prevent free movement of the tongue? Do malpositioned teeth or dental appliances restrict tongue activity?

The Lips. Is the size of the mouth opening within normal limits? Are the lips full and flexible? Does scarring prevent free movement on protrusion? Is the function of the lips symmetrical? Do the lips retain adequate tonus during articulation of lip sounds, or are they too flaccid? Do the lips meet in an edge-to-edge relationship, or is the contact on the lingual surface?

The Velum. Is the velum of adequate length? Does it elevate symmetrically? Does it elevate sufficiently? Is the arch of the velum within normal limits?

Evaluation of the Valving Function. Early writings in the field of speech often compared the speech mechanism to a musical wind instrument. That analogy is tremendously oversimplified, yet the speech system is highly dependent on its structures and its valving. The necessity of maintaining proper flow paths and establishing needed pressure, and the reliance of the mechanism on the valving system to produce distinctive aspects of sound, are common both to the vocal apparatus and an instrument. In fact, deviations in air flow, air pressure, and distinctive effects (phonemes) reveal whether or not the valving system is functioning properly. Since aspects of the system have been previously described, and some form of study of the articulatory valves is a basic part of every diagnosis, they need not be repeated here.

When velopharyngeal closure is not possible, aberrant valving patterns can develop. They may occur at the glottis, producing glottal stops or catches; at the valve created by the back of the tongue and pharynx, producing pharyngeal hisses or fricatives; and at the valve formed by the back of the tongue and the palate, producing palatal fricatives. Nasal snorts may also be considered a form of improper valving when substituted for fricatives or, occasionally, for plosives; and some people have even been observed producing these sounds on inhalation. The undesirable solutions people devise to compensate for the inability to use standard valving patterns are ingenious and take forms too varied to be described in their entirety. However, the clinician should be on the alert for them.

Evaluation of Auditory Factors. In a population badly in need of acute hearing to assist in perfecting speaking skills, poorer auditory function is common. The importance of detecting a hearing loss and of continuously studying hearing acuity in children with cleft palates is obvious, as is the need for otological care. The exact type of care to be provided, however, is not so obvious. The speech-language pathologist is frequently asked whether adenoid tissue, which appears to be interfering with acuity because of the aural pathology it is causing in the middle ear, should be removed. This is a difficult decision, for the choice often involves the possible improvement of hearing at the sacrifice of velopharyngeal efficiency, and we can only hope that advances in otological care and maxillofacial surgery will make it possible not to have to sacrifice speech or hearing. At present, it is a decision each management team has to make, according to the needs of the particular individual.

Auditory discrimination can be measured by the Templin Speech Sound Discrimination Test (Templin, 1943), the Boston University Speech Sound Discrimination Test (Pronovost and Dumbleton, 1953), and tests by Wepman (1958) and Goldman, Fristoe, and Woodcock (1969). All of these tests will permit assessment of the subject's ability to discriminate differences among consonant sounds. None of them, however, tells much about his or her ability to assess the accuracy of production of the sounds in his or her own speech or the ability to distinguish between oral and nasal voice quality. To measure these, the speech-language pathologist must rely on tailor-made testing, such as that described by Johnson, Darley and Spriestersbach (1963), or on his or her own ingenuity. One method is to have the patient record a set of phonetically balanced (PB) words (Egan, 1948; Hirsch et al., 1952) and then write down what is heard when the same list is played back after a day or two. Having recorded the material should make the auditory task somewhat easier, but it frequently does not. Moreover, the task is motivating for some subjects but discouraging for others; the clinician will have to decide on the procedure's applicability for each subject individually.

Another way of measuring both articulation and voice quality discrimination is to have the patient rate the speech of other people with cleft palates in terms of these characteristics. The practice can yield interesting information, besides serving as good therapeutic procedure.

Evaluation of Social, Emotional, and Intellectual Factors. Much of the information on how the prognosis is affected by social, emotional, and intellectual factors is provided by the psychologist or social worker, or it is obtained from school or clinic records. With children, it is well to supplement this information with answers to the following questions: (1) can the child and her or his family carry out treatment plans?; (2) does the family accept and help the child?; (3) does the family overprotect or overindulge the child?; (4) is the child self-conscious or self-critical?; (5) do the child and the family have good insight into the problems associated with her or his cleft palate and into their role in habilitation?

Interpretation of the Data. After the data are accumulated, the clinician has the task of attempting to derive meaning from them; that is, the evaluation of the relationship between speech problems and physiological, oral, and valving problems, and the direct and indirect relationships of the deficiencies to the speech of the individual with a cleft palate.

In relating the speech problems to the valving deficiencies identified in the testing programs, the speech-language pathologist is concerned with the following kinds of questions: Can therapy be successful with the existing structures? What type of therapy is needed? Are referrals indicated? What suggestions, from a speech stand-point, can be made to medical and dental specialists?

As far as speech problems totally unrelated to the cleft are concerned, they should be examined as thoroughly as if the cleft were not present. The same can be said about defects only indirectly related to the cleft palate.

Making Appropriate Referrals. The clinician is responsible for improving the communication skills of the person with a cleft palate. To fulfill that responsibility he or she must supply those services which his or her training included and of which he or she is capable. Beyond that, it must be seen that the patient receives any other measures and services that will assist in developing the best possible communication. The speech-language pathologist thus must make appropriate referrals and follow them up. The specialist must make certain that the program of habilitation is moving ahead and be prepared to defend his or her judgment and present rationale.

To diagnose, to prognose, to refer, and to follow up other measures of habilitation are all extremely important responsibilities. But the prime responsibility is communication therapy. If it is not successful, the other measures have little meaning.

PRINCIPLES OF COMMUNICATION REMEDIATION

Total habilitation of communication for the person with a cleft palate is directed toward helping achieve the best possible structure, function, and use of the oral mechanism, with the ultimate end of assisting toward realization of physical, emotional, social, and educational goals consistent with interests and abilities. Further, to repeat, development of the client's verbal communication skills to their maximum potential is the particular concern of the speech-language pathologist.

Because the problems of verbal communication in the population with cleft palates are so varied, it is not possible to develop a single treatment plan. Instead, as noted earlier, remediation must be tailored to the specific needs of each individual, as determined by the diagnosis. Moreover, specific remedial methods must be appropriate not only to the objectives of the remedial program, but also to the patient's interests, age, and capabilities. After therapeutic goals have been set, the clinician must select and develop the practices necessary to accomplish them.

There are, however, certain principles basic to habilitation practices that are applicable to the cleft-palate population as a group and on which an individual program should be based.

1. The success of speech therapy is primarily determined by the anatomical structures.

Clefts of the face and palate, organic disorders, are basically medical problems. The surgical creation of a speech mechanism, protection of health, preservation of hearing, and achievement of a satisfactory cosmetic image are all medical responsibilities. The success of speech remediation depends largely on the structure the surgeon creates. In fact, the speech-language pathologist cannot and should not accept the responsibility for the speech of children whose structures are totally incapable of adequate speech. The clinician must recognize the limits of his or her ability to assist, and this factor should be considered in the diagnosis, although it may be difficult to determine. Prognosis is uncertain in any event, considering that a child with nearly normal structures may fail to respond to therapy, and one with a relatively wide-open cleft may produce nearly normal speech.

On the other hand, the speech-language pathologist must recognize the problems confronting the surgeon, who often works with minimal tissue and performs early surgery on structures that are so small and delicate that any repair is commendable. But a difficult situation sometimes arises when the surgeon advises the parent, "My surgery is completely successful. Now, a little speech therapy is all that's needed." The clinician must handle such situations diplomatically, with a realistic appraisal of speech needs. Seldom does "a little therapy" accomplish anything, and the parents must be realistic in their expectations concerning the length and results of speech therapy.

When the patient lacks minimal organic requirements for speech, therapy will only increase frustration, and lead to a belief that he or she cannot communicate adequately, leading to the distrust of the clinician's ability to help. When in doubt, a trial period of therapy with stated limits is the wisest course.

2. The earlier the treatment, the better the prognosis.

Language and speech development cannot wait for physical habilitation to begin or be completed. The infant begins learning verbal communication at birth. If a cleft palate is present, assistance is needed to stimulate and direct this development so that the child can learn to cope with the abnormalities of the oronasal mechanism. The sooner assistance is provided, the less undesirable compensations are likely to be learned to use in coping with speech. An early program of stimulation may rule out, and certainly reduce, the need for remediation in later years. When speech remediation is not begun until later, it will necessarily emphasize corrective procedures rather than stimulation, making the program more difficult and time consuming. However, until a sufficient number of preschool facilities are available, corrective therapy will continue to receive major emphasis.

3. Parental counseling, guidance, and participation are important.

In studying habilitation programs for people with cleft palates, the need is consistently evident for parental counseling, parental guidance, and parental involvement. Although clefts may have existed in a family's history, they often have not, and many parents are completely unfamiliar with the condition. Frequently, there may have been no history of difficulty during gestation, nor any episode, such as birth injury, to explain what has occurred. Moreover, the experts to whom the parents turn for explanations may either give them no explanation at all or one that is vague or otherwise unsatisfactory. Some parents, in search of a reason, blame themselves or their spouses for what they consider to be an "imperfect child." It is not unusual for them to express feelings of guilt over past conduct or try to "make it up" to their child by being oversolicitous or permissive. This tendency is strengthened as their child undergoes operations and other treatment at hospitals and clinics. It is not uncommon to hear them say, "He's been through so much," or "I feel so sorry for her."

Thus, the problem of cleft palate is a total family problem which calls for professional assistance. This assistance should begin with an explanation of the problem as soon after the child's birth as practicable, assuming that the parents are ready for such counseling. To reassure anxious parents, many programs show slides of children who have been successfully treated. This showing takes place in the mother's room before she leaves the hospital. Educational materials such as *Bright Promise* (McDonald, 1959) and *Understand Those Feelings* (McDonald, 1962) are also effective in assisting parents at this stage. Counseling should be continued on the first visit to the clinic, and should be given at least once every six months during the habilitation program. Parents should be told about the timing of treatment, the nature of the treatment process, and their role in the overall program. Hill (1956) supported this view in a study that revealed a positive relationship between information given the parents and the attitudes they reflected.

The parents also need guidance in helping their child with pre-speech activities by encouraging development of labial and lingual contact and oral activity. In effect, the mother and/or father is the child's first clinician, a role for which the parent requires basic information about the timing of speech and language development in children and about providing the child with the daily stimulation needed for verbal development. Involving the parents in this way not only helps the child; it also helps allay anxieties by giving the parents the feeling that they are "doing something." A later discussion on assisting parents with the cleft-palate child deals with these matters in greater detail.

4. Language needs early and continuing attention.

For some children with cleft palates, delays in language development persist into the primary school years, and can be detrimental to their emotional, social, and educational adjustment. Thus, despite the defectiveness of a child's early speech, and the fact that it may be easy to forget to provide stimulation if the child is not verbally responsive, stimulation should not be neglected. The clinician must not only counsel and advise the parents, but must also demonstrate procedures for language stimulation. In many instances, help must be given the parents in recognizing their child's first words.

5. The individual must experience success in therapy and be convinced that the production of acceptable speech is possible.

Attempts to compensate for structural deficiencies by adjustments in speech, commonly observed among persons with cleft palates, may be avoided if early guidance is given; but otherwise they are likely to be present in people who reach school age with moderately or severely defective speech. As a rule, most of these compensations end in failure. The person has difficulty being understood, may be mimicked, and cannot correct his or her speech in ways that those around him or her suggest. Thus, a *resignation to failure* may develop and the person may become convinced that he or she cannot produce normal speech. This attitude may result in halfhearted articulatory attempts, rapid speech, slurring of words, omission of sounds or parts of words, totally inappropriate substitutions, lack of verbal responsiveness, and many other forms of negative speech behavior. A patient must be helped to overcome such feelings and develop positive attitudes toward speech in general, his or her speech in particular, and his or her ability to produce adequate speech. He or she must experience success.

6. Exercises should not require strenuous activity that cannot be adapted to the rapid transition required for speech.

Exercises should be designed to achieve optimum tonus in the speech mechanism and optimum expenditure of air. Otherwise an improvement in one area may simply produce undesirable habits in other areas. Facial grimaces, constriction of the nares, nasal snorting, and rapid arrhythmic speech may all result from undesirable speech exercises.

7. Auditory acuity and auditory discrimination must be as nearly normal as possible.

The ability to monitor one's own speech and language, important for all speakers, is particularly important for the speaker with a cleft palate. Therefore, continuing medical supervision is needed to minimize recurrent episodes of middle ear disease and fluctuating hearing levels, which are physically debilitating and hinder verbal development.

The parents should be alerted to the symptoms of middle ear disease, and educated in its significance and remediation. Children with cleft palates may not be as reactive to pain from middle ear disease as other children; therefore, parents cannot rely on being alerted to the condition by complaints of earaches. They must watch for signs of inattentiveness, inappropriate responses, and unusual irritability. Sometimes, the only evidence of middle ear disease is provided by audiometric examination or impedance measurements. Thus, auditory acuity should be tested frequently, using air- and bone-conduction testing and impedance assessment.

When an auditory problem arises, the speech-language pathologist must be prepared to accommodate the objectives and procedures of therapy. If a hearing loss is present, amplification may be a part of the therapy program if indicated. If diagnosis reveals that auditory discrimination is not functioning within normal limits, it, too, must be emphasized in therapy.

8. The single most important factor is velopharyngeal function.

Complete closure of the velopharyngeal opening may not be necessary—as research evidence seems to indicate, but the person with a cleft palate must be able to direct most of the air flow and acoustic energy through the oral cavity and impound or constrict air at the valves of articulation without having the air escape through the nose. And while therapy may improve valving function that is defective through misuse or disuse, and may minimize the influence of inadequate closure, it cannot lengthen the palate nor restore neuromuscular function when it is inadequate.

9. The air stream must travel along an open and relatively unencumbered path.

The tongue must not be an obstacle to the passage of the air stream, and the oral opening should be wide enough to permit air and sound energy to exit efficiently. This suggests low and forward tongue placement and good action of the mandible and lips. Action of the articulators should be as precise and rapid as possible. Tight contacts or narrow strictures should be avoided.

The closure of the vocal tract during the production of plosive consonants or the constriction of the vocal tract during the production of fricatives may force air through the nasal cavity. Loose articulatory contacts, similar to those advocated in some stuttering activities, may result in relaxing the closure or stricture, thus reducing the amount of air forced through the nasal cavity and lowering the air need, so that there is less likelihood of excessive air use. The articulators are kept in motion, and words are easier to produce.

Blowing exercises, aimed not at increasing muscle function or improving velopharyngeal closure, but at directing the air stream through the oral cavity, are still desirable. Blowing exercises, however, have recently been questioned by some researchers on the ground that, requiring sustained muscle activity rather than the light and rapid movements of speech, they do not appropriately reflect speech production. This is partially true. Some of the blowing exercises in current use require excessive air and can result in poor respiratory habits and facial grimaces. Directional blowing exercises, however, are for a different purpose. Besides being helpful, these exercises provide an enjoyable experience for children if used in games.

Blowing exercises can also improve muscle function, if used with reason and for a specific purpose. It is the indiscriminate use of blowing exercises or the careless assignment of undesirable and perhaps even harmful exercises that must be avoided.

10. Occasionally the success of therapy is related to the person's ability to control his or her rate of speech.

When therapy is begun early and restorative measures are excellent, this point may not be applicable. But, for patients whose articulators and velopharyngeal mechanisms function only marginally, rate may be a critical factor. Many people with cleft palates, who can produce good speech in isolated words but cannot sustain it at conversational rates, must learn to slow down their rate of speaking, at least initially. Later, it may be possible to increase it.

11. The greatest improvement in communication will come from improved precision of articulation.

Improved articulatory ability will result not only in better intelligibility, but also in less perceived nasality, which is a highly desirable goal of therapy. Since many patients find it easier to learn to produce a consonant than to improve voice quality, an emphasis on the former will result in faster and more noticeable gains—a reinforcing factor in any training situation.

12. Tactile and visual stimulation may be of as much help as auditory stimulation in developing acceptable production of speech sounds.

In the presence of velopharyngeal inadequacy, emphasis should be placed on the development of correct placement for speech sound production. To accomplish this, it is sometimes more efficient to direct attention to visual and tactile cues as the various phonemes are taught. For example, with young children, the /f/, rather than being the "angry cat sound," might be labeled the "bite-your-bottom-lip" sound. Models to show how the sound is produced and descriptions of placement and production may also be helpful.

13. Mental health is a desirable and necessary consideration in habilitation.

Whatever the clinician can do to help the patient improve as a person or improve feelings about himself or herself will contribute materially to the habilitation program. Involving the parents in the habilitation program and building on success experiences are important ways of contributing to a patient's mental health. Particularly helpful with other children and adults is the practice of promoting a study of cleft palate, as this often reduces anxiety and helps patients understand themselves and their problems better. In addition, an attractive appearance is very beneficial; surgeons report that children frequently say, "I don't care how I sound. Just make me look good."

The above list of principles is neither universally applicable nor all-inclusive. Some will not be appropriate for given individuals, and some that may be critical for other persons may not have been mentioned. With such a varied population, however, it is impossible to cover every contingency. It is hoped that the clinician will find in this overall statement of principles a sound basis for planning a habilitation program.

REMEDIAL PRACTICES

Too often, therapy for speech-language disorders resulting from cleft palate is delayed until school age or even later, but—as emphasized throughout this chapter—it should begin shortly after the birth of the child and last until all procedures have been completed and the child or adult is judged either to have acceptable speech and language or to have reached the limits of his or her ability. A child should continue to be seen periodically until adulthood has been reached, because changes in structure and function associated with maturation may cause a deterioration in speech performance, necessitating additional therapy. One of the first steps in assisting the child is attention to the needs of the parents.

Assisting Parents of Children with Cleft Palates

Concern for the well-being of persons who are parents of children with cleft lips and palates as well as recognition of the parents' role in the psychosocial development of their children has led to increased interest in aiding parents. Recognition of the desirability of parental involvement has focused attention of professionals on the wide variety of parents who are responsible for the upbringing of children with cleft palates and the consequent wide variety of attitudes and information and the intellectual, social, emotional, and financial resources which these persons possess. Professionals are more sophisticated than in the past, when the simplistic approach was to have the parent "accept the child as he or she is"—as the solution to all aspects of parental handling. It is a tribute to parents of children with handicaps that they did not respond en masse, "that's easy for you to say."

Parents' Self-Study. Although the need for objectivity on the part of professionals is desirable, some degree of subjective empathy is also needed. Far more parents complain about seeming lack of real caring than of lack of objectivity in the professionals with whom they have been associated. One way for professionals to achieve greater empathy is to attempt to understand more clearly what it is that the parents are really experiencing. From the time each person reaches a level when being a parent is first considered, each person often fantasizes about "my child." Whatever direction this fantasizing takes, aspirations are almost invariably high. This continues until marriage, often including discussions of "how many children," "boys or girls," "what will they be like," and so forth. Then, when pregnancy occurs, the entire focus is on the birth of the child. Few parents, other than offering the usual, almost automatic statement, "I hope the baby will be all right," seriously consider the possibility of their child being handicapped. Thus, in one announcement by the physician, who is often too harried to display complete understanding or compassion or to engage in discussion of prognosis and planning, all the dreams of a lifetime are altered. Bewilderment, resentment, fear, anger, hostility, martyrdom all may be hidden behind the facade of "I have to accept my child" or "there's really nothing wrong with my child" or "everything is going to be all right" or "I must be brave" or the many other faces professionals may see.

The first step is to allow the parents to be themselves. If they can verbalize their disappointment, possible feelings of guilt, and concerns, they are on the road to better relations with themselves and with their child. In some instances it is easier for parents to write down their feelings than to say them. Prompt them with such questions as, "What were your aspirations for this child?" "How do you think these aspirations will be affected?," "Specifically, what do you believe is wrong with your child?," "What can be done to assist your child?," "What are the time frames for treatment and habilitation?," "How expensive do you think this will be?," "Will expenses present a major problem?," "What are your greatest concerns regarding the planning?," "What concerns do you have about your ability to be an effective parent for this child?" After reviewing the information received from parents, there should be clues as to how to proceed. It is helpful to have individual assessments of each of the two parents. It is not unusual to find that each parent has an entirely different view of the situation. Sometimes parents have diametrically opposing views. Fathers often seem to have more difficulty in accepting the presence of a problem. Also, even if the parents' views are compatible, the presence of a child with a handicap places an additional burden on a marriage. If the professional can aid the parents to work together as a team, the marriage, each parent, and the child will be helped.

Parents should be assisted to understand that whatever their feelings, they are not uncommon and are understandable. They should be encouraged to continue to look at their feelings honestly and realistically. They should develop habits of being able to verbalize feelings, to put emotions into words, to assess their accuracy, and to be able to share with their mate and professionals. Any feeling, no matter how unwarranted, is not ridiculous, humorous, or unimportant if it is important to the parent. The fact that many concerns are genuine should not be avoided. There *will* be problems, there *will* be financial burdens, there *will* be confusion as to how to proceed. However, many of these things can be anticipated and planned for with flexibility for change, which is totally predictable in all human activity.

Understanding the Child. Parents should be encouraged to view their child as a child with a cleft palate rather than as a handicapped child. The difference is subtle but important. A child with a cleft palate is more child than cleft palate. He or she has much in common with other children and much that is normal. Parents have ideas of what to do with a child, it is the other part that is confusing to them and difficult to deal with. The focus should be on using accepted methods of parenting and then on making alterations and allowances to accommodate the handicapping condition.

It is likely that the greatest assistance that can be provided the parents in counseling is helping them to develop an objective understanding of their child. If, in even a small way, the total subjectivity of parents can be altered and objectivity developed, to some degree, this will aid immeasurably. The first step in this process is to help each parent describe the child as realistically as possible. Where is the child in development? What is the rate of growth? What can the child do and what can't the child do? Keeping a log of the child's activities can serve as a medium of helping the parents understand the difference between fact and inference. This is a critical part of the process. All professionals are familiar with the "halo effect," in which parents adopt a prideful, protective, and unrealistic positive assessment of their child's abilities and potential. For most parents this poses no serious problem. For the parents of a child with a cleft palate it may provide a barrier for objective understanding. This is not to suggest that we must be "brutally frank." Consideration must be given the parents' readiness to accept information. Devastating them will not be productive. The sympathetic professional will understand the difference between realistic appraisal and unnecessary frankness. Helping parents to be able to realistically describe their child and his or her needs takes a little longer, but pays dividends in increased parental acceptance.

Planning is very helpful in aiding parents. Knowing the "what," "when," "how," and "why" is a very positive aspect. Physicians seldom have the time or have taken the time to inform parents about future plans. Other professionals do not have particularly good records in this area either. Parents need to have someone provide more than a cursory overview of the future. Certainly their plans will be altered. However, to know what to expect based on available information is highly desirable.

Understanding Professionals. Parents often view professionals as being super-human. This has some advantages because it engenders faith and hope. However, over time, negative effects may occur. Failure to deliver on promised gains, professional disagreements, changes in plans—all may lead to confusion and other ill effects for parents' well-being. It is better that parents understand that professionals are human and that each attempts to do what he or she thinks is best. This may lead to conflicting views. This does not necessarily mean that one professional is "right" and another is "wrong." Sometimes parents create negative feelings by their excessive demands on the professionals. It is difficult to assist parents to understand the difference between a crisis in their child's life and their own over-concern in reaction to a particular occurrence.

Most parents are aware that there are some incompetents, even charlatans, in every profession. However, by far, most professionals are competent, are attempting to provide the best services of which they are capable, are sincere in what they say and do, and want to be of assistance. It has been said so often that it is trite, but the parents are part of a team. They must develop the best team possible and then themselves be cooperative and contributing team members.

Understanding the Community. Finally, the parents should attempt to analyze and assess the particular community in which they live. Are adequate resources available? Can improvements be made in resources and can parents assist in this process? Are the parents equipped to assist not only their own child but others as well? There are many satisfactions in aiding children. Developing methods for assisting parents to realistically analyze and assess themselves, their children, professionals, and their community can provide even greater satisfaction to the professional. Even more importantly, it can lead to better lives for children and their families.

The Remedial Program

Stages of the Program. Approximately four stages can be differentiated in the total remedial program based on the age of the child. These stages delineated by ages approximate the stages in the evaluation of the individual with a cleft palate.

Stage one—The prelinguistic period. This period occurs from birth until eighteen months, during which the parents provide stimulation to the child with suggestions from the professional.

Stage two—Development of basic speech-language skills. This period, from eighteen months until three years, involves the cooperative efforts between the speech-language pathologist and the parents. The clinician provides therapeutic intervention and advises the parents on follow-up in the home environment.

Stage three—The preventative-corrective period. From three to five years the clinician continues to attempt to prevent the development of aberrant speech and language patterns and to correct or minimize existing auditory and/or speech-language errors.

Stage four—The corrective stage. This period, from five years on, unfortunately is the period during which therapy is often begun. It should not be, since preventative

Figure 6–6. Sequencing of Remedial Measures.

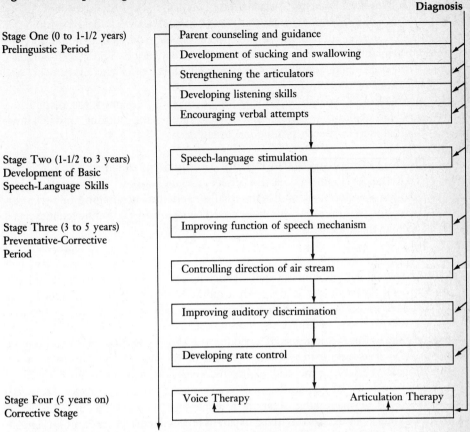

Diagnosis

Stage One (0 to 1-1/2 years) Prelinguistic Period	Parent counseling and guidance
	Development of sucking and swallowing
	Strengthening the articulators
	Developing listening skills
	Encouraging verbal attempts

| Stage Two (1-1/2 to 3 years) Development of Basic Speech-Language Skills | Speech-language stimulation |

Stage Three (3 to 5 years) Preventative-Corrective Period	Improving function of speech mechanism
	Controlling direction of air stream
	Improving auditory discrimination
	Developing rate control

| Stage Four (5 years on) Corrective Stage | Voice Therapy   Articulation Therapy |

measures will yield better results than will attempts to correct the "bad habit" aberrant patterns that have developed in efforts to compensate for inadequate oral structures and functions. However, the clinician should be prepared to assist the child when she or he first sees the child, regardless of age level.

Steps in the Remedial Program. If several experts were asked to sequence therapy for an individual with a cleft palate it is likely that each would present a different model. Some would include items others omitted, and the order of attention would be varied. This would be due to differing philosophies and the differing needs of each individual with a communication deficit. Thus, figure 6–6 is less an exact order of presentation than a general guide for consideration in developing a remedial program for each individual. There is no such thing as a specific guide; the diagnosis prescribes the therapy.

The steps in therapy must be juxtaposed with the previously mentioned stages. Steps in the remedial program are dependent on the age level when the individual is first seen for therapy. It is hoped that this will be early in the child's development. If this is so, the first step will be aimed at parental counseling as previously described. Another mental health measure for the parents is involvement in the preventative-remedial process. As previously stated, since parents feel they participated in the creation of the child's problems, most parents want to be part of the solution. Not all parents handle this well and the specialist must carefully assess the parents' ability to be of help to the child. Not only does this benefit mental health, but early stimulation throughout the entire day is important to speech-language development and only the parents are available to carry this out over so extended a period. The speech-language pathologist should make suggestions, provide guidance, offer encouragement, and share evaluations of success.

The production of speech is dependent on systems designed for respiration, mastication, and deglutition. Thus, development of chewing, sucking, and swallowing is an initial step in speech production in children.

Stage One—The Prelinguistic Period. During the prelinguistic period, attention is paid to the development of such skills as sucking, swallowing, strengthening of the articulators, development of listening skills, and the encouraging of verbal attempts. Attention to these areas should be based on need and some children may need no assistance in these areas.

Sucking. Sucking is initially reflexive in each child. For the first few weeks after birth almost any taste, touch or temperature will elicit a sucking response. If the child feeds at the mother's breast or can nurse from a nipple without the holes enlarged, it is likely that sucking is adequate. A normal nipple can be roughly defined as one that will allow twenty drops of liquid per minute when the bottle is held upside down. When the child is not feeding, use of a pacifier can provide additional lip and tongue exercises as well as aiding in the development of sucking. Although children are weaned usually between nine and eighteen months, it may be helpful to delay weaning as long as the physician feels this is acceptable, to promote sucking activity.

Efforts should be made after weaning to encourage the child to suck through a straw. Wrapping a plastic straw with transparent tape will enlarge the straw and make it easier for the child's lips to adapt to it. As time goes by, the size of the taping can be reduced. Liquids used should be cool, sweet, and have a pleasant odor. Where liquids do not have prominent odors the rim of the glass can be rubbed with small amounts of ammonia, mint, oil of cloves, or some other scent. This entire sucking practice should be a leisurely one, and only encouraging, approving sounds should be made. If the child has difficulty drawing liquid through a straw, the teeth should be brought together by the parent's direction and manipulation and the straw placed between the lips just touching the teeth. After the child can do this, some pleasant tasting liquid should be drawn into the straw by immersing the straw and then closing one end with a finger to hold the liquid in about one-third to one-half the length of the straw. The straw is then placed between the lips so that the child tastes the liquid. Most often this will assist the child in beginning to swallow and, after added trials and encouragement, the child will usually begin to suck. Initially, the task should be made as easy as possible for the child by the tilt of the glass. As the child succeeds the task should be made more difficult. Sucking a stick candy, popsicles, or suckers can also be helpful.

Swallowing. Swallowing may also need attention. Difficulty may be evidenced by drooling. Normal neuromuscular maturation usually eliminates drooling by the end of the first year. Delay beyond a year may suggest that the child is having difficulty in using the tongue to propel foods posteriorly. Giving the child small amounts of liquids he or she enjoys on a spoon and then tilting the head slightly backward may be of assistance initially. Care must be taken not to use excessive amounts which may cause the child to choke. The child next should be encouraged to accomplish a swallow without tilting the head. The next step is to have the child take several small sips from a glass, swallowing strongly. After swallowing appears adequate, the child should be advanced through foods as normally as the mechanism permits. The physician's recommendations should be followed in moving from liquids to baby foods, to junior foods, and to table foods. The child should learn to eat more than soft foods and should be taught to chew deliberately and completely.

Strengthening the Articulators. In addition to sucking and swallowing, the infant should have other experiences in strengthening the articulators. Lip-smacking and loud pressure sounds made by drawing the lips in and then releasing them also are helpful. Playing follow-the-leader with lip protrusions and retractions, smiles and frowns, tongue activity and jaw movements encourages exercises. A mirror should be used so the child can observe herself or himself as well as the parent. The child should be held whenever possible in following these exercises. At times imitation can take place while both child and parent are looking in the mirror. Effort should be rewarded more than success, and activity should be filled with joy and laughter. The child can be encouraged to blow bath bubbles off the mother's or father's hand and to blow out matches or blow on candle flames. The child may be able to blow a bubble pipe or blow feathers across the high-chair tray. Tissue can be blown across an area. When the child has a little more blowing strength, balloons can be blown up, preferably after a parent has first done so. The clinician should aid the parent in evaluating all blowing exercises to make certain that they are within the capabilities of the child. The child should not become frustrated, and exercises should afford success.

Jam, jelly, and peanut butter can be placed in the corners of the mouth and on the upper and lower lips for the child to lick off. The substance can gradually be moved a little farther outward so that slightly greater effort is required. Holding a sucker outside the child's mouth for the child to lick also can be useful.

Listening Skills. Developing listening skills is important. Careful attention should be given to the child's hearing, and frequent checks are necessary. In addition, efforts should be made to have the child make full use of the auditory skills available. The child should listen to the activity around the house and have attention drawn to it by verbal labels. "What's that?" should be a common phrase when a new sound is heard. Saying, "Shh," with a finger over the mouth will serve as an alert for the child to listen carefully. Not just loud sounds but softer sounds such as a bird call or the steam from a cooking utensil should be identified auditorily. "Where is it?" can be played by having the child point to the source of sound. Whistles, horns, and other noisemakers can be used to maintain the child's interest. Commercial records or the use of an inexpensive cassette recorder with sounds recorded can be helpful. After the sound is heard, the parent and child can look through books and magazines to find pictures of the sound source. Stories can be embellished by making the sounds the animals make, or the car or truck makes, or the boat, and so forth. The child's world should be filled with sound, and the parent should see if the child can match sounds, or the sound maker to the sound, or whether the child can begin to note differences in sounds (higher or lower, louder or softer, nearer or farther away). Maintaining adequate auditory acuity and developing good listening skills can pay good dividends in the development of adequate speech and language.

Encouraging Verbal Attempts. The parents should engage in daily sound play with the child—talking to him or her, fondling the child, and babbling with him or her. Since their early attempts will likely elicit little response, they will need encouragement to continue. Later the baby should begin to attend, and later still, to imitate. In their activities with the baby, the mother and father should describe what they are doing in soft, cheerful tones and short and simple language patterns. Also, they should reward the baby's babbling and early speech attempts by fondling, smiles, and pleasant vocal tones.

Although the child's first words may be nasal and imprecise, the parents should accept them and work for language development and more speaking attempts. They will need reassurance that the child's speech will improve if they are patient and confident. They must be urged to respond positively to the child's verbal attempts and provide recognition and feedback stimulation. They should verbally describe for the child objects, people, and actions, using simple words and phrases. They should discourage the child's use of gesture substitutes for language either by not responding or by using talk that parallels the indicated message. Their awareness of the child's verbal activity can be fostered by having the parents keep, for discussion with the clinician each week, a list of the words they hear their child use.

Even after the child begins to produce words, the sound play between the parents and the child should continue. They should encourage the child to use strong jaw activity and wide-open lip positions in the production of such sounds as the /a/ in /ap/. To accomplish this, yawning or sighing can be used. Playing "open wide" during meal time is another enjoyable activity which can produce similar results, with a variation in the form of chewing vigorously and "making a big cave" of the mouth and then closing it.

Lowell and Pollack also describe early stimulation activities in chapter 9; although the activities are designed for the deaf or hearing-impaired child, many of them can be used with the child with a cleft palate, and the reader may find it useful to refer to that discussion. Particular reference might be made here, however, to the practice of naming objects for the child and telling him or her what sounds they make, as well as of taking him or her for trips to the zoo or a farm and later looking for pictures of the animals, naming them, and imitating their sounds. Speech efforts should be rewarded for their presence, not their perfection. Because the parents should accept what the child has to offer, they must tolerate noise and even encourage it—rewarding humming, singing, reciting, and echoing. Again, the child's world should be filled with sound. He or she should be talked to and listened to. Speech should be both pleasurable and necessary.

The parents should acquire an understanding of prelinguistic development, knowing which sounds to expect early and which to expect later. They should also understand the essential elements of the speech process and the effects of the cleft palate on the child's speech. If assisted in gaining this understanding, they can give their child the kind of encouragement and support required.

Stage Two—Development of Basic Speech-Language Skills. When the child is eighteen months old, several words have emerged and direct assistance from the clinician is desirable. The early sessions, held once or twice a week, should be very informal play situations, with the speech-language pathologist using the child's interests and activities to accomplish specific goals. At this level, individual, in addition to group, sessions are preferable. The parents should watch the clinician working with the child and should also be involved in the activity; they should be taught along with the child and be observed working with the child. This process is somewhat variable, and they may have to watch from an adjacent room rather than participating directly in the session. At times, they may control the activity, with the clinician observing from another room and counseling them later.

Speech-Language Stimulation. The actual stimulation in speech and language development, more formal than the play sessions, begins when the clinician feels that the child is ready, and is then conducted on a regular basis. It should follow a sequence such as—

1. encouraging the child in play activity and gradually interacting with him or her;
2. using imitation, with the child being imitated first and then being the one who imitates;
3. having the child name things—objects first and then activities—with the process of identifying things common to the child's environment being guided by such considerations as what an object is, what it does, and what sound it makes;
4. engaging in describing, an extension of the naming process, in which words are acted out and pictures are described and the child's increasing continuity of expression is encouraged, thus leading to a more complex use of language;
5. engaging in dramatizing, which enables the child to use speech and language for expression, along with gestures and bodily movement; and
6. using riddles and nursery rhymes toward the end of this period, when the child is three years old.

The speech-language pathologist should have available many materials and resources to add to this list and implement its use. The general goals are to expand vocabulary, develop syntax, and stimulate the development of correct sounds and articulatory patterns consistent with the child's age level. Additional suggestions can be found in chapter 2 on language.

Stage Three—The Preventative-Corrective period.
Language stimulation activities should continue and advance to the remediation of specific deficits found in the evaluation. In addition, more emphasis should be given to correcting the function of the velopharyngeal mechanism, directing the air stream, placement of the articulators, and achieving optimal voice quality and articulation. Specific techniques can be taken from the suggestions given below.

Improving the Function of the Speech Mechanism. The following techniques should not be used routinely, but only to meet the specific needs of individual patients. A better method of exercise for the articulators is provided by working on defective sounds.

(a) *The lips.* Because surgery of the upper lip may make it immobile or inflexible, some physicians have recommended that parents massage the operative area with cocoa butter. In addition, protruding and retracting the lips four or five times, several times a day, can aid flexibility and tonus. Berry and Eisenson (1956) have also suggested changing from a smile to a whistle with exaggerated lip movements, chewing bubble gum, and blowing bubbles with vigorous lip-smacking.

Blowing out a lighted candle which is held at several positions—first under the chin, then near the bridge of the nose, and then to the right and left of the mouth—gives the individual practice not only in blowing but also in exercising the lips.

(b) *The tongue.* The patient must learn to use forward tongue placement and good tongue tip activity. The exercises recommended previously for children, in which jam, jelly, or honey is placed in the corners of the mouth and on the upper and lower lip, can be used for older persons too, as can the practice of placing peanut butter behind the central incisors. Other helpful exercises involving retrieving a toothpick half an inch from the mouth by curling the tongue tip and drawing it in, and rolling a toothpick across a table with the tongue.

Berry and Eisenson (1956) have recommended the following exercises. Have the patient:

1. Point the tongue straight out of the mouth. The tip should deviate neither to right nor to left and should have a fine point.
2. "Dot" the lips with the point of the tongue "up, side, down, side"—doing this first on the inside of the lips and then on the outside. Repeat the exercise, sweeping the lips with the tongue tip in rhythmic action.
3. "Dot" the palate with the tongue from front to back in four steps, then sweep the palate with a backward and forward movement of the tongue tip and blade.
4. Place the tongue tip behind the lower teeth and bulge the blade and dorsum, alternately relaxing and bunching the tongue.
5. Push the tongue tip against the alveolar ridge as for /t/, increasing the pressure noticeably before exploding the sound.
6. Groove the tongue along the median raphé with a slender stick and ask the individual to curl the tongue around the stick.
7. "Suck" the tongue up against the palate, and then release it. The same result may be obtained by asking the person to raise the whole tongue high and "past" the sides against the premolar and molar teeth, leaving only the tongue tip free.

(c) *The jaw.* Have the patient chew two pieces of bubble gum once a day, chew food long and vigorously, and chew against self-imposed pressure by holding the jaw shut with one hand while trying to chew.

(d) *General exercises.* Once a day, have the patient drink liquid during a meal through a straw. Also, have the patient pretend to drink a thick malted through a straw and thus be required to suck vigorously.

If the patient is old enough to read, read aloud for five-to-ten minutes a night—articulating as clearly as possible—while holding a pencil between the teeth. This exercise forces exaggerated lip and tongue movements.

Controlling the Direction of the Air Stream. The ability to direct the air stream through the oral cavity may explain why some people with wide-open clefts can manage to achieve acceptable articulation and voice quality. Many of the following blowing exercises can be done at home as well as in the clinic setting; and, as emphasized previously, their purpose is not to build up muscle strength but to control the direction of the air. The patient should always breathe deeply, remain relaxed, and blow directionally.

A candle on a saucer provides several good blowing exercises. To begin with, the patient should blow just to bend the flame from a near distance, and then increase the distance until he or she is about fourteen inches from the candle. Next, the patient should try to bend the flame by blowing while not disturbing a small piece of tissue placed on a tongue depressor or butter knife, held just under the nose. Feathers can be used in a similar manner: a feather can be glued to the bottom side of a three-by-five-inch card, and another feather laid loosely on top. The person can try to blow the bottom of the feather without disturbing the top one. Observing himself or herself in a mirror aids in the performance of this exercise. If there is difficulty at first directing the air stream, the person can blow through a straw; this will provide lip as well as blowing exercise if the straw is held in the lips.

Another good exercise is to blow a Ping-Pong ball across a table, or play Ping-Pong soccer with another player, each trying to blow the ball off the opponent's side of the table through a twelve-inch medially located space. Other possibilities include blowing feathers in the air and trying to keep them aloft, or blowing through a straw into colored liquid.

If the patient can do none of these exercises successfully, he or she or the speech-language pathologist should hold the nostrils shut with the fingers, but frequent checks should be made to see whether the patient has reached a stage where this is not necessary.

Again, the clinician is cautioned against blowing which becomes too strenuous. If any facial grimaces are observed, the exercise should be stopped.

Improving Auditory Discrimination Ability. These exercises are directed at improving the patient's ability to discriminate nasality from non-nasality and to distinguish among different speech sounds.

(a) Nasality discrimination. Helping the patient learn to distinguish between acceptable and unacceptable voice quality can be accomplished in several ways. First, the person can judge the adequacy of samples which the clinician demonstrates beginning with speech of grossly defective quality and gradually moving toward minimally defective quality. When the individual can make these judgments successfully, he or she can begin to judge actual samples of speech that the clinician has previously recorded, rating them on a five-point scale from "normal" to "severely defective." After becoming adept at making these judgments, the patient can demonstrate various levels of defectiveness for the clinician and compare judgments with the clinician's. Evaluation of his or her own voice quality during speaking attempts should continue.

(b) Discrimination of speech sounds. Many exercises are available for developing auditory discrimination in articulation. The clinician can use them, or he or she can use the programs that are now becoming available in tape form.

Developing Rate Control. Rate control, which has been mentioned frequently, is a vital part of therapy for some clients. If possible, the parents should demonstrate an appropriately slower rate for the child to imitate, but this is not always successful. Other techniques involve the use of a metronome, with one method aiming at gradual reduction of the child's rate of speech by setting the device's speed back bit by bit as the child becomes able to adjust the rate of speech to it. In another method, the metronome is set considerably below the child's speaking rate and the child is asked to attempt a more marked adjustment of rate all at once.

The child's speaking rate also can be slowed down through suggestions to "talk like an old man or old woman," engaging him or her in playacting, or having vowel sounds prolonged in speech. At an appropriate age, the child can learn poetry that suggests a slow rate of speech, but conversational speech is a superior form of exercise.

For older subjects, practice in rate control at therapy sessions, and reminders at other times, may be helpful. Mechanical devices such as metronomes are commercially available and may be helpful with some individuals.

Stage Four—The Corrective Period. The steps described are not mutually exclusive. For example, during the same therapy session, the clinician may work on rate control and auditory discrimination successively. Also, even though articulation is described as the more important aspect of therapy, voice quality may be worked on, first, because consonants usually cannot be produced in isolation—the syllable being the basic unit of speech. Thus, auditory discrimination of orality-nasality and two vowels, the /a/ and the /æ/, are worked on first in order to supply vowels for consonant drills.

Voice Quality Therapy Techniques. Success in voice quality therapy is important in itself, but it also is basic to success in the articulation therapy program. It is hoped that previous work in directing the air stream, in keeping the tongue low and forward, and in ear training has met with success. The speech-language pathologist should have the patient phonate the vowel /a/, and provide intensive training in producing it non-nasally. The tongue should be checked to see if it is low; if it is not, a tongue depressor may be used to hold it down. A dramatic reduction in nasality sometimes occurs when the tongue is held down during phonation of /a/. If palatal movement is still minimal and the patient cannot achieve non-nasal vowel production, three other possibilities exist—all of which should have the approval of the physician.

Stroking the palate with a small paint brush can be tried to develop awareness of the palatal area. If the patient does not have this awareness, the stroking can be done farther back until it elicits a gag reflex. The patient should be instructed to be aware of the feeling of the palatal area and the movement that occurs during gagging and swallowing. Also, the person should "get the feel" of sucking and swallowing.

If the above measures are not successful, more attention can be given to the sequence of movements in swallowing. The patient uses a mirror to observe swallowing, and may find it helpful to take small sips of water from a glass. After learning to swallow with the mouth open, he or she begins the swallow but interrupts it at the point of maximum palatal movement. The sequence to this point is: (1) begin to swallow; (2) hold the muscle set for a second or two; and (3) release it. After practicing this for some time, begin to swallow, then from the muscle set to phonation of /a/. The vowel /æ/ can be added when sufficient practice with /a/ has been completed.

Third, there is another method that can be tried if the above attempts are unsuccessful, but it must be done carefully. Paraffin is built up into a half-inch ball around the unpointed end of a knitting needle; the ball is inserted into the patient's mouth and used to carefully lift the velum. It is best to have the patient insert and lift the wax ball, since he or she knows how far to proceed with it and is more secure when he or she controls the activity. The patient should be asked to elevate the velum and phonate /a/ as before. After practicing this, see if he or she can do it successfully without using the paraffin ball. If this is possible, work first on phonating the /a/ non-nasally, and then the /æ/.

After the patient can produce the /a/ and the /æ/ non-nasally, work should begin on other vowels, going from low to high, and front to back sounds. The patient should continue trying for good action of the articulators in maintaining as wide an oral pathway as possible.

If none of the techniques described are successful, the prognosis for therapy must be considered questionable, although some patients who experience minimal results from voice quality therapy can show improvement after intensive articulation therapy.

Articulation Therapy Techniques. The techniques described here should be used when velopharyngeal function is a minor problem and is likely to improve significantly. (If velopharyngeal function and the resulting flow and pressure patterns are adequate, the usual articulation therapy techniques such as those presented by Sommers in chapter 3 can be used.)

(a) *Vowel and consonant productions.* To achieve early success, it is best to start with the continuants, which are least frequently defective, and proceed from them into drills on more difficult phonatory and articulatory patterns. In other words, therapy might begin with /w/, /l/, /r/, /j/, and /h/, in combination with the least nasalized vowels, /a/, and /æ/. In this program, the technique of using loose contacts should be remembered, as should the practice of initially pinching the nostrils to aid in non-nasal vowel production.

Since not all of the sound combinations can be covered in detail here, the sequence involving the correction of the /a/ by using the /w/ and /p/ will serve to illustrate the technique. The drill sequence is as follows:

1. Practice /awa/ until minimal nasality is obtained. Use exaggerated lip and jaw movements.
2. Practice /æwæ/, as in item 1.
3. Practice /wawæ/ and /wæwa/.
4. Practice /awa/, /apa/—using very loose contact on the /p/ initially and gradually tightening the contact until the /p/ is recognizable, though still not a tight contact.
5. Practice /apa/.
6. Practice /ap/. Prolong the /a/ before the loose contact in /p/—that is, /a::p/.
7. Practice words such as the following, with /ap/ in the initial position:
   opera
   operate
   opposite
8. Practice these words in short phrases.
9. Practice words such as the following, with /ap/ in the final position:
   cop   pop   top   bop
   sop   shop   lop   hop
10. Practice these words in short phrases.
11. Practice words such as the following, with /pa/ in the initial position:
    pot   pod
    pop   palm

12. Practice these words in short phrases.
13. Practice words such as the following, which introduce the /p/ sound into drill on longer words:

   possible pollen part
   pocket   park   possum

14. Practice these words in short phrases.
15. Follow the sequence described in items 1 to 14 with /æ/ and /p/.
16. Follow the same sequence with other vowel sounds and /p/. Begin with the low front vowels and progress gradually to the high back vowels.
17. Prepare sentences and then short paragraphs incorporating the words used in drills.
18. Practice monitoring conversational speech, in the clinic and then outside.
   (Work on /b/ should follow the same sequence as that outlined for /p/.)

Using the above sequence as a model, similar ones can be set up on which /l/ is used in drills to assist in the correction of /t/ and then /d/; /j/ is used with /k/ and then /g/; and /h/ is used with /s/ and then /z/. From /s/ and /z/, the sequence proceeds to /ʃ/ and /ʒ/, then /tʃ/ and /dʒ/, then /θ/ and /ð/, and finally /f/ and /v/.

(b) Glottal stops, and pharyngeal and palatal sibilants. The best way to deal with errors of substitution is to work on producing the sounds correctly. Pinching the nostrils or holding the tongue forward may help in the beginning.

SUMMARY

This chapter has suggested that there is no simple nor single way to improve the communication of the person with a cleft lip or palate. The variability and complexity of the problems associated with cleft palate mitigate against this, and imply that therapy must be tailored to meet the needs of each client.

In the ideal therapeutic situation, the speech-language pathologist begins the program of habilitation shortly after the birth of the infant and follows her or him to adulthood—first counseling, then guiding, providing remedial assistance, and following up to ensure the client's continuing habilitation. Along the way, a number of other specialists cooperate in the therapy process, and hopefully, the result is a successful total habilitation program.

Unfortunately, however, the speech-language pathologist does not always find this to be true. Often, he or she is not brought into a therapy process early enough. When the speech-language pathologist is brought in, a number of obstacles may be present, which are thought to impair successful habilitation. But the speech-language clinician has the responsibility to take the patient as presented and perform the most thorough and accurate diagnosis that clinical skills and the available professional facilities will allow, then use therapeutic ability to the fullest and, when it appears insufficient, seek additional assistance. If all attempts fail, the patient should return to the medical and dental specialists for further velopharyngeal assistance in repairing the cleft and/or the improvement of oral function. The sooner it can be determined that this is necessary, if it is to be, the more frustration will be spared the patient and the clinician.

The patient and the patient's family should receive, in effect, an ongoing course in speech, language, and cleft lip and palate: they should receive available information on the cause of the cleft, embryology, and treatment; how speech and language are produced and developed; and the aims of speech-language therapy. While the parents are the child's first clinicians, eventually the patient assumes a clinician's role—monitoring his or her own speech and daily attempting to meet communication goals. Better mental health and improved communication ability will result if the individual is equipped with information essential to this task.

BIBLIOGRAPHY

Alt, A., Heilunger Taubstummheit erzielte durch Beseitigung einer otorrhoe und einer angebornen Gaumenspalte. *Arch. Augen. Ohren*, **7**, 211–218 (1878).

Berlin, A. J., Classification of cleft lip and palate. In W. C. Grabb, et al., (Eds.), *Cleft Lip and Palate*. Boston: Little, Brown and Company (1971).

Berry, M. F., Lingual anomalies associated with palatal clefts. *J. Speech and Hearing Dis.*, **14**, 359–362 (1949).

Berry, M. F., and Eisenson, J., *Speech Disorders: Principles and Practices of Therapy*. New York: Appleton-Century-Crofts, Inc. (1956).

Brooks, A. R., Shelton, R. L., and Youngstrom, K. A., Compensatory tongue-palate-posterior pharyngeal wall relationships in cleft palate. *J. Speech Hearing Dis.*, **30**, 166–173 (1965).

Buck, M., Velopharyngeal movements and tongue carriage during speech in adults with unrepaired incomplete cleft palates. *Cleft Palate Bull.*, **10**, 8–10 (1960).

Bzoch, K. R., Articulation proficiency and error patterns of preschool cleft palate and normal children. *Cleft Palate J.*, **2**, 340–349 (1965).

Bzoch, K. R., *Communicative Disorders Related to Cleft Lip and Palate*. Boston: Little, Brown and Company (1979).

Clifford, E., Psychological aspects of cleft lip and palate in K. R. Bzoch (Ed.), *Communicative Disorders in Cleft Lip and Palate*. Boston: Little, Brown and Company (1979).

Dickson, S., Barron, S., and McGlone, R., Aerodynamic studies of cleft-palate speech. *J. Speech Hearing Dis.*, **43**, 160–167 (1978).

Dunn, L. M., *The Peabody Picture Vocabulary Test*. Circle Pines, Minn.: American Guidance Service, Inc. (1980).

Egan, J. P., Articulation testing methods. *Laryngoscope*, **58**, 955–991 (1948).

Fletcher, S. J., Cleft palate: a broader view. *J. Speech Hearing Dis.*, **31**, 3–13 (1966).

Fraser, F. C., Etiology of cleft lip and palate. In W. C. Grabb et al. (Eds.), *Cleft Lip and Palate*. Boston: Little, Brown and Company (1971).

Goldman, R., Fristoe, M., and Woodcock, R. W., *Goldman-Fristoe-Woodcock Test of Auditory Discrimination*. Circle Pines, Minn.: American Guidance Service, Inc. (1969).

Graber, T. M., Bzoch, K. R., and Aoba, T., A functional study of palatal and pharyngeal structures. *Angle Orthodontia*, **29**, 30–40 (1959).

Hanson, M. L., A study of velopharyngeal competence in children with repaired cleft palates. *Cleft Palate J.*, **1**, 217–231 (1964).

Hardy, J. C., and Arkebauer, H. J., Development of a test for velopharyngeal competence during speech. *Cleft Palate J.*, **3**, 6–21 (1966).

Heller, J. C., Hearing loss in patients with cleft palate. In K. R. Bzoch (Ed.), *Communicative Disorders Related to Cleft Lip and Palate*. Boston: Little, Brown and Company (1979).

Hess, D. A., Pitch, intensity, and cleft palate voice quality. *J. Speech Hearing Res.*, **2**, 113–125 (1959).

Hess, D. A., The TOM puffed cheeks test of velopharyngeal competence. Unpublished manuscript (1970).

Hess, D. A., A new experimental approach to assessment of velopharyngeal adequacy: Nasal manometric bleed testing. *J. Speech Hearing Dis.*, **41**, 427–443 (1976).

Hess, D. A., and McDonald, E. T., Consonantal nasal pressure in cleft palate speakers. *J. Speech Hearing Res.*, **3**, 201–211 (1960).

Hill, M. J., An investigation of the attitudes and information possessed by parents of children with clefts of the lip and palate. *Cleft Palate Bull.*, **6**, 3–4 (1956).

Hirsch, I. J., Davis, H., Silverman, S. R., Reynolds, E. G., Eldert, E., and Benson, R. W., Development of materials for speech audiometry. *J. Speech Hearing Dis.*, **17**, 321–337 (1952).

Hochberg, I., and Kabcenell, J., Oral stereognosis in normal and cleft palate individuals. *Cleft Palate J.*, **4**, 47–57 (1967).

Holm, V. A., and Kunze, L. H., Effect of chronic otitis media in language and speech development. *Pediatrics*, **43**, 833–839 (1969).

Isshiki, N., Honjow, I., and Morimoto, M., Effects of velopharyngeal incompetence upon speech. *Cleft Palate J.*, **5**, 297–310 (1968).

Isshiki, N., and Ringel, R., Air flow during the production of selected consonants. *J. Speech Hearing Res.*, **7**, 233–244 (1964).

Johnson, W., Darley, F. L., and Spriestersbach, D. C., *Diagnostic Methods in Speech Pathology*. New York: Harper & Row (1963).

Kernahan, D. A., and Stark, R. B., A new classification for cleft lip and cleft palate. *Plastic and Reconstructive Surgery*, **22**, 435–441 (1958).

Lee, L., *The Northwestern Syntax Screening Test*, Evanston, Ill.: Northwestern University Press (1969).

Lerea, L., Assessing language development. *J. Speech Hearing Res.*, **1**, 75–85 (1958).

Lipmann, R. P., Detecting nasalization using a low-cost miniature accelerometer. *J. Speech Hearing Res.*, **24**, 314–317 (1981).

Loeb, W. J., Speech, hearing and the cleft palate. *Arch. Otolaryngol.*, **79**, 4–14 (1964).

Lubker, J. J., An electromyographic-cinefluorographic investigation of velar function during normal speech production. *Cleft Palate J.*, **5**, 1–18 (1968).

Mazaheri, M., Millard, R., and Erickson, D. M., Cineradiographic comparison of normal to non-cleft subjects with velopharyngeal inadequacy. *Cleft Palate J.*, **1**, 199–209 (1964).

McDonald, E. T., *Bright Promise for Your Child with a Cleft Lip and Palate*. Chicago: National Society for Crippled Children and Adults (1959).

McDonald, E. T., *Understand Those Feelings*, Pittsburgh: Stanwix House (1962).

McDonald, E. T., and Koepp-Baker, H., Cleft palate speech: an integration of research and clinical observation. *J. Speech Hearing Dis.*, **16**, 9–20 (1951).

McWilliams, B. J., Some factors in the intelligibility of cleft palate speech. *J. Speech Hearing Dis.*, **19**, 524–527 (1954).

McWilliams, B. J., Articulation problems of a group of cleft palate adults. *J. Speech Hearing Res.*, **1**, 68–74 (1958).

McWilliams, B. J., Communication problems associated with cleft palate. In R. J. Van Hattum (Ed.), *Communication Disorders: An Introduction*. New York: Macmillan Publishing Co., Inc. (1980).

McWilliams, B. J., and Bradley, D. P., Ratings of velopharyngeal closure during blowing and speech. *Cleft Palate J.*, **2**, 46–55 (1965).

McWilliams, B. J., Musgrave, R. H., and Crozier, P., The influence of head position upon velopharyngeal closure. *Cleft Palate J.*, **5**, 117–124 (1968).

McWilliams, B. J., and Musgrave, R. H., Psychological implications of articulation disorders in cleft palate children. *Cleft Palate J.*, **9**, 294–303 (1972).

McWilliams, B. J., and Philips, B. J., Velopharyngeal Incompetence. In H. K. Cooper et al. (Eds.), *Cleft Palate and Cleft Lip: A Team Approach to Clinical Management and Rehabilitation of the Patient*. Philadelphia: W. B. Saunders Co. (1979).

Mecham, M. J., *Verbal Language Development Scale*. Circle Pines, Minn.: American Guidance Service, Inc. (1958).

Moll, K. L., A cinefluorographic study of velopharyngeal function in normals during various activities. *Cleft Palate J.*, **2**, 112–122 (1965).

Moll, K. L., and Shriner, T. H., Preliminary investigation of a new concept of velar activity during speech. *Cleft Palate J.*, **4**, 58–69 (1967).

Morris, H. L., Spriestersbach, D. C., and Darley, F. L., An articulation test for assessing competency of velopharyngeal closure. *J. Speech Hearing Res.*, **4**, 48–55 (1961).

Nation, J. E., A comparative study of comprehension and usage vocabularies of normal and cleft palate preschool children. University of Wisconsin dissertation (1964).

Olson, D. A., A descriptive study of the speech development of a group of infants with unoperated cleft palates. Northwestern University dissertation (1965).

Paradise, J. L., Bluestone, C. D., and Felder, H., The universality of otitis media in 50 infants with cleft palate. *Pediatrics*, **44**, 35 (1969).

Philips, B. J., and Bzoch, K. R., Reliability of judgments of articulation of cleft palate speakers. *Cleft Palate J.*, **6**, 24–34 (1969).

Pitzner, J. C., and Morris, H. L., Articulation skills and adequacy of breath pressure ratios of children with cleft palate. *J. Speech Hearing Dis.*, **31**, 26–40 (1966).

Powers, G. R., Cinefluorographic investigations of articulatory movements of selected individuals with cleft palates. *J. Speech Hearing Res.*, **5**, 59–69 (1962).

Pronovost, W., and Dumbleton, C. A., A picture-type speech sound discrimination test. *J. Speech Hearing Dis.*, **18**, 258–266 (1953).

Schneider, E., and Shprintzen, R. J., A survey of speech pathologists: Current trends in the diagnosis and management of velopharyngeal insufficiency. *Cleft Palate J.*, **17**, 249–253 (1980).

Shames, G. H., and Rubin, H., Psycholinguistic measures of language and speech. In W. C. Grabb, et al. (Eds.), *Cleft Lip and Palate*. Boston: Little, Brown and Company (1971).

Shelton, R. L., Brooks, A. R., and Youngstrom, K. A., Clinical assessment of palatopharyngeal closure. *J. Speech Hearing Dis.*, **30**, 37–43 (1965).

Shelton, R. L., Chisum, L., Youngstrom, K. A., Arndt, W. B., and Elbert, M., Effect of articulation therapy on palatopharyngeal closure, movement of the pharyngeal wall, and tongue posture. *Cleft Palate J.*, **6**, 440–448 (1969).

Simpson, R. K., and Colton, J., A cephalometric study of velar stretch in adolescent subjects. *Cleft Palate J.*, **17**, 40–47 (1980).

Smith, J. O., and Smith, D. D., *Peabody Articulation Decks*. Circle Pines, Minn.: American Guidance Service, Inc. (1975).

Smith, R. M., and McWilliams, B. J., Psycholinguistic considerations in the management of children with cleft palate. *J. Speech Hearing Dis.*, **33**, 26–32 (1968).

Spriestersbach, D. C., Darley, F. L., and Morris, H. L., Language skills in children with cleft palates. *J. Speech Hearing Res.*, **1**, 279–285 (1958).

Spriestersbach, D. C., Darley, F. L., and Rouse, V., Articulation of a group of children with cleft lips and palates. *J. Speech Hearing Dis.*, **21**, 436–445 (1956).

Spriestersbach, D. C., Moll, K. L., and Morris, H. L., Subject classification and articulation of speakers with cleft palates. *J. Speech Hearing Res.*, **6**, 362–371 (1961).

Spriestersbach, D. C., Moll, K. L., and Morris, H. L., Heterogeneity of the "cleft palate population" and research designs. *Cleft Palate J.*, **1**, 210–216 (1964).

Spriestersbach, D. C., and Powers, G. R., Nasality in isolated vowels and connected speech of cleft palate speakers. *J. Speech Hearing Res.*, **2**, 40–45 (1959a).

Spriestersbach, D. C., and Powers, G. R., Articulation skills, velopharyngeal closure and oral breath pressure of children with cleft palates. *J. Speech Hearing Res.*, **2**, 318–325 (1959b).

Spriestersbach, D. C., and Sherman, D. (Eds.), *Cleft Palate and Communication*. New York: Academic Press (1968).

Subcommittee on Cleft Lip and Palate Nomenclature, International Confederation for Plastic and Reconstructive Surgery (1968).

Subtelny, J. D., Koepp-Baker, H., and Subtelny, J. D., Palatal function and cleft palate speech. *J. Speech Hearing Dis.*, **26**, 213–224 (1961).

Subtelny, J. D., Kho, G. H., McCormack, R. M., and Subtelny, J. D., Multidimensional analysis of bilabial stop and nasal consonants—cineradiographic and pressure-flow analysis. *Cleft Palate J.*, **6**, 263–289 (1969).

Subtelny, J. D., Worth, J. H., and Sakuda, M., Intraoral pressure and rate of flow during speech. *J. Speech Hearing Res.*, **9**, 498–518 (1966).

Templin, M. C., A study of sound discrimination ability of elementary school pupils. *J. Speech Dis.*, **8**, 127–132 (1943).

Travis, L. E. (Ed.), *Handbook of Speech Pathology*. (Rev. ed.) New York: Appleton-Century-Crofts (1971).

Van Denmark, D. R., Misarticulation and listener adjustments of the speech of individuals with cleft palates. *Cleft Palate J.*, **1**, 232–245 (1964).

Van Denmark, D. R., A factor analysis of the speech of children with cleft palates. *Cleft Palate J.*, **3**, 159–170 (1966).

Van Denmark, D. R., and Swickard, S. L., A pre-school articulation test to assess velopharyngeal competency: Normative data. *Cleft Palate J.*, **17**, 175–179 (1980).

Van Denmark, D. R., and Van Denmark, A., Misarticulations of cleft palate children achieving velopharyngeal closure and children with functional speech problems. *Cleft Palate J.*, **4**, 31–37 (1967).

Van Hattum, R. J., Articulation and nasality in cleft palate speakers. *J. Speech Hearing Res.*, **1**, 383–387 (1958).

Van Hattum, R. J., *Communication Disorders: An Introduction.* New York: Macmillan and Company, Inc. (1980).

Van Hattum, R. J., and Worth, J. H., Air flow rates in normal speakers. *Cleft Palate J.*, **4**, 137–147 (1967).

Van Riper, C., *Speech Correction: Principles and Methods.* (6th ed.), Englewood Cliffs, N.J.: Prentice-Hall, Inc. (1972).

Van Riper, C., and Irwin, J., *Voice and Articulation.* Englewood Cliffs, N.J.: Prentice-Hall, Inc. (1958).

Veau, V., *Division Palatine.* Paris: Masson (1931).

Warren, D. W., and Mackler, S. B., Duration of oral port constriction in normal and cleft palate speech. *J. Speech Hearing Res.*, **11**, 391–401 (1965).

Wepman, J. M., *Auditory Discrimination Test.* Chicago: Language Research Associates (1958).

7 Communication Therapy for Problems Associated with Cerebral Palsy

Louis M. Di Carlo
Walter W. Amster

THE CEREBRAL PALSY DISORDER

Introduction

Of the many catastrophies that affect living none proves more devastating than forced isolation imposed by communication constraints or failure. Language provides the most economical and least fragile interface between nonverbal cognition and informed verbal communication. For the verbal non-cerebral palsy population these behaviors follow a developmental pattern sequence. The verbal mode precedes reading and writing subsystems, requiring no formal instruction. For many individuals with cerebral palsy, acquisition of competent verbal communication becomes an unachievable, costly, intellectual, emotional, and social purchase.

The literature during the past decade has become rather extensive representing the contributions of many varied professionals. This ever increasing number of inquiries, investigations, and studies of cerebral palsy reflects the magnitude and complexity of problems articulating from and associated with this sensorimotor neurological deficit. Reports frequently appear to disagree, but a careful evaluation of them reveals that the differences are superficial, lie chiefly in ambiguity of definition, elaboration of classification, diversity of examination, variety of diagnostic and habilitation procedures, and the specific sample employed. All investigators strongly advocate the multidisciplinary approach in assessment, diagnosis, and habilitation, stressing the

Grateful acknowledgment and appreciation is expressed to Dr. G. Robert Hopper and Dr. Judith B. Amster for their careful reading and suggestions. Acknowledgment is also extended to Carol G. Cohen for helpful advice relating to augmentive aids for non-speaking children with cerebral palsy and to Sally J. Volk and Beth C. Babok for assistance in the preparation of the Bibliography.

use of basic developmental principles in evaluating the behavior of individuals with cerebral palsy.

Excellent overall accounts of cerebral palsy, dealing with definition, classification, etiology, diagnosis, and habilitation may be explored in the works of Cruickshank and Raus (1955), Denhoff and Robinault (1960), Cruickshank (1966), Keats (1968), Holt and Reynell (1967), and Mysak (1971).

The communication processes of children with cerebral palsy are abundantly stressed in the publications of DiCarlo and Amster (1955), Mecham, Berko, and Berko (1960), McDonald and Chance (1964), Lencione (1966), McDonald and Schultz (1973), DiCarlo (1974), Lencione (1976), and Mysak (1980).

Definitions, Classification, and Epidemiology

Cerebral palsy presents a nonspecific description of a chronic nonprogressive set of neurophysical symptoms such as paralysis, weakness, and incoordination associated with central nervous system deficits. Nevertheless, despite this emphasis on the neurological and physiological aspects, it must be clearly understood that these processes may not only influence, but also contaminate and interfere with the progress of the psychological modalities of audition, vision, perception, intelligence, emotion, and personality in the developing organism (Milner-Brown and Penn, 1979).

Statistics on the incidence of cerebral palsy vary according to the time period in which they are accumulated. Nevertheless, recurrent figures report 7 of every 1,000 new births in the United States each year are cerebral palsy babies. The United Cerebral Palsy Association (1977) estimated the current population of cerebral palsy individuals to be 750,000, at least a third of whom are under twenty-one years of age.

Different authors have classified the conditions associated with cerebral palsy consistent with their predictions for logical meticulosity. A careful study of the various classification systems suggests that the cerebral palsy constellation may be categorized into six principal symptom areas: (1) spasticity, (2) athetosis, (3) cerebellar ataxia, (4) rigidity, (5) tremors, and (6) flaccidity. Other classifications are on the basis of anatomic site of brain lesion, topographic involvement of extremities, degree of muscle tone, severity of involvement and pathology (Perlstein, 1949, 1952; Phelps, 1950; Abbot, 1953; Anderson et al., 1978). These six principal symptom areas may be described as follows:

1. *Spasticity* is characterized by hyperactivity of the stretch reflex, whereby a muscle stretched by the action of its antagonist contracts maximally and therefore cannot perform its release function. It is secondary to a lesion in the cerebral cortex which causes loss of control and differentiation of fine voluntary movements with increased muscle tone. (See figure 7–1.)

2. *Athetosis* is involuntary writhing or squirming movements that are irregular, coarse, relatively continuous, somewhat rhythmic and consist of twelve different types: nontension, tension, rotary, tremor, shudder, emotional release, cerebellar release, deaf athetoid, arm and neck, hemiathetoid, dystonic, and flair. It is secondary to a disturbance in the extrapyramidal system, usually in the basal ganglia. (See figure 7–2.)

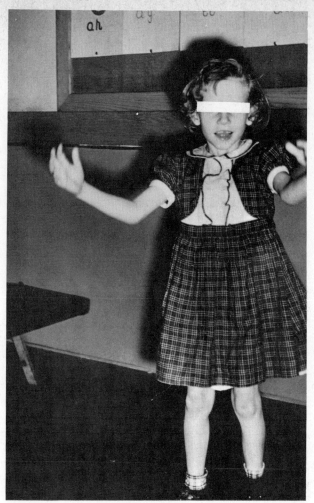

Figure 7–1. A Case with Spasticity of Both Arms and Both Legs (Spastic Quadriplegia). Note the walking posture assumed with reduced sensation in both arms and legs.

3. *Cerebellar Ataxia* is a primary incoordination due to a disruption of the kinesthetic sense and may involve loss of the sense of balance due to cerebellar dysfunction. (See figure 7–3.)

4. *Rigidity* is a "lead-pipe" character of the muscles without any change in the reflexes. If a limb is moved passively, it bends slowly and with difficulty, and when released it does not return to the initial position. Rigidity resembles severe spasticity except in the lack of the stretch reflex.

5. *Tremors* are of two types, athetoid tremor and rigidity tremor, differing in that the second involves a greater tension in the muscles. The picture of tremor is one of a generalized trembling of the extremities involving both the flexors and the extensors. Athetosis, rigidity, and tremors are frequently classified under the term dyskinesia.

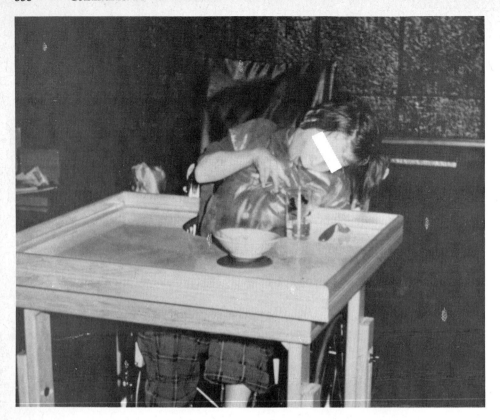

Figure 7–2. A Case with Athetosis. Note the involuntary movement when attempting to sip fluid through a straw.

6. *Flaccidity* in cerebral palsy is usually due to damage to the sensorimotor cortex. The flaccid muscle cannot be contracted voluntarily, although atrophy is not present and the muscle will still respond reflexively.

Ninety percent of the different system constellations are distributed as follows:

Spastic	65 percent
Athetoid	20 percent
Ataxic	5 percent

Denhoff (1976) also includes the mixed category which involves combinations of athetosis, spasticity, rigidity, and ataxia.

Another manner of classifying cerebral-palsied patients stresses the site of the pathology. Those with pyramidal tract lesions include the spastics, who have marked difficulty in executing movement. Lacking inhibitory control over their musculature, they are extremely labored and slow in muscular coordination. A second category, extrapyramidal tract disturbances, accounts for failure of voluntary control over muscular activity. These individuals have motor disturbances characterized by athetosis, rigidity, and tremor. A third category, impairments localized in the cerebellum includes individuals, described as ataxic or atonic, who are unable to synchronize fine

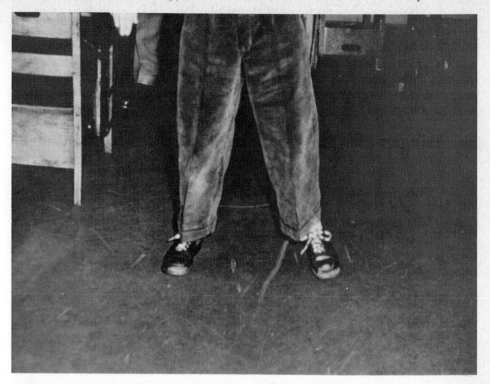

Figure 7–3. An Example of an Ataxic Gait. Note the wide-spreading of the feet when walking.

movements, such as those needed for speech. The impairments in their kinesthetic systems, which signal and coordinate intermuscular feedback relationships are the chief causes of their motor disabilities.

Additional classification schemes, which may be less useful diagnostically but may serve to increase the accuracy of describing the cerebral-palsied patient, differentiate between forms of the disorder according to the number of limbs involved (hemiplegia—one side of body, arm, and leg; paraplegia—legs; diplegia—legs and, to some extent, the arms; and quadriplegia—impairment of both arms and legs). Other classification systems concern the individual's mobility, and the degree of muscle tonus.

Many cerebral-palsied individuals do not show single pure syndromes, although the literature suggests that spasticity and ataxia are less contaminated by the other symptom complexes. Spasticity and athetosis are thought to account for eighty to ninety percent of the cerebral palsied population, with rigidity, tremor, and ataxia accounting for the rest.

Etiologies

Cerebral palsy may result from prenatal, perinatal, and postnatal factors. Among the first group are heritable disorders such as hereditary athetosis, familial tremors, familial spastic paraplegia, Rh factor, infections, prenatal anoxia, placental pathology, maternal anemia, prenatal cerebral hemorrhage, maternal bleeding, and metabolic disturbances. The perinatal factors include all of the conditions and constitutional factors that may obstruct respiration and cause anoxia, such as placenta praevia, breech deliveries, cerebral hemorrhage, contusions, sudden pressure changes and damage from obstetrical intervention. The postnatal factors include cerebral trauma, infections, vascular accidents, anything resulting in anoxia, and any other factors that may affect the central nervous system.

Cerebral palsy is found to be three times greater in premature high-risk infants because of unavoidable intracranial hemorrhages. In full-term babies difficult labor and traumatic deliveries precipitate conditions that may result in cerebral palsy.

Multidisciplinary Considerations

Early intervention embracing the team discipline approach should begin shortly after birth as soon as habilitation measures can be instituted. The first crucial prerequisite in successful management of individuals with cerebral palsy depends on immediate correct medical diagnosis, which embraces the complex expertise and procedures of the different specialties. Fifteen disease entities mimic cerebral palsy and may be misdiagnosed as cerebral palsy. Myopathies, poliomyelitis, myotonic dystrophy, muscle weakness, and delayed motor development are among the possible sources for error (Boyer and Symonds, 1978).

The habilitation process begins even before the individual's birth if the prenatal medical examinations reveal danger signs. Orienting the fetus' parents of the possible complications and preparing them for their roles becomes the responsibility of the team captain. Orthopedic and neurosurgical intervention are carefully and cautiously evaluated and utilized where and when indicated. Sterotaxic neurosurgery, relieving contractures, increasing gamma system activity, tympanic neurectomy to correct drooling, and other procedures to improve function in the habilitation hierarchy may provide some degree of independence for the cerebral palsy person (Vining et al., 1976; Friedman and Kaplan, 1975; Gornall, Hitchcock, and Kirkland, 1975).

In the proper time frame implanted electric stimulation may be selected for certain individuals. Moreover, possible improvement through drug therapy has been explored. Both these approaches have not proved entirely productive. In the therapy programs where implanted electric stimulators were employed in double blind studies, the results revealed that while no deleterious effects were observed, neither was clinical efficiency demonstrated. Sodium dantrolene and diazepam as well as other drugs produced varied results contingent on experimental design, criterion, and controls. These two treatment methodologies are still experimental and need further careful study (Denhoff et al., 1975; Ratusnik et al., 1978; Bensman and Szegho, 1978; Marquis, 1979; Whittaker, 1980; Keats, Morgese, and Nordlund, 1963).

This chapter will concern itself with cerebral palsy as it relates to communication, language and speech impairment, and specifically to the manner and methods of alleviating effects of the disorder in the development of communication abilities in children with cerebral palsy. Variables which contribute to communication difficulties in these children are explored in the opening section, while the balance of the chapter is devoted to a presentation of diagnostic and habilitative procedures.

SPEECH AND LANGUAGE PROBLEMS

Variables Related to Impairment of Language Development

The variables operating to impair language development in the child with cerebral palsy may cover a broad spectrum of interrelated factors. Important in the stages of the child's receptive, associative, and expressive speech and language development include such determinants as possible hearing impairment, visual abnormalities, psychological impairments, sensorimotor integration difficulties, lack of motivation, and reduced physical stamina. In the present context the terms *language* and *speech* as expressive forms must be defined in the broadest possible terms, because they embrace all behaviors, verbal and nonverbal, that link the cerebral-palsied child communicatively with the environment.

Hearing Impairment. Discrepancies exist among many studies reporting incidence, type, and degree of hearing impairment to be found among children with cerebral palsy. The final statistics in any study will be contingent on the definition of hearing impairment, manner of collecting data, methodologies, test material, criteria employed, and sample selected. One survey reports an incidence of 13.4 million people in the United States with some degree of hearing impairment (Schein and Delk 1971). Of these 13.4 million, the authors report 1.8 million deaf of whom 400,000 are prevocationally (under age nineteen) deaf. In addition to being the largest handicapped group, 33 percent of the hearing handicapped have additional handicaps. This survey calculated 6.6 percent of the total population in the United States to have hearing impairments. Stewart (1978) employing a formula derived from an earlier census (Schein and Delk, 1971) estimated 50,965 hearing-impaired, cerebral-palsied persons. A review of the literature verifies the hypothesis that children with cerebral palsy, particularly athetotic, have higher auditory detection thresholds, poorer speech reception thresholds, and discrimination than children without cerebral palsy. Notwithstanding, the possession of normal audiograms does not guarantee adequate auditory functioning. The auditory process develops through the combined influences of maturation and experience, indispensable for speech and language acquisition, but their efficacy is too complex to be assessed by the usual audiometric tests. Assessing the integrity of auditory recognition, auditory memory span for immediate and delayed content, auditory recall, auditory discrimination, synthesis, and closure on the basis of reduction, fractionation, contamination, auditory monitoring, storage and retrieval, all of which are contingent on the efficient functioning of the auditory processes, requires the use of more sophisticated tests.

The important people in the cerebral-palsied child's environment must continue to stimulate the individual to prevent perceptual atrophy through disuse. The child must receive constant auditory stimulation as a pleasant experience, conditioning the individual with a desire for repetition. The parent's voice in the ear while playing with and caressing the child stimulates a powerful incentive to attend. Regardless of the child's responses, audition must continue to be stimulated and integrated with other modalities. It should especially be reinforced with amplification when appropriate and administered within the framework of a systematic auditory training program, resulting in selection of an appropriate amplifying prosthesis.

Visual Impairments. That vision contributes significantly to the development of communication is demonstrated by the speech reading and manual systems of the deaf. In addition, vision permits linguistic decoding when speech utterances are produced concomitantly in environmental noises. Vision also contributes to the fundamental requirements of overall readiness (Barrett, 1965; Betts, 1969; Dechant, 1970; Ekwall, 1978), and numerous studies have emphasized the role of vision and visual perception in reading readiness. The child with cerebral palsy, because of the nature of his or her motor disability, is necessarily restricted in the exploration of his environment. Wolfe (1950) reported 26 percent of his fifty cerebral palsied children had strabismus. He also indicated that this estimate was higher than that found in the normal population but stressed the difficulties involved in testing the visual acuity of these children. His results suggested visual difficulties may be reconciled with the organic involvement for both hemiplegics and triplegics, and permitted him to hypothesize that the injury occurred in that area of the brain located near the one where injury would cause corresponding hemianopsia. Westlake (1951) reported the visual acuity of cerebral palsy children manifested a number of inadequacies, among them near point vision, fusion, and vertical movements of the eyes. The involuntary movements of athetosis interfere with fixation patterns. Palmer (1943, 1949, 1954) also observed that vision as well as auditory phenomena may be replete with distortion, which may interfere with the child's readiness development.

Hopkins, Bice, and Colton (1954) report the vision status of 1,297 children with cerebral palsy. Of these, 21.4 percent had defective vision while 6.2 percent had questionable vision. When the two figures are combined, the percentage of children with defective vision was 27.6 percent. The spastic group comprised 641 individuals, while 328 were classified as athetoid, 176 as rigid, and 152 as ataxic. Of these children, 144 spastics had definite defective vision with 31 questionable, 57 athetoids had defective vision with 10 questionable, and 47 of the ataxics exhibited defective vision with 18 questionable. While a greater number of the spastic individuals had defective vision, the ataxic group had a much larger proportion, almost 43 percent with defective vision.

Dunsdon (1952) reports that of 575 children with cerebral palsy, nearly one third of them exhibited visual defects. She was interested in implications of visual defects for reading and also postulated that the prevalence of convergent defects among these children might in part account for their general poor spatial ability.

Duckman (1979) investigated the incidence of visual abnormalities in a population of cerebral palsy children. An earlier study (Breakey, Wilson and Wilson, 1974) investigating 120 children with cerebral palsy, 60 quadraplegia athetoids and 60 spastics, found 9 visual anomalies: refractory errors, acuity at $^{20}/_{40}$ or less, optic atrophy amblyopia, muscle imbalance, visual field defects, less than 60 percent fusion on the Wirt Dot Test, gaze palsy or paresis, and rotational abnormalities. In only one category, fusion, the spastics' errors exceed those made by the athetoids. Both groups made errors in tracking, accommodation, refraction, ocular posture, eye-hand coordination, visual acuity, and ocular motor dysfunction, and both reflected poor directional concepts and visual perceptional dysfunction. These deficits certainly influence perception and cognitive development and mandate integrated programs negating or minimizing these deleterious effects. Programs that integrate the interdisciplinary contributions of the different specialties should be designed to promote stimulation, motivation, and facilitation among the modalities.

Tactual and Kinesthetic Impairments. Likewise, the refinement of tactual experiences may provide further essentials for overall perceptive development leading to "readiness." Dolphin and Cruickshank (1952) observed that tactual motor perception for children with cerebral palsy was poorer than for non-cerebral palsied children. Westlake (1951) suggests that while children with cerebral palsy may be aware of tactual sensation they experience difficulty in pinpointing the source and consequently are unable to capitalize on these sensation cues in the organization of their motor behavior.

Speech development proceeds sequentially and efficiently if the total sensorium becomes integrated as part of the learning process. Wherever the sensorium fails to facilitate discrimination and differentiation in the communication network, acquisition of speech is delayed or arrested. Speech in a communication framework functions as adjustment stimuli whose effects are circulatory.

Intellectual Impairments. Besides encountering speech and language problems associated with their sensorimotor deficits, children with cerebral palsy may share the learning difficulties of the mentally retarded. A study by Hopkins, Bice and Colton (1954), in fact, found that half of one group of 933 cerebral palsied children had IQs below 70.

More recently Capute (1974) reports 50 to 60 percent of the cerebral palsied population to be retarded while the remaining 40 to 50 percent that possess normal intelligence evidence a learning disability due to the presence of perceptual-cognitive deficiencies. But even without mental retardation, if the motor involvement is severe enough, a cerebral palsied child may have trouble with the development of receptive and expressive language, thereby resulting in deficit intelligence scores on standardized tests. This does not mean, however, that the child's decoding will have no incoming linguistic competence or performance. All individuals conceptualize latent grammatical forms before expressing them in speech. For example, when a mother feeds her infant, the milk or formula may be said to represent a semantic content, while the actual feeding may be called a syntax, since it involves a subject (the mother) administering to an agent (the infant). All such actions, as well as the infant's indications of discomfort and the mother's resulting relieving behaviors, may be viewed as having a linguistic form and communicative effect.

In attempts to distinguish between communication disorders of mentally retarded and non-mentally retarded cerebral-palsied children, psychometric evaluation of very young children has not proved reliable. Psychologists, therefore, have tried to refine the test situations and materials over the past few years, concentrating on the use of sensorimotor, nonverbal behavior tasks. Each improvement in validity and reliability has led to a higher estimate of the incidence of mental retardation among the cerebral palsied. The problem, of course, is complicated by the finding that while mentally retarded children with cerebral palsy tend to show the same kind of speech development behavior as non-cerebral-palsied mentally retarded children, other children with cerebral palsy (non-mentally retarded) also tend to show some delay in speech development. Once the developmental process has begun, however, their speaking rate and growth profiles resemble those of normal children.

Socio-Emotional Factors. Even with children who do not suffer from cerebral palsy, the development of receptive and expressive language may be thwarted by such environmental factors as insufficient stimulation and motivation, improper teaching methods, unrealistic aspirations for them, excessive parental or environmental pressures, bilingual conflicts, emotional trauma, lack of good speech models, parental rejection, overprotection, and ambivalence (Palmer, 1943; Hood, Shank and Williamson, 1948).

The cerebral-palsied child may be subject to all of the above influences and more. Where the non-cerebral-palsied child tends to move away from his parents in a quest for psychological freedom, the cerebral-palsied child, because of his limited mobility, must undergo a prolonged period of infantile dependency, during which time parental conflicts of rejection and overprotection prevent their recognition of the child's needs. To forestall harmful effects on the child's personality and communicative development, training efforts in the home should begin early to foster the family's understanding and acceptance of the child's principal deficit (Johnson, 1956). The parents, therefore, must become integral members of the multidisciplinary team. Through conferences and training, parents learn to manipulate the environment conducive to learning and adjusting. Parents sophisticated through interdisciplinary conferences modify the environment by the knowledge transmitted and team participation. Under these conditions psychological cohesiveness and integration will result and a trust bond between child and parent will eventually permit the child to accept himself or herself with persistent satisfaction, be accepted by peers, and function within self-imposed, rather than externally imposed, achievement levels. Child-parent relationships will circumvent destructive self-pity, foster learning and adjustment, reinforce a worthy self-concept, and move toward a happy, contributing life.

Readiness Factors. The concept of readiness pertains to the fact that children normally appear to acquire particular behaviors at specific stages of development. Only when they have mastered certain prerequisite skills and behaviors can they begin to learn new ones. The speech readiness period, defined by Stinchfield-Hawk and Young (1938), Johnson et al. (1967), Berry (1969), Menyuk (1974), and Muma (1978) as occurring in normal children from twelve to eighteen months, may actually extend to forty-two months. The beginning of this period depends partially on the child's physiological, social, and psychological development. If the child does not develop speech within or shortly after this period, he is considered to have delayed speech.

If a child is pressured into trying to learn speech before he is ready, the tensions produced by the frustrating attempt may interfere with his later, satisfactory learning; or it may produce partial learning, which leads to inadequate responses to communication. This observation is particularly apt in relation to the cerebral-palsied child, whose motor deficit retards the usual maturation processes. Where normal children lay the groundwork for adequate speech and language development by integrating hearing, vision, touch, and movement through their explorations of the world around them, the cerebral-palsied child, being severely restricted in his exploratory activities, does not readily acquire the necessary skills of stimulus generalization and discrimination. The situation is not improved by the losses in auditory, visual, and tactile perception that so often accompany cerebral palsy.

Why some cerebral-palsied children seem able to develop receptive and expressive language without training, while others have difficulty despite long training periods, depends not only on environment, mental ability, hearing, and readiness, but also on such additional factors as how much control they have over their muscles of speech and associated movements, how ambidextrous they are, how many seizures they have, and the function of their oral speech structures. Specific disorders, however, can be treated with dental appliances and certain aids for helping a child obtain control over involuntary behavior.

Variables Related to Impairment of Speech Production

An examination of the literature reveals that about 70 percent of children with cerebral palsy have speech impairments with even higher incidences among athetoids and ataxics (Wolfe, 1950; Dunsdon, 1952; Hopkins, Bice and Colton, 1954). However, there appears to be insufficient evidence for the notion that these impairments are so distinctive as to justify the concept of a specific, distinctive "cerebral-palsy speech."

The idea that the utterances of individuals with cerebral palsy can be identified by their prosodic linguistic features of loudness, pitch, rate, rhythm, and quality has prompted a number of investigations. In an early study, Rutherford (1940) concluded that, in general, the utterances of children with cerebral palsy did not differ significantly in these features from those of non-cerebral-palsied children, but she did think that the productions of athetoids were somewhat slower and more jerky than those of spastics. Differences in communication characteristics were noted by Hyman (1952), who measured and compared the relative sound pressure levels and durations of the speech responses of spastic, athetoid, and non-cerebral-palsied children to oral stimuli. He reported that the athetoids spoke more slowly than spastics and responded to intensity levels, whereas the spastics responded to the duration of stimuli. On the basis of his findings he advocated the use of different therapy approaches for the different groups of children with cerebral palsy.

The opinion that the speech of athetoids is slower, more labored, and more arhythmic than that of spastics still persists to some degree. Shapiro (1960), in a carefully designed investigation, could not confirm that concept. In fact, his research strongly suggested that no distinctive "cerebral-palsy speech" truly exists, in terms of quantity and type of errors or manner of production. Hopper (1968) studied the speech sound learning ability of a selected group of cerebral-palsied children and compared their efforts with a control group. The children were selected on the basis of range of intelligence, age, language abilities and speech intelligibility. Both groups were taught three unfamiliar phonemes not found in their native language, English. Results indicated that the two groups learned the sounds with equal facility.

Research into the speech production impairments of the cerebral palsied has centered upon the variables of respiration, phonation, and articulation.

Respiration and Phonation. Hull (1940); Perlstein and Shere (1946); Gratke (1947); Palmer (1949, 1950); Wolfe (1950); Rutherford (1950); Westlake (1951) and

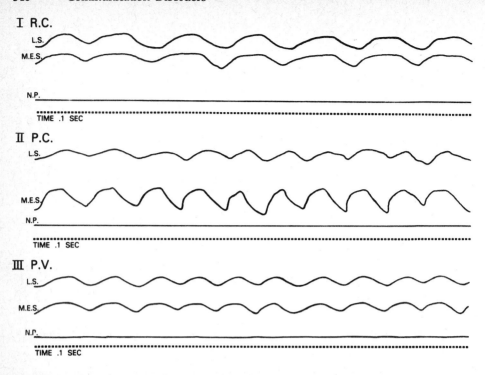

I R.C.
L.S.
M.E.S.
N.P.
TIME .1 SEC

II P.C.
L.S.
M.E.S.
N.P.
TIME .1 SEC

III P.V.
L.S.
M.E.S.
N.P.
TIME .1 SEC

Figure 7–4. Sample of One-Minute Kymograms of Silent Breathing for Three Normal Children. Pneumographic tracings of chest movements in the three subjects are shown by the L.S. (lower sternum region) lines in each set, and of abdominal movements, by the MES. (mesogastric region) lines. The N.P. (negative pressure) lines record syllable pulse movements taken at the epigastric region. Since there are no chest pulses in silent breathing, the N.P. lines are smooth. The chief difference in the three kymograms is in the greater amplitude of abdominal wall movement in the center set.

others imply a relationship between speech inadequacy and breathing abnormalities among the cerebral palsied. Hull (1940) studied the respiratory behavior of fourteen cerebral-palsied children classified as spastics. She obtained kymograph recordings during silent and speech breathing. Her analysis of the results revealed that the silent breathing of the children in her experiments deviated from that of children without cerebral palsy. Under speech situations the breathing anomalies increased. Increasing the complexity of the speech materials did not affect the breathing abnormalities. During speech her children exhibited unusual amounts of thoracic expansion. During breathing her children maintained the position of thorax for an unusually long portion of the respiratory cycle. Out of phase thoracic-abdominal movements occurred both during silent and speech breathing. Palmer (1949, 1950) reports the presence of breathing problems including gross deviations from the predictable time and amplitude of the inspiratory-expiratory movements, shallow breathing, thoracic-abdominal opposition, and little or no abdominal excursion.

Cypreanson (1953) studied the breathing and speech coordinations of twenty-five cerebral palsied and twenty-five non-cerebral-palsied children and the relationship of the breathing movements to speech intelligibility. Her cerebral palsy sample comprised ten spastics, thirteen athetoids, and two ataxics. Her criteria for the selection of

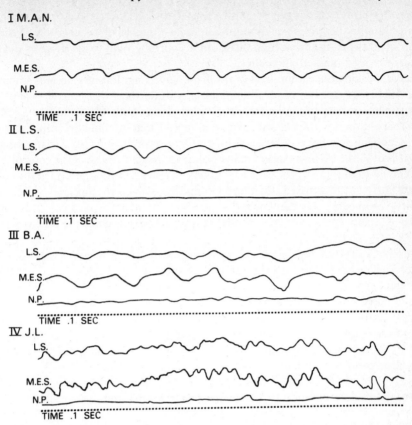

Figure 7–5. Sample of One-Minute Kymograms of Silent Breathing for Four Cerebral-Palsied Children. The first subject, M.A.N. (triplegia spastic, moderate extent), is the best speaker of the four. The second one, L.S. (athetoid quadriplegia, moderate extent), is a fair speaker. Her tracings reveal less abdominal than chest amplitude and a slight indication of the syllable pulse. Sharp contrasts are shown in the kymograms of the third and fourth subjects. B.A. (athetoid quadriplegia, severe extent) recorded irregular chest and abdominal cycles, with slight ripples in the former indicating the possibility of the athetoid movement. As noted by the N.P. line, there was an excursion of the chest pulse, indicating the use of muscles ordinarily applied in speaking. J.L. (athetoid quadriplegia, moderately severe extent), is the poorest speaker of the four. Excessive chest and abdominal movements, out of phase at many points, indicate difficulty in silent breathing and poor speech.

the cerebral palsy sample included an age range of eight to twelve years, exhibition of speech impairments, possession of normal intelligence, and normal hearing, and the ability to read second-grade material. These children were examined and diagnosed by a certified member of either the American Academy of Cerebral Palsy or the American Board of Orthopedic Surgeons. The non-cerebral palsy samples were matched in age, sex, intelligence, hearing, and reading level. Silent and speech breathing records were obtained by means of a variable speed kymograph as illustrated in figures 7–4 and 7–5. Samples of speech were recorded on a Magnecorder and audited by trained listeners.

Cypreanson's results for silent breathing revealed that the cerebral palsy group had a greater number of cycles per minute than the controls. The kymograph configuration for good speakers approached those of the control group, while those of the poor speakers revealed marked anomalies.

During speaking the cerebral palsy group employed significantly greater amount of time, number of phrases, and abdominal amplitude than the control group. Her findings with respect to abdominal amplitude concur with Westlake's observations (1951) that children with cerebral palsy tend to maintain infantile breathing patterns. When Cypreanson analyzed her speech breathing records, she found that configuration patterns of the better speakers in her group approached those of the control group more closely than those of the poorer speakers. Analysis of the speech rhythm of the cerebral palsy group stressed the interrelationship between rhythm and speech intelligibility. Moreover, she emphasized that time, number of phrases, and rhythm correlated significantly with speech intelligibility. The speech of the athetoid group was the least intelligible.

Not only is rhythm dependent upon breath control, but phonation is as well. (See chapter 5.) The control of the air column affects the action of the vocal cords and the glottis, and laryngeal adjustment and phonation must be integrated with the movements of breathing and synchronized with the syllable pulses. Cerebral palsied children may not be able to sustain phonation long enough for adequate phrasing, and they are vulnerable to vocal abuse in their struggling attempts at voice production. Wolfe (1950) reported a high incidence of breathing anomalies and rate difference for his cerebral palsy subjects.

Articulation. Intelligibility is the chief criterion for judging the speech production of cerebral-palsied children as well as of other groups. Speech is a dynamic process requiring highly skilled coordination of the articulatory movements in the production and sequencing of sounds into words and sentences. Analysis of consonant and vowel production and other variables has revealed that the consonants are most important to the intelligibility of a speaker, especially if the rhythm of the sentence preserves its contextual integrity.

Heltman and Peacher (1943) investigated misarticulation and diadochokinesis among 102 children with spastic paralysis with an age range of four to twenty-five years and compared them with 159 non-spastic individuals with speech difficulties with an age range of eight to fifteen years. They found the paralysis of the articulatory mechanism accounted for approximately 50 percent of the speech difficulties. They reported greater significant differences for spastics between rate of lips and tongue movement when phonating than when not. They also found the lingual-rugal sounds most difficult for them and recommended a program of exercises for the tongue, lips, jaw, and velum. Wolfe (1950) evaluated the involvement of the peripheral speech mechanism for 50 cerebral palsy children and reported that the involvement of lip musculature to be greatest with respiration, tongue, velum, larynx, and mandible following in that order. Of these subjects 70 percent had articulatory difficulty. Rutherford (1944) evidenced interest in the analysis of the frequency of articulatory substitution in children with cerebral palsy. She reported definite and persistent sound substitutions for speech-impaired children. She found the sounds [s], [z], [l], and [θ] were misarticulated most frequently. Dunsdon (1952) reported a high incidence of articulatory difficulty in her study. Among the athetoids she described, speech was often accompanied by facial grimacing and movements from other parts of the body. Beginning and controlling movements of the articulatory musculature may be associated with abnormalities of swallowing.

Corroborating these essential findings of articulatory difficulty in children with cerebral palsy are investigations by Irwin (1972), Iandoli (1958), Byrne (1959), Hardy (1961), Hixon and Hardy (1964), Netsell (1969), Kent and Netsell (1978), and Love, Hagerman, and Taimi (1980). In addition, recent investigations of articulatory difficulties in adults with cerebral palsy indicated that such disorders continue into adulthood (Platt et al., 1978; Platt et al., 1980).

Other Related Factors. Rutherford (1944) conducted a comparative investigation of loudness, pitch, rate, rhythm and quality of speech for cerebral and non-cerebral-palsied children. Her cerebral palsy sample contained forty-eight children classified as athetoids and seventy-four as spastics. Her control contained sixty-nine children.

She rated the speech status of her children and classified them into two subgroups, one having good speech, and the other defective speech. She concluded from her study that in general the trends in loudness, pitch, rate, rhythm, and quality for the cerebral palsy group resembled those of her control group. She carefully stressed that her study did not reveal a specific type of speech production which could be labeled as cerebral palsy speech. Nevertheless, her investigation provided her with some cues for differentiating between the speech of the athetoid and spastic groups. The athetotic cerebral-palsied in her group used "slower, more jerky speech" than the spastic children. In the athetoid group there also appeared to be more loud voices, more low-pitched voices, more monŏtonous, and more breathy voices. The differences between the groups were attributed in part to the control and function of the breathing mechanism.

Palmer (1953) suggests that laryngeal blocks might interfere with adequate phonation. He calls attention to the proper functioning of the intrinsic laryngeal structure in consummating the delicate adjustment of the vocal cords for satisfactory glottal vocal attack for speaking. Westlake (1951) noted variation among the cerebral palsied in their ability to phonate and to prolong phonation. There is a manifest need for further specific information concerning the coordinated role of respiration, phonation, and articulation, as well as information on resonance and cerebration in the communication process and performance of children with cerebral palsy.

THE DIAGNOSTIC PROCESS

The speech and language habilitation program for the cerebral-palsied child should have clearly defined general and specific objectives, based upon the child's communication potential. It should be coordinated and integrated with other therapeutic programs, such as physiotherapy and occupational therapy, and it should be a "team" effort. That is, the therapists in charge of the individual programs should discuss the child's status and progress among themselves in order to direct their efforts toward the common goal of helping the child realize the maximum potential for growth.

The objectives, of course, should not be chosen arbitrarily. They should be rooted instead in the diagnostic assessment—a necessarily global evaluation of the child's motor impairment, intelligence, hearing, speech, language, social, and educational potentials. In particular, the specific concomitants of cerebral palsy (deafness, mental retardation, congenital aphasia, and emotional maladjustments) require meticulous assessment and clarification. This process has been assisted by the implementation of PL 94–142 in 1974 which, through the Individual Educational Plan (IEP), provides a defined structure for this approach.

The process of diagnosis and therapy are interrelated in that, though they may be considered as separate aspects of a single dynamic phenomenon, it is often difficult to tell where the one ends and the other begins. Evaluation and reappraisal are continuous and include an ongoing reorganization of experience. If the continuity of a diagnostic-therapeutic continuum is lost, so that diagnosis and evaluation only precede the actual formulation and initiation of a therapeutic program, the ability to anticipate and predict frustrating situations is lost, and the program may become too rigid to permit satisfactory learning for the child. Ideally, the diagnostic-therapeutic continuum should provide a matrix within which the child's aspirations and achievements may be reconciled, maturation may be stimulated, and self-concept may be sufficiently developed to permit the child to help establish learning goals. Such an orientation minimizes conflict between the aspiration levels of the child, the clinician, and the parents.

Evaluation of the communicative status of children with cerebral palsy requires an analysis of factors that both arrest and facilitate speech behavior. Evaluation procedures should use multisensory, motor, psychological, and sociological developmental cues within the framework of differential diagnosis. When an adequate evaluation of the cerebral-palsied child's motor impairment has been completed and case-history and data has been placed in the most useful perspective, the analysis should present a realistic profile of the child's developmental status and needs.

The following case study, by way of negative example, points up the importance of a realistic and adequate evaluation. On the positive side, it shows the value of ongoing diagnostic review.

R. M. K., a three-year-old girl enrolled in a Head Start program, was shown, in a complete physical and neurological examination, to be a cerebral-palsied child with athetosis with a moderate degree of involvement and a good prognosis for functional movement. But clues to hearing and learning difficulties were apparently obscured by the "halo effect"; the child's attractiveness and her membership in a very prominent family interfered with an unbiased assessment of her competence and performance, and consequently prevented the development of an adequate training approach.

Although the child could not be formally tested for intellectual capacity, her performance on several developmental scales and her failure to have developed any significant vocabulary or linguistic ability did alert the psychologist to the possibility of reduced intellectual potential. His report, however, was not consulted in the planning of the habilitation program.

In tests of the child's hearing, formal audiological procedures were unsuccessful, and informal techniques employing physiological cues (acoustic reflex, startle reflex, localization, and observation of response to auditory stimulus) suggested that she might possess satisfactory detection thresholds. On the basis of the administered tests and observations, it was concluded that she had normal hearing. Electrodermal Response (EDR) and Electroencephalographic (EEG) audiometry were not used.

The subsequent habilitation program did not emphasize a systematic and concentrated auditory training approach, and when the child did not appear to develop speech and language commensurate with the time devoted to instruction, she was referred to a diagnostic center for evaluation. Extensive and sophisticated testing confirmed her possession of normal auditory detection thresholds, but it unequivocally demonstrated serious deficits in all of the auditory processes.

Because the auditory processes had not been suspect, two years of habilitation efforts had shown no maturation or improvement in any spontaneous linguistic behavior.

R. M. K. had improved in motor behavior, but her language development had not kept pace.

At five years of age, R. M. K. was transferred to a training center, but without any further evaluation until one was initiated three years later because of a change in the center's administrative staff. At this time the disturbances in the child's auditory processes, and her linguistic, memory, and general learning deficits were explicitly demonstrated and diagnosed. To complicate the problem in the meanwhile, the child had developed serious behavior problems. Her achievement level was inconsistent with expectations for her. She began withdrawing, developed enuresis, and showed anxiety reactions to test situations. She was uncooperative, and destructive, and distracting to classmates and others.

A program, constructed within the framework of the child's limitations and proper diagnosis, was inaugurated. Although the early insufficient diagnosis and inadequate planning had resulted in seven unremunerative years—years of learning disability and unadjustive habit formation—the new habilitation program began to lead to improved communication behavior and a more satisfactory emotional adjustment. The professional staff felt that the prognosis for further improvement, despite the years of delay, was much more encouraging.

Audiological Evaluation

As the preceding case of R. M. K. has illustrated, more is needed for a child's proper auditory functioning than just normal sound detection thresholds. That is, even when their hearing thresholds fall within normal limits, children with cerebral palsy may present speech perception problems, for, being easily distracted by high environmental noise levels (at or above 70 dB), they develop selective listening habits to exclude as well. The possibility of serious learning disabilities that are concomitant with disturbances of the auditory processes thus require that tests of the cerebral-palsied child's hearing embrace all of the other developmental variables. The testing should be undertaken as early as possible in the child's development because of its implications for speech and language performance.

Research has revealed that reflex and startle cues can be used early in the appraisal of a child's hearing acuity, for if unexpected or loud sounds evoke automatic motor responses, the child may have functional hearing. Furthermore, if the child looks or moves toward sound, these cues may be interpreted to mean that the child has a useful level of auditory acuity. The introduction of sounds in different frequencies and intensities in a sound field, with the child resting in the mother's lap, may also elicit responsive behavior.

Many of the procedures employed in testing the hearing of non-motor-handicapped children can be used with cerebral-palsied children if adapted to offset the effects of motor impairment on their responses. Such adaptations usually center on increasing attention to acoustic events by making the testing experience as pleasurable as possible and on forcing the child to make discriminatory responses to auditory stimuli by appropriately structuring the didactic-diagnostic situation.

Parents often must be asked to take part in the testing situation and instructed sufficiently in the procedure to provide the observer of the parent-child communication patterns with useful diagnostic cues. This technique may provide more useful information than any other in assisting the examiner to estimate the child's mental and social levels through his responses, adaptation, and learning performance.

In testing the auditory perception of the child who exhibits delayed speech, such as the cerebral-palsied child, significance should be attached to the presence or absence of gesture interaction, facial expression, unintelligible vocalization, and stereotyping of response. Children whose speech development is still delayed at five years of age or more may seem to be able to hear because they respond to speech. In identifying words, however, they may capitalize on such cues as the more intense vowel sounds, and they may fail to perceive the consonants, even the voiced ones. Unless the testing materials are so structured that the phonetic contours of the test words are similar except in the one element which carries the meaning, these children may be misclassified. If the failure of consonant perception is due to a moderate or severe hearing loss—and the distinction may be a difficult one for the examiner to make—the child may develop serious habits of inattention since the few acoustic cues which remain may interfere with the association of meaning to auditory symbols.

Discrepancies exist among the many estimates of incidence, magnitude, and type of hearing impairment found among children with cerebral palsy, but a careful comparison of criteria, methodologies, and test material employed by various investigators permits the hypothesis that some children with cerebral palsy, particularly the athetoids, have distinctly poorer auditory thresholds, as mentioned earlier. Many of these findings have been postulated on the basis of tests that require subject motor participation and qualitative judgment by the examiner of the subject's responses to pure tones, speech, and environmental noises, employing locational and play audiometry techniques.

In many of the children with cerebral palsy, the apparent auditory deficits represent failure of the functioning of information transmission, assembly orientation, coding, storage, organization, and retrieval at different levels because of the more intense attention the child with cerebral palsy must devote to kinesthetic sense demands in order to maintain equilibrium and achieve homeostasis. Hearing and listening become fleeting phenomena that do not appear to operate within the modern learning paradigm. Auditory fixations are too infrequent and evanescent to permit the establishment of conditional behavior clusters indispensable for normal language and speech acquisition.

For difficult to test subjects, especially children with cerebral palsy, a search for objectivity fostered the development of electrodermal, and electroencephalic audiometry (DiCarlo, Kendall, Goldstein, 1962). Although not all investigators agree on its efficacy, electrodermal (EDR) audiometry, has been used for testing hearing acuity where regular audiometry is not successful. However, electrodermal audiometry has not proved productive for children with cerebral palsy because of their neurophysiological disability.

As in the case of electrodermal audiometry, cortical electroencephalic audiometry (EEA) or the Cortical Evoked Response was used rather extensively during the 1960s. While initially promising, these measures have not proved sufficiently reliable. The inherent problems in administration and interpretation have negated the use of EEG procedures for auditory assessment with difficult-to-test populations. By the early 1970s using procedures which transcend the limitations of earlier EEG auditory assessment techniques, investigators succeeded in specifying more accurate organic hearing configuration levels through the use of brainstem response to acoustic stimuli.

Spastic and athetoid cerebral palsy children's violent stretch reflexes and involuntary movement to auditory stimulation provide problems but do not preclude use of these techniques for auditory diagnosis.

In investigations of the difficulties in assessing the auditory status of children with cerebral palsy, Haberfellner and Müller (1976a) examined the influence of tonic reflex patterns on the auditory evoked potential (AEP) in normal adults and normal-hearing cerebral palsy children. The normal subjects adopted postures which correspond to tonic reflex patterns in the cerebral palsied. In a related investigation (Haberfellner and Müller, 1976b), these authors pursued the effect of Bobath's reflex inhibiting patterns (r.i.p.), a key procedure in Bobath therapy, on the processing of acoustic stimuli. Their findings revealed changes in amplitude and suppression of evoked potential responses possibly leading to false responses. It is important to note, however, that the slow auditory evoked potential may be recorded from any part of the skull. It is nonspecific, demands alertness, and strict attention, and is probably not productive with difficult-to-test subjects. Moreover, movement may displace the electrodes introducing degrading conditions. Abnormality of cortical evoked potential response may be generated by non-auditory stimulation. Cochleography and brainstem audiometry, especially with sedated subjects, provides a useful approach. Furthermore, latency, rather than amplitude, may be a better criterion for normality. The authors report significant differences in dB between induced and relaxed positions. However, the actual dB difference is less than 5 dB which is accepted as a tolerance limit for nonsignificant change. The values presented offer no pragmatic significance. The authors further report significant improvement in cerebral palsy children, attributing the improvement to the Bobath therapy reflex inhibiting patterns. Whether the gains have practical significance, and whether the influence of the r.i.p.'s alone actually influence central processing, requires further research involving a larger population and control of all but the independent variable. Also, the contribution of threshold in central processing needs clarification.

The research on evoked potential responses by different investigators and the continuous sophisticated update of equipment favors this procedure as the one of choice for the early detection of thresholds among difficult-to-test individuals, including cerebral palsy children.

Language Evaluation

Comprehension of language, as the precursor of speech, may be estimated during the administration of any testing procedure that requires the child to identify objects with or without background figures, follow directions, comprehend language, make discriminatory responses, exhibit recall, and indicate generalization of experiences which do not require verbal output. As stated earlier in this chapter, for the cerebral-palsied child, language and speech must be viewed as including all behaviors that link him communicatively with his environment.

That careful evaluation can delineate between groups of cerebral-palsied was demonstrated by the work of Myers (1965), who used the Illinois Test of Psycholinguistic Abilities (Kirk, McCarthy and Kirk, 1968) in a study of the language disabilities of thirty-eight spastics, twenty-four athetoids, and thirty-two normal subjects. On the basis of his findings, Myers reported that the subscales of the ITPA differentiated between the three groups. That is, the spastic children performed more adequately than the athetoid children on the automatic sequential tasks, while the athetoids were better than the spastics at representational tasks, and the normal subjects performed more adequately on all subtests. These results should be compared with Love's (1964) finding that when the linguistic skills of cerebral-palsied children are measured when they are older, they tend to approximate those of normal children of the same age and intellectual capacity.

To test comprehension ability, items may be drawn from a number of sources for testing performances at different ages. Such sources include the Stanford-Binet (1972), the Wechsler Intelligence Scale for Children (Wechsler, 1974), the Wechsler Preschool and Primary Scale of Intelligence (Wechsler, 1967), and others. Information concerning comprehension of more specific linguistic aspects can be obtained from measures such as the Test for Auditory Comprehension of Language (Carrow, 1973), which does not require verbal output by the child. Certain subtests of the Test of Language Development (Newcomer and Hammill, 1977) are also of value in assessing language ability as well as the phonological skills of word discrimination and articulation. The Callier-Azusa Scale (Stillman, 1976), developed for multi-handicapped children, assesses a wide range of behavior including receptive and expressive language, as does the Developmental Potential of Preschool Children (Haeussermann, 1958), which was specifically designed for use with cerebral-palsied children. Wiig and Semel (1976) provide a well-organized review of cognitive and linguistic instruments.

The examiner using these measures should be aware of the normal verbal output and comprehension levels for various age groups, and should be prepared to modify the tests so that the child's handicaps will not penalize him. Even then, the test results should be regarded as rough estimates, to be interpreted with great caution. The enactment of PL 94–142 legally mandates nondiscriminatory evaluation for the handicapped, necessitating even greater attention to removal of bias in the testing situation for the cerebral-palsied child. Presentation and response modalities of all instruments used must be evaluated and modified as required if results are to be considered useful.

The comprehension measures obtained in the testing situation should further be compared with the parents' reports of their child's performance at home. This comparison should throw some light on parent-child adjustment and on the child's motivation, mode of communication, functioning in the home situation, and social adjustment. The Parent-Child Communication Inventory (MacDonald, 1973) not only permits language assessment in the home setting but serves to involve parents in the diagnostic process. The Vineland Social Maturity Scale (Doll, 1965) or the Cain-Levine Social Competency Scale (1964) may profitably be used at this point to amplify other data.

The child's acquisition of semantic distinctions or features of language, by which he or she is able to express needs and manipulate and control the environment, may be tested by developmental scales. In particular, the receptive semantic level may be evaluated with vocabulary tests, although Menyuk (1971) has cautioned that these instruments may not yield adequate measures for the language-impaired child, who may follow different semantic rules than the normal child.

An examination of the child's verbal output may reveal the fluency in formulating levels of abstraction consistent with group norms, the inflexibility or flexibility in language use, and semantic ability as related to the environment. Methods suggested by Lee (1974) and Menyuk (1971) for eliciting language are relevant. Principles developed by Hayakawa (1949) and Johnson (1946) may prove worthwhile in analyzing the cerebral-palsied child's use of language, both in terms of its semantic level and its implications concerning the child's readiness for further learning. Chapter 1 and chapter 2 include a review of some language scales designed to assess different language parameters.

Speech Evaluation

The ultimate aim of speech is intelligible communication. Verbal output which is so distorted that it does not unite the speaker with the listener fails to achieve this objective and may even militate against it. Consequently, it becomes imperative for the examiner to weight the effectiveness of the child's speech production. Such evaluation of speech production must consider at least the three basic processes of respiration, phonation, and articulation. Westlake (1951) suggests a breakdown of these processes for the cerebral-palsied child into certain "critical skills: breathing, phonation, chewing, closing the mouth, elevating the tip of the tongue, and peristaltic movement," and sets up minimum quantitative rates and measures for speech musculature movement. He further discusses the acts involved in speaking as patterns of continuous movement rather than isolated behavior acts. He emphasizes the vital importance of initiating and sustaining tone for adequate breathing patterns and the early solicitation of the physical therapist in the preparatory activities of head and feet balance, and strengthening of the arms and shoulders. Rutherford (1950) employed an examination format for assessing the speech act of cerebral-palsied children. In her examination, Rutherford was concerned with certain aspects of phonation, voice quality, volume, and pitch rate. She also concerned herself with the effects of rhythm on intelligibility, as well as with the distractive effects of extraneous movements. Cass (1951) attempted to develop a diagnostic framework which would provide cues for "motor re-educational speech therapy." She was interested in rate, range and strength of function in her quest for residual speech abilities.

Speech Coordinations. Speech consists of a series of rapid, highly skilled movements of the breathing and articulatory muscles. The speed of normal speech tends toward high speed, during which the units cluster about minimal limits. Speech movements progress on the expiration phase of respiration and involve all of the articulatory musculature, which are finely integrated into a unitary culminative movement. Speech movements, like all highly skilled movements, have thresholds of maximum physiological limits and rates.

The ballistic movements of the chest muscles produce the syllable pulse, which Stetson (1951) demonstrated to be the fundamental unit of speech, while the larger abdominal muscles support the action of the chest musculature in producing a series of syllables and fusing these syllables into a single breath-group or phrase on the expiratory phase of respiration. These coordinated speech movements of the expirative phase of respiration offer some cues for the analysis of speech among cerebral-palsied children.

Respiration. Before the speech act can be effective, it must be based upon adequate breath control (Stetson, 1951). Stetson pioneered in clarifying the relationship between silent breathing and speech breathing. By refining and perfecting the kymographic methods of recording the breathing and speech movements, he was able to indicate that breathing and speaking occur as a single unitary process and that the musculature involved followed the behavior of all muscles in general.

Rutherford (1950), Westlake (1951), Palmer (1950), Hull (1940), and others in early research and clinical observation have indicated that cerebral-palsied children manifest irregularities of breathing patterns. They do not all differentiate between silent breathing and speech breathing. No general agreement of criteria exists nor does a standardization of measuring instrumentation.

Hull (1940) and Cypreanson (1953) suggested the use of the kymograph for distinguishing between silent and speech breathing and evaluating the total speech process with respect to respiration. Where the kymographic facilities are available they should be employed as a clinical tool throughout the entire diagnostic-therapeutic continuum. The kymograph gives information on breathing cycles, time of respiration cycles, configuration of respiration cycles, and whether the patterns of muscle behavior have the proper phase relationship. In speech breathing the kymograph gives an indication of the number of phrases, the time, and the configurations of the speech breathing with respect to phase. Kymographic recordings require careful interpretations and children usually need a period of training before the results can be considered reliable. It is especially helpful in evaluating silent and speech breathing patterns of cerebral-palsied children. Where the kymograph is not part of the clinical facilities a good deal of this information may be obtained through clinical observation and methods which may be adapted for this purpose.

Phonation. Phonation is a part of the speech breathing process. The control of the air column for proper use in speech provides the basis for adequate vocal-glottal-laryngeal adjustment. In the production of phonation, the vocal cords are brought into play and the speech process becomes one of considering adjustments above and below the glottis. Laryngeal adjustment and phonation are integrated in the speech breathing movement and also synchronized with the syllable pulses. For adequate speech there must be adequate voice production as well as breath control. Sustained voice production must be integrated in the speech breathing coordinations for intelligibility. Experimentation has not yet decided minimum phonation time necessary for speech by cerebral-palsied children, but Westlake (1951) suggests that the cerebral-palsied child should be able to sustain voice on an exhalation phase for ten seconds. Rutherford (1950), in early investigations, extended her examination and adapted certain procedures to include volume, pitch, rate, and quality of phonation. Cerebral-palsied children who require too many intakes of breath for sustaining the life processes may not be capable of sufficient sustaining phonation for adequate phrasing and consequently need to develop breath control and voice production long before the actual production of speech. The vital capacity of cerebral-palsied children was measured at pre- and post-stages during a breathing exercise program in which increases were noted for the experimental group of 31 percent over pretest values (Rothman, 1978). Furthermore, these children are vulnerable to vocal abuse in their struggled attempts at voice production. Tension produced in situations or tension produced by motor deficiency may interfere with the phonation process. Phonation is most efficiently produced when the breathing and speech organs economically participate in the process (Palmer, 1953; Westlake, 1951). Ease of production leads to the best results. Examination procedures should not only include early otological appraisal but also complete laryngoscopic workup for determining the possible existence of laryngeal pathology. A complete laryngological workup should provide cues for any organic bases for voice quality disturbances. Standard clinical procedures for examining voice quality, rate, pitch, and loudness should be adapted to the testing of cerebral-palsied children, as described in chapter 5.

Articulation. In addition to the breathing apparatus, the peripheral-oral mechanism must function adequately for the child to achieve intelligible speech. The activities of sucking, swallowing, and chewing become important functions in the development of speech among cerebral-palsied children and historically have received considerable attention. These activities are integrated into the breathing patterns. Palmer (1947) discusses application of chewing, sucking, and swallowing to speech disorders. He also indicates some of the implications of chewing, sucking, and swallowing in the development of speech among cerebral-palsied children. Froeschels (1943) has constructed elaborate therapy procedures employing the concept of chewing as a basic act in the speech process. His methodology may provide the hearing and speech therapist with cues concerning muscle conditions that may have a predictive value for therapy. Sittig (1947), adapting Froeschels' chewing method for the cerebral-palsied child, suggested that it improves the functions of the mouth and the speech organs as well as the voice. Furthermore, chewing enhances swallowing and may decrease salivation and drooling. Westlake (1951) stresses analysis and suggests techniques for improving "chewing and closing the mouth, elevation of the tip of the tongue, and peristaltic movement." He further observes in his work with children with cerebral palsy, that in many of these children the ability to raise the tip of the tongue is either absent or inadequate. He was also interested in all various types and degrees of lip and tongue movements, and differentiating the manner in which similar activities were completed under conditions of voluntary and involuntary control. The importance of sucking, swallowing, and chewing for speech production remains a viable concern in both the evaluation and habilitation processes for the cerebral-palsied child (Kamalashile, 1973; Palmer, Thompson and Linscheid, 1975; Love, Hagerman and Taimi, 1980).

Examination of the peripheral speech organs in terms of muscular function may indicate the extent, range, and degree of involvement, but may not be directly correlated to the production of specific speech sounds. Wolfe (1950) ranked movements of the speech organs in order of involvement without relating them to specific sound production. This concept of muscle involvement and its relationship to speech-sound production requires clarification. The movement of the speech organs as isolated physiological activities simulating speech movements without production of speech, and movements of the speech organs in the production of speech may represent highly differentiated coordination. Stetson (1951) attempted to obtain complete diagnostic profiles of muscle movements. Speech may necessitate analysis of movement patterns. The production of speech sounds in isolation and the production of speech in larger units (phrase) do not utilize the same coordinations. In larger speech units the elements fuse, telescope, shift, change, and assimilate dynamically. Certain speech sounds produced in "isolation" may require more skillful coordination and may represent difficulty of production, whereas the same sound used in larger speech units may represent much less difficulty.

The concept of sound complexity or difficulty level cannot be generalized for either handicapped or non-handicapped speakers. Tapping pressures in the mouth, outside the mouth, and recording tongue and lip movements through kymographic instrumentation may provide satisfactory cues for the analysis of speech behavior. Kymographic recording of mouth and nasal pressures and tongue and lip movements may be difficult to establish with cerebral-palsied children but experimentation to adapt such methods may prove profitable.

Speech intelligibility depends upon the proper coordination of consonant functions in the syllable movements and also upon larger phrase coordinations. Analysis of speech production should be based upon the primary concept of intelligibility. Many variables contribute to intelligibility. Among them are the general factors of rhythm and the specific factors of accuracy of the function of the consonants and vowels in the syllable structure, the way these phonemes combine and fuse into speech units, and the coordination of the breathing and speech apparatus in producing and controlling the air column (Hudgins and Numbers, 1942).

Redundancy in the speech of cerebral-palsied children might prove helpful in understanding them, but even the redundancy in their speech may be so faultily produced that intelligibility may still suffer. Speech distortions of children with cerebral palsy may still be intelligible, if the distortions do not occur in those words which require the preservation of integrity for understanding. Since understanding may occur even with distortion, intelligibility cannot be rigidly restricted in its use for diagnostic purposes. For research and clinical purposes verbal output for children with cerebral palsy may be recorded and studied for intelligibility. Individuals in the child's environment can judge the child's speech operationally on a rating scale basis (Beach, 1953; Cypreanson, 1953). Superfluous, extraneous, and grimacing movements may influence the production of the speech and consequently its intelligibility. These movements may also influence the judge's rating of the intelligibility performance. The effects of these movements should be considered in the intelligibility judgments. In evaluating the cerebral-palsied child's speech performance for articulation proficiency, the clinician is concerned with the frequency of occurrence of the different sound-error categories and the various types of errors occurring within these categories. Speech errors may be generally classified according to the place and manner of articulation, and by the presence or absence of voice. The traditional methods of classification may be adapted and applied in the examination of the speech proficiency of children with cerebral palsy.

In a comprehensive study Irwin (1972) provided a major contribution with respect to the communication variables of the cerebral-palsied with specific in-depth attention to articulation. Kent and Netsell (1978) reported large ranges of jaw movement, inappropriate tongue position, difficulties in velopharyngeal closure, and prolonged transition times for articulatory movement for their athetoid sample. Andrews, Platt and Young (1977) found more errors on word-final consonants than on word-initial consonants. Extraneous vocal behavior in cerebral-palsied speakers was examined by Farmer and Lencione (1977). Prevocalization was prevalent with relatively intact control over phase of articulation, but temporal incoordination was evidenced for manner of speech production. Further research is necessary to clarify the interrelationship between sound production and muscular involvement.

In the past decade, the investigations of Darley, Aronson, and Brown (1975) in motor speech disorders have elaborated on the various dysarthrias as they relate to lesions of the motor systems. These investigators examined various clusters of certain deviant speech dimensions, including imprecise consonantal production, breathiness of voice quality, nasal emission, audible inspiration, harsh voice quality, use of short phrases, and monotony of pitch and loudness. The application of such an approach appears to be beneficial in the task of assessing and describing the dysarthrias and other speech disturbances seen in the cerebral-palsied individual which involve respiration, phonation, and articulation.

Research indicates the high incidence and the complex nature of speech impairments among the cerebral-palsied. Poor coordination between the functions of respiration, phonation, and articulation figures in the basic impairment, on which other variables have a compounding effect, adding to the necessity for careful diagnostic assessment and a total habilitation effort.

The literature reveals considerable agreement concerning abnormalities of respiration, inadequacies of phonation, and incidence of articulatory impairments among cerebral-palsied children. There is a manifest need for further specific information concerning the coordinated role of respiration, phonation, and articulation as well as some information on resonance and cerebration in the communication process and performance of children with cerebral palsy.

THE HABILITATION PROCESS

Sensorimotor Integration

Sensorimotor integration results from the process of receiving sensory information by an organism. This information is synthesized and integrated with the organism's competency to accommodate input information and finalize a response (Gilfoyle and Grady, 1971). Sensorimotor integration culminates in neurodevelopment and proprioceptor neuromuscular facilitation, which locks and synthesizes input, transmission, association and output sensory and neurological systems. Temporal and place neurological integration proceeds not only as a result of maturation but also because of learning (Miller and Goldberg, 1975; Neman et al., 1974).

Campbell (1974) describes an infant stimulation program for children with central nervous system dysfunction based on Piaget's cognitive growth theory which emphasized the importance of early reflexes and sensorimotor patterns in the development of intellectual behavior. Mysak (1980), in discussing the speech habilitation process for the cerebral-palsied child, refers to a form of treatment which he terms, "neurospeech therapy." In so doing, he attempts to relate the concerns of his approach with phylo-ontogenetic factors as well as with the integration centers of the central nervous system. Mysak further describes neurospeech therapy as neuroeclectic in nature in that it involves both neuroevolutional and neurointegrative parameters and indicates that the basis of this therapy approach stems from the previous work of Rood, Fay and, most specifically, the Bobaths. Neurospeech therapy is involved with three areas: evaluation of basic and skilled speech movements and stimulation of such movements as they relate to speech development. Mysak elaborates the goals of neurospeech therapy as integration and elaboration of lower-center listening behaviors, lower-center tone, posture and movements (TPM) patterns, and lower-center TPM patterns by centers that mediate skilled speech movements. Mysak states that the

> goals of neurospeech therapy reflect what may be called the vertical-lateral dominance theory of speech central nervous system (SCNS) maturation. The theory is based on the progressive and successive integration of lower sensorimotor integration centers by higher centers and, finally the integration of the right hemisphere by the left hemisphere (Mysak, 1980, p. 184).

Notwithstanding the approach used, certain areas basic to all therapies must be addressed in the habilitation of the child with cerebral palsy.

Coordinated Team Approach

The habilitation hierarchy selected for the child with cerebral palsy exfoliates as each coordination blends into global behavior. The combined roles of the pediatrician, orthopedist, neurologist, otolaryngologist, surgeon, psychiatrist, psychologist, nurse, and the physical, music, occupational, vocational, and educational therapists in conjunction with the audiologist and speech pathologist are made explicit from the beginning. Each service, while planning and executing its functions in the assessment, diagnosis, and treatment protocols and charting daily progress on its specifically developed formats, contributes to the coordinated team approach. Anderson et al. (1978) describes an effective coordinated care program of this nature.

The interdisciplinary treatment program examines the individual, submits a total diagnosis, outlines a long-term treatment plan, and assigns priorities on the basis of needs, readiness, and feasibility. Continuous on-going appraisal of results will dictate administration, type, and time of different therapies, and monitor progress for modification if indicated.

In the present context the coordinated team approach integrates the activities of the different therapies in a matrix of interrelated objectives (Bobath and Bobath, 1967). Although individual therapies possess autonomy in the execution of the therapy program, they are nevertheless part of an interdependent, ongoing assessment process. In the total program leading to the acquisition of communicative skills, all therapies contribute in some way to pre-speech behavior. Each therapy may be designed to develop motor behaviors which establish appropriate posture patterns and eliminate prolonged infantile and pathological reflexes (Mysak, 1980). Similarly, activities producing adequate feeding conditions are active precursors to verbal communication (Jones, 1978; Haberfellner and Rossiwall, 1977; Love, Hagerman and Taimi, 1980).

In addition the activities of physical, occupational, and music therapists all contribute to proper breath support. Specifically, music therapy has additional value in both the pleasure derived and motivation. Consequently, compartmentalization in which any one therapy functions without constant interaction with other therapies seems to have lost its appeal as a standard operating procedure. Because each therapy is in daily communication with all other therapies the cerebral palsy child's program will be constantly modified based on the impact of the other specialties.

Specific Habilitation Concepts

Developmental phenomena, such as speech readiness and sensory development, must underlie the planning and administration of the habilitation program. If readiness behaviors are not at adequate levels, the program should be first directed toward improving them. At the same time, early habilitation procedures must include attempts to coordinate breathing and articulatory muscle movement, laryngeal adjustments for phonation, and rhythm of speech utterances, for adequate breath control is essential for effective and intelligible speech production. In addition, procedures to coordinate overall motor skills with speech development should be included.

Another integral part of the habilitation program should be the presentation of sound stimuli in a context of easy, effortless productions, since learning to discriminate speech sounds is essential to communication proficiency. Amplified sound stimulation may be needed to establish meaningful values for the auditory stimuli and promote the development of semantic levels of communication behavior, essential for the consistently appropriate use of language.

In the classroom, a major objective of the educational process should be the minimization of the motor disability as much and as early as possible by the adequate manipulation and structuring of environmental factors, for example, by constructing ramps and runways with proper support for the child's continuous mobility and maximum freedom. In addition, there must be a satisfactory reinforcement schedule to ensure the transfer of training. Under these optimum conditions, motor, perceptual, and cognitive development will proceed uniformly. Such a program requires active contributions from all of the individuals in the educational environment, and—most important—active participation by the child himself.

More specifically, the techniques that assist in the speech and language habilitation of the cerebral-palsied child fall into the areas of (1) psychological adjustment; (2) readiness techniques; (3) preauditory training; (4) speech and language development; (5) methods of relaxation; (6) coordination of breathing and speech; and (7) adapting methods to individual needs.

Psychological Adjustment. From the very beginning of the assessment process strong efforts will be exerted to assess the cerebral palsy child's potential for developing the necessary skills for adjustment. The child's psychological adjustment will be contingent not only upon the degree of the impairment but also on the interaction between the child and the important people in the environment, specifically the parents. Consequently, the key people in the environment need to become an integral part of the team for orientation and education relative to the cerebral-palsied child's problem. A review of the literature by Knott (1979) indicates the primary areas of concern for parents of cerebral palsy children to be (1) causes and effects of cerebral palsy; (2) family dynamics and counseling; (3) availability of educational and vocational programs; and (4) possible employment opportunities. The need for psychotherapeutic intervention for the family of children with cerebral palsy has been stressed by a number of investigators (Heisler, 1974; Zisserman, 1978; Park, 1979).

The first reaction of the cerebral palsy child's parents may prove to be devastating and catastrophic with the strong possibility of rejection and withdrawal occurring. Therefore, it is mandatory that parents become a part of the team in order that they be vitally involved in the establishment of goals, and actively participate in the therapy program itself. This particular adaption may expedite acceptance of the child. Moreover, a comfortable relationship established between parents and child becomes an incentive towards a unified pleasurable relationship which provides security and trust for both child and parents. This relationship may prevent future emotional frustration and intellectual disillusionment. Such an environment will help the parents and the child accept themselves with some persistent satisfaction and minimize attitudes of maladjustment (Podeanu-Czehofsky, 1975; Seidel, Chadwick, and Rutter, 1975; Andrews et al., 1977; Minde, 1978).

The motor impairment of a cerebral-palsied child restricts his mobility and consequently the number of educational experiences he can have. Parental overprotection or rejection—either of which may induce in the child feelings of conflict or ambivalence over his attempts to adjust—may further restrict his experiences and may, as mentioned above, interfere in other ways as well. If, however, the parents can be helped to look at the motor impairment as a neutral condition, they may be able to see that their child, though impaired, still has some potential for learning. This point of view can foster their early participation in a remedial program for which the objective is the extension and enrichment of the child's experiences, particularly through the development of language and speech skills.

Readiness Techniques. The nonhandicapped child acquires his readiness for learning certain tasks from informal experience, not from consciously structured learning activities. Maturation and learning supplement each other as the child learns to listen and, eventually, to discriminate between auditory experiences, thus becoming better able to learn and understand. Cerebral-palsied children, however, show a lag in the developmental process. Their communication deficiencies may be prolonged unless the clinician initiates readiness-promoting activities, such as exercising the muscles and improving neural control in such behaviors as sucking, chewing, and swallowing—perhaps through exaggerating the movements involved, as by chewing gum or by sucking through a straw (Palmer, 1947), or by putting bits of food at different places in the mouth so that the lips, tongue, and jaws can work together in a coordinated effort. By thus extending the range and strength of the movements used in speech and increasing the dexterity so necessary for adequate articulation, such activities will, particularly if carried out from infancy, facilitate the cerebral-palsied child's speech development (Jones, 1978; Haberfellner and Rossiwall, 1977).

The necessary growth in concept formation and motor auditory-linguistic skills may be promoted by activities that prepare the child to use his skills in realistic problem-solving situations. Every child should have daily practice in language comprehension and response, for example, so that he can integrate his experiences and proceed to abstractions and generalizations. Banham (1972) has proposed that the treatment team is responsible for developing an orientation program that will permit carrying out readiness activities in line with child development principles. The speech and language development activities should be structured in a sequential framework geared to the child's needs, as expressed in his relationship with his parents.

From the beginning, the child's environment must be saturated with all kinds of speech and language stimuli, though they need not be formally structured. The child may then come to understand some speech and may attempt to communicate. Any act, whether employing gesture or sound, which the child indicates as having a communicative value should be accepted by the parents. His attempt to communicate implies that he is attending to differential stimuli in his environment and that he is aware of the use of communication in manipulating his social environment. His efforts to communicate will be facilitated by readiness activities that are designed to refine the interpretive process and concomitant speech motor skills.

Preauditory Training. In the habilitation of hearing-impaired children without motor handicaps, the educational process is often devoted to accelerating the tendency to compensate through the other sensory modalities. Since this emphasis favors visual and tactile stimulation, the development of language habits and abilities which depend on the sense of hearing proceeds slowly, unless patient and skillful attention is given to preauditory training (DiCarlo, 1964; Mavilya and Mignone, 1977). Similar preauditory training will help the cerebral-palsied child develop satisfactory listening habits and attention. If irrelevant and competing environmental noises are minimized and speech is focused to compel the child's attention, the words he hears may become capable of releasing their meaning to him.

In previous publications, DiCarlo (1948, 1954, 1964) suggested methods for building sound awareness and attempted to set training principles in a sequential pattern for children with impaired hearing. With some modification, that basic outline may be applied to building sound awareness in cerebral-palsied children. The clinician should basically approach the goal of listening by making it a pleasurable, continuous activity. The clinician should see that auditory experiences are structured around the child's own physical, social, emotional, and intellectual needs in order to foster the association of stimuli with experience.

As training comes to deal with sound as a part of a larger, meaningful whole, the child will learn to attribute correct meaning to specific auditory stimuli. Work with all auditory stimuli must still, of course, occur, but it can now move toward developing listening acuity for speech sounds. The child must learn to discriminate between speech sounds, note contrasts, detect similarities in speech spectra, and recognize accent and rhythm patterns, inflection, and the multiple complexities of speech. The next aspect of training deals with teaching the child to listen to speech and other sounds as adjustment stimuli within a group framework. The clinician now should provide practice with all kinds of speech material, so that the child can achieve optimum understanding and interpretation.

It is at this last stage that greater demands are made of the child to capitalize on, and refine interpretations of, auditory experiences. The child learns to use vision as well as hearing, for, though sounds may be difficult to hear, their printed symbols are easy to see and contain obvious and significant clues to meaning. The acquisition of speech is thus facilitated by making clear the connection between printed and spoken language, giving hearing practice through listening to music, to speech, and to stories read by parents and other adults, and through taking part in group activities entailing conversation. These activities, none of them so artificial that they are not found in the child's everyday experiences, permit the child to improve ability to concentrate on sounds which have meaning and to disregard sounds which do not contribute to the semantics of the situation.

It should be pointed out that, in the diagnostic-therapeutic continuum, the realization that a child with adequate potential is not functioning at optimum level requires an investigation of the possible causes of the delay. For children who exhibit developmental lag because of multiple impairments, the program of early stimulation advocated above may demand additional supports in the way of modified materials and methodology.

Speech and Language Development. For the normal child with adequate potential for learning speech and language, the period of spontaneous vocalization begins at birth and continues with a steady increase in comprehension and number of utterances. An awareness of the semantic features of language develops as the child notes, and aligns horizontally, expressions with similar properties, and as the child arranges them vertically into categories of complexity. As vocabulary increases, these deep-structure components of language filter through to the surface units—the terminal strings. In the process, the child projects rules for acquiring semantic distinctions that bring verbal and nonverbal language into a mutual correspondence. McNeill (1966, 1972), Menyuk (1971, Crystal (1973), Muma (1978) and others have demonstrated that children respond to intonation as semantic content long before they begin to produce meaningful utterances; they can discriminate voices as early as four months of age, and their random utterances and babbling are precursors of linguistic production. Crystal (1973) doubts that the prelinguistic child even exists and that the onset of language has its beginnings in speech perception and comprehension. From this early stage, a child moves toward the stabilization of the linguistic univerals; the first holophrastic (one-word) sentences, occurring at about the ninth to the eleventh month, are the beginnings of a pragmatic grammar. The progression from one-word to five-word utterances occurs between eleven and fifteen months; a period of scarce production follows the child's first one-word utterances, but between eighteen and twenty-four months the child shows a development of some linguistic competence, with a definite grammar and a variation of grammatical and semantic markers. (Whether this competence is innate or learned still remains unresolved.) By twenty-four months, the child's linguistic repertoire contains nouns, verbs, pronouns, phrases, and sentences—a complete grammar, similar in function but somewhat different in complexity and total structure from that of adults—and linguistic competence includes projection rules for producing well-formed utterances. Thereafter, vocabulary multiplies rapidly until by the age of six the child has more than 2500 words at his command.

Since research on the development of language in children without motor handicaps has shown that their first words, generally nouns, may connote complete single actions or ideas, the same early ideation should be sought in building up the vocabulary of cerebral-palsied children with delayed speech and language. The words presented to them for learning should include nouns, verbs, and all other parts of speech. If this vocabulary is presented unambiguously and proceeds from simple concepts to more complex ones, it will meet the functional requirements of communication and endow language with problem-solving characteristics.

In the early instructional periods, objects should be presented visually, tactually, and auditorially for concept formation and vocabulary development. Pictures, objects, and all kinds of live representations should be included in the development of the conceptual process, and each word, when spoken in the child's hearing, should always be employed in complete, simple sentences. Verb forms should be presented by having the parent or the clinician and the child act them out. Adjectives and adverbs should be introduced early as qualifiers. Bates (1976) presents evidence that early speech acts develop from precursors (action, sound, and gestures) in the pre-linguistic period. For the cerebral palsy child, whose movements and sensorimotor experiences may be restricted, careful attention to such training activities is of great importance. The procedures developed by Schiefelbusch and Lloyd (1974) and Muma (1978) offer general guidelines for language intervention. Specific and relevant instructional techniques for enhancing language growth in young children are presented by Engel (1968) and Bangs (1968).

The variations and combinations of materials to be employed are limited only by the clinician's ingenuity in adapting and timing them to the child's needs and progress and in functioning with the parents in building key forms, commands, and expressions to carry the child through the process of developing language behavior.

Methods of Inducing Relaxation. Relaxation, variously conceived as the achievement of "optimal tonicity" or the reduction of tension conducive to appropriate muscle tone for conducting and managing daily activities, appears to be a necessary condition for the development of adequate speech. Its role in the treatment of cerebral-palsied children is to prepare them for attending to learning tasks by stabilizing their bodies and freeing them from the attention-binding effects of stimuli. Only by attending can they interact with their environment, and the proper induction of relaxation within the framework of a carefully designed habilitation program should facilitate and expedite learning and adjustment.

Relaxation is a state that the cerebral-palsied child must particularly strive for during the speech learning period. The literature contains few explicit definitions or methods for achieving the ideal relaxation state, but Jacobson (1938) did introduce exercises for "progressive relaxation," whereby an individual induces relaxation at some point in his body and allows it to spread progressively until total relaxation has been achieved, and Korzybski (1948) introduced the idea of "semantic relaxation," a procedure which produces relaxation as a result of the logical and accurate use of language to make the verbal and nonverbal universes correspond. Ortega (1978) investigated the effects of Jacobson's progressive relaxation training in the treatment of cerebral palsy adults finding that the overt spastic symptoms of cerebral palsy may be reduced through relaxation training.

Within the last decade increasing emphasis has been given to behavior modification theory and practice, which offers several methods of inducing relaxation. Wolpe (1969), for example, presents the concept of reciprocal inhibition as a major approach to the achievement of relaxation; Eysenck and Beech (1971) favor counterconditioning and related methods for stabilizing the individual; the Bandura (1971) approach employs modeling principles to achieve relaxation; and still others suggest the value of biofeedback procedures. The central concept in biofeedback is that the individual can use input from bodily processes in a correction system which permits the modification or change of the psychophysiological factors governing behavior. For instance, Leaf and Gaarder (1973) demonstrated that the use of electromyographic feedback can achieve significant relaxation for the individual.

The use of chemotherapy (medication) to promote relaxation in the treatment of individuals with cerebral palsy continues to be investigated. However, reports of its efficacy have been contradictory. Some of the many variables affecting medication dosage, schedule, and change of medication itself, remain to be examined.

Coordinating Respirations and Speech. Despite the early promotion of sensory and motor readiness, some cerebral-palsied children may still experience respiration difficulties. And, as was noted in a preceding section of this chapter, these difficulties are significantly related to speech intelligibility. The treatment of improper breathing requires an accurate identification of the specific nature of the difficulty, as by a kymographic study (Stetson, 1951). The measures of timing, phrasing, and phasing so obtained may offer essential clues for establishing more satisfactory breathing patterns. The treatment approach need not, however, focus only on speech; James, Hardy, and Shipton (1963) met with some success in modifying the breathing patterns of two athetoids by electrical stimulation.

Improvement in Breathing. Proper breathing can be promoted by several techniques. Using the Bobaths (1952) method of "reflex inhibiting postures" to "disassociate" respiration and speaking from body movements, Marland (1953) reported that not only do grimacing and drooling decrease, but babbling noises and even simple words appear as the child feels new sensations in the "reflex inhibiting posture." Phonation and babbling can be further promoted by hand manipulation, wherein the consequent ease of production leads to better inflection and articulation.

Lefevre (1952) tried to improve "weak" respiration behavior by providing direct resistance for the child to overcome in breathing. She suggested forcing the child's elbows over his chest, exerting downward pressure on the expiration phase, and securing the child sufficiently to make him or her uncomfortable and force deep breathing. As the child's breathing improves, resistance can be coordinated with arm movements to full extension.

Dixon (1955) studied the effects of a chest-abdominal respirator on the breathing and speech coordinations and on the judged speech and time needed for speaking. Although all changes observed were not significant statistically, the author notes that periodic application of the respirator resulted in some desirable changes.

Westlake (1951) suggested techniques designed to shift breathing activity from the abdomen to the chest and to improve the function of the chest and neck muscles. He also pointed out that breath control and phonation can be better accomplished by "prolonging phonation" than by "prolonging blowing." Others, such as Froeschels (1943), Cass (1951), Rutherford (1965), and Mysak (1980) have also suggested procedures that might help improve the cerebral-palsied child's breathing.

Voice Training. The hypersensitive stretch reflex of the spastic with the resulting imbalance in the speech muscles, the lack of position coordination of the ataxic, the hyperactivity of the athetoid's muscles, rigidity, and tremor—all interfere with achieving proper balance between respiratory and phonatory forces. Such conditions require early training devoted to establishing the best possible movement of total musculature, with various muscle activities being differentiated into a series of movements and with phonation occurring on the expiration phase of respiration. The clinician's early efforts to obtain adequate laryngeal adjustments for vowel prolongation by the child may include induction of laughter and babbling, and various voice training methods may be modified to meet the child's needs. Proper breathing habits and adequate voice control, once achieved, should eliminate vocal abuse produced by slow, labored speech, and tension-reducing conditions reinforced through auditory perception should bring about improvements in pitch, loudness, and phrasing.

Berg (1970) found that simple physical training improved the oxygen intake and physical capacity of cerebral-palsied children. Efforts to increase vital capacity and expiratory volume using exercise and Bobath techniques were shown to be successful by Rothman (1978). The physical therapist may also orient the parents to the necessity of establishing good breathing coordinations early, and in this connection Cardwell (1947) and Brunyate (1949) have offered helpful instructions to parents for physical and occupational therapy which remain relevant.

Articulatory Training. Articulatory movements should be trained while phonation takes place, even if their range, strength, and speed are limited. Their inclusion in a dynamic pattern may result in some improvement, for coordinated muscle training may cause a decrease in such abnormalities as the production of extraneous syllables and the failure to produce releasing and arresting consonants. Also, it may lead to a decrease in grimacing and facial distortion.

Improvement of sucking, swallowing, and chewing activities must also be coordinated with the function of the breathing apparatus because proper breath control and adequate voice production are not sufficient in and of themselves for intelligible speech. The basic tongue, jaw, and lip movements must function at least minimally in altering cavity shapes for vowel production and for interrupting the breath and voice stream to produce the consonants. Heltman and Peacher (1943) recommended a program of tongue, lip, jaw, and velum exercises to achieve this minimal function in cases of paralysis of the articulatory mechanism.

Froeschels (1943), Kastein (1948), and Sittig (1947) advocated the chewing method for developing proficiency of the articulatory organs. They also indicated that chewing reduces grimacing and drooling behavior. The chewing method, however, proved useful only for children who possessed some residual efficiency or who could be trained to regain the chewing movement; athetoids tended to exhibit only limited improvement. Froeschels (1943), dealing with unilateral paralysis of the tongue and associated grimacing behavior in the production of speech, manipulated the tongue away from the weaker side in an attempt to relieve the pressure from the stronger side. He reported that this method reduced grimacing and strengthened control of the tongue. Westlake (1951) discussed the acts involved in speaking as patterns of continuous movement rather than as isolated acts. In that context, he emphasized the vital importance of adequate breathing patterns for initiating and sustaining tone and the early involvement of the physiotherapist in teaching the child how to balance his head and feet. He observed that, because movements that cannot be produced voluntarily may often be produced by inducing movements in other organs, "confused motion" of the lips, tongue, and jaw may be treated through formal muscle training exercise. Hardy (1965) indicates that the total dynamics of the speech physiology mechanism must be considered in order to understand the dipathic aspects associated with cerebral palsy. Dorinson (1954) introduced an anti-drool mask, designed to enhance swallowing patterns with the mouth closed while breathing through the nose. He claimed that successful achievement of this coordination stopped the drooling. Shavell (1977) discusses several approaches to the alleviation of drooling and concludes that oral surgery should be used for patients not responding to other methods.

Since the consonants have no independent existence in the stream of speech and cannot be learned "in isolation," the cerebral-palsied child must, in learning these sounds, develop ballistic strokes of the tongue, lips, and jaw that are adequate in terms of speed, strength, and range. Hardy (1965) supports the concept that careful assessment and remediation of restrictions of motility of the speech mechanism may best be accomplished by utilizing the movements of those structures during the speech act.

Work reported by McDonald and Solomon (1967) suggests the dependence of oral motor function on stereognosis which is linked to articulation proficiency. Mysak (1980) discusses stimulating feedback and movement facilitation maneuvers as well as movement exercises in facilitating articulation development and remediation. On the other hand, a study of velopharyngeal closure by Hardy et al. (1969) suggests that the procedure of choice in managing some articulation problems, such as palatal paresis, may often be surgery or, more often, prosthesis.

Development of Rhythm and Phrasing. The rhythm of speech, so essential to intelligibility, can only be produced by syllabic production—the sounds accented and grouped into units—but imparting it may require the use of techniques that do not depend upon speech materials. In other words, the concept of rhythm may best be imparted through music, where the clinician taps out a rhythm and the child responds with movements he can easily execute. Singing, also, can be employed in introducing rhythm and phrasing. A dynamic approach to the use of this method might involve starting the muscle movement on a best phase as a means of inducing the back phase, although Fothergill and Harrington (1949) were unable to accept this notion of a "controlled" ballistic movement. Instead they sought a "controlled movement" equated with a slower, more precise articulation. Their method was intended to "push back" the stretch reflex threshold and permit greater articulation adequacy.

Other studies include those by Palmer (1948), who emphasized the correction of the mandibular-condyle relationship as a prerequisite to improving the speech of the cerebral-palsied, and by Westlake (1951), who outlined training procedures for accelerating the coordinated movements in opening and closing the mouth and suggested techniques for stabilizing the extensor thrust of the jaw. Negative practice in eliminating excessive extraneous movement from the act of speaking has proved effective, and the use of distractive techniques for channeling muscle overflow during phonation has also been suggested (Wepman, 1943).

Adapting Methods to Individual Needs. When a child's speech intelligibility has reached a level of minimal social adequacy, people will barely be able to understand the communication intended. At this stage in the learning continuum, work must proceed on refining consonant articulation through the use of stimulation procedures and phonetic placement methods are used. They should be taught as movements rather than as positions; motokinesthetic methods in general use by speech pathologists may be modified and adapted for the cerebral-palsied child. Whatever the method used, the production of speech sounds should meet the minimum criteria for continuous speech rather than for individual sounds, and the common goal of all methodologies should be the ability of the child to evaluate and correct his or her own speech behavior. Instructions, varying according to the needs of the child, should be provided individually, but, whenever and as soon as possible, group work should also be provided because of its socialization value.

Where cerebral-palsied children are concerned, speech development trends and norms that have been based on studies of normal populations of children should serve as useful guides rather than as authoritative rules. Moreover, while a given educational scheme may present a logical consistency, these cases reveal psychological and physiological differences that may make some modification of the schemes necessary. Thus, in the motor training of cerebral-palsied children whose speech development fails to follow normal development principles, a special methodology must often be adapted to meet the specific motor, intellectual, emotional, and social needs of the child, as identified in the diagnostic-therapeutic process.

Augmentative Aids For Nonspeaking Children With Cerebral Palsy

For those children whose prognosis and training for verbal communication appears to be nonproductive, evaluation of his or her communication skills should be matched to available augmentive telecommunication instrumentation at the appropriate performance level. Training at the simplest levels may facilitate and lead to more complex communication skills at the next communication hierarchy. As each step in the communication process is mastered the child's total communication increases and the complexity of the symbolic interaction is increased. Failure at communication, rather than disabilities, creates isolation, misery, and rejection. Before the advent of telecommunication science, nonspeaking individuals existed in a universe of marked deprivation. Noncommunicative children with cerebral palsy endured an existence of desolate monotony.

In 1973, McDonald and Schultz described how communication for speechless children with cerebral palsy might be improved by the employment of communication boards. Davis (1973) formulated a sentence construction board that outlined procedures for acquiring generative grammar concepts in the learning of language. As the number of publications multiplied and interest in telecommunication application increased, the question of terminology became manifest as evidenced by the American Speech-Language-Hearing Association's publication of a position paper, "Non-Speech Communication" (1980). Chapter 8 reviews some of those communication aids used with aphasics.

Laurentana (1960) and Hunsinger (1976) suggested the optical bead pointer or simple headstick might prove functional for expediting the communicative process for cerebral-palsied children with severe motor disabilities. Telecommunication scientists and educators interested in pragmatic application cooperated interactively in the development of an array of both simple and highly sophisticated instruments and programs employing microprocessors, integrated circuitry, and educational and psychological learning principles (Silverman, 1980). Interested industrial units have and are devoting talent, energy, and financial resources in the development and modification of augmentative communication instrumentation.[1] Although technology and

[1] Information relative to instruments and prostheses may be obtained from United Cerebral Palsy Association, 66 East 34th Street, New York, New York 10016.

theory relative to non-speech communication have cooperated, theory has not accommodated totally to available technology. Interdependency between device and user has not been completely resolved. Nevertheless, continued research will arrive at a solution for matching individual capacity and prosthesis capability.

Among the present instrumentation three basic device categories exist:

1. Direct selection where communication is effected by specific input and single movement selection on a one-to-one correspondence between individual and device. The device provides feedback and is faster than scanning because it does not demand operations to arrive at the target transformations. The operation does require adequate motor control of at least one of the extremities.
2. Scanning units organize each communication segment into several time or combined sequences, and may be operated at a single source with less motor skill but slow in output.
3. Encoding involves selection of context material represented by characteristic codes available by recall or listings. Encoding devices, because of complexity, demand higher level functioning.

Materials, method of operation, and input and output display considerations contribute to the total communicative process, but the most crucial element in the procedure remains the decision in the selection of the prosthesis. The system encompasses two types of materials: symbol selection (software), displays (hardware). The symbol system comprises picture words, letters, sentences, traditional orthography, signs ASL, SEE, AmerInd, speech, Blissymbols (Vanderheiden and Grilley, 1976; Archer, 1977; Vanderheiden, 1978). Hardware includes augmentative displays: electronic, nonelectronic, indicating characteristics, output modality, auditory, visual, and proprioceptive displays.

A most crucial factor in the total process remains the selection decision paradigm which matches the user's talents with the device's capacity to perform specific operations (Shane and Bashier, 1978). Both users' and prostheses' capacities are analyzed and evaluated within the selection decision matrix to insure optimum communication efficacy. Individual evaluation ascertains cognitive functions, educational level, sensorimotor dexterity, communication ability (linguistic competency and performance), learning potential, and personality assessment. Instrument evaluation includes determination of cost effectiveness, accessibility, portability, control complexity, flexibility, ease of operation, size, weight, and input-output characteristics. The final prosthesis selection will be contingent on the task the instrument must perform and the competencies of the individual. The interface of time and spatial relationships must lock both individual and prosthesis into a compatible functioning whole. The limited observation the authors have monitored with nonspeaking individuals using these prostheses promises a freedom from isolation, deprivation, misery, and despondency not yet realized. The cost of administering such a program, while in some cases high, may still be negligible in terms of total budget. Nevertheless, in terms of salvaging human self-esteem through realistic self-appraisal of both limitations and potentialities, eliminating human suffering and misery, and providing opportunities for intellectual, physical, emotional, educational, social, and civic growth, there can be no greater remuneration, a noble task worthy of our great democracy.

SUMMARY

Cerebral palsy is not a disease, nor an ailment, but a neurophysiological disorder that may generally improve within the framework of a systematically planned habilitation program. In the final analysis, the major goal for habilitation or rehabilitation time tables for children with cerebral palsy is not the acquisition of perfect hearing skills and speech performance but rather the improvement of their learning ability so that they may continuously reorganize their experiences and refine their intellectual, emotional, and social values and improve the quality of their living. In our democratic society two basic principles operate to formulate care and educational programs: (1) preservation of individual integrity; (2) the guarantee of equal opportunity before the law.

Communication provides the indispensable, fundamental artery to the achievement of these goals. For those children who do not succeed in acquiring verbal communication modern science has designed, assembled, and made available microelectronic integrating circuitry that enhances and expedites communication with or without verbal speech production so that communication may no longer be denied cerebral-palsied children. Habilitation and educational programs should provide for basic activities, but also for the cultivation of all experiences: educational, social, and vocational pursuits. It also should constantly monitor, reappraise, and ascertain that progress is commensurate with potential and prevent the formation of unrealistic goals and aspirations which could seriously impede the habilitation efforts. Mastery of earlier skills should prepare and eventually lead to learning of higher and more complex behavior.

Emphasizing the child's abilities rather than his or her disabilities reflects the view that impairments do not directly determine personality development. Whatever effects impairment may have on personality growth are a function of his or her interaction with influences in the environment, and improving that interaction will foster personality development. With such an orientation, the team effort merges as a total contribution that is greater than the sum of individual efforts. Open channels of communications between team members provide for participation and sharing; and while all contributions are unique and necessary, the role played by the communication clinician is perhaps the most crucial in planning and monitoring the progressive stages in growth and development.

Early diagnostic-therapeutic appraisal of the cerebral-palsied child's abilities by a professional team is the necessary first step in charting an educational program suited to his or her needs and abilities, and should consist of a thorough and comprehensive assessment which does not focus only on the child's impairments in an isolated and unrelated fashion. It should instead seek ways of integrating the child's abilities in a total educational continuum which includes early and continuing prevocation and vocational pursuits which will help placement and success in gainful employment. For those who cannot achieve this goal, the habilitation program should permit individuals to adjust to a sheltered environment where they can make a contribution within their achievement level and derive feelings of self-worth and security.

Research into cerebral palsy and its effect on communication has been extensive and has produced some results holding promise for treatment of the many problems. Investigation is continuing into almost every aspect of cerebral palsy, particularly into the nature and function of the sensory and neurophysiological mechanisms involved, the related psychomotor ramifications, the effect of the impairment on personality, and the best employment of learning theory in devising communication habilitation programs. This need will continue to challenge our knowledge and technology, yet every new discovery will contribute to a greater understanding of this perplexing problem and to more successful methods of salvaging and educating children with cerebral palsy.

BIBLIOGRAPHY

Abbot, M., *A Syllabus of Cerebral Palsy Treatment Techniques*. New York: American Occupational Association (1953).

American Speech-Language and Hearing Association, Nonspeech communication: A position paper. *ASHA*, **22**, 267–272 (1980).

Anderson J. T., Comfort, T. H., Strand, P. J., and Winter, R. B., Coordinated care for cerebral palsy. *Minnesota Medicine*, **61**, 161–164 (1978).

Andrews, G., Platt, L. J., Quinn, P. T., and Neilson, P. D., An assessment of the status of adults and cerebral palsy. *Develop. Med. Child Neurol.*, **19**, 803–810 (1977).

Andrews, G., Platt, L. J., and Young, M., Factors affecting the intelligibility of cerebral palsied speech to the average listener. *Folia phoniat*, **29**, 292–301 (1977).

Archer, L. A., Blissymbolics—a nonverbal communication system. *J. Speech and Hearing Dis.*, **43**, 568–579 (1977).

Bandura, A., Psychotherapy based upon modelling principles. In A. E. Bergin and S. L. Garfield (Eds.), *Handbook of Psychotherapy and Behavior Change*. New York: John Wiley and Sons, Inc. (1971).

Bangs, L., *Language and Learning Disabilities of the Pre-Academic Child*. Englewood Cliffs, N.J.: Prentice-Hall, Inc., (1968).

Banham, K. M., Progress in mental development of retarded cerebral palsied infants. *Exceptional Child*, **39**, 240 (1972).

Barrett, T. C., Visual tasks as predictors of first grade reading achievement, *The Reading Teacher*, **18**, 276–282 (1965).

Bates, E., Pragmatics and sociolinguistics in child language. In D. Morehead and A. Morehead (Eds.), *Normal and Deficient Language*. Baltimore: University Park Press (1976).

Beach, M. N., An investigation of some of the factors which may influence the development of speech and language in cerebral palsied children. Unpublished master's thesis, Syracuse University, New York (1953).

Bensman, A. S., and Szegho, M., Cerebellar electrical stimulation: A critique. *Arch. Phys. Med. Rehabil.*, **59**, 485–487 (1978).

Berg, K., Effect of physical training of school children with cerebral palsy. *Acta Paediatrica Scandinavica*, 204, Suppl. 7t (1970).

Berlin, C. I., and Dobie, R. A., Electrophysiologic measures of auditory function via electrocochleography and brainstem evoked responses. In W. F. Rintelmann (Ed.), *Hearing Assessment*. Baltimore, Md.: University Park Press (1979).

Berry, M., *Language Disorders of Children*. New York: Appleton-Century-Crofts (1969).

Betts, E., Reading: Perceptual learning. *Education*, **89**, 291–297 (1969).

Blood, G. W., and Hyman, M., Dichotic listening in cerebral palsied and normal children. *J. Auditory Research*, **17**, 139–144 (1977).

Bobath, B., and Bobath, K., The neuro-developmental treatment of cerebral palsy. *Physical Therapy*, **47**, 1039–1041 (1967).

Bobath, B., and Bobath, K., A treatment of cerebral palsy. *Brit. J. Phys. Med.*, **15**, 1–11 (1952).

Boyer, M. G. and Symonds, M. E., Conditions which masquerade as cerebral palsy. *Develop. Med. Child Neurol.*, **20**, 230 (1978).

Bradford, L. T., Respiration Audiometry. In L. J. Bradford (Ed.), *Physiological Measures of the Audio-Vestibular System*. New York: Academic Press (1975).

Breakey, A. S., Wilson, J. J., and Wilson, B. C., Sensory and perceptual functions in the cerebral palsied: III some visual perceptual relationships. *J. Nerve. Ment. Dis.*, **158**, 70–77 (1974).

Brunyate, R. M., O. T. means freedom for parents. *The Crippled Child*, **26**, 11–13, 28–29 (1949).

Byrne, M., Speech and language development of athetoid and spastic children. *Journal of Speech and Hearing Research*, **24**, 231–240 (1959).

Cain, L., Levine, S., and Elzey, F., *Cain-Levine social competency scale*. Palo Alto: Consulting Psychologists Press (1963).

Campbell, S. K., Facilitation of cognitive and motor development in infants with central nervous system dysfunction. *Physical Therapy*, **54**, 346–353 (1974).

Capute, A. J., Developmental disabilities; an overview. *Dent. Clin. North Am.*, **18**, 557–577 (1974).

Cardwell, V. E. (Ed.), *The cerebral palsied child and his care in the home*. Revision of Pamphlet No. 1. New York: Association for the Aid of Children (1947).

Carrow, E., *Test for Auditory Comprehension of Language*. Austin, Texas: Learning Concepts (1974).

Cass, M. T., *Speech Habilitation in Cerebral Palsy Children*. New York: Columbia University Press (1951).

Cruickshank, W. M., and Raus, G. M., *Cerebral Palsy: Its Individual and Community Problems*. (2nd ed.) Syracuse: Syracuse University Press (1966).

Crystal, D., Linguistic mythology and the first year of life. *British J. of Dis. of Commun.*, **8**, 29–36 (1973).

Cypreanson, L. E., An investigation of the breathing and speech coordination and speech intelligibility of normal speaking children and of cerebral palsied children with speech defects. Unpublished doctoral dissertation, Syracuse University, Syracuse, New York (1953).

Darley, F. L., Aronson, A. E., and Brown, J. R., *Motor Speech Disorders*. Philadelphia: W. B. Saunders (1975)

Davis, G. A., Linguistic and language therapy: the sentence construction board. *J. Speech Hearing Dis.*, **48**, 205–214 (1973).

Dechant, E. V., *Improving the Teaching of Reading*. Englewood Cliffs, N.J.: Prentice-Hall (1970).

Denhoff, E., Medical aspects. In W. M. Cruickshank (Ed.), *Cerebral Palsy: A Developmental Disability*. (3rd ed.) New York: Syracuse University Press (1976).

Denhoff, E., Feldman, S., Smith, M. G., Litchman, H., and Holden, W., Treatment of spastic cerebral palsied children with sodium dantrolene. *Develop. Med. Child Neurol.*, **17**, 736–742 (1975).

Denhoff, E., and Robinault, I. P., *Cerebral Palsy and Related Disorders*. New York: McGraw Hill (1960).

DiCarlo, L. M., Hearing aids for hearing handicapped children. *Hearing News*, **16**, 1–2, 19–20 (1948).

DiCarlo, L. M., Research trends and present applications. *Volta Rev.*, **56**, 351–353 (1954).

DiCarlo, L. M., *The Deaf*. Englewood Cliffs, N.J.: Prentice-Hall, Inc. (1964).

DiCarlo, L. M., Communication therapy for problems associated with cerebral palsy. In S. Dickson (Ed.), *Communication Disorders: Remedial Principles and Practices*. Glenview, Ill.: Scott, Foresman and Company (1974).

DiCarlo, L. M., and Amster, W. W., Hearing and speech behavior among children with cerebral palsy. In W. Cruickshank and G. Raus (Eds.), *Cerebral Palsy: Its Individual and Community Problems*. Syracuse: Syracuse University Press (1955).

DiCarlo, L. M., Amster, W. W., and Herer, G. R., *Speech After Laryngectomy*. Syracuse: Syracuse University Press (1955).

DiCarlo, L. M., Kendall, D. C., and Goldstein, M. A., Diagnostic procedures for auditory disorders in children. *Folia Phoniatrica*, **14**, 206–264 (1962).

Dixon, R. F., An exploratory investigation of the effects of the chest-abdomen respirator on the breathing and speech coordinations and the judged speech coordinations and the judged speech intelligibility of children with cerebral palsy who display abnormal breathing patterns and speech difficulties. Unpublished doctoral dissertation, Syracuse University, Syracuse, New York (1955).

Doll, E., *Vineland Social Maturity Scale*. Minneapolis: Educational Test Bureau (1965-Rev.).

Dolphin, J. E., and Cruickshank, W., Tactual motor perception of children with cerebral palsy. *Journal of Personality*, **20**, 446–471 (1952).

Dorinson, M., Antidrool mask for children with cerebral palsy. *J.A.M.A.*, **155**, 439–440 (1954).

Duckman, R., The incidence of visual anomalies in a population of cerebral palsied children. *J. American Optometric Assoc.*, **50**, 1013–1016 (1979).

Dunsdon, M. I., *The educability of cerebral palsied children*. London: Newnes Educational Publishing Co., Ltd. (1952).

Ekwall, E., *Diagnosis and Remediation of the Disabled Reader*. Boston: Allyn and Bacon, Inc. (1978).

Engel, R., *Language Motivating Experiences for Young Children*. Sherman Oaks, Calif.: Rose C. Engel (1968).

Eysenck, H. J., and Beech, R., Counterconditioning and related methods. In A. E. Bergin and S. L. Garfield (Eds.), *Handbook of Psychotherapy and Behavior Change*. New York: John Wiley and Sons, Inc. (1971).

Farmer, A., and Lencione, R. M., An extraneous vocal behavior in cerebral palsied. *British Journal of Disorders of Communication*, **12**, 109–118 (1977).

Fothergill, P., and Harrington, R., The clinical significance of the stretch reflex in speech re-education for the spastic. *J. Speech Hearing Dis.*, **14**, 353–355 (1949).

Friedman, W. H., and Kaplan, B., Tympanic neurectomy. *N.Y.S.J. Med.*, **75**, 2419–2422 (1975).

Froeschels, E. A., A contribution to the pathology and therapy of dysarthria due to certain cerebral lesions. *J. Speech Dis.*, **8**, 301–321 (1943).

Gilfoyle, E. M., and Grady, A. P., Cognitive-perceptual-motor behavior. In H. S. Willard and C. S. Spackman (Eds.), *Occupational therapy*. Philadelphia: J. B. Lippincott Company (1971).

Gornall, P., Hitchcock, E., and Kirkland, I. D., Stereotaxic neurosurgery in management of cerebral palsy. *Developmental Med. Child Neurol.*, **17**, 279–286 (1975).

Gratke, J. M., *Help Them Help Themselves*. Dallas, Texas: Society for Crippled Children (1947).

Haberfellner, H., and Müller, G., Sequelae of head and neck positions on auditory performance. *Neuropadiátrie*, **7**, 373–378 (1976a).

Haberfellner, H., and Müller, G., Bobath-therapy, tonic reflex-activities and processing of acoustic stimuli. *Neuropadiátrie*, **7**, 379–383 (1976b).

Haberfellner H., and Rossiwall, B., Treatment of oral sensorimotor disorders in cerebral-palsied children: preliminary report. *Develop. Med. Child Neurol.*, **19**, 350–352 (1977).

Hardy, J. C., Research in speech problems associated with cerebral palsy and implications for the young cerebral palsied child. In W. T. Daley (Ed.), *Speech and Language Therapy with the Cerebral Palsied Child*. Washington: The Catholic University of America Press, Inc. (1965).

Hardy, J. C., Intra oral breath pressure in cerebral palsy. *J. Speech and Hear. Dis.*, **26**, 309–319 (1961).

Hardy, J. C., Netsell, R., Schweiger, J. W., and Morris, H. L., Management of velopharyngeal dysfunction in cerebral palsy. *J. Speech Hearing Dis.*, **34**, 123–137 (1969).

Hayakawa, S. I., *Language in Thought and Action*. New York: Harcourt, Brace and Co. (1949).

Heltman, H., and Peacher, G., Misarticulation and diadokokinesis in the spastic paralytic. *J. Speech Dis.*, **8**, 137–145 (1943).

Hixon, T. J., and Hardy, J. C., Restricted mobility of the speech articulators in cerebral palsy. *J. Speech and Hearing Dis.*, **29**, 293–306 (1964).

Holt, K. S., and Reynell, J. K., *Assessment of cerebral palsy: II*. London: Lloyd-Luke (Medical Books) Ltd. (1967).

Hood, P. N., Shank, R. H., and Williamson, D. B., Environmental factors in relation to the speech of cerebral palsied. *J. Speech Hearing Dis.*, **13**, 325–331 (1948).

Hopper, G. R., Speech sound learning ability in cerebral palsied children. Unpublished doctoral dissertation, Indiana University, Bloomington (1968).

Hopkins, T. W., Bice, H. V., and Colton, K. C., *Evaluation and Education of the Cerebral Palsied Child*. Washington: International Council for Exceptional Children (1954).

Hull, H. C., A study of the respiration of fourteen spastic paralysis cases during silence and speech. *J. Speech Dis.*, **5**, 275–276 (1940).

Hunsinger, K. W., A simple headstick for cerebral palsied children. *Amer. J. Occup. Therapy*, 30, 506 (1976).

Hyman, M., An experimental study of sound pressure level and duration in the speech of cerebral palsied children. *J. Speech Hearing Dis.*, **17**, 295–300 (1952).

Iandoli, E. W., An analysis of the articulatory errors and voice quality characteristics and their relationship to intelligibility of children with cerebral palsy. Unpublished doctoral dissertation, Syracuse University, Syracuse, New York (1958).

Irwin, O. C., *Communication Variables of Cerebral Palsied and Mentally Retarded Children*. Springfield, Ill.: Charles C. Thomas (1972).

Jacobson, E., *Progressive Relaxation*. Chicago: University of Chicago Press (1938).

James, E. I., Hardy, J., and Shipton, H. W., Development of electrical stimulation in modifying respiratory patterns of children with cerebral palsy. *J. Speech Hearing Dis.*, **28**, 230–238 (1963).

Johnson, W., *People in Quandaries*. New York: Harper and Brothers (1946).

Johnson, W., Adjustment problems of the cerebral palsied. *J. Speech Hearing Dis.*, **21**, 12–17 (1956).

Johnson, W., Brown, S. F., Curtis, J. F., Edney, C. W., and Keaster, J., *Speech Handicapped School Children*. New York: Harper Row (1967).

Jones, A. M., Overcoming the feeding problems of the mentally and the physically handicapped. *Journal of Human Nutrition*, **32**, 359–367 (1978).

Kamalashile, J., Speech problems in cerebral palsy children. *J. Lang. Speech*, **18**, 158–165 (1973).

Kastein, S., Speech therapy in cerebral palsy. *J. Rehab.*, **14**, 17–20 (1948).

Keats, S., Morgese, A., and Nordlund, T., The role of diazepam in the comprehensive treatment of cerebral palsied children. *Western Medicine*, 4, Special Supplement (1963).

Keats, S., *Cerebral Palsy*. Springfield, Ill.: Charles C. Thomas (1968).

Kent, R., and Netsell, R., Articulatory abnormalities in athetoid cerebral palsy. *J. Speech Hear. Disorders*, **43**, 353–377 (1978).

Knott, G. P., Attitudes and needs of parents of cerebral palsied children. *Rehabilitation Literature*, **40**, 190–195 (1979).

Korzybski, A., *Science and Sanity: An Introduction to Non-Aristotelian Systems and General Semantics*. (3rd ed.). Lakeville, Conn.: The International Non-Aristotelian Library Publishing Co., The Institute of General Semantics (1948).

Leaf, W. B., and Gaarder, K. R., A similified electromyograph feedback apparatus for relaxation training. In C. M. Franks and G. T. Wilson (Eds.), *Annual review of behavior therapy: theory and practice*. New York: Brunner/Mazel, Inc. (1973).

Lee, L., *Developmental Sentence Analysis*. Evanston, Ill.: Northwestern University Press (1974).

Lefevre, M. C., A rationale for resistive therapy in speech training for the cerebral palsied. *J. Exceptional Children*, **19**, 61–64 (1952).

Lencione, R., Speech and language problems in cerebral palsy. In W. M. Cruickshank (Ed.), *Cerebral Palsy—A Developmental Disability*. (3rd ed.) Syracuse: Syracuse University Press (1976).

Love, R. J., Oral language behavior of older cerebral palsy children. *J. Speech Hearing Ed.*, **7**, 349–359 (1964).

Love, R. J., Hagerman, E. L., and Taimi, E. G., Speech performance, dysphagia and oral reflexes in cerebral palsy. *J. Speech Hear. Disorders*, **45**, 59–75, (1980).

MacDonald, J. D., *Parent-Child Communication Inventory*. Columbus, Ohio: Nisenger Center (1973).

Marland, P. M., Speech therapy for the cerebral palsied based on reflex inhibitions. In C. Van Riper (Ed.), *Speech Therapy: A Book of Readings*. New York: Prentice-Hall, Inc. (1953).

Marquis, P., Therapies for cerebral palsy. *Amer. Fam. Physician*, **19**, 101–105 (1979).

Mavilya, M., and Mignone, B., *Educational Strategies for the Youngest Hearing Impaired Children*. New York: Lexington School for the Deaf (1977).

McDonald, E. T., and Chance, B., *Cerebral Palsy*. Englewood Cliffs, N.J.: Prentice-Hall, Inc. (1964).

McDonald, E. T., and Schultz, A. R., Communication boards for cerebral palsied children. *J. Speech Hearing Dis.*, **38**, 73–88 (1973).

McDonald, E. T., and Solomon, B., Oral sensorimotor function in athetoids. *Developmental Med. Child Neurol.*, **9**, 119 (1967).

McNeill, D., Developmental linguistics. In F. Smith and G. A. Miller (Eds.), *The Genesis of Language*. Cambridge, Mass.: The M.I.T. Press (1966).

McNeill, D., *Acquisition of Language*. New York: Harper and Row (1972).

Mecham, M. J., Berko, M. J., and Berko, F. G., *Speech Therapy in Cerebral Palsy*. Springfield, Ill.: Charles C. Thomas (1960).

Menyuk, P., *The Acquisition and Development of Language*. Englewood Cliffs, N.J.: Prentice-Hall, Inc. (1971).

Menyuk, P., Early development of receptive language from babbling words. In R. Schiefelbusch and L. Lloyd (Eds.), *Language Perspectives: Acquisition, Retardation and Intervention*. Baltimore: University Park Press (1974).

Miller, T. G., and Goldberg, K., Sensorimotor integration: An interdisciplinary approach. *Physical Therapy*, **55**, 501–504 (1975).

Milner-Brown, H. S., and Penn, R. D., Pathophysiological mechanisms in cerebral palsy. *J. Neurol. Neurosurg. Psychiatry*, **42**, 606–618 (1979).

Minde, K. K., Coping styles of 34 adolescents with cerebral palsy. *Am. J. Psychiatry*, **135**: 11, 1344–1349 (1978).

Muma, J., *Language Handbook: Concepts, Assessment, Intervention*. Englewood Cliffs, N.J.: Prentice-Hall, Inc. (1978).

Myers, P., A study of language disabilities in cerebral palsied children. *J. Speech Hearing Res.*, **8**, 129–136 (1965).

Mysak, E. D., Cerebral palsy speech syndromes. In. L. E. Travis (Ed.), *Handbook of Speech Pathology and Audiology*. New York: Appleton-Century-Crofts, Inc. (1971).

Mysak, E. D., *Neurospeech Therapy for the Cerebral Palsied: A Neuroevolutional Approach*. New York: Teachers College Press (1980).

Neman, R., Roos, P., McCann, B. M., Menolascino, F. J., and Heal, L. W., Experimental evaluation of sensorimotor patterning used with mentally retarded children. *American Journal of Mental Deficiency*, **79**, 372–384 (1974).

Netsell, R., Changes in orapharyngeal cavity size in dysarthric children. *J. Speech Hearing Dis.*, **12**, 646–649 (1969).

Newcomer, P. L., and Hammill, D. D., *The Test of Language Development*. Austin, Texas: Empiric Press (1977).

Ortega, D. F., Relaxation exercise with cerebral palsied adults showing spasticity. *Journal of Applied Behavior Analysis*, **11**, 447–451 (1978).

Palmer, M., Similarities of the effects of environmental pressures on cerebral palsy and stuttering. *Journal of Speech Disorders*, **8**, 155–160 (1943).

Palmer, M., Studies in clinical techniques: II. normalization of chewing, sucking and swallowing reflexes in cerebral palsy: A home program. *J. Speech Dis.*, **12**, 415–418 (1947).

Palmer, M., Studies in clinical techniques: III. mandibular facet slip in cerebral palsy. *J. Speech Hearing Dis.*, **13**, 44–48 (1948).

Palmer, M., Speech disorders in cerebral palsy. *The Nervous Child*, **8**, 193–202 (1949).

Palmer, M., Speech disorders in cerebral palsy. In Marguerite Abbot (Ed.), *Proceedings Cerebral Palsy Institute*. New York: Association for the Aid of Crippled Children, Inc. (1950).

Palmer, M., Laryngeal blocs in the speech disorders. In C. Van Riper (Ed.), *Speech therapy, a book of readings*. New York: Prentice-Hall, Inc. (1953).

Palmer, M., Recent advances in the scientific study of language disorders in cerebral palsy. *Cerebral Palsy Review*, **15**, 3–6 (1954).

Palmer, S., Thompson, R. J., and Linscheid, T. R., Applied behavior analysis in the treatment of childhood feeding problems. *Develop. Med. Child Neurol.*, **17**, 333–339 (1975).

Perlstein, M. A., The current status of drug therapy in cerebral palsy. *The Crippled Child*, **27**, 8–10 (1949).

Perlstein, M. A., Infantile cerebral palsy: Classification and clinical correlations. *J.A.M.A.*, **149**, 30–34 (1952).

Perlstein, M. A., and Shere, M., Speech therapy for children with cerebral palsy. *American Journal of Diseases of Children*, **72**, 389–398 (1946).

Phelps, W. M., Etiology and diagnostic classification of cerebral palsy. In M. Abbot (Ed.), *Proceedings of the Cerebral Palsy Institute*. New York: Association for the Aid of Crippled Children, Inc. (1950).

Platt, L. J., Andrews, G., Young, M., and Neilson, P. D., The measurement of speech impairment of adults with cerebral palsy. *Folia Phoniat.*, **30**, 30–57 (1978).

Platt, L. J., Andrews, G., Young, M., and Quinn, P. T., Dysarthria of adult cerebral palsy: intelligibility and articulatory impairment. *J. Speech Hearing Res.*, **23**, 28–55 (1980).

Podeanu-Czehofsky, I., Is it only the child's guilt? some aspects of family life of cerebral palsied children. *Rehabilitation Literature*, **36**, 308–311 (1975).

Quinn, P. T., and Andrews, G., Cerebral dominance for language in cerebral palsy. *J. Neurol. Neurosurg. Psychiatry*, **40**, 608–610 (1977).

Ratusnik, D. L., Wolfe, V. I., Penn, R. D., and Schewitz, S., Effects on speech of chronic cerebellar stimulation in cerebral palsy. *J. Neuro. Surg.*, **48**, 876–882 (1978).

Rothman, J. G., Effects of respiratory exercises on the vital capacity and forced expiratory volume in children with cerebral palsy. *Physical Therapy*, **58**, 421–425 (1978).

Rutherford, B. R., The use of negative practice in speech therapy with children handicapped by cerebral palsy, athetoid type. *J. Speech Dis.*, **5**, 259–264 (1940).

Rutherford, B. R., A comparative study of loudness, pitch, rate, rhythm and quality of the speech of children handicapped by cerebral palsy. *Journal of Speech Disorders*, **9**, 263–271 (1944).

Rutherford, B. R., Speech and language therapy for the cerebral palsied child. In W. T. Daley, *Speech and Language Therapy with the Cerebral Palsied Child*. Washington: The Catholic University of America Press, Inc. (1965).

Rutherford, B. R., *Give Them a Chance to Talk*. (Rev. ed.) Minneapolis, Minn.: Burgess Publishing Co. (1950).

Schein, J., and Delk, M., *The Deaf Population in the United States*. Silver Springs, Md.: National Association of the Deaf (1971).

Schiefelbush, L., and Lloyd, L., *Language perspectives—acquisition, retardation and intervention*. Baltimore: University Park Press (1974).

Seidel, U. P., Chadwick, O. F. D., and Rutter, M., Psychological disorders in crippled children: A comparative study of children with and without brain damage. *Develop. Med. Child Neurol.*, **17,** 563–573 (1975).

Shane, H. C., and Bashier, A. S., Election criteria for determining candidacy for an augmentive communication system: Preliminary considerations. Paper presented at American Speech-Language and Hearing Association Convention, San Francisco, California (1978).

Shapiro, I., An investigation of the ability of auditors to assess athetoid and spastic cerebral palsy by listening to speech samples. Unpublished master's thesis, Syracuse University, Syracuse, New York (1960).

Shavell, A., Drooling in cerebral palsy. *South African J. Commun. Dis.*, **24,** 76–87 (1977).

Silverman, F. L., *Communication for the Speechless*. Englewood Cliffs, N.J.: Prentice-Hall, Inc. (1980).

Sittig, E., The chewing method applied for excessive salivation and drooling in cerebral palsy. *J. Speech Dis.*, **12,** 191–194 (1947).

Stanford-Binet, *Intelligence Scale, Revised Form L-M*, Norms Edition. Boston: Houghton Mifflin (1972).

Stetson, R. H., A motor theory of rhythm and discrete succession. *Psychological Review*, **12,** 250–270, 293–350 (1905).

Stetson, R. H., *Motor phonetics: A Study of Speech Movements in Action* (2nd ed.) Amsterdam: North-Holland Publishing Co. (1951).

Stewart, L. G., Hearing-impaired developmentally disabled persons in the United States: definitions, causes, effects and prevalence estimates. *Annals of the Deaf*, **28,** 488–494 (1978).

Stillman, R., *The Collier-Azua Scale*. Dallas: The University of Texas at Dallas (1976).

Stinchfield-Hawk, S. M., and Young, E. H., *Children with delayed or defective speech*. Stanford, Calif.: Stanford University Press (1938).

United Cerebral Palsy Association, *Facts and Figures*. New York: UCPA, Inc. (1977).

Vanderheiden, G., *Nonvocal Communication Resource Book*. Baltimore: University Park Press (1978).

Vanderheiden, G., and Grilley, K. (Eds.), *Non-vocal Communication Techniques and Aids for the Severely Physically Handicapped*. Baltimore: University Park Press (1976).

Vining, E. P. G., Accardo, P. J., Rubenstein, J. E., Farrell, S. E. and Roizen, N. J., Cerebral palsy: A pediatric developmentalist's overview. *Amer. J. Dis. Child*, **130,** 643–649 (1976).

Wechsler, D., *Wechsler Preschool and Primary Scale of Intelligence*. New York: The Psychological Corporation (1967).

Wechsler, D., *The Wechsler Intelligence Scale for Children*. (Rev. ed.) New York: The Psychological Corporation (1974).

Wepman, J., A speech correction technique. *The Crippled Child*, **21,** 75–83 (1943).

Westlake, H., *A System for Developing Speech with Cerebral Palsy Children*. Chicago: National Society for Crippled Children and Adults (1951).

Whittaker, C. K., Cerebellar stimulation for cerebral palsy. *J. Neursurg.*, **52,** 648–653 (1980).

Wiig, E. H., and Semel, E. M., *Language Disabilities in Children and Adolescents*. Columbus: Charles E. Merrill Publishing Co. (1976).

Wolfe, W. G., A comprehensive evaluation of fifty cases of cerebral palsy. *Journal of Speech and Hearing Disorders*, **15,** 234–251 (1950).

Wolpe, J., *The Practice of Behavior Therapy*. New York: Pergamon Press (1969).

8   Aphasia Rehabilitation

Joyce Fitch-West

INTRODUCTION

The term *aphasia* implies a constellation of linguistic deficits which result from damage to one of the cerebral hemispheres of the brain. In this chapter we shall define what is meant by this term and describe the language and behavior typical of aphasic patients. As we do this, a classification system will emerge. Although the system described here evolved in the late eighteenth century as scientists began to localize language in the brain, it has reemerged today as one of the most widely used classification systems (Goodglass and Kaplan, 1972). Since classifying a patient as to the type of aphasia displayed can be an important feature of diagnosis and treatment planning, even the early history of aphasia could have direct relevance to you as you face a particular patient. It is the intent of this chapter to show how each facet of the phenomena of aphasia might relate to the management of the patient as is seen by you in your clinical work. It continues with a brief review of classification systems other than that described by Goodglass and Kaplan (1972), provides a description of some of the variables that affect a patient's ability to respond to stimuli, reviews various treatment approaches used today, and concludes with a description of the process of becoming an aphasia therapist. What we hope you will gain from reading this chapter is an appreciation for how the history of aphasia, the characteristics of the patient, the diagnostic and treatment approaches selected, and your own attitudes will impact upon the patient you treat.

CHARACTERISTICS OF ADULT APHASIA

Etiology and Classification of Aphasia

The term *aphasia* refers to language disturbances caused by lesions (damage) to one of the hemispheres of the brain, usually the left hemisphere. Any process that interferes with the transport of oxygen to the cells of the brain may produce these lesions: trauma, brain tumors, certain inflammatory processes and degenerative diseases may have as their sequelae, brain damage, and resulting aphasia. The vast majority of

378

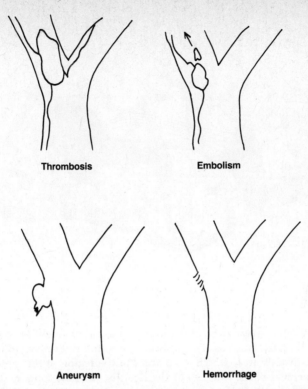

Figure 8–1. Schematic of an Artery Showing the Four Major Processes That Result in Stroke. Note that changes occurred in the walls of the artery which contribute to the formation of the plaque.

aphasias, however, are the consequence of *cerebrovascular accident* (CVA) or stroke. Stroke is typically the outcome of *arteriosclerosis* (commonly referred to as hardening of the arteries) which has spread throughout the vascular system. Arteriosclerosis is a condition marked by loss of elasticity, thickening, and hardening of the arteries. *Atherosclerosis* is an extremely common form of arteriosclerosis in which lipid and cholesterol deposits accumulate in the blood vessels, damaging their walls and accelerating the formation and the adhesion of blood clots. *Hypertension* (high blood pressure) and *high cholesterol* levels in the blood contribute to an increase in atherosclerotic plaque, but the exact nature of the process that changes a healthy artery into one with the potential for a stroke is not precisely known. Stroke occurs when the deposits have accumulated to the point where (1) an artery is occluded (blocked) by a blood clot that stays at its point of origin *(thrombosis)*; (2) a bit of the plaque or a clot or other deposit breaks off and travels from a large artery to a smaller one *(embolism)*; or (3) an artery ruptures because of an aneurysm or because of the deterioration in its wall causing a cerebral *hemorrhage* (see figure 8–1). The stroke thus causes a sudden interference to the arterial system that brings blood (and thus oxygen and other nutrients) to the brain; this deficiency of blood is referred to as *ischemia*. When brain tissue is deprived of oxygen, the cells die *(necrosis)* and an area of cell death *(infarct)* is created. Infarcts in particular areas of the brain result in specific kinds of language disorders, but "it is the

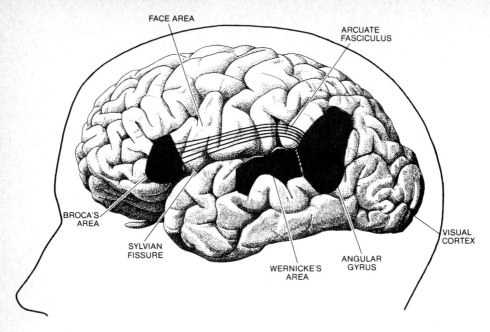

FACE AREA

ARCUATE
FASCICULUS

BROCA'S
AREA

SYLVIAN
FISSURE

WERNICKE'S
AREA

ANGULAR
GYRUS

VISUAL
CORTEX

Figure 8–2. Primary language areas of the human brain are thought to be located in the left hemisphere, because only rarely does damage to the right hemisphere cause language disorders. Broca's area, which is adjacent to the region of the motor cortex that controls the movement of the muscles of the lips, the jaw, the tongue, the soft palate and the vocal cords, apparently incorporates programs for the coordination of these muscles in speech. Damage to Broca's area results in slow and labored speech, but comprehension of language remains intact. Wernicke's area lies between Heschl's gyrus, which is the primary receiver of auditory stimuli, and the angular gyrus, which acts as a way station between the auditory and the visual regions. When Wernicke's area is damaged, speech is fluent but has little content and comprehension is usually lost. Wernicke's and Broca's areas are joined by a nerve bundle called the arcuate fasciculus. When it is damaged, speech is fluent but abnormal, and patient can comprehend words but cannot repeat them.

neuroanatomic location of the brain damage, not the causative agent, that is the key to the symptomatology" (Benson, 1979, p. 18).

Aphasia results from damage to the hemisphere that is dominant for language and is often associated with *contralateral hemiplegia* (paralysis of the opposite half of the body). For most individuals, regardless of their handedness, the dominant hemisphere for language is the left hemisphere. Left-handed people complicate the picture somewhat, but more than half of them also have their language organized in the left hemisphere; the remaining presumably have language either in the right hemisphere, or, more probably, some language represented in both hemispheres (Springer and Deutsch, 1981). Thus, aphasia in most individuals is caused by lesions in the left hemisphere; it is often associated with right hemiplegia, for the left side of the cerebral hemisphere controls the right side of the body, and vice versa. Lesions in the left hemisphere will almost always produce some degree of aphasia (Boller and Vignolo, 1966). The severity will vary a great deal, from minimal, temporary

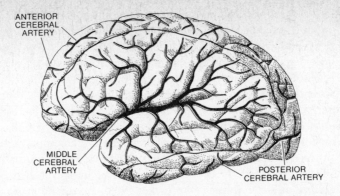

ANTERIOR
CEREBRAL
ARTERY

MIDDLE
CEREBRAL
ARTERY

POSTERIOR
CEREBRAL ARTERY

Figure 8–3. Cerebral areas are nourished by several arteries, each supplying blood to a specific region. The speech and auditory region is nourished by the middle cerebral artery. The visual areas at the rear are supplied by the posterior cerebral artery. In patients who suffer from inadequate oxygen supply to the brain the damage is often not within the area of a single blood vessel but rather in the "border zones." These are the regions between the areas served by the major arteries where the blood supply is marginal.

dysfunction, to almost total and permanent inability to understand spoken language, speak, read, and write.

Lesions in areas along the Sylvian fissure of the left hemisphere (the *perisylvian* region) produce the more common types of aphasia (see figure 8–2). The Rolandic fissure or central sulcus is also an important anatomical guidepost. Lesions in front of the fissure, (see figure 8–2) *pre-Rolandic* lesions, produce a nonfluent aphasia *(Broca's* aphasia), while post-Rolandic lesions, those occurring behind the fissure, produce fluent aphasias (such as *Wernicke's*, conduction, or anomic aphasias). These areas are served by the middle cerebral artery; thus, aphasia is most often caused by involvement of some branch of the middle cerebral artery. (See figure 8–3.)

Aphasia is without a doubt one of the most devastating impairments that can happen, for it strikes at the essence of what it is to be human, the ability to use and understand language. From the earliest days, aphasiologists have reserved the term aphasia for language disorders, contrasting it with those speech impairments that are primarily related to the production of speech. Hughlings Jackson in 1874 said "to speak is not simply to utter words it is to propositionize" (p. 159). In the case of aphasia, the disorder is one that involves the ability to conceptualize, to propositionize, to use language in creative, human ways. Disorders of speech, on the other hand, impair the ability to articulate words but do not affect the underlying ability to use and understand language.

Views of aphasia have tended to reflect the changing philosophical stance of the field of neurology. When the disorder was first described, it triggered much enthusiasm for localizing all mental functions within circumscribed areas of the brain. Broca in 1861 had declared that he had identified the center of articulated language and since it had not been clear to this point just what the neurological substratum for language might be and where it might lie, Broca's discovery was greeted with great excitement among most neurologists and anthropologists. Unfortunately, the enthusiasm for localization frequently exceeded what could be scientifically documented, and there were attempts to localize all of man's intellectual abilities and his emotions such as love, charity, honor, and the like, in delineated areas of the brain. But the excesses of his colleagues should not be allowed to detract from Broca's contribution, for it indeed had a profound impact on the history of neurology and science in general. Broca (1861) identified the third left frontal convolution as the center of articulated language; the center for the *production* of language (see figure 8-2). When, in 1874, Wernicke described a center in the temporal lobes of the left hemisphere as the site for the *comprehension* of language, the logic and simplicity of viewing aphasia and ultimately language in terms of a motor/sensory dichotomy or an input/output schemata became very attractive. The two types of aphasia were viewed as mutually exclusive. Thus, the aphasia described by Broca (which he had initially called *aphemia*) was variously described as *motor* aphasia (Wernicke, 1908), *expressive* aphasia (Pick, 1913; Weisenburg and McBride, 1935), an *encoding* deficit (Osgood and Miron, 1963), and *efferent* aphasia (Luria, 1964), while that of Wernicke was labeled as *sensory* aphasia (Wernicke, 1908; Goldstein, 1948), *receptive* aphasia (Wernicke, 1908; Goldstein, 1948), a *decoding* deficit (Osgood and Miron, 1963), or *afferent* aphasia (Luria, 1964). The impact of the view that there is an opposition between the functions of language input and language output has affected the classification of aphasic disorders from the beginning to the present. The advantages that such systems have of simplicity and a certain scientific logic do not outweigh their potential for detriment to the patient, however. For example, clinicians who used the Weisenburg and McBride (1935) system all too frequently ignored their structure that "the disorders are only *predominantly* [their italics] expressive or receptive, the other processes in either case are always more or less affected. . . ." (p. 144).

Early aphasiologists tended to extrapolate directly from behavior to brain center. That is, they would identify a patient with a specific language disorder, let us say, for example, a remarkable impairment in writing. When the patient died they would examine his brain at autopsy. Finding pathology in a focal area of the brain, the conclusion drawn would be that they not only had discovered the causative lesion, but the brain center for writing as well. Although good scientific practice would dictate that more than one such patient and brain be observed before generalities were drawn, discrepancies and exceptions among patients were frequently overlooked in the rush to prove the existence of specialized brain centers.

From the beginning, however, there were those neurologists who fought against localizing mental phenomena with such all-encompassing exactness. Jackson (1874) said "to locate the damage which destroys speech and to locate speech are two different things" (p. 130). Marie (1903) reacted vociferously to the localizationists with a paper entitled "The third frontal convolution does not play any special role in the function of language" and declared that there was but one true aphasia, the sensory aphasia described by Wernicke. Henry Head, Jackson's student, wrote most disparagingly of the earlier "diagram makers" (1926, p. 54), those individuals who had attempted to locate all of man's intellectual and emotional capabilities in circumscribed areas of the brain. Head felt that language functioning was too complex for one part of the process to be disturbed in isolation. Following Head, the prevailing theories of aphasia emphasized the holistic nature of the language impairment. Kurt Goldstein's view (1948) was that the altered language behavior of the aphasic patient could only be understood in relation to the total cerebral disorganization created by the brain injury.

As we review the history of aphasia, which, unlike many other areas of our discipline, has a long and varied history, we see that at any point in time there were those who argued from a localizational point of view and those who adopted a more holistic approach. If you were a localizationist, you were more or less obligated to acknowledge that there could be relatively "pure" disorders. If you believed that an isolated center for writing existed, for example, the conclusion would follow that a lesion could be restricted to that particular area and would produce a "pure" agraphia (writing impairment). If, on the other hand, you argued from a holistic point of view, you would be much less inclined to believe such a pure disorder could exist in isolation and argue that most, if not all, aphasics would have language impairment in all language modalities. Speaking, understanding spoken language, reading, and writing would be impaired. Pure disorders from this point of view were suspect; more remarkable deficits in writing might occur because the lesion impinged upon an integration area necessary for writing (Luria, 1964, 1966), but the disorder would occur against a background of aphasia, however subtle.

Observation of aphasic patients leaves little doubt that most have impairment in all language modalities. They have difficulty producing language orally or in writing, and they have difficulty comprehending spoken or written language. Hildred Schuell and her associates (1964) based their classification system upon this observation. They considered aphasia "a general language deficit that crosses all language modalities and may or may not be complicated by other sequelae of brain damage" (p. 113). Brown (1968) has a similar viewpoint that strongly emphasizes the "one aphasia" concept (Benson, 1979, p. 59).

On the other hand, when classic examples of Broca's or Wernicke's aphasia appear in a clinician's office, one cannot help but be impressed with the validity of the anatomically based concepts, particularly when modern-day CAT (computerized axial tomography) scan confirms the localization. In truth, as Benson (1979) has pointed out, "while it is accurate to divide prevailing approaches to aphasia into the anatomically based localizers and the psychologically based holists, most investigators utilize material from both approaches to a greater or lesser degree" (p. 16).

Perhaps the best marriage of the two points of view has evolved in recent years at the Veterans Administration Medical Center in Boston where researchers in the aphasia unit (Geschwind, 1965; Goodglass, Quadfasel, and Timberlake, 1964; Benson, 1967; Goodglass and Kaplan, 1972) have revitalized the use of the classical system based upon anatomical site of lesion, while at the same time vigorously investigating the neurolinguistic[1] characteristics of the patients studied, and integrating these characteristics into the description of each syndrome. Their classification system will be discussed in depth as we pursue the neurolinguistic characteristics of aphasia.

Why should classification issues be of importance to a clinician about to embark upon a treatment program for a particular patient? As Goodglass (1981) has noted "the neurolinguistic features that distinguish individual patterns represent the *minimal* repertory of dimensions of aphasia to which the clinician should attend—*minimal* because there are many other features that are important to the understanding of aphasic patients' functioning and that are common to many forms of aphasia" (p. 2).

---

[1] Neurolinguistics is the application of the methods and models of linguistics to the study of disturbances of the realization of speech caused by cortical lesions (Lebrun, 1976).

Types of Aphasia and Their Neurolinguistic Features

The Types of Aphasia. Although a review of the history of aphasia leads to the conclusion that there are dozens of terms used to classify the disorder, in reality most investigators describe the same four or five major groups: Broca's, Wernicke's, conduction, anomic, and global aphasic. For our purposes, these five groups will suffice to provide an adequate picture of the types of aphasia a clinician is most likely to see. Other types such as the transcortical aphasias or modality specific syndromes are rare or less generally described (Kertesz, 1979). Since our concern is aphasia rehabilitation, our emphasis will be on the neurolinguistic aspects that are outstanding features of a particular type of aphasia; we will then explore in more depth how some of these features impact on treatment planning. Broca's, Wernicke's, conduction and anomic aphasia figure prominently in the classification system used by Goodglass and Kaplan (1972); Kertesz (1979) emphasizes Broca's, Wernicke's, anomic, and global aphasia. Table 8–1 lists the major characteristics of each of these aphasias.

A lesion in Broca's area produces a nonfluent aphasia. The Broca's aphasic may be so severely impaired as to be speechless, or reduced to one-word utterances, often laboriously produced; if sentences are produced they are typically agrammatic: the substantives may be present, the little words signaling the syntax of the utterance lacking. Speech sounds dysfluent and effortful. Comprehension is almost always relatively mildly impaired. It is this observation alone that makes a strictly localizational point of view hard to reconcile, for Broca's area is some distance away from Wernicke's area. Unless one argues for an integrative concept of the language areas functioning together, it is difficult to explain why the Broca's aphasic has comprehension problems of any sort, although the reading centers are now thought to be multiple (Levine and Calvanio, 1982). Indeed, such comprehension deficits were frequently overlooked by individuals who were zealous about their anatomical models. Comprehension for the Broca's aphasic, though, is usually better preserved than production or, on a relative scale, mild compared to his limited verbal output. There are a number of investigators (Zurif, Caramazza, and Myerson, 1972; Zurif and Blumstein, 1978; Schwartz, Saffran and Marin, 1980) who today argue that there is a general deficit which affects syntactic processes in production as well as in comprehension. Reading parallels the auditory comprehension deficits the patient experiences and writing, the productive difficulties (Albert, Goodglass, Helm, Rubens, and Alexander, 1981).

The following is an excerpt from an interview with a twenty-eight-year-old veteran who suffered left brain damage and consequent Broca's aphasia after being hit by a helicopter blade in Vietnam. He is describing photographs he took of horses grazing near an abandoned stable.

> *Therapist:* "What pictures did you take?"
> *Patient:* "uh . . . uh . . . the uh . . . the . . . the . . . three
> uh . . horse . . . no horses . . . uh . . in barns . . in
> barns?"
> *Therapist:* "three horses in barns?"
> *Patient:* "no . . . three barnhorses . . . uh . . . barnhorses."
> *Therapist:* "*stable horses?*"
> *Patient:* "stable horses . . . stable horses . . . and. . . uh . . .
> then torn down. No, not torn down, but abandoned."

Broca's Aphasia	Wernicke's Aphasia
prosodic alterations	normal melody
limited verbal output	copious verbal output
impaired articulatory agility	normal articulatory agility
reduced rate of speaking	normal or supra-normal rate of speech
short phrases	normal or supra-normal phrase length
limited grammatical forms	full range of grammatical forms
telegrammatic, agrammatic	syntax preserved
comprehension relatively intact	comprehension definitely impaired with semantic paraphasias occurring primarily

Conduction Aphasia

fluent, paraphasic speech, primarily literal paraphasias
outstanding number of literal paraphasic errors
repetition disproportionately impaired
near normal auditory comprehension
acute awareness of errors; rejects incorrect efforts

Anomic Aphasia	Global Aphasia
fluent speech, good articulation, appropriate grammatical forms	severe loss of all receptive and expressive modalities
severe word finding deficits	speech almost totally absent
comprehension relatively intact	recurring stereotypic utterances often occur
unusual circumlocutions for words that cannot be recalled	may use a normal melody and intonation with stereotypic utterances such that normal comprehension is often mistakenly inferred
writing content often unclear and sterile	
literal and semantic paraphasic errors minimal	

Table 8–1. Characteristics of Broca's, Wernicke's, Conduction, Anomic, and Global Aphasia.

Therapist: "Did you get any good shots?"
Patient: "Yes. And then the . . . the . . . the trees. And the and the and old trees . . . and . . . no . . . uh . . . no . . . uh . . . uh."

Another patient who had a CVA at age forty-nine following a long-standing history of hypertension, described the comprehension problems he experienced as a Wernicke's aphasic:

Well, after when I sit home or just take my time and n' just look at what it is and I'll take time and I'll take it over again, do this an then, this here I'll know I'll know exactly what it is, y'know. But if I'll take my time I can do this and do this n' do this n' do this and take my time (unintelligible) right away, right away I'll I'll forget it. I'll get the long. I'll, I'll get the I'll put, I'll put them down, but it be not.

As we can see, the Wernicke's aphasic contrasts quite sharply with the Broca's aphasic (see table 8–1). The patients with Wernicke's aphasia produce fluent, well-articulated speech that is made with little effort. They are often too loquacious, producing speech that may be at a supranormal rate or of a supranormal phrase length. Their speech, however, is typically quite empty and seems devoid of meaning. The patients are circumlocutory and tangential, unable to keep to the point. Comprehension is moderately to severely impaired in most instances. The patients are sometimes unaware of their deficits and have little feedback as to what their own speech sounds like. Reading comprehension may be severely impaired but because the written symbol is present and stable rather than fleeting, reading comprehension may be somewhat better preserved than auditory comprehension. Writing is often produced effortlessly but typically is as empty as the oral speech; it is not unusual to ask a patient to write his name and have him produce an entire page of empty speech. The words produced may be true words, or they may be *neologisms*, words that appear to be invented. These patients make many paraphasic (substitution) errors, both *phonemic* or *literal* (sound) and *semantic* or *verbal* (word-meaning) substitutions, although semantic substitutions are typical of all types of aphasia.

The conduction aphasic first described by Wernicke is another classic type of aphasic from an anatomical point of view, for these patients should, by definition, have lesions in the conducting pathway, the *arcuate fasciculus*, (see figure 8–2) connecting Broca's and Wernicke's areas. According to Wernicke's model, comprehension should be normal or nearly normal in such patients. Speech output is fluent and characterized by many literal paraphasic errors. Speech tends not to be as empty as that of the Wernicke's aphasic, but they do have difficulty repeating words or phrases. In theory what is heard in Wernicke's area cannot be transmitted to Broca's area and this accounts for the repetition deficit. (See table 8–1.)

Describing his efforts to complete the *New York Times* crossword puzzle (which would be an extraordinary feat for an aphasic of any type), one of our patients said:

Ah tee, ah tee I da dese do ah ats in der wad in da oderwa I do na know. Ah da dis ma n' da ma ba I dan not ge da for the life of me.

[I think, I think I got these two but what's in the one in the other one I do not know. I got this one and that one but I cannot get that for the life of me.]

This sample was spoken at an extremely rapid rate. It was, as we can see, all but unintelligible yet there was a run of five words, the cliché "for the life of me" that was easily and correctly produced. Such samples are typical of this patient and of conduction aphasics in general. The extreme number of literal paraphasic errors is a distinguishing feature of conduction aphasia. Our patient's comprehension of spoken language was excellent. Asked to repeat "No ifs ands or buts about it," however, produced "no iffle, no eifel"; most efforts to repeat produced only articulated struggle with no real words resulting. This patient's success at the *New York Times* crossword puzzle was limited, but he was able to do simpler crosswords and his reading was enough unimpaired to enable him to read for pleasure.

The outstanding feature of the syndrome called anomic aphasia is the severe word-finding deficits these patients exhibit. Conversational speech typically sounds dramatically empty, for the patient uses many indefinite words such as "thing" or "one" as substitutes for words that cannot be recalled. Confrontation naming (requiring the use of specific words) is often quite impaired, but there are anomic patients who have confrontation naming preserved in spite of dramatic difficulties in free speech. Speech is fluent, well-articulated, with preserved grammatical form. Comprehension is typically quite good, and repetition often excellent. Reading and writing may vary as to the degree of impairment; writing very often is as empty as oral language. Literal and semantic paraphasic errors are minimal, but the patient may make rather bizarre circumlocutions for words he or she cannot recall.

In an interview where the patient was describing his childhood stuttering problem, the following was transcribed:

Therapist: "Where did you have therapy for it?"
Patient: "Oh, I had it in all kinds of places."
Therapist: "Well, for example . . . "
Patient: "Well, it's . . it's hard to tell you which one it is.
    Because I couldn't do it. Because I'm not I'm not not
    uh in the uh . . Oh, let's say in the right place . . to
    tell you."
Therapist: "I didn't quite understand that."
Patient: "No . . . I . . . I . . . I couldn't say where."
Therapist: "Why?"
Patient: "Actually, I . . I don't know why, really."
Therapist: "Now, is it because you don't remember, or because
    you can't find the word . . . or what?"
Patient: "Maybe . . . the word . . . and the remembering, too."

When another therapist apologized for mixing up his name, he said, "One more time, you know. You're gonna to get something in your house then which will say, 'he is not what he says.' "

In response to a test item on the Boston Diagnostic Aphasia Examination (Goodglass and Kaplan, 1972), "Where do we go to buy medicine?," the patient said, "I've never done that. My wife buys everything and that's not fooling you either." "Well, where does she go?," asked the therapist. "She's in Pennsylvania and always goes to the other . . . you know, the other one . . . the one over there . . . but we never buy medicine." The latter statement would be true for a Veterans Administration patient, since medicine is typically provided by the hospital pharmacy, but it still begs the question!

Schuell (1965) described global aphasia as an irreversible aphasic syndrome characterized by almost complete loss of functional language skills in all modalities. The term thus implies severe involvement of all receptive and expressive modalities. Speaking, comprehension, reading, and writing are each seriously compromised and none serve as an adequate mode of communication. Speech is either almost totally absent or characterized by recurring stereotypic utterances; that is, utterances that are constantly repeated but without linguistic meaning. Very often these are single phonemes such as "wu-wu-wu" or phrases such as "one-uh-one-uh-one-uh." Global aphasics may inflect these stereotypies with such variety and feeling that the listener feels a conversational exchange has occurred. Similarly, because such patients seem to be alert to the nonverbal nuances in a conversation, their comprehension seems much better than objective test data would indicate, and the untrained listener is frequently convinced that much more has been understood than in fact has been. Family members often claim that the patient understands almost everything said to him. "Even though Norm doesn't really speak to me, I can speak to him, and I more or less can understand what he wants to tell me most of the time, and we kid around and we joke a lot, and we just make the best of it," said the wife of one of our very alert but globally impaired patients.

The following is a conversation between a visiting clinician and a global aphasic:

Therapist: "How are you today?"
Patient: "Two. O.K., but two-two. Two. Come on, but (sniff) two, two" (shakes head negatively).
Therapist: "You don't feel well?"
Patient: "Two. And two. Two-two" (nods head affirmatively).
Therapist: "You have a bad cold?"
Patient: "Two. But, O.K., two."
Therapist: "Does your wife have a cold, also?"
Patient: "Yeah . . . here. Two. See, eh, two (sniffs), yeah, two. (Nods head affirmatively and looks intently at the therapist) . . . two?"
Therapist: "Oh, I'm sorry to hear that."

The visiting therapist concluded that the patient's wife had a cold and was pleased that she understood the transaction. In fact, the patient's wife did *not* have a cold, although he did, and that part of the transaction he was able to successfully convey, but not with language. His gestures, his facial expressions, and particularly his "sniff" were what contributed to his listener's comprehension of his share of the conversation.

Many who came into contact with this patient assumed that his comprehension was normal, for he truly maintained his share of the conversational burden. Communication occurred, but the informational exchange could be spotty.

The five aphasia types discussed thus far should be considered as reference points to help define how neurolinguistic features cluster into patterns following brain damage. As Goodglass (1982) has noted, "aphasic syndromes are not 'real' entities; the syndromes represent 'modal' patterns of response to injury in certain zones within the language area. "Fewer than half of the patients with aphasia can be assigned with confidence to one of the standard syndromes" (p. 2). A majority of aphasic patients *can*, however, be validly classified as "fluent" or "nonfluent" (Benson, 1979). Broca's aphasics are nonfluent; Wernicke's, conduction, and anomic aphasics are fluent. In terms of localization, pre-Rolandic lesion patients, those with lesions in Broca's area, are nonfluent, while post-Rolandic lesion patients, those with lesions in the temporal and temporoparietal regions, are fluent. The former group are the Broca's aphasics, the latter, the Wernicke's, conduction, and anomic aphasics. One important aspect of the fluency dimension is phrase length. The nonfluent aphasic rarely exceeds four-word groupings; the fluent aphasic may have runs of six or more words (Goodglass, 1981). Nonfluency is associated with impaired articulatory agility (laborious articulation), effortful speech that lacks grammatical structure, alterations in the prosody of speech, and reduction in the flow of speech. Fluency is associated with normal articulation, preserved prosody and grammatical structure, ease in producing a flow of speech, and a preponderance of paraphasic and anomic word-finding problems (Goodglass, 1981). We shall, accordingly, discuss some of the neurolinguistic features in further detail using the nonfluent/fluent dichotomy as a useful reference point in differentiating what consequences these features have on patient management.

The Impact of Certain Neurolinguistic Features of Aphasia on Patient Management

Both the fluent and the nonfluent aphasic make paraphasic errors, but there is a sense, a quality, that is different in the way each type makes an error (Albert, Goodglass, Helm, Rubens and Alexander, 1981). Paraphasic errors are errors of substitution. They may be on the phonemic level, *phonemic paraphasias*, also referred to as *literal paraphasias*, or on the semantic level, *semantic* or *verbal paraphasias*. Paraphasic errors made by the Wernicke's aphasic seem effortless, without struggle. They are typically made in the context of clearly articulated utterances. The Broca's aphasic, on the other hand, may make the same error, yet it seems to be made with struggle and effort. Identifying an object, the Broca's and conduction aphasic may struggle, "it's a fork . . . no, no, a-a-a-sork . . . no . . . no, a nork . . . no, no, a f- f-, a fort," while the Wernicke's aphasic names the fork rapidly, "that's a fort," and goes on with little awareness of the error he's made. The anomic aphasic's speech is characterized by circumlocutions, generalizations, and word-finding pauses, but relatively few paraphasias. In the case of the Broca's aphasic, the final misnaming of the fork as "fort" seems to come from some sort of mis-targeting in the articulation, while the way the Wernicke's aphasic makes his phonemic paraphasic error seems freer and more clearly produced as an obvious phonemic substitution. Paraphasias abound in the speech of the Wernicke's and conduction aphasic, and important diagnostic distinctions can be made among the types of fluent aphasics. A prevalence of semantic paraphasias suggests Wernicke's aphasia, a prevalence of literal paraphasias, a conduction aphasia, and the absence of either semantic or literal paraphasias suggests an anomic aphasia (Benson, 1979).

In evaluating a patient for treatment it is important to analyze how the search for the correct word occurs. Capitalizing on a patient's existing strategy at word retrieval and helping him refine that strategy rather than creating a new one may be a more efficacious approach. Thus, a patient who says, "cut . . . no . . . cutter . . . no . . . no . . . kif . . . knife," may be revealing something about the strategy with which he is approaching word retrieval. Working with the action imagery of cutting to help him visualize the act of cutting with a knife may help him retrieve the word *knife*. In other words, visual imagery could serve as a strategy for word retrieval (West, in press). Asking the Wernicke's aphasic to pause and listen to what he has just called an object, to repeat it aloud, may help him begin to develop the feedback necessary to begin self-correction.

The substitution errors may be so extreme as to sound like invented new words or *neologisms*. Thus, when asked what he does with a comb, one of our fluent aphasics said, "Well, it's a good thing for taking the nits out of your riggy." One could argue that both "nits" and "riggy" were neologisms, but because this patient went on to self-correct, "I mean, the knots out of your hair," it seems clear that "nits" was probably an example of a literal paraphasia, while "riggy" was more clearly a neologism.

When the paraphasias become so extreme as to produce unrecognizable utterances, the speech output is referred to as *jargon*. The jargon may be fluent, well-articulated words that mean nothing, add up to little if any meaning—*semantic jargon*—or there may be strings of sounds that are spaced together like words in an utterance, but the words have been so altered by phonemic substitutions as to change their composition—*phonemic jargon*. The two may coexist in the same patient. We treated a patient with a wonderful flow of inflected phonemic jargon and a very outgoing, cheerful personality. So engaging was our patient that people assumed that he was speaking some language to them that they didn't understand. There were those who swore it was Yiddish, others said, no, a Norwegian dialect. But, no one, it turned out, could translate this flow, and, in fact, the patient had spoken only English prior to his stroke. Another patient with semantic jargon was asked to tell us what he did that day. "Well, if of wak, and I sought for the way, for riching, and is nordic and it's cameron and nornon and finally now."

Virtually all aphasics show some degree of *anomia*, word-retrieval difficulty, and it is often the only obvious remaining deficit in recovered aphasics. Benson (1979) suggests the following tests provide useful diagnostic information:

"1. Auditing conversational speech for word-finding problems to determine whether the defect stems from word production problems (faulty articulation, paraphasia) or an inability to retrieve the correct word;
2. Testing the ability to name items by visual presentation from the following categories: objects, parts of objects, body parts, colors, geometric shapes, numerals, letters, and actions;
3. Testing the ability to name items on tactile presentation;
4. Testing the ability to name from auditory stimulation;
5. Testing the ability to name objects from a verbal description of their function;
6. Testing the ability to name illness-oriented items;
7. Monitoring the ability to benefit from cues (prompting) when naming is failed;
8. Testing the ability to produce words from a given category (animals, articles of furniture, words beginning with the letter "R," etc.)" (p. 35)

One should carefully assess each patient's word-finding ability in each of the above areas, for there may be contexts or situations in which word-finding ability is relatively better preserved. Not only does it help in therapy to have, for example, a category of names one can be assured of for success, but useful treatment strategies may become apparent from how the patient succeeds or fails on each of the above tests. Certainly, knowing the types of cues that help a patient retrieve a name can be important diagnostic information.

Some patients respond readily to a phonemic or semantic cue supplied by the examiner; "it's a f . . . " or "knife and _____," to cue *fork*, but other patients seem completely blank and no cue helps. Nonfluent aphasics respond well to cuing as a rule, but fluent aphasics often are unable to recognize the correct word even if they have said it correctly themselves or the examiner has supplied it. Holding a knife one of our patients said "knife?, knife?" and echoed it again when the examiner said, "yes, knife." And then he finally put the knife down saying, "I don't know what you call it." Anomia is perhaps the one aphasic deficit with which the normal speaker may feel a personal identity, for we have all suffered breakdowns in our ability to retrieve the name of someone, a place, or even an object. The "tip of the tongue" phenomenon so often felt by normal speakers is frequently true of aphasics (Goodglass, Klein, Weintraub, and Ackerman, 1976), and this is diagnostic information important to treatment planning.

Grammatical errors are made by both fluent and nonfluent aphasics, but again, how the errors are made seems totally different in the two types of aphasics. The speech of the nonfluent aphasic will convey much more information than that of the fluent aphasic; the words the Broca's aphasic produces are usually nouns, action verbs, adjectives, or adverbs, usually referred to as the *substantives* or *content* words. These are produced with such effort that one could conclude that the reason for the omission of the grammatical units of language, the *agrammatism*, is an effort to conserve energy, although since it seems clear that similar errors are made in some comprehension tasks, energy conservation could be only part of the story. This alteration in the grammatical structure of speech was referred to as *telegrammatic* speech, for it sometimes resembles the speech one would use in a telegram. The strategy appears to be to delete the "little" words of the language, the prepositions, articles, many adjectives and adverbs, and preserve the most meaningful units. It is characteristic of the nonfluent aphasic to have great difficulty comprehending and using relational words (tall-short, nearer-farther), as well as morphological endings (plurals, possessives, tense) (Goodglass and Berko, 1960) and syntactically complex encoded sentences (Schwartz, et al., 1980).

The empty, loquacious speech of the fluent aphasic is often described as *circumlocutory*: such patients seem to circle around the topic with lengthy utterances and never get to the point. Asked on the Porch Index of Communicative Ability (PICA) (Porch, 1981) to "tell me what you do with each of these" one of our fluent aphasics said about the toothbrush, "Actually, after I eat, I need a whatever. After I eat, I get something proper and I can smell pretty good and I need them more than tum-tum-tum. Or when I wake up and I feel yuk and then I wash." Some fluent aphasics make errors in the use of grammatical structures, and these are referred to as *paragrammatisms*. Most, however, produce utterances that are grammatically correct, but devoid of substantives. The circumlocutions are typical of the diffuse, tangential behavior seen in fluent aphasia, and it is often a first goal of therapy to stop this flow of words so that the patient can begin to listen and develop feedback. On the other hand, some fluent aphasics can learn to use their circumlocutions to effectively overcome their word-finding disabilities. "It's, well, it's one of those things that lots of people use," is not very informative and yet a typical response from such a patient. If the utterance could be extended to "it's one of those things that lots of people use for cutting," or the gesture added, then the circumlocutions may serve to facilitate the listener's comprehension of the target word.

All aphasics will show deficits in comprehending what is spoken (*auditory comprehension disorders*) or written (*alexia*); these deficits may be very subtle or quite profound. As we've discussed previously, the auditory comprehension disorders seen in the Broca's aphasic are typically milder than their verbal output deficits and the reverse may be true for the Wernicke's aphasics: their comprehension of auditory stimuli may be remarkably impaired even though oral output, at least at first blush, could appear relatively intact. The auditory comprehension deficits may be very much dependent on such variables as length (Siegel, 1959), frequency of occurrence (Howes and Geschwind, 1964), vocabulary difficulty (Shewan and Canter, 1971), imageability (Paivio, 1971; West, in press), and syntactic complexity (Levy and Taylor, 1968; West, 1968; Baker and Holland, 1971; Levy and Holland, 1971; Goodglass, et al., 1979).

In single word contexts, e.g., "point to the dog," one aphasic patient may perform relatively well, but another, equally impaired patient may profit from more redundancy, "let's now point to the *dog* that barks, the *dog* that's man's best friend." Under controlled experimental conditions, Gardner, Albert, and Weintraub (1975) demonstrated that speed and redundancy exert a potent effect on comprehension, independent of the particular form of aphasia. These researchers advise that both in therapy and during bedside examinations, more attention should be directed to the rate at which messages are transmitted and to the particular context in which the target word is spoken. They recommend the following sequence in therapy: begin with the word alone, move next to the word in a slowly enunciated, semantically-redundant utterance, then gradually eliminate redundant semantic cues and increase the rate of speaking.

Reading disturbances, *alexia*, are also present in most aphasics. The existence of multiple, specific areas to mediate reading has been confirmed by studies of changes in cerebral blood flow during reading (Lassen, Ingvar, and Skinhj, 1978). The nature of the aphasic alexia does not seem to vary systematically with the location of the lesion, however. Error profiles do differ among alexic subjects, but it may be the case that "differences in error profiles reflect varying degrees of severity along a unidimensional continuum with a predominance of visual errors indicating a less severe problem, semantic errors, a more serious impairment, and perseverations representing the most extreme" (Levine and Calvanio, 1982, p. 385).

For all of the current research on alexia, there are still aphasic patients whose behavior does not fit an experimental paradigm. We see patients who continue to act as if they can read newspapers, magazines, or novels, even though our test data would indicate that reading comprehension even at the simple sentence level is severely impaired. For example, one of our fluent aphasics had been the type of reader who always had a thriller at hand. He continued to carry such books around with him and seemed quite surprised that anyone would question his ability to read them. Even though our testing had revealed marked deficits in reading comprehension, he did indeed seem to grasp something from the thrillers he was reading, for he could tell us bits about their plots. On the other hand, it could be argued that the plots were the same from one thriller to the next, so he had the advantage of familiarity.

The writing impairment (*agraphia*) seen in aphasic patients parallels their speech output. Nonfluent patients write in a manner similar to the way they speak, if they are able to write at all. These patients typically can only write single words; attempts at anything longer is usually met with failure or at best remarkable agrammatic output. Spelling is quite impaired and one sees letter reversals and perseveration (repetition of the same letters or words). The deficit may be so severe as to affect copying and it is also present when the patient attempts anagrams or typing. The written output of the Wernicke's aphasic is also similar to verbal output: the written product is produced effortlessly and with ease but is empty and lacking in substantives. It is often garrulous: the patient will produce pages when a line or two would be adequate. One of our fluent aphasics once wrote an essay as one of his self-imposed homework assignments and mailed it to his therapist. Reviewing it with her, he was quite amused to agree that it was "a nothing of the nothings", his phrase that roughly meant that it didn't make sense to him either.

Hughlings Jackson (1879–80) was one of the first to describe *stereotypies* or *recurring utterances*. Jackson's theory was that these were utterances the patient was making or thinking at the time of onset. He described a woman patient who was taken ill while riding on a donkey, and, hence, her recurring stereotypy was "Gee-Gee." Jackson postulated that these utterances came from the right brain. There is some modern evidence that this might be so; patients who have had left hemispherectomies typically have stereotypies, and the right brains of split brain patients seem to use and comprehend expletives and automatic speech. We have a series of rather remarkable videotapes of a patient whose stereotypy was "thrill-thrill-thrill." He had had much of his left hemisphere removed after sustaining severe head injury following a fall down a flight of stairs. He was a global aphasic with no testable language skills in any modality. And yet, with his "thrill-thrill-thrill" he managed to convey a great deal of emotion and content and was able to set up truly communicative situations with his therapists and his family. He quite clearly tells us on the videotape that he is fed up with being treated as if he were a child; intoning his "thrill-thrill-thrill," he mimics how others talk down to him. Questioned by his therapist, he indicates that not only had his wife visited him the past weekend, but that he has had too many other relatives visiting for his taste. Language in all modalities remained unfunctional for this patient from the point of view of our test data, yet he was able, following discharge, to care for himself at home while his wife worked and to convey basic wants and emotions to sympathetic family members.

Impaired articulatory agility is characteristic of Broca's aphasics. There appears to be a loss and precision of accuracy in forming individual sounds. This may be a part of the general nonfluency and effort involved in producing speech which is characteristic of these patients. *Dysarthria*, on the other hand, is an articulation disorder resulting from neuromuscular disturbance. It often occurs with aphasia, but it should be viewed as concomitant to aphasia and considered a speech disorder rather than a language disorder. Dysarthria is present in many Broca's aphasics, but is relatively rare in fluent aphasia, although the literal paraphasic errors of a conduction aphasic may sound like dysarthria.

A distinction should be made between the dysarthrias caused by cortical lesions (affecting the *upper motor neuron* system) and those caused primarily by damage to the cranial nerves (affecting the *lower motor neuron* system). The oral musculature is innervated bilaterally by the cranial nerves. Those cranial nerves (see figure 8-4) serving speech have their neurons located in the medulla and pons of the brain stem. The fifth cranial nerve (trigeminal) supplies the muscles of mastication; the seventh (facial) innervates the muscles of the face. Motor axons of the tenth (vagus) travel with the ninth (glossopharyngeal) to serve the stylopharyngeus muscle; other motor axons of the tenth join sensory and autonomic fibers to form the vagus nerve and supply the muscles of the soft palate, pharynx, and larynx. Finally, the twelfth (hypoglossal) nerve supplies the intrinsic and extrinsic muscles of the tongue. When the lower motor neuron system is impaired, there is weakness, loss of muscle tone, reduced reflexes, and consequent flaccidity or paralysis. Muscles not receiving cranial nerve innervation atrophy and develop tiny twitches (fasciculations).

Unilateral (on one side) lesions of the upper motor neuron system should cause only

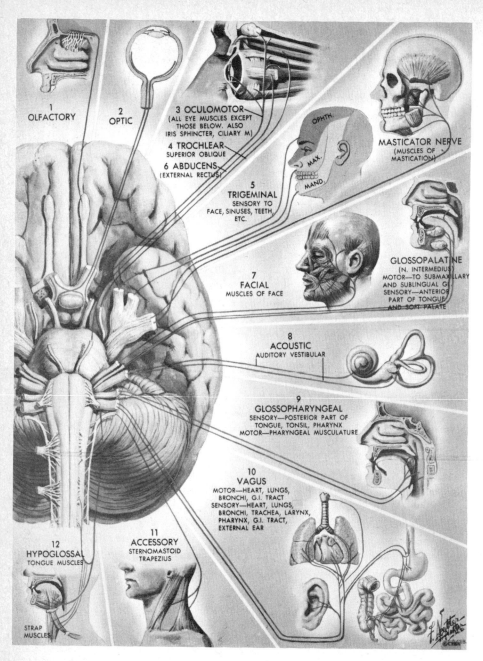

Figure 8–4. The Cranial Nerves

fleeting if any dysarthria because the oral musculature is bilaterally innervated. Consequently, persisting dysarthria in a patient diagnosed as having a unilateral lesion should be a red flag that something else has occurred in the patient's neurological history. Either he has had a previously undetected lesion or more extensive damage occurred during the most recent episode.

Bilateral lesions of the corticobulbar tract (pathways connecting the cortex with the "bulb" or brain stem) produce *pseudobulbar palsy*. Swallowing and articulation are affected because the oral musculature's innervation is bilaterally affected. Reflexes normally inhibited by the cortex such as the sucking reflex or the jaw jerk are released. In addition, the patient has episodes of *emotional lability*, outbursts of crying or laughing that become inappropriately excessive for the minimally humorous or sad situation that triggered the response. Upper motor neuron lesions produce a *spastic dysarthria* which is characterized by slow rate, low pitch, harsh quality, imprecise articulation, and effortful phonation (Darley, Aronson, and Brown, 1975).

Another speech disorder often associated with aphasia is *apraxia*. Apraxia is viewed as a motor programming disorder. Liepmann (1900) defined it as a disturbance of purposeful movement distinguishing it from other motor disorders resulting from paralysis, ataxia, or pathologies affecting muscle tone. Many forms of apraxia have been described in the literature, and it is a disorder fraught with controversial issues. It seems clearest in those instances described as *motor apraxia* or *ideomotor apraxia*. Here the patient is unable to carry out a motor act voluntarily that he is able to perform involuntarily. For example, the patient may be unable to scratch his head, or smile upon command, and yet be able to perform such motions spontaneously. In *ideational apraxia* the patient seems unable to conceptualize the idea of the act itself. We once had an instance of two aphasics sharing a room together. The one patient complained to us of the other: "I don't know; the guy is funny. He gets up and he holds his head, holds his head. And I says, 'Lou, don't hold your head.'" Asked why Lou might be holding his head, Jack, our complainer, who was a mildly impaired fluent aphasic, said,

> Well, the radio was on and Lou, he don't know how to turn it off! So I says to him, 'Lou turn off that damn radio; don't hold your head!' So Lou goes over to the radio, but he can't seem to figure out how to turn the radio off. And I show him the knob, and I says, 'Here, Lou, this turns off the radio, see.' But Lou, he don't seem to know how to turn the knob.

In fact, Lou no longer seemed able to conceptualize many such acts. Even putting toothpaste on his toothbrush seemed beyond him unless we started him out on the sequence of steps leading up to brushing his teeth. In another instance one of our patients was unable to show his therapist how to wave good-bye, but as she left his bedside, he spontaneously waved good-bye.

The types of apraxia most often associated with aphasia have been called *verbal apraxia* or *apraxia of speech*, and *oral apraxia*. Darley and his associates (Johns and Darley, 1970; Deale and Darley, 1972; Darley, et al., 1975; Johns and LaPointe, 1976) believe that apraxia of speech may exist as an entity distinct from aphasia, whereas Martin (1974) argues that since the errors the apractic patient makes are linguistically based, the disorder must be considered as part of a higher order language disorder, that is, aphasia. Darley and his associates would argue that apraxia could occur as a pure disorder, Martin that it could not. Most aphasiologists would agree, however, that there is a symptom complex that exists in some patients, sometimes to such a remarkable extreme as to be the patient's most striking disorder. The patient seems unable to remember the positioning for the articulators or the sequence of movement necessary for the voluntary production of sequences of speech sounds. These errors are highly variable and inconsistent: an error made in one context may not occur in another similar context.

In oral apraxia the patient seems unable to make voluntary nonspeech movements with his articulators. For example, he may be unable to stick out his tongue when asked by an examiner, yet does so spontaneously when the examiner approaches with tongue blade in hand. Asked to whistle, the patient may begin the attempt, then puff out his cheeks and exhale. The classic example is that of a patient who is asked to cough. He seems genuinely puzzled by his inability to perform the act, attempts to do so, and ends with a triumphant rendering of the words, "cough, cough."

Dysarthria and apraxia complicate the picture of aphasia insofar as treatment is concerned. For example, aphasia with persisting dysarthria implies that the neurological involvement that has occurred is either a consequence of bilateral cortical lesions or involves sites in addition to the cortical lesion causing the aphasia. The more extensive or widespread the neurological damage, the less optimistic is the prognosis for recovery. Apraxia can be an almost intractable syndrome to overcome and patients often make considerable progress in other modalities and yet remain virtually speechless because of the apraxia.

There are many other variables that influence recovery from aphasia; we shall now consider some of the more important ones.

Variables Influencing Recovery from Aphasia

At least eight variables have been identified that can influence recovery from aphasia: severity of the aphasia and comprehension deficit at onset, type of aphasia, etiology, age, handedness, onset of therapy, intellectual level, and personality characteristics. A description of each follows.

Initial *severity* predicts recovery from aphasia perhaps better than any other variable (Kertesz, 1979). Schuell (1953) and Smith (1971) found that the severity of the comprehension deficit was a good prognosticator of recovery. When the patient makes errors on subtests requiring the act of pointing to single words, the prediction for recovery of functional language was poor (Culton, 1969; Schuell 1953).

Kertesz (1979) examined the relationship of *type of aphasia* to recovery in sixty-seven patients who had had an initial examination as well as a follow-up test at least one year later (Kertesz and McCabe, 1972). Progress for almost all of the global aphasics remained poor, whereas Broca's and Wernicke's aphasics showed a wider range of outcome. The Wernicke aphasics' recovery curves seemed to be bimodal: some doing fairly well, others poorly. The Broca's aphasics seemed about evenly divided between fair and good recovery. Anomic, conduction, and transcortical aphasics all had a uniformly good prognosis, the majority of cases showing excellent recovery. Kertesz (1979, 1981) presented evidence to show that aphasic symptoms evolve from one clinically distinct group into another as recovery occurs. The patterns of evolution are: global aphasia recovers toward Broca's aphasia; Broca's aphasia shows good recovery with resulting deficits of word-finding difficulty and dysfluency; Wernicke's aphasia often persists, but if recovery occurs it evolves toward conduction or anomic aphasia; conduction aphasia recovers toward anomic aphasia or recovers completely;

anomic aphasia often shows complete recovery; anomia is a common end-stage for all types of aphasia.

Etiology is another very significant variable. In general, trauma patients do much better than vascular or neoplastic (tumor) patients. This may be confounded by the *age* factor since trauma patients tend to be younger than patients with vascular etiologies. Younger patients as a rule do better than older patients, presumably because younger brains show more plasticity. Vascular lesions, of course, occur in older populations, usually against a background of widespread cerebrovascular disease. The stroke is but the culmination of insidious changes in the vascular system. Many of the studies of penetrating head wounds, of course, were of young war casualties. It is an interesting and rather frightening observation, however, that autopsies on the Vietnam War casualties showed widespread cerebrovascular changes even in so young a population. There are several studies (Culton, 1971; Sarno and Levita, 1971; Smith, 1971), however, which found no significant correlation between age and recovery. As Kertesz (1979) points out, "clinicians will observe remarkably good recovery in elderly patients while some of the young will remain severely disabled" (p. 268).

Handedness appears to be another important variable affecting recovery. Left-handed patients are reported to have a better prognosis than right-handed individuals (Gloning, Gloning, and Haub, 1969; Subirana, 1969; Luria, 1970). On the other hand, left-handed individuals are more likely to become aphasic regardless of which hemisphere is damaged. This suggests that left-handed people show bilateral language representation.

Onset of therapy may be a factor, and many aphasia therapists believe that aphasia therapy should begin as soon after onset as possible for best results. The Wertz et al. (1981) study, a Veterans Administration Cooperative Study with five hospitals participating, substantiated this observation. Recovery occurred throughout the twelve-month period that patients were treated, but the rate of recovery was greatest in the early months. Earlier studies (Butfield and Zangwill, 1946; Wepman, 1951; Vignolo, 1964; Sands, Sarno, and Shankweiler, 1969) also concluded that those patients who received treatment before six months had elapsed showed the most significant gains in treatment. Although the rate of recovery dropped off beyond six months, gains were continuing to be made in the VA study.

It has been our observation that we see significant consolidation of language skills in the second year post-onset. Aphasics who have continued in our outpatient groups have continued to show specific language gains several years beyond their initial insult. Smith (1971) reported recovery in aphasics who received their first aphasia therapy at a point several years post-onset. Most aphasia therapists can think of examples of patients who began treatment several years after their stroke and made astonishing gains very rapidly. Some of these gains may be spurious, to be sure. A patient several years post-onset has not had experience with the clinical routine, and may, in fact, be responding better at the second examination because he has adapted to the testing situation. On the other hand, the gains may be real and occur because the therapist has facilitated consolidation of language skills. That is not to say, however, that the patient would not have shown even greater gains had treatment begun sooner. Such patients have very often adopted strategies for coping with their language problems on their own, and treatment that evolves from what the patient brings to the therapeutic situation can be highly effective. It often takes simply a refinement in, let us say, a patient's word retrieval strategies to see significant changes.

Intellectual level and its correlates of education and socioeconomic background are presumed to influence recovery in a positive manner, but there is not much hard evidence to substantiate that clinical belief. Darley (1972) concluded that the higher the original IQ, the greater the gains in therapy. Clinical experience with highly intelligent patients substantiates Darley's observations. One frequently sees remarkable language changes in such patients. They, however, may have much higher expectations and have, presumably, lost much more. What might be adequate reading level for a recovered aphasic from a working-class background who did little reading would hardly be adequate for a patient whose profession required reading skills. We treated a patient in our clinic who was a lawyer with a prosperous practice. At initial evaluation, he was minimally impaired by our standards, but his minimal impairment on standard aphasia batteries was maximal impairment for a practicing lawyer. Although our patient regained much functional reading ability, even to the point of being able to absorb the *New York Times*, he never was able to return to his law practice. Our view of his complete recovery was not his view. On the other hand, we have had patients who have viewed themselves as quite adequately recovered even though we continued to find significant reading and writing impairment. As the wife of one of our patients put it, "he never was one for much reading or writing, anyway."

The intangible, unmeasurable *personality* variables are perhaps among the most important in determining recovery from aphasia. Every clinic has remarkable instances of patients who have continued to improve beyond anyone's expectations, except possibly their own. Some patients seem to have drive and determination that is unexplainable, whereas other patients seem to embrace their illness and give up too easily.

The kind of processing strategies that patients bring to language tasks may be among the most important variables affecting outcome. Variables such as motivation, insight, self-corrective behavior and the like are all important in determining recovery.

The patient's response to how people react to him can be important, too. Stand near an aphasic patient sitting in a wheelchair and observe the reaction of people passing by. As soon as they realize that the patient cannot talk, the typical reaction is to talk to the patient as if talking to a child. This is infuriating to some patients and one of the sparks that drives them to work for recovery. Others seem to adapt all too readily to being treated as a child and become child-like in their docility.

Perseveration, the tendency to repeat an act once it has occurred, is readily observed in the verbal output of many aphasics. It is particularly evident in testing situations when the patient is under stress. A response is given, sometimes the correct one, sometimes an incorrect one, and then that response is repeated for several subsequent responses unless something happens to intervene, to disrupt the process. Naming objects on the PICA, one of our patients said, "that's a *cigarette, comb, comb, comb, comb,*" briskly itemizing each object, being unaware that following his one correct identification of the comb he had continued to call the fork, knife, and matches "comb" as well. Similar responses were evoked when he attempted to write the names of objects. He wrote pen, "pene" and then continued to write "pene" for the next three objects. The perseveration seemed to break up on its own with an apparent misspelling, "pene" becoming "pan." Thereafter, however, the remaining responses were meaningless combinations of letters until he correctly wrote "key" and then "comb." It was our observation that perseverative responses with this patient occurred when the task was beginning to be beyond his capabilities. Similar observations have been made by Albert et al., (1981).

Perseveration is an obvious phenomenon in the verbal output of aphasic patients, but it probably occurs in comprehension tasks as well. Thus, it would often seem that although the therapist may have continued on with a therapeutic task, the patient remains locked into a previous stimulus/response combination and is focused in two or three steps behind the therapist. In conversation, the patient sometimes seems to remain with an idea or concept long past the time that is appropriate. Thus questions or responses that seem to come from left field may, in fact, occur because the patient is continuing to perseverate on an idea presented earlier in the conversation.

Goldstein (1948) believed that perseveration was a way for the organism to avoid a *catastrophic response*. Catastrophic responses are normal reactions to situations that seem to go out of control. They are extreme emotional responses and indicate that the patient is under stress. Thus, a patient may begin to laugh at a situation that is humorous, and continue to laugh beyond a point appropriate. Or he may feel saddened at a reminder of his past and find that he is out of control, weeping uncontrollably. Such emotional roller coastering is called emotional *lability*. Persisting lability is indicative of release phenomenon: lack of integrated cortical control over the emotions and thus a sign of bilateral brain damage. The best way to deal with such reactions is to be matter-of-fact, to discuss the impact and the embarrassment to the patient that this outburst may have, and to move on to another, less stressful topic. Lability can usually be managed in the therapeutic situation by being sensitive to the patient's vulnerability to stress and fatigue.

Many brain-damaged patients show increased thresholds: it seems to take them longer to absorb a stimulus and then muster a response. Hence, pacing in terms of delivering stimuli may be critical. They also show a tendency to lock into a set and persist or resist change. They tend to be concrete and are unable to assume an "abstract attitude" (Goldstein, 1948, p. 6). Such patients are often extraordinarily egocentric: able to understand concepts only in terms of themselves. Thus, the patient may not be able to tell you what he does with a cigarette because he's not allowed to smoke. The patient may seem to be uninterested in other family members; it is almost as if people do not exist if they are not within his immediate environment.

The entire hospital stay for patients, however, very often reinforces and sets up these egocentric behaviors. The patient may be critically ill during the early phases of his hospitalization, all concerned with his survival attempting to reduce stress and anxiety. Everyone during these early stages focuses entirely on the patient's well-being. He is anxious and fearful of dying, and every breath may be examined and fretted over. Infantilization may occur; some patients rebel against it, but many seem to embrace the attitude all too readily. Thus, by the time rehabilitation is ready to begin, the patient's personality is altered from what it was prior to onset of the stroke.

Personality changes in patients with unilateral lesions are usually temporary. A stroke doesn't make an individual's character better, and it may make it worse. Major personality changes usually occur following bilateral brain damage. Persisting dysarthria, lability, and concreteness are all signs that the neurological damage may be more widespread than first assumed. This is a fairly frequent occurrence. The patient's stroke has been an obvious event; minor strokes in the past may have gone undetected. Thus, it is almost as if there is a synergistic effect; the little undetected strokes now loom with much more behavioral significance and the patient presents with bilateral signs. Bilateral brain damage does not mean that there cannot be significant recovery in language functions, but it does complicate the picture and limits the prognosis. What we might see in a single patient are the behavioral characteristics associated with right brain damage, that is, visuospatial deficits, and the linguistic deficits associated with left brain damage. In addition, since recovery may hinge on tapping into right hemisphere functions, there are obvious limitations if there is also right brain damage. And the personality characteristics we have previously described such as lability, concreteness, catastrophic reactions, and the like persist rather than abate.

If there is nothing else medically wrong, it is fairly predictable that an aphasic patient will get better. Even globally impaired patients become more alert, more responsive to the environment as recovery takes place. The period following the stroke when this recovery is occurring most rapidly is called the period of *spontaneous recovery*. It seems to be a period of physiological restitution, when the brain is recovering from the impact of the stroke or trauma. Von Monakow (1914) referred to the process that was occurring during this period as *diaschisis*. He theorized that damage to parts of the nervous system cuts off other areas from stimulation and creates a state of shock. Undamaged sections of the brain become nonfunctional. As the shock of diaschisis subsides, the brain begins to resume function. Undamaged parts begin to function without the input from the damaged areas and regrouping and reorganization occurs. Thus, we may see substantial language changes. Culton (1969) suggested that the period of spontaneous recovery may be over at two months. Most clinicians would agree that spontaneous recovery occurs in a rather limited time period, but that therapy extends the recovery curve so that the rate of recovery appears to reach a plateau at about six to nine months post-onset (Davis, 1983). Physicians have tended to attribute all recovery from aphasia to spontaneous recovery, but speech pathologists are beginning to demonstrate that therapeutic intervention speeds recovery at all stages (Basso, Capitani, and Vignolo, 1979; Wertz, Collins, Weiss, et al., 1981).

Darley (1975) concludes that there is no single factor that is of such a strong negative influence as to preclude at least a trial of therapy. Experienced clinicians would certainly grant that. An example of a patient whose recovery exceeded all expectations is an elderly Armenian patient we worked with. He had no immediate family, some difficulty speaking and writing English premorbidly, but was nonetheless determined to recover. He was virtually speechless when we first began to work with him, a severely impaired Broca's aphasic. He was in poor health, over sixty when he had his stroke, had had no formal education, and was a difficult and demanding patient. Yet he was also one with courage and drive that inspired all who worked with him.

He would spend hours painstakingly writing poetry "to make my mind work." It would appear at first draft (see figure 8–5) to be almost jargon, for he could not spell at all. By spending hours pouring over a dictionary (since he couldn't spell he had great difficulty finding words in the dictionary), making numerous telephone calls to friends asking them how to spell a given word, his poems would gradually assume some semblance of English. At that stage his therapists would help him polish and refine them (see figure 8–6). He certainly was an example of a patient with a poor

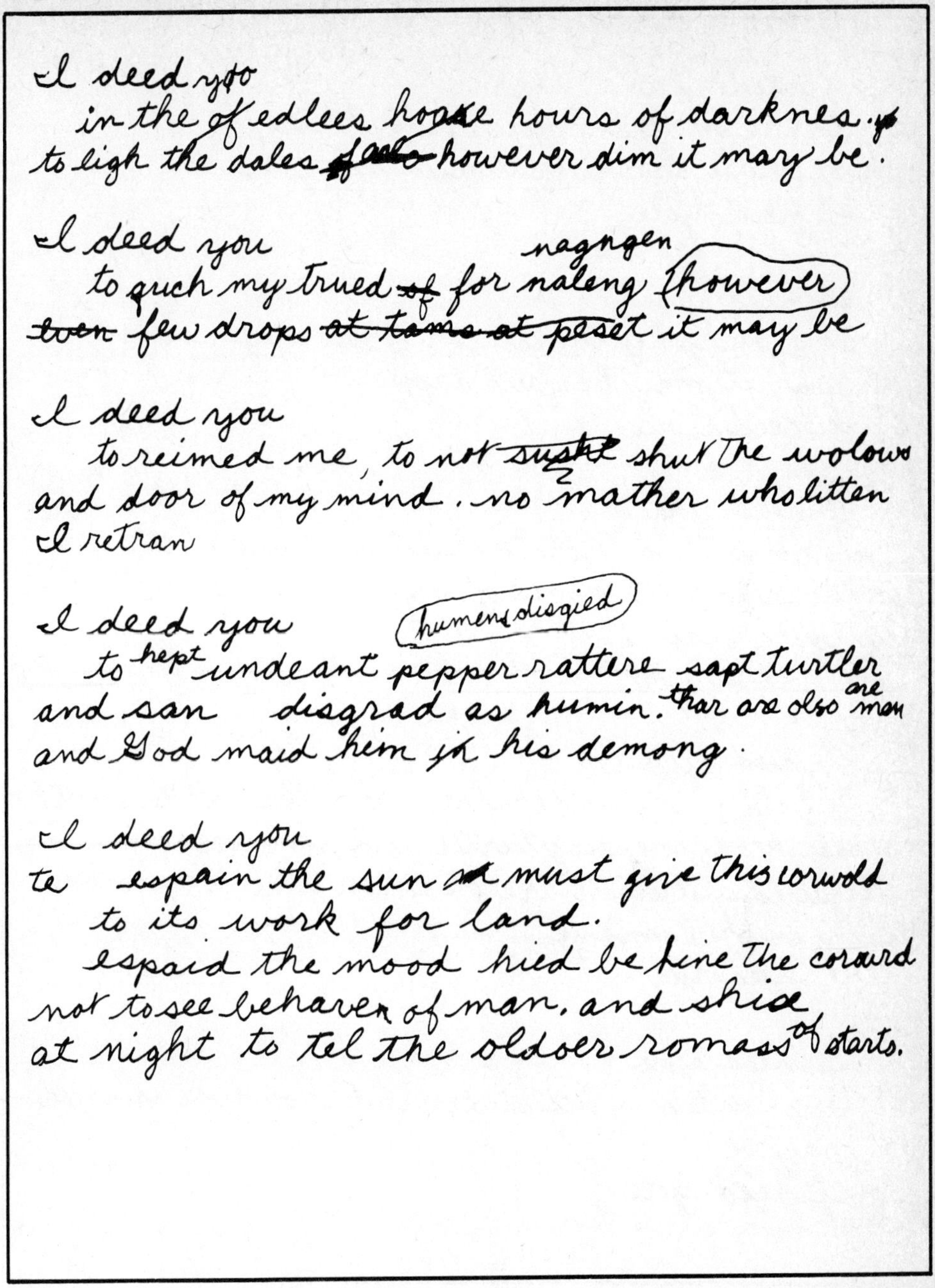

I deed you
in the of edlees hoase hours of darkness.
to ligh the dales ~~face~~ however dim it may be.

I deed you
            nagngen
to quch my trued ~~of~~ for naleng (however)
~~even~~ few drops ~~at tams at peset~~ it may be

I deed you
to reimed me, to not ~~sugtt~~ shut the wolows
and door of my mind. no mather who litten
I retran

I deed you   (humens disqied)
to hept undeant pepper rattere ~~sapt~~ turtler
                                           are
and san   disgrad as humin. thar are olso man
and God maid him jr his demong.

I deed you
te espain the sun se must give this corwold
to its work for land.
espaid the mood hied be fine the corard
not to see beharer of man. and shise
at night to tel the oldoer romass starts.

Figure 8-5. First Draft of the Poetry of a Sixty-Three-Year-Old Broca's Aphasic

I need you
In the endless hours of darkness, to light
the condle, however dim it may be.
I need you

I need you
To quench my thirst for knowledge, even
though it may be few drops.
I need you

I need you
To remind me not to shut the shade of the
windows and the doors of my mind, no matter how
little it retains.
I need yoo

I need you
To help me to understant that the rattle smake,
copper head, snapping turtle, and the scorpion
disguised as human are olsomen, and God made
men in his image.
I need yoo

I need you
To mend my deflated mind, how ever damaged
it may be.
I need you.

Figure 8–6. Polished Version of the Poetry Seen in Figure 8–5

prognosis who proved us all wrong; language in all modalities showed remarkable increases over time. Perhaps the intangible personality element that matters most is "true grit"!

The neurolinguistic features we have considered thus far are important in forming a diagnostic impression of the patient and in helping to classify as to type of aphasia; other variables that might influence recovery, such as those noted in this section, should also be considered. But prognosis for recovery from aphasia is best determined following formal assessment, as much depends on the severity of the aphasia. Without question, effective treatment planning depends on a thorough review of all language modalities. In the next section we shall review the more popular assessment batteries. Additional assessment tests not reviewed here are mentioned in chapter 1.

FORMAL ASSESSMENT

Introduction

Formal assessment serves many purposes. It helps delineate the nature and the extent of the linguistic impairment, the severity of the aphasia, and, in some instances, the predicted course of recovery. It examines each language modality systematically to determine where the patient experiences difficulty producing and understanding language, and it serves to provide baseline data to measure therapeutic change. Assessment can also serve as a means of communicating to the patient and family the nature and extent of the aphasic impairment.

The patient and the family may be unaware of the extent of the impairment. In a hospital setting, for example, a patient may not have attempted to read or write. While puzzled by the incomprehensibility of what others say, the patient may not have been aware to this point that the problem extends to such a level as to be unable to understand the names of simple objects. Knowing perfectly well what each of the pictures on the test cards represents, the patient may be astounded to find that the names of these objects are unrecognizable when the examiner names them, even though on another level, it does seem that the correct word is being said. Imagine the frustration that the testing situation creates for such a patient!

On the other hand, there are many patients who are enormously relieved to have their language deficits highlighted in a systematic manner. That someone knows to probe into just where the difficulty occurs is comforting and helps build confidence that what has once been revealed may also be treatable.

The goal is to assess the patient's strategies as well as weaknesses. The clinician will wish to know how a patient arrived at successes as well as how and where failures occurred. It is the examiner's observation of the patient's strategy as he or she approaches each test item, as well as the interpretation of performance within given modalities, that leads to effective treatment planning.

Test items, of course, should be administered according to the test protocol. But the examiner should make notes for further exploration to determine whether behavior observed during the testing situation can be further delineated. In some patients, for example, repeating what the examiner has said, although unsolicited, improves performance on auditory comprehension tasks. For other patients, such repetition interferes with performance, particularly if the repetition is erroneous. Making note of this, the therapist would explore this phenomenon in more detail informally as therapy begins. As another example, the examiner might have noted that when stimulus items in the test battery are polysyllabic, performance is better, suggesting that comprehension is improved with longer stimuli. Yet the reverse might be true for other patients: performance being better on monosyllabic stimuli. Administration of a formal battery is but a beginning to the diagnostic workup that should be completed on a patient for effective treatment planning, yet it is an essential first step, for in addition to delineating the nature and the extent of the aphasia, it will provide baseline data to document recovery as it occurs.

The following aphasia batteries will be described: the Minnesota Test for Differential Diagnosis of Aphasia (MTDDA), the Boston Diagnostic Aphasia Examination (BDAE), the Porch Index of Communicative Ability (PICA),—two tests of functional language, the Functional Communication Profile (FCP), the Communicative Abilities in Daily Living (CADL), the Token Test. Other tests such as oral peripheral speech mechanism examinations, tests for apraxia and dysarthria, reading batteries, and the Coloured Progressive Matrices will be briefly mentioned.

The Minnesota Test for Differential Diagnosis of Aphasia (MTDDA).

The Minnesota Test for Differential Diagnosis of Aphasia (Schuell, 1965) has since its inception been a great favorite with those speech pathologists who, upon finishing the formal assessment of a patient, expect to initiate a treatment program. Schuell believed that aphasia affects all language modalities and thus her test battery provides a clinician with a fairly comprehensive assessment of a patient's disturbances in auditory comprehension, visuospatial processing, speech and language, visuomotor skills and writing, and some evaluation of disturbances of numerical relations and arithmetic processes. Items are scored on a plus or minus basis, but the insights the therapist gains that are most helpful in treatment planning come from observations and notes made as the patient progresses through the test, rather than from a test item profile. A sense of what a patient can do readily, where he fails yet almost succeeds, and where he absolutely fails is not expressed in the MTDDA's scoring system, yet it is this information that one gains from the MTDDA that is so helpful in treatment planning.

Because of the way test items and subtests are arranged, it is clear when the patient makes more errors as the stimulus items become longer or more complex. More severely impaired patients experience difficulty sooner than the less severely impaired. A sense of where the patient lies on various continuums of difficulty can be derived from the MTDDA as well as how breakdowns can translate into a starting point for therapy.

The patient is classified according to the severity of language disturbance and related central sensory or motor impairments into one of five possible groups. These groups are:

• Group 1. Simple aphasia
• Group 2. Aphasia with visual involvement
• Group 3. Aphasia with sensorimotor involvement
• Group 4. Aphasia with scattered findings—visuomotor involvement
• Group 5. Global aphasia

Thus, for example, if the patient made many errors on the visual and reading disturbances section of the test, the patient would be classified as being in group 4:

Aphasia with Visual and Motor Involvement. The classification system may not be very helpful and is seldom used by the clinicians who use the test in our program. It certainly cannot be translated to others within the medical profession and it does not improve communication to indicate in a medical chart that the patient is a group 4 aphasic. But what the test does provide in terms of useful medical chart information is its emphasis on the fact that aphasia affects all language modalities. Diagnostic reports can say, "the patient shows a moderate aphasia, characterized by impairment in all language modalities; auditory comprehension, speaking, reading, and writing are all moderately impaired," and then go on to describe the deficits in each modality in more detail. It brings home sharply to all who deal with the patient the reality that aphasia is truly a comprehensive disorder, for, however often it is demonstrated to the contrary, the myth still persists that a speechless aphasic patient should be able to write what he or she cannot say. The MTDDA lends itself remarkably well to description of the aphasic impairment rather than mere labeling, and that fact always contributes to better patient management.

The Boston Diagnostic Aphasia Examination (BDAE). The Boston Diagnostic Aphasia Examination (Goodglass and Kaplan, 1972) is one of the most widely used tests for aphasia. The patient's speech is rated (see table 8–2) and then classified according to neurological models that date back to the late 1800s. The site of the lesion producing the aphasia can sometimes be inferred, and the terminology used in classification can be readily communicated to the medical profession. The classification system works well when the patient's aphasia is classic, as we've noted, but fewer than half can be assigned to a syndrome (Goodglass, 1981).

In addition to an evaluation of the patient's spontaneous speech and his description of a picture, the BDAE assesses auditory comprehension, oral expression, the ability to understand written language, and writing ability. Subtests within a modality are scaled for difficulty, so that the clinician can determine how complex or lengthy a stimulus item must be before the patient experiences difficulty.

Since the BDAE assesses conversation as well as item-specific responses, studying the patient's responses to the two types of items on the BDAE can give insight into the discrepancies observed between relatively poor performance on a diagnostic test and quite adequate performance in a nontest situation.

The Porch Index of Communicative Ability (PICA). The Porch Index of Communicative Ability uses a multi-dimensional scoring system (see tables 8–3 and 8–4), a forty-hour training course for test administration, and a rigid testing protocol to assure a high degree of testing reliability. With high reliability, the variability observed in patient behavior from one test to another can be assumed to be due to changes occurring within the patient (i.e., he is getting better) and not due to changes within the testing situation (i.e., a different examiner, variability in the way a given bit of behavior is scored, and so forth).

With the multidimensional scoring system each bit of behavior is rated on a sixteen-point scale, allowing the behavior observed to be quantified more precisely than on any other aphasia battery. Because each point assigned implies differences among responses, a great deal of qualitative information can be gained when the PICA scores are perused. The scoring system thus provides more depth of information than does a plus/minus scoring system.

Patient's Name _____ Date of rating _____
                                                              Rated by _____

APHASIA SEVERITY RATING SCALE

0. No usable speech or auditory comprehension.

1. All communication is through fragmentary expression; great need for inference, questioning and guessing by the listener. The range of information which can be exchanged is limited, and the listener carries the burden of communication.

2. Conversation about familiar subjects is possible with help from the listener. There are frequent failures to convey the idea, but patient shares the burden of communication with the examiner.

3. The patient can discuss *almost all everyday problems* with little or no assistance. However, reduction of speech and/or comprehension makes conversation about certain material difficult or impossible.

4. Some obvious loss of fluency in speech or facility of comprehension, without significant limitation on ideas expressed or form of expression.

5. Minimal discernible speech handicaps; patient may have subjective difficulties which are not apparent to listener.

RATING SCALE PROFILE OF SPEECH CHARACTERISTICS

	1 2 3 4 5 6 7		
MELODIC LINE intonational contour	Absent	limited to short phrases and stereotyped expressions	runs through entire sentence
PHRASE LENGTH longest occasional (1/10) uninterrupted word runs	1 word	4 words	7 words
ARTICULATORY AGILITY facility at phonemic and syllable level	always impaired or impossible	normal only in familiar words and phrases	never impaired
GRAMMATICAL FORM variety of grammatical construction (even if incomplete)	none available	limited to simple declaratives and stereotypes	normal range
PARAPHASIA IN RUNNING SPEECH	present in every utterance	once per minute of conversation	absent
WORD FINDING informational content in relation to fluency	fluent without information	information proportional to fluency	speech exclusively content words
AUDITORY COMPREHENSION converted from objective z-score mean	absent $(z=-2)$	$(z=-1.5)(z=-1)(z=-.5)(z=0)(z=+.5)$	normal $(z=+1)$

Table 8–2. Aphasia Severity Rating Scale and Rating Scale Profile of Speech Characteristics from the Boston Diagnostic Aphasia Examination.

Table 8-3. A Sample of a PICA Score Sheet

SCORE SHEET

Name C.T.   Onset 8-21-68   No. L-53

Date 10-8-80   By BEP   Time 9:47 to 10:35   Total Time 48

Test Conditions STANDARD

Patient Conditions GOOD, COOPERATIVE   △ = SPANISH

Glasses: YES   Hearing aid: No   Dentures: NO   Hand Used: R

ITEM	I	II	III	IV	V	VI	VII	VIII	IX	X	XI	XII	A	B	C	D	E	F
1. Tb	7	13	13	7	12	6	12	15	7	15	15	△14	⑤	6	6	6	13	14
2. Cg	11	9	11	12	11	15	12	15	△7	15	15	15	⑤	6	6	6	15	12
3. Pn	11	11	11	10	12	15	12	15	13	13	15	15	⑤	6	6	6	6	14
4. Kf	11	7	7	15	12	13	12	15	15	13	15	15		6	6	6	15	15
5. Fk	11	9	7	(13)	12	15	12	15	15	13	15	15		6	6	6	15	12
6. Qt	11	11	7	9	12	15	12	15	12	15	15	15	6	6	6	7	11	
7. Pl	7	11	11	15	12	13	12	15	7	15	15	15		6	6	6	7	12
8. Mt	7	7	11	15	12	15	12	15	11	15	15	15		6	6	6	15	12
9. Ky	7	7	11	10	12	15	12	15	15	15	15	10		6	13	6	15	14
10. Cb	7	9	11	15	12	15	12	15	15	15	15	15		15	6	10	15	12
TIME	:51	:56	:01	:03	:05	:06	:07	:08	:09	:10	:11	:12	:14	:20	:25	:31	:33	:35
MINUTES	4	5	5	2	3	1	1	1	1	1	1	1	2	6	5	6	2	2
MODALITY	VRB	PTM	PTM	VRB	RDG	AUD	RDG	VIS	VRB	AUD	VIS	VRB	WRT	WRT	WRT	WRT	CPY	CPY
MEAN SCORE	9.0	9.4	10.0	12.1	11.9	13.7	12.0	15.0	11.7	14.4	15.0	14.0	5.0	6.9	6.7	6.4	12.3	12.8
%ILE	54	36/37	31	59	58/59	44	50/58	34↑	55	48/54	18↑	59/62	20/52	57	49	43	63	46/48
VARIAB.	20	36	30	29	1	13	0	0	33	6	0	6	0	81	63	36	27	22

MPO	OVERALL	WRITING	COPYING	READING	PANTOMIME	VERBAL	AUDITORY	VISUAL
13 yrs.	11.04	6.25	12.55	11.95	9.70	11.80	14.05	15.00
%ile	52	52	57	58	33	56	46	52↑
Variab.	403	180	49	1	66	88	19	0
Mean Var.	22.4	45.0	24.5	.5	33.0	22.0	9.5	0

	Gestural	Verbal	Graphic	9 HI	9 LO	HOAP	Correction	Target
Score	12.68	11.80	8.35	13.52	8.56	11.36	0	
%ile	43	56	52	54	51	56	0	56%

Score	Category	Dimensional Characteristics
16	COMPLEX	Accurate, responsive, complex, prompt, efficient
15	COMPLETE	Accurate, responsive, complete, prompt, efficient
14	DISTORTED	Accurate, responsive, complete or prompt, distorted
13	COMPLETE-DELAYED	Accurate, responsive, complete or complex, delayed
12	INCOMPLETE	Accurate, responsive, incomplete, prompt
11	INCOMPLETE-DELAYED	Accurate, responsive, incomplete, delayed
10	CORRECTED	Accurate, self-corrected
9	REPEATED	Accurate, after instructions are repeated
8	CUED	Accurate, after cue is given
7	RELATED	Inaccurate, almost accurate
6	ERROR	Inaccurate attempt at the task item
5	INTELLIGIBLE	Comprehensible but not an attempt at the task item
4	UNINTELLIGIBLE	Incomprehensible but differentiated
3	MINIMAL	Incomprehensible and undifferentiated
2	ATTENTION	No response, but patient attends to the tester
1	NO RESPONSE	No response, no awareness of task

Table 8–4. The PICA Categories for Scoring Responses of One of the VA Patients

Porch (1981) directs treatment at improving processing ability rather than at the more traditional content-type goals. He feels that treatment should begin at the point where the patient first begins to have processing difficulties. The multi-dimension scoring system is readily adaptable to treatment, as well. For example, stimuli for a task can be selected, the dimensions of the task determined, and the therapist can then sample the patient's performance on those items, using the multi-dimensional scoring system, before therapy begins. Sampling performance after treatment can provide a sensitive daily indicator of how effective a treatment approach has been. LaPointe (1977) has designed score sheets to facilitate adapting this method to treatment.

Tests of Functional Language. The *Functional Communication Profile* (Sarno, 1969; Taylor, 1965) uses a nine-point subjective scale to assess forty-five behaviors that index the aphasic patient's communicative ability. The test is specifically designed for use by the experienced aphasia therapist, and Sarno (1969) reports high inter-rater reliability when the scale is appropriately used. The patient's ability to use residual communication skills in common everyday situations is rated relative to his or her premorbid level of ability.

The Communicative Abilities in Daily Living (CADL) (Holland, 1980) evaluates the aphasic's communicative ability in sixty-eight different tasks using interview and role-playing situations. Responses are scored on the basis of the success of the patient's attempts to communicate: an adequate response is scored as 1 point, an inadequate response as 0, while a correct response with some elaboration is scored as 2 points. Holland (1980) reports high inter-examiner reliability and good concurrent validity (performance on the CADL correlates highly with performance on other tasks).

Both the FCP and the CADL, then, can be used as indicators of how well the patient functions in practical, everyday situations (i.e., using "yes" or "no" appropriately, making change, asking for or imparting information, and so forth). Both tests will highlight the discrepancies so often observed between performances in functional situations and performance during formal testing. While the behavior observed on the FCP or the CADL may affirm a family's assertion that the patient is functioning better than a test such as the BDAE might indicate, the FCP and CADL can also be useful tools to use in counseling families as to the extent to which aphasia impairs functional language. Demonstrating very specific situations in which communication breaks down may be more helpful to the family than telling them about the performance differences observed across semantic categories.

Both scales will help the clinician focus in on functional language skills that could be improved. From either assessment, the therapist can determine behaviors that are just on the margin of being truly functional and work to improve the patient's underlying skills. In other words, the functional language skills emphasized in treatment can be prioritized. While aphasia therapy does not necessarily always focus on functional language situations, the consequences of that therapy should generalize to functional situations. Repeated measurement with either or both the FCP and the CADL should help the clinician determine that that goal is being approached.

The Token Test (DeRenzi and Vignolo, 1962; DeRenzi and Faglioni, 1978) was designed to reveal subtle receptive deficits that might be overlooked upon cursory examination. It uses progressively longer, nonredundant phrases that ask the patient to point to or manipulate tokens that vary according to shape, size and color. The phrases are nonredundant because each word must be decoded in order for the response to be correct. The syntactic complexity of the command itself is also varied in the final subtests, that is, "put the green rectangle away from the yellow rectangle." It has often been said that there are as many versions of the Token Test as there are examiners using it. The commands are readily adaptable from the two Italian versions, the original described by DeRenzi and Vignolo in 1962 and the shortened version presented by DeRenzi and Faglioni in 1978. In addition, there are published variations of the Token Test (McNeil and Prescott, 1978; Spreen and Benton, 1977). Most clinicians have their tokens made locally although they are now commercially available in both the McNeil and Prescott test, the Spreen and Benton battery, and through Teaching Resources (1982).

Boller and Vignolo (1966) report that virtually all patients with left hemisphere lesions will experience comprehension deficits on the Token Test. In fact, clinical experience would indicate that aphasia can be ruled out when a patient does *not* experience difficulty with the Token Test. Conversely, the Token Test is such a difficult test of auditory comprehension that administering it to aphasic patients with moderate to severe impairment may be futile, for their performance will be only minimal and such failure can be an extremely frustrating experience for the patient.

Treatment programs that extrapolate directly from the Token Test have been designed to improve auditory comprehension for aphasic patients (West, 1972; Holland and Sonderman, 1974). The Token Test seems to favor processing strategies that are specific to the left hemisphere. The patient must process commands that are presented in a very specific time frame, the commands as given are linear and sequentially arranged in time, and the patient must use analytic skills in order to decode their meaning. The nonredundancy of the Token Test commands does not allow for a holistic grasp of the overall meaning; the patient must decode each lexical unit in the command and then unify those units into some sort of conceptual whole before responding. West (1973) found that training on items similar to those in the Token Test resulted in significant generalization to other auditory comprehension skills such as those evaluated in the MTDDA or the patient's subjective impression of improved functional comprehension, for example, the ability to follow a movie.

Other Tests. Depending upon the patient's specific problems, the clinician may wish to evaluate other behaviors. Most would administer an examination of the oral peripheral speech mechanism to patients who show any dysarthria or apraxia, for these deficits will interfere with the patient's speech output during therapy. Several studies (Schuell, 1965; Vignolo, 1964; Keenan and Brassell, 1974) have indicated that concomitant dysarthria and apraxia are negative prognosticators.

Commercial test batteries for apraxia and dysarthria are available (Dabul, 1979; Yorkston and Beukelman, 1981), but most clinics have developed their own version, typically adapted from the work of Darley and his associates (Darley, Aronson, and Brown, 1975; Wertz and Rosenbek, 1971).

A comprehensive evaluation of reading impairment may also be warranted. The Reading Comprehension Battery for Aphasia (RCB) (LaPointe and Horner, 1979) is designed specifically to evaluate the kinds of reading problems aphasics will experience and has been standardized on an aphasic population. An analysis of the extent of the reading impairment and the patterns of deficit noted would be useful in determining a starting point for therapy, as well as its focus, if the goal is to work on reading, per se. Even in those aphasics for whom reading comprehension seems less vital, the visual modality may be a very effective means of assuring that auditory input is comprehended, the theory being that multi-modality stimulation (e.g., combined auditory and visual input) is cumulatively more effective than stimulating one modality (e.g., the auditory) only. Hence the analysis of the reading impairment provided by the RCB may have particular relevance.

In our clinic we routinely administer the Coloured Progressive Matrices (CPM) (Ravens, 1962). While the CPM is a test of visuospatial ability and requires no verbal response, most individuals would use verbal strategies to solve some of the more advanced matrices problems, which probably explains why aphasics do poorly on the CPM. We have long felt that good CPM performance was an indication of a good prognosis for recovery. Certainly, poor performance usually indicates a poor prognosis. The CPM may be tapping right hemisphere functioning; those patients who perform well may be those without lesions in both hemispheres, while those who perform poorly may have undetected right hemisphere lesions.

Most of our patients are also routinely evaluated in a neuropsychology clinic where, in addition to the standardized aphasia batteries, a wider variety of visuospatial skills are assessed. Again, good performance on this battery may be indicative of good right hemisphere functioning. Many aphasic patients continue to struggle to use verbal strategies to solve visuospatial problems and thus score poorly, while others seem to adapt rapidly to the right hemisphere's processing strategies that remain available to them.

Evaluation is essential to treatment planning. In the next section we will examine various approaches to treatment, first, with a review of the two major theoretical points of view about aphasic rehabilitation, and then with a review of specific therapeutic techniques.

TREATMENT APPROACHES

The Stimulation Approach

Hildred Schuell is identified with a treatment approach that is usually labeled "the stimulation approach." She and her co-writers (Schuell, Jenkins, and Jiménez-Pabón, 1964) stated "it would seem that sensory stimulation is the only method we have for making complex events happen in the brain. All evidence suggests that auditory stimulation is crucial in control of language processes" (p. 338). As Duffy (1981) points out, it was Schuell's sound foundation in the areas of theory, evaluation, methods of observing and categorizing behavior that helped develop the rationale for the stimulation approach. But there was something more about her writing that made it especially compelling to the clinician. In the book she wrote with Jenkins and Jiménez-Pabón (1964) and in some of her articles (Schuell, 1953; Schuell, Carroll and Street, 1955), we see the depth of her concern and insight for the aphasic patient. She describes the treatment of a severely impaired physician who suddenly questions his therapist as to whether she is going to continue to treat him:

> She said some days were still better than other days, and she did not always know why. He was still regarding her searchingly. She asked "is it because you think it's no use?" He made an affirmative gesture, then began to sob painfully. He tried to apologize, but the clinician said, "It's all right. You needed to do this. You've been holding it in too long."
>
> This was not emotional lability. It was long-restrained grief for the loss of his profession; and pent-up resentment at being a patient and helpless instead of a doctor doing his work in the hospital. This is grief that is hard for a man to express. He tries to shield his family from knowledge of it, and he does not find it easy to share with anyone. Even the clinician must wait until a question is asked in some way. Usually when the patient can ask the question, he knows at least part of the answer, and has begun to make the hard adjustment (1964, p. 280).

Strong, controlled, intensive auditory stimulation was the method Schuell used to facilitate language recovery, but she also advocated combining visual and auditory stimulation, manipulating that stimulation at progressive levels of complexity, until the patient could respond to each modality alone on any given level of complexity.

Beginning therapists often make mistakes when working with an aphasic patient, she states:

"1. They tend to talk around the patient, instead of to him simply and directly.
 2. They fail to appreciate the patient's need for strong stimulation to compensate for his own defective feedback processes, and so do not succeed in making materials meaningful to the patient.
 3. They do not make adequate use of the principle of repeated stimulation.
 4. They do not elicit an adequate number of responses from the aphasic patient.
 5. They tend to overcorrect and overexplain. In general, the clinician should restimulate until a maximal response is obtained rather than try to elucidate errors.
 6. They tend not to be evaluative enough of what happens in therapy. Probably the best way to acquire this facility is to record and study patient responses consistently." (Schuell, et al. 1964, p. 348)

Seven positive rules for increasing clinical effectiveness follow from the theory:

"1. Talk simply and directly to the patient, eliminating extraneous noise that has no communicative value.
2. Control stimulation to elicit maximal response.
3. Control amount of material used to make it meaningful.
4. Use the principle of repeated stimulations to facilitate discrimination and recall.
5. Work to elicit a maximal number of responses. The patient should be responding continuously throughout the clinical period.
6. In general, restimulate, rather than explain or correct.
7. Evaluate the effectiveness of each procedure for each patient." (Schuell, et al., 1964, p. 349)

Every aphasia therapist should read Schuell's chapters on aphasia treatment, for more than any other writing, they catch that intangible that is the essence of the therapeutic process. Schuell provided techniques, but she said, "we tend to feel that all techniques should be stored in bottles marked: *Poison: Use only for good reason*, since any technique is ineffectual if used indiscriminately" (1964, p. 348).

The Programmed Learning Approach

The term *operant conditioning* came from B.F. Skinner's (1961) emphasis on the study of behavior that operates upon the environment in order to produce some outcome. A *verbal operant* was defined as a dependency relation between a verbal response of some sort and some antecedent condition. Speaking could be considered a conditioned operant response to some internal or external stimuli. According to Skinner (1957, p. 190), "the aphasic has lost some of the functional relationships which control his behavior." Therapy, then, would aim to restore those lost relationships. Defining the relationships between stimuli and responses, specifying and measuring carefully defined behaviors as they change over time, and applying operant procedures systematically to modify behavior characterizes the programmed operant approach. Programmed instruction represents the application of the operant condition paradigm (Goldfarb, 1981). Costello (1977) defines it succinctly, "the term 'programmed instruction' is intended to mean a systematically designed remediation plan which specifies a priori the teaching and learning behaviors required of both the teacher and the learner" (p. 3).

LaPointe (1978, p. 144) outlines the following major steps in a programmed learning approach:

1. Obtain baseline measures, defining the patient's behavior precisely in operational terms, the rate at which the behavior occurs before treatment begins, and the stimulus conditions that control the responses;
2. Apply behavior-modification procedures, first specifying a precise operational definition of the terminal behavior, then selecting procedures designed either to change the response rate or establish new responses. Attention must be paid to the type of reinforcer used and the schedules of reinforcement adopted. The terminal behavior is then shaped by the use of small controlled steps or by changing the stimulus conditions surrounding the desired response;
3. Extend stimulus control to assure carry over or transfer of training from the highly controlled clinical setting to more spontaneous and natural situations of communication.

Remedial Variables and Techniques Affecting
Comprehension and/or Production

If a therapist controlled for every variable known to affect an aphasic's response to stimuli, the therapist would undoubtedly spend so much time organizing material that there would be little time left to plan meaningful treatment. Indeed, the danger of emphasizing the importance of the variables that we will be discussing is that their control may become an end in and of itself, and the fact that language usage is a creative, evolving process overlooked. Nonetheless, as we shall see, the characteristics of the stimulus materials used in therapy do matter.

The obvious, most basic variables to control are those of frequency of occurrence or word familiarity, concreteness, imageability, complexity, redundancy, length, age of acquisition. These variables affect learning for any human population. Normal adults' learning curves are affected by them as are those of children. Aphasia does not alter the basic human response to these primary variables, and inasmuch as there has been substantial research on their effect on a variety of normal and pathological populations, it is probably trivial at this point to verify to any further extent their effect on an aphasic population. Further, a decade ago there was a substantial body of research to substantiate the fact that some of the primary variables such as frequency of occurrence had, if anything, an even more profound effect on aphasic's responses than on normal speakers (cf., Thurston, 1963; Wepman, et al., 1956; Siegel, 1959; Bricker, et al., 1964; Schuell, and Jenkins, 1961; Howes and Geschwind, 1964).

Occurring as single words in auditory comprehension tasks, or in visual comprehension tasks (reading), or in copying and writing tasks, highly frequent words that are concrete, imageable, acquired early in life, and familiar to the subject will be better recognized, recalled, or learned, than a word that is less frequent, abstract, not imageable, or part of a more mature vocabulary.

In sentences, the effect of each of these variables becomes more complicated, for the meaning of a sentence is much more than the sum of the individual words. Thus, the idea conveyed in a sentence could be more familiar or concrete to a given patient, while the individual words less so. But, in general, controlling for frequency of occurrence, imageability, concreteness/abstractness, and so on, of the individual words in a sentence also has an effect. In addition, numerous studies (Levy and Taylor, 1968; West, 1968; Baker and Holland, 1971; Levy and Holland, 1971) have demonstrated that as the syntax of sentences increases in complexity, the aphasic's performance or comprehension decreases. Finally, most therapists know, and most families rapidly discover, that being redundant helps aphasic patients to comprehend, and research, such as that by Gardner and his associates (1975) and Wiig and Globus (1971) experimentally substantiate this observation.

Length is known to affect aphasic responses, and with sentences the matter is quite clear: the longer the sentence, the more the stimulus overload (Darley, 1982). With single words, however, the issue of length becomes a bit murkier. Highly frequent words are typically shorter words, and for that reason might be more desirable as stimulus items. On the other hand, shorter words by definition occur very quickly in time and may be too short for an aphasic to "tune into"; thus a slightly longer word would allow for more processing time and better comprehension.

With a more severely impaired patient, the therapist might wish to assure that stimuli selected for, let us say, an auditory comprehension task, are also gesturable, if for no other reason than that the therapist could fall back on the gesture to assure comprehension. But there is additional evidence to indicate that words that represent manipulable objects are better recognized or recalled than those that do not. The act of manipulation is the gesture typically used to represent a word (i.e., the motion of writing for the word *pencil*, the motion of the arms rocking to represent the word *baby*). The literature on children's learning (Wolff and Levin, 1972; Wolff, Levin and Longobardi, 1972, 1974) demonstrates that children learn better when they have been allowed to manipulate or see manipulated the stimuli they are later to remember. Furthermore, research with normal subjects indicates that action imagery results in better learning than does static imagery (Paivio, 1971, 1975). Since acting out words or phrases heightens visual imagery, including action in the form of action words or gestures may facilitate the aphasic's comprehension (West and Grossman, 1980; Grossman, 1979).

Another reason why action verbs should be integrated into treatment programs comes from the observation that some severely impaired aphasic patients respond best to whole body commands (Boller and Green, 1972; Grossman, 1979). Such movements primarily involve midline bodily structures which are centered along the axis of the body and are bilaterally innervated. Examples of verbs encoding this type of movement are *turn*, *jump*, and *run*. In contrast, another major category of verbs can be isolated which encode discrete movements involving the individual limbs. Such unilateral movements receive their innervation from contralateral pathways. Examples of individual limb or distal verbs are *kick*, *scratch*, and *throw*.

Concrete nouns have repeatedly been shown to be the easiest word category for either hemisphere to recognize (Sperry and Gazzaniga, 1967; Paivio, 1971; Seamon and Gazzaniga, 1973; Ellis and Shepherd, 1974; Hines, 1976). Furthermore, Goodglass and his associates (1966) concluded that the pattern of differences in naming and auditory discrimination among words of various semantic categories such as objects, letters, colors, actions, geometric forms, and body parts varies predictably with the major clinical types of aphasia.

Thus, we must conclude that controlling the nature of the stimulus materials used in treatment will make a difference in how an aphasic patient responds to what we've selected. As we indicated at the start of this section, it would seem that controlling for all the variables that affect response could be overwhelming. Fortunately, many of these variables interact. Highly imageable nouns are typically also concrete and frequent in the language. Action verbs also occur frequently, and they, as we've seen, are highly imageable. Pictures used in treatment paradigms are by definition pictureable and will be accordingly more imageable than a word that is not pictureable. Redundancy can be built into the way the therapist uses the stimuli presented and the sentence length of the stimulus items appropriately controlled.

What we have done in our clinic is to alphabetize our stimulus materials, indicate their frequency of occurrence (see Thorndike and Lorge, 1944; 1972), their imageability (if available) (Paivio, Yuille, and Madigan, 1968), and file them in boxes so that a variety of frequencies are readily available. Word or sentence lists showing other stimuli that are equivalent in frequency of occurrence but varying in imageability are also available. Other file boxes hold the duplicates of our picture stimuli arranged by semantic categories. While the initial organizing work was very time-consuming, the effort pays off daily. And, as a matter of fact, a group of minimally impaired aphasics used the alphabetizing activities as part of a very effective treatment program and were invaluable in helping us initiate our organizational efforts as well as contributing to their own treatment programs.

How material is presented will make an inordinate difference in how readily the aphasic patient responds, how accurate the response will be, and the influence that response has on future responses. Again, there is nothing so unusual about the aphasic patient. The variables we will be discussing affect normal adults and children in the same manner that they affect aphasics. But with the aphasic patient the impact of these variables is much greater and very often much more devastating.

It should be obvious that material presented at rapid rates will have a negative effect on response. Much of normal adult conversation rates of speech are too rapid for aphasics to comprehend. The research evidence is more suggestive than it is definitive (Parkhurst, 1970; Gardner, et al., 1975), but in general, slowing down the rate of delivery, and interspersing pauses between phrases to reduce the length and/or number of units of information that a patient must retain at once will have a positive effect on comprehension (Ebbin and Edwards, 1967; Liles and Brookshire, 1975; Lasky, Weidner, and Johnson, 1976). Virtually all brain-damaged patients show an increased reaction time to stimuli presented in any modality. DeRenzi and Faglioni (1965) suggest that reaction time is proportional to the extent and severity of a cerebral lesion irrespective of its focus. One might expect that as a patient improves, his reaction time might improve accordingly; clinical experience would suggest that patients who function well also learn to adopt compensatory strategies in difficult listening situations. For example, many patients repeatedly ask for processing time. One of our fluent aphasics described previously analyzed his problems in the following manner:

> Well, after when I sit home or just take my time n' just look [listen] at what it is and I'll take time and I'll take it over again, do this an then, this here I'll know, I'll know exactly what it is, y'know . . . but right away, right away, I'll, I'll forget it. I'll not get the long. I'll put them down, but it be don't. It be all, it'll be five or seven. And me ten, you know. I know it'll be here but I want to take my time, and, see [listen], then it's all.

What he's saying is that when he's alone or has plenty of time he's able to determine what's been said, but when something's said "right away," then he'll not be able to hold onto it and will forget what was said. By "I'll put them down, but it be don't," he meant that he'd get the individual words as they were stated, but he would forget them by the time the utterance was completed and hence be unable to comprehend overall meaning. "It'll be five or seven. And me ten . . . ." is the essence of his problem. I judge that he means that on a hypothetical time scale if the speaker is at a five or seven unit rate, he would need ten units of processing time in order to understand what was said. And he was quite correct in his diagnosis of his problems. On a one-to-one basis his comprehension was nearly adequate, but under any pressure his performance deteriorated rapidly, and he, unfortunately, interpreted most business or social interactions as pressure situations.

Aphasics experience stimulus overload very rapidly, so that the total time of a message may have a deleterious effect as well. Clearly, the patient described above would experience information overload very rapidly if as he says information is coming in at a five or seven unit rate and his auditory processing system needs ten units of time. Aphasics are much better at handling shorter information units than longer (West, 1968). Introducing delay between the stimulus and the response required can be helpful (Yorkston et al., 1977) if the delay is used by the patient to process what has been said. On the other hand, since virtually all aphasics show a deficit in short-term memory processing, the effect of delay may simply add more time and thus be negative. Most normals would use a delay period to rehearse, code, or plan retrieval strategies for what is to be remembered, but aphasics seem very often to bring no strategy at all to bear on to-be-remembered information, or at least, a very altered one (Swinney and Taylor, 1971; Tillman and Gerstman, 1977). Comprehension is an active cognitive process; perhaps the most serious consequence of left brain damage is not the loss of linguistic skills per se but rather the dimunition of the ability to use the cognitive processing skills associated with the left hemisphere.

We have used the classic short-term memory (STM) and paired associated learning (PAL) paradigms very effectively in therapy (West, 1970) to work on some of these processing problems our patients experience. Their advantages as a therapeutic tool lie in the ease with which variables such as those described in the previous section can be controlled, the fact that specific strategies can be taught that will help the patient overcome his deficits, and that variables such as *delay* and *interference* can be introduced so that a task that might begin at a lower level can be progressively elevated in a learning hierarchy. Let us use as an example the patient whose stereotypy is "two." As we noted, his is a very expressive "two" and he manages to convey a great deal of the emotional content of what he intends to communicate. Such a stereotypy in a chronic patient is intractable, but we have begun to help him make some modifications in its use. The theory is that if the patient can begin to check his involuntary utterance then we have the first signs of the breaking down of the stereotyped condition (Alajouanine, 1956). Even though every verbal response our patient made was "two" or "two-two," he was unable initially to repeat "two" on command. But after several trials he was able to repeat "two" immediately after the therapist, and then to say it two or three times at her request. Our next step was to introduce delay in order to make the task somewhat less automatic and move the use of the stereotypy closer to voluntary control. Could he wait two seconds after the examiner had said "two" and then say it? Initially, he couldn't, but eventually he was able to successfully repeat after as long as a five-second delay. When we found that he was beginning to have more control over the involuntary utterance of "two" we introduced *interference*, the examiner saying "two," counting aloud to five and then asking the patient to repeat "two." This, of course, made the repetition task more difficult, but it also made "two" that much less automatic.

Delay can be introduced in a variety of verbal learning tasks. In a memory task, for example, three words might be presented, "dog-grass-boy," followed by a delay period. The patient is required either to repeat the words that were read to him after the delay period has elapsed, or, if repetition is not possible, to perhaps sequence word cards in the order that the words were read. Now, if the patient used the delay period to rehearse, presumably he could improve his performance. Unfortunately, an aphasic very often gets himself into paraphasic boggles as he tries to rehearse. Attempting to recall "dog" he retrieves "cat," "grass" triggers "green," but "green" triggers "grass" so that instead of recalling "dog-grass-boy," he recalls "cat-green-grass." On the other hand, from a therapeutic standpoint, that's not so far off target. Our approach is to teach him a coding strategy that will help him retrieve the words more accurately. We might use a sentence, "the dog plays on the grass with the boy," knowing that it's well documented that using such a verbal coding strategy improves performance for normal subjects and children (Levin and Rohwer, 1968). On the other hand, using a verbal coding strategy for a patient with aphasia may simply compound the problem. If the word lists were longer, we might teach the patient to cluster words from the same category, for clustering by category is a major strategy used by normals in the free recall learning (FRL) of lists of words (Bousefield, 1953). Tillman and Gerstman (1977) found aphasics remarkably deficient in their ability to use the clustering technique for FRL, but found great variability in their ability to be trained to use the technique.

Introducing delay or interference in any learning task for aphasics will make the task more difficult, but it should perhaps be the first parameter manipulated. To use the most basic therapeutic activity as an example, let us say that you are asking a patient to point to pictures after you name them. You have been using high frequency, concrete, highly imageable nouns with success and you want now to increase the difficulty of the task. Adding delay periods and then interference would induce the patient to begin to use coding strategies, and thus be more effective therapeutically than starting to increase the difficulty of the task by first decreasing the frequency, imageability, or concreteness of the words used as stimuli. Learning to adopt verbal coding or visual memory strategies can produce rehabilitation outcomes that generalize. Since very often verbal strategies are severely depressed, using visual imagery strategies is perhaps the favored approach, for visual imagery is largely mediated by the right hemisphere, and the right hemisphere in left brain-damaged subjects presumably remains intact. Imagery, according to Paivio (1971) is specialized for the symbolic representation of concrete situations and events, whereas the verbal system is characterized by the capacity to deal with more abstract stimulus information. Even though our aphasic patients may be unable to code or retrieve verbally, the potential for using the visual symbolic code may remain. The visual symbolic system could serve as an alternative means of symbolically representing events in the world. In normal populations, pictures and highly imageable words are most likely to be dually coded (i.e., visually and verbally) and consequently stored in and retrieved from memory more readily than other stimuli (Paivio, 1965, 1966; Paivio and Csapo, 1969; Katz and Paivio, 1975). According to theory since both codes can function independently, either code can be activated depending upon the stimulus attributes of the recall or recognition tasks. In a study by Edelstein (1977), it was found that when aphasic subjects were given a description that enhanced visual imagery, learning a list for later recognition memory was improved. The aphasic subjects were shown lists of words or pictures, simultaneously hearing a verbal description of the picture, which was composed either to enhance the imageability of the item or to be neutral in its ability to arouse an image. For example, as the picture of a "bird" was shown, the relevant verbal description was "See the feathered body. It has wings." A nonrelevant description was "I've seen one. That's what it is." Or, "There it is. It is very familiar." Following the presentation of the study lists, the patient's task was simply to indicate whether or not each stimulus item shown had appeared in the previous study list. Our results demonstrate that it is possible to heighten visual imagery in aphasic patients; the relevant verbal descriptions written to heighten visual imagery produced the best recall for almost all patients (West, 1977).

The paired associate learning (PAL) paradigm lends itself well to the therapeutic situation. The patient is shown two items. Let us say, two objects, a *can of soup* and an *ashtray*. His task is to remember that the two objects go together, so that when he is shown the stimulus *can of soup*, he'll remember the response, *ashtray*. The research on visual imagery has repeatedly demonstrated (see Paivio 1971, 1975; Levin, 1976) that one of the best ways to remember the pair is to form an image that links the two together and research on children has demonstrated that imagery is further facilitated if the objects are actually manipulated (Wolff and Levin, 1972). During the study trial, then, we help the patient form the image by placing the ashtray on top of the can of soup, thereby creating a bizarre image, because it's also documented that "bizarreness" also improves a subject's ability to recall images (Wollen, Weber, and Lowry, 1972; Senter and Hoffmann, 1976). The research (Edelstein, 1977; Altman, 1977) and our clinical experience (West, 1977) suggest that aphasics are able to profit from using imagery strategies. Because the right hemisphere is undamaged in most patients, an argument can be advanced (West, in press) that we should place more emphasis on heightening its cognitive strategies.

In general, the more modalities stimulated in aphasia therapy, the better the responses. If you can say the name of an object, show a printed word that identifies it as you show the object or its picture, give the object's gesture, and help create an image of the object for recall, then response will be maximized. As Schuell et al. (1964) put it "sensory stimulation is the only method we have for making complex events happen in the brain" (p. 338). They believed that auditory stimulation in particular was crucial in the control of language processes, but since feedback from more than one sensory modality may contribute to behavior, they felt there was no rationale for using this mode exclusively. They also advanced the theory that "repeated sensory stimulation is essential for organization, storage, and retrieval of patterns in the brain" (p. 338). They proposed that auditory stimuli presented to the aphasic be massed, hypothesizing that auditory comprehension or naming ability would improve as the number of consecutive presentations of a stimulus increased. They note that a patient who "could name five or six out of twenty pictures after twenty-four hours when he had received ten successive auditory stimulations for each word, was able to recall from fifteen to twenty words the next day when he received twenty successive stimulations on each word" (p. 341). Although there is some evidence (Weigel-Crump and Koenigsknecht, 1973) to support the Schuell hypothesis, the technique of distributed presentation (DP) produces better learning in normal subjects (see Underwood 1961, 1969, 1970) and, for the most part, our research with aphasic subjects indicates that distributed practice results in better free recall learning and naming. We asked sixteen aphasic subjects (West, 1971) to name forty-four pictured nouns which were then divided into two sets of twenty-two words each. One list was presented under a massed presentation (MP) schedule so that the multiple occurrences of a word occurred together, the other under a DP schedule in which the multiple repetitions of the word were randomly dispersed throughout the list. The patients were asked to recall as many of the words as they could. What we found was that recall of words heard under DP was much higher than those heard under MP. Similar results were obtained by Shapiro and West (1976), who asked aphasic subjects to subsequently name pictures that had been presented under an MP or DP schedule. The subjects were able to name significantly more of the pictures presented under DP than those under MP. This is not to say that Schuell and her co-workers (1964) were incorrect in their hypothesis that aphasics require massive doses of stimulation, but rather that those doses need not be massed. If, for example, you are naming five pictures for the patient to later point to in an auditory recognition task, it is better to name each picture successively, finish the list, and then repeat the list, rather than to say each name repeatedly until you think it has "registered."

Positive reinforcement doesn't seem to hurt anyone, and it does seem to help aphasic performance. The problem is that beginning therapists very frequently fall

1. Count from one to ten.
2. What do you put in a fountain pen?
3. What is the opposite of big?
4. What color hair do I have?
5. What do you do on the telephone?
6. Where does milk come from?
7. What is soap for?
8. Name one animal you would find on a farm.
9. What do you put on corn flakes?
10. Which is the warmest season of the year?

Table 8–5. Examples of the Rapid Alternating Questions (RAQs)

into the trap of saying "good," "O.K.," "terrific," to the patient's correct responses and then are dismayed at having to imply "bad" when the patient responds incorrectly. What we have done in this regard is to redefine our goals. A technique worked out in our clinic by A. Damien Martin is called Rapid Alternating Questions (RAQs) (see table 8–5). The point of our RAQ therapy is that any response is "correct" as long as the patient delivers it quickly, promptly, and is prepared to move on to the next item almost immediately. There are no "right" answers, and the patient is encouraged to give the first response that he retrieves. We are trying with this technique to avoid the "locking in" behavior that is so typical of the Broca's aphasic; we try to eliminate struggle, and we're prepared to settle for semantically related responses, approximations, nearly correct responses, and so forth from these patients, who under other circumstances will struggle and struggle for the correct response. It is also a good task for the fluent aphasic, but for other reasons. Fluent aphasics need the constant input, the repeated "shift of gears." They are not going to "lock in" but are so tangential and fragmentary in their ability to comprehend that this technique encourages them to exploit what listening skills are intact, allowing for the opportunity to zero in on one sentence, tune out, and zero in again. In general, this technique facilitates the kind of underlying listening strategy that we want the patient to employ. In this sense, the technique provides a great deal of positive reinforcement, for any response is OK as long as the patient has attempted to respond. And in general we find that this is a much healthier attitude for treatment than trying to work with a patient for the one perfectly correct response, for that is absolutely not the point of aphasia therapy. I recall with distress a story told to me by a colleague. "Oh," she said, "I had such a good day! One of my aphasic patients said 'bus' today and we haven't even worked on "s" in the final position!" Every aphasia therapist has a story about the patient who creates his own impossible situation. We had such a patient who thought that it would be a wonderful Christmas gift to his wife to be able to say her name. She would arrive to take him home for the holidays, and he'd say, "Hi, Alice." Since we support the concept of patients helping to define treatment goals, we complied with his decision and every session included some drill on Alice's name. "My wife's name is_____" the therapist would say and our patient would say, "Alice." "Hello,_____" and our patient would fill in "Alice." When Alice showed up for the holidays, our patient greeted her by saying, "Hello, Mary," thereby calling Alice, his second wife, by the name of his much maligned first wife, Mary. So much for precision drill work with aphasics! The point is that one simply does not drill meaningful language into an aphasic patient. What we hope to do is facilitate the use of available linguistic or nonlinguistic strategies that will enable the patient to use language creatively, or, at least, to participate in the communicative act. For the most part, few of our patients are going to recover to the point where they are "letter-perfect"; they have to be able to substitute, to circumlocute, to work around a point, to find alternate ways to communicate their point, for definitive word retrieval is not going to be available to even the most recovered aphasic patient. For that matter, it's not available for nonaphasic normal patients, either.

All of this is not to say that material presented to the aphasic patient should not be graded in difficulty, that as much success as possible shouldn't be experienced during treatment, that difficult tasks shouldn't be interspersed with easier tasks, and the like. These are obvious learning principles, and they should apply to aphasia treatment even more so than they might apply to any other learning situation. But we do not advocate setting up treatment programs so that the aphasic never "fails." Failure is simply not a term to be used or thought of in aphasia therapy. There are tasks that are more or less difficult, and it is the therapist's responsibility to predict their level of difficulty for a given patient and adjust accordingly, but aphasics are adults, and they will accept the parameters set by the therapist if it's done in an adult-to-adult manner. "Look, let's not try to name these pictures just yet; let's try instead to match the name of the picture and then see how your naming goes."

Should you talk louder when you talk to an aphasic? No. As Darley (1982) says, "we do not help them understand better by simply presenting the message more loudly." It must be one of the terrible burdens of being aphasic that everyone shouts at them, thinking that raising one's voice will improve comprehension. It seems to be a universal trait, and one that not only aphasics must suffer through. I once had an experience with a concierge in a small Paris hotel who was convinced that if she only shouted loudly enough at me I'd comprehend her French. The louder she shouted, the less I understood. The same holds true for aphasics. Aphasia is a lot like becoming a non-native speaker in one's own country.

Intonation may be a very important variable in the sense that this may be what the severely impaired aphasic is responding to in conversational speech and may explain why the patient seems to comprehend better in such situations. Ask a globally impaired patient a question, and you may well get an answer. Not an intelligible one, but the answering intonation will be appropriate to your questioning intonation. Boller and Green (1972) found that severely impaired aphasics were able to discriminate meaningful sentences from nonsense, and even though they could not respond correctly to meaningful questions and commands, they nonetheless were able to distinguish in some way the syntactic forms of the test items. In another study, Boller and his associates (1976) found that increasing the emotional content of the auditory input appeared to increase the patients' responsiveness; emotional arousal was seen to have an effect on reception as well as expression of language.

Intonation contours seem to be processed by the right hemisphere (Blumstein and Cooper, 1974), which may explain why patients with massive left lesions respond so well to it. Furthermore, such globally impaired patients are often able to use intonation to convey meaning very effectively. We once had such a run of patients who had only the stereotypy "one-one" or "one-two-three" that a puzzled foreign resident in physical medicine asked if this were a characteristic of American aphasics. Our patient who intoned "one-two-three" managed to keep his entire ward and his family in tip-top shape simply by intoning "one-two-three." He wanted his socks lined up and color coded in his drawer, his bedstand arranged very precisely, and his family to be at his beck and call, and he was quite effective in achieving his ends with just "one-two-three." He was yet another example of a difficult personality that was made only more difficult by the onset of brain damage. Although his wife complained about how controlling and difficult he'd become, when she was counseled as to how to deal with these problems, she'd respond "oh, well . . . he was always like this." And, indeed, this was a case where the recurring utterance seemed to have some relationship to our patient's past, for he was a retired drill sergeant who'd always run his family as if they were a military unit, and he'd have been very happy to run our clinic in the same way if we'd only done what was best for us!

We have talked in passing about the information load. One can easily overload even the most minimally impaired patient with a barrage of linguistic material. Fatigue and irritability are usually the consequence. Our patients are operating under enormous constraints and the efforts they expend to understand and speak are inordinate compared to what we as normal speakers/listeners might experience. It is as if they must struggle to comprehend against a background of overwhelming noise. One reason for working on all language modalities during a given therapeutic session is to allow for changes in the nature of the information processing. Auditory comprehension tasks can be very difficult for a patient. Switching off to a quiet, unstressful reading task might be what's needed to assure adequate performance on more difficult auditory tasks later in the therapy session. We maintain our patients in forty-five minute treatment sessions and usually find that that's not overtaxing, but it does depend upon the therapist being able to plan a variety of tasks that alternately expand and contract the processing demands placed on the patient.

Among the simplest of auditory recognition tasks would be that of verification (see Clark and Chase, 1972; Carpentar and Just, 1975). We use this technique as an initial step in our attempts to build auditory processing ability; it is in many respects one of the "easiest" tasks available. As a treatment paradigm, it has the advantage that many of the variables affecting the stimulus or the response can be readily manipulated to make the task easier or harder according to the patient's needs. With this technique, the therapist says a word or sentence, simultaneously showing its picture; the patient has simply to indicate whether or not the word spoken goes with the picture shown. The therapist shows a picture of a cat and says "dog." The patient is to indicate "Yes," it is a dog, or "No," it is not a dog. This ostensibly "simple" task is truly quite complicated, and the processes underlying normal subjects' ability to judge whether the sentence is true or false with regard to the picture have been extensively studied. As Clark and Chase (1972) point out:

> the main *a priori* requirement of any theory of sentence-picture comparison is that for a sentence and picture to be compared they must be represented, ultimately, in the same mental format. One cannot, for example, compare the printed word *orchestra* directly with a picture of an orchestra and judge them to "mean" the same thing, for there are no properties intrinsic to the graphemic and pictorial modes to indicate that the word and picture represent the same concept. (p. 473)

To compare a sentence (or word) against a picture, people must at some stage represent the sentence and picture in a compatible mental format. Since it is the interpretation, not the direct perceptual characteristics, of the picture or object that is the basis for the verification, it is the interpretation that must be coded and compared against the picture. Clark and Chase (1972) identify four stages in this comprehension process: the sentence (in the case of aphasics, usually a word) and then the picture (or vice versa) are encoded into abstract mental representations; they are then compared bit by bit to see if they match each other; a response is then produced, "true" if the two representatives match, "false" if they do not. Thus, we can see that even this simple processing task can be quite difficult, and the presence of aphasia would complicate its operation even more. Aphasic difficulties might well occur at any stage: at the beginning when the sentence and the picture are put into comparable mental formats, at the comparison stage when short term memory deficits might interfere, at the productive stages, and so forth (West, Gelfer, and Rosen, 1978). How much more complicated, then, the task becomes when one asks the patient to point to one picture in an array, for then the characteristics of the other pictures in the array will also be a major factor. Let us suppose that the task at hand is for our patient to point to one of five pictures after the therapist has said its name. The therapist will have in front of the patient the correct response and four alternative choices. If alternatives are used that are in any way related to the word that is being said, the difficulty of the task has been increased. If, for example, the words being said are "man," and the response alternative array has a picture of a "man" along with "boy," "woman," and "can," the therapist has stacked the deck against the patient, for the task becomes more difficult as the relatedness among the items increases. Thus, "man" and "can" show *phonemic similarity*. If the task were a reading task, then *visual similarity* would also affect response: words that look alike such as "horse" and "house" or "bank" and "bark" are confused. Schuell and Jenkins (1961) found these variables to affect response regardless of whether the aphasic patient was asked to recognize spoken words, to name, to match printed words to pictures, to match printed to spoken words, or to write words to dictation. They considered this evidence of a language deficit independent of modality and of the recurring patterns of clinical symptoms found in aphasic patients.

The number of items in the response array will also influence performance, for the more items the patient must scan in order to select a correct response, the more difficulty will be experienced. As we mentioned earlier, that is one of the reasons why the initial subtests of the auditory comprehension section of the BDAE are difficult, for there are three categories and eighteen items on each stimulus card that the patient must scan in order to find a correct response.

The obvious therapeutic strategy is to gradually increase the number and extent of the associations among the items in the response array. We have organized many of our therapy materials with this goal in mind. The practical application of these principles can perhaps best be illustrated with some of the materials from our patient-directed treatment programs. We program time for our patients to work on their own with the notion that this fosters independence and a sense that the commitment to continued therapeutic gain lies as much with the patient as with the therapist. Consequently, we've organized our standard materials into workbooks so that the patient either uses the material in the notebook on its own, or the notebook can be combined with a language master or tape recorder if auditory stimulation is needed. We consider our GAR (General Auditory Recognition) program the easiest program from the point of view of having little if any semantic or phonemic association among the items. The patient hears "owl" and circles the picture of the owl choosing it from any array *wallet, owl, sailor*, or he might be asked to write the name of the picture if he were working at another level. At a later stage, the patient might use a notebook with semantic associations among the items in the response array: *house, church, garage, school, barn.* An array with phonemic similarity includes *net, nest, nuts* in one row, *yard, yawn, yarn* in another. A reading task includes phonemic similarity (*rail, bail, fail, tail*) and semantic similarity (*laser, razor, shave, blade*). Another reading task with semantic similarity has *mad, hate, anger, rage* and *scared, brave, frightened, afraid* as choices. Word association norms (Toglia and Battig, 1978) were used to determine the relatedness among the items.

If an auditory stimulus is presented, for example, "toe" and the aphasic's response array includes only pictures, the task is quite difficult, for there is no verbal label present for the patient to compare with the auditory stimulus. Having the word written under each picture would facilitate response. If the therapist said the word and showed the printed word as well, and the patient selected from an array that included the picture and the word that identifies it, then performance would be maximized. Another variation would be for the therapist to show the word alone, the patient being asked to select the correct picture from the array. A direct word-to-word match could be effected as well, or the "reading" task could be made more difficult by showing a phrase such as "show me what you listen with." Controlled auditory stimulation is closely identified with Schuell's approach to treatment (1964), but most aphasiologists, regardless of their theoretical persuasion, would use a great deal of auditory stimulation when treating an aphasic. In general, multimodal presentation facilitates the best response: if you can say the name of the object, show a printed word that identifies the object, give the object's gesture, and help create an image of the object for recall, then response will be maximized in an auditory recognition task, particularly if there is no semantic, phonemic, or visual similarity among the items in the response array.

Most auditory comprehension tasks demand at least a pointing response. Yet one must not lose sight of the fact that pointing is *a response* and as such will be affected by variables that affect the aphasic's productive abilities. What happens within the organism to effect a pointing response? The auditory stimulus must be decoded, some sort of cortical integration must occur for the stimulus to be understood and acted upon cognitively, and then a response must be encoded. Much must happen within the "black box" of the brain before even a simple response such as pointing to an object can be organized and effected. It is for this reason alone that one can say categorically that there is no modality-pure stimulus or response. One of the reasons why aphasics seem to comprehend so well in conversational settings is that comprehension can be indicated even though specific responses are not required, and one can evaluate the patient's grasp of the total gestalt of the communicative process as it occurs. This is probably as valid, albeit unreliable, an assessment of his or her comprehension ability as any other, yet it is one to which we seldom give official credence and there have been few attempts to measure it.

A widely used technique both in therapy and in diagnostic tests are tasks that require pointing span. Pointing span entails a great deal of production, as it is necessary to reproduce at an inner level the words just heard in order to point to them in the correct order. The patient is asked to "point to the ceiling, then to the floor" (BDAE, Goodglass and Kaplan, 1972). In such commands as "put the pencil on top of the card, then put it back" (BDAE, Goodglass and Kaplan, 1972), the complexity of the syntax also affects response. Such commands overtax the memory load for most aphasics; they simply are unable to handle the increasing number of words in the utterances. Other aphasics will echo the command, yet be unable to comprehend it. Still others seem to understand the command; they glance fleetingly at the correct objects or pictures, yet they seem unable to encode the response. Goodglass, Gleason, and Hyde (1970) reported that pointing span for the best of the aphasic groups they studied was below the average level of normal six-year-old children. This deficit in pointing span was particularly severe in the Broca's aphasic group, even though they were at the same time able to comprehend quite long and involved sentences.

In this section we reviewed a variety of variables that will influence comprehension and/or production of language. Included are such variables as frequency of occurrence, word familiarity, concreteness, imageability, complexity, redundancy, and length of words. In addition a variety of remedial techniques influencing the learning process for the aphasic were also presented. Included were rate of teaching, learning delay and learning interference, paired associate learning, modality stimulation, positive reinforcement techniques, voice and intonation characteristics, association and verification techniques, and pointing techniques. Therapists should consider the utilization of these variables and techniques as a means of facilitating language recovery.

Specific Treatment Approaches

Hundreds of specific intervention techniques for aphasia rehabilitation are cited in the literature (Sarno, 1981). It is interesting to note, however, that many of the more recent approaches combine stimulation with a hierarchical arrangement of steps, so that behavior modification principles such as gradual shaping of behavior are incorporated. In other words, stimulation approaches incorporate the pedagogy of behavior modification, and behaviorally oriented therapies emphasize the nature of the stimulation. For example, Helm-Estabrooks (Albert et al., 1981; Helm, 1977) views her approach as one which stimulates the patient to improve his accessing or retrieval strategies, yet she says, "it is axiomatic in dysphasia rehabilitation that one begins where the patient has the greatest chance of success and progresses in small steps" (Albert et al., 1981, p. 154). LaPointe (1978) believes that his Base-10 Programmed Stimulation approach combines behavioral modification features, such as clearly defining the task, measuring baseline performance, and plotting progress session by session with many of the features of the stimulation approach, such as controlling the amount of stimulation, requiring continuous responding by the patient, allowing for restimulation, and the like. He questions the assumed dichotomy between stimulation and programmed approaches, stating that many similarities and areas of overlap exist between the two.

Even Schuell, (1964), the advocate of the stimulation approach, said,

> it is always necessary to begin at the level where language breaks down for each patient, and to proceed systematically from easier to more difficult tasks. A good method may fail if materials are too easy or too difficult at a given time. The patient should build from success to success at gradually increasing levels of complexity (p. 353).

The sections that follow discuss a few of the more innovative specific therapeutic approaches developed in recent years. In most instances these are old ideas in new bottles; that is, the techniques themselves have been around in individual therapist's clinical armamentarium, but they are now presented within a theoretical framework and systematized so that the results of the therapeutic intervention can be communicated. Most do, in fact, combine features of the stimulation approach and behavior modification.

Melodic Intonation Therapy. It has long been noted that some aphasics can not only sing the melody of a popular song, but sometimes articulate the words as well. Jackson (1875–1958) assumed that the more automatic speech processes were more equally and fully represented in each half of the brain than were the higher forms. The role of the right hemisphere in the processing and perception of intonation suggests that it is this hemisphere's participation that explains the aphasic's preservation of familiar songs and thus leads to the hope that melody might be a means of tapping the undamaged right hemisphere's potential. Indeed, nurses or family members may note the amazing phenomenon of the otherwise speechless patient singing, and ask why if the patient can articulate the words of a familiar song so well, words in conversational speech cannot be articulated equally as well. In fact, most aphasics can carry the melody of popular songs and *some* patients can sing the words as well, but the latter phenomenon is rarer than the former. Very often when one listens carefully to what has been described as singing, it is observed that singing occurs fairly well in unison, but when accompaniment fades out, the patient reverts to stereotypic utterances. Most therapists and families discover that attempts to extend the nonpropositional language heard in the patient's song to propositional language are futile. Melodic Intonation Therapy (MIT) grew out of such an attempt. It is an approach that uses intoned utterances which are based on the melody pattern, the rhythm, and the points of stress of a spoken model (Sparks, 1981). However, the melody patterns of familiar songs are avoided. The utterances used in MIT should have a slower and more lyrical tempo than speech, with more precise rhythm and more accentuated points of stress (Sparks and Holland, 1976). Experience with MIT has shown that when sentences were adapted to familiar melodies the patient would revert to the lyrics associated with the melody rather than the intended phrase. Thus, MIT avoids any distinct melody even reminiscent of a popular song or jingle (Sparks, Helm, and Albert, 1974).

The first level of MIT includes unison recitation of the sentence by the patient and the therapist. Simultaneously, the rhythm of the utterance is tapped out, the therapist holding the patient's hand. As the patient's intonation becomes successful, the therapist gradually withdraws stimulation. Progression of the program leads eventually to repetition of the sentence in normal speech prosody (Albert, Sparks, and Helm, 1973). As the patient improves, the melodic aspects of the program are faded, and confrontation questions are introduced. The MIT program, then, is one of gradual progression. The aphasic patient is guided through a sequence of steps which increase the length of the units, diminish dependency on the clinician and reliance on intonation (Sparks and Holland, 1976). Details of the program's sequence are presented in Sparks and Holland (1976), Albert et al. (1981), and Sparks (1981). MIT is effective for only about one fourth of the aphasic population (Sparks, 1981), specifically those with severe output limitations including oral apraxia and/or a restricted phonemic stereotypy, relatively preserved auditory comprehension, and poor repetition (Helm, 1978).

Promoting Aphasics' Communicative Effectiveness (PACE). Another new approach to aphasia rehabilitation which extends an established therapeutic technique is PACE (Wilcox and Davis, 1978; Haire and Davis, 1979; Davis and Wilcox, 1981). It incorporates a technique long used in a game-like group therapy situation. The PACE technique is placed into a theoretical framework and a treatment approach that uses components of face-to-face conversation. The theoretical foundation for PACE grows from Davis and Wilcox's interest in pragmatics, the study of how language is used in context. The interaction in PACE is based on the reciprocity of speaker and listener roles. The aphasic and the therapist alternate between these roles in as natural a setting as possible.

The technique is as follows: both patient and therapist have a stack of pictures lying face down on the table. Taking turns as the sender, each selects a picture and keeps it from view of the receiver. The goal of the sender is to convey to the receiver what the picture depicts. The pictures may be of objects, actions, or stories, depending on the patient's interest and communicative abilities. PACE is based on four interdependent principles:

1. There is an exchange of new information between the clinician and the patient.
2. The patient has a free choice as to which communicative channels he or she may use to convey new information.
3. The clinician and the patient participate equally as senders and receivers of messages.
4. Feedback is provided by the clinician in response to the patient's success in conveying a message (Davis and Wilcox, 1981).

The communicative value of residual speech is heightened in PACE, for even with minimal verbal output a patient can convey a variety of messages when able to utilize nonverbal channels and contextual information.

Visual Communication Therapy (VIC). Globally impaired patients are those who are unable to use any form of natural language successfully. Visual Communication Therapy (VIC) (Gardner, et al., 1975) is an experimental technique designed to teach the global aphasic artificial language using a system of arbitrary symbols. It grew from the work of Premack (1971) who had successfully taught a simple communication system to chimpanzees. With VIC, eight globally impaired patients were taught to recognize symbols and then manipulate them to (a) carry out commands; (b) answer questions; (c) describe actions; (d) describe events; (e) express feelings and desires or other emotions. The findings support the notion that some globally impaired patients can master an alternate communication system and that some of the cognitive operations necessary for natural language are preserved despite severe aphasia (Sarno, 1981).

Visual-Action Therapy (VAT). A related technique for the globally impaired patient is called Visual-Action Therapy (VAT) (Helm and Benson, 1978; Albert, et al., 1981). VAT uses eight real objects. In series of hierarchically arranged steps, the patients are taught that the line represents the real object, and that the object and the drawing can also be represented by a gesture. Later, the patient is taught to produce these gestures in response to the presentation of the object. Comparison of pre- and posttreatment scores indicates that the patients completing the program show significant improvement in auditory comprehension and gestural pantomime. More importantly, Helm-Estabrooks feels that patients successfully completing the program are then able to profit from more linguistically oriented therapeutic techniques.

Amer-Ind. Amer-Ind (Skelly, 1979) is another approach that uses gestures, but gestures modified from American Indian hand talk. The system is said to be 80 to 90 percent understandable by untrained listeners, making it particularly attractive as an alternate system for the speechless patient, for he or she can thus communicate to strangers to the system. It is, however, highly symbolic in the sense that a sign stands for an object or concept, and as such is difficult for aphasic patients to learn, but Amer-Ind is reported (Skelly, et al, 1974) to have been successfully used with patients having long-standing severe apraxia of speech.

Deblocking. Another technique which incorporates old ideas into a new theoretical framework is that of "deblocking" described by Weigl (1968). The deblocking technique makes systematic use of a patient's intact language modalities by evoking a response in an intact channel (such as recognition of a printed word), just before presenting the same stimulus to a blocked channel (i.e., the same word presented through the sense of hearing).

The Preventive Method. Beyn and Shokhor-Trotskaya (1966) attempt to prevent telegraphic speech (which often seems inevitable in a nonfluent aphasic) from developing by teaching at first only the simplest possible words which could express whole ideas, such as "no," "oh," "myself," "good," "thanks." At a later stage phrases such as "I want" or "I shall" are combined with predicates such as "eat," "sleep," "walk." Nouns are introduced only when they appear spontaneously in the patient's speech. The authors report that the telegraphic speech which they feel is inevitable with other methods of aphasia rehabilitation did not emerge in any of the twenty-five patients trained with the preventive method.

The Helm Elicited Language Program for Syntax Stimulation (HELPSS). The Helm Elicited Language Program for Syntax Stimulation (Estabrooks, 1981) is an approach designed to stimulate the agrammatic or paragrammatic aphasic's access to syntactical knowledge. It uses the story completion technique accompanied by a single action drawing to elicit verbally eleven sentence types, each at two levels of difficulty. At Level A, the patient produces a delayed repetition of the target sentence:

Probe: I see a shooting star, so I tell my friend, "Look up." What do I tell him?
Target Response: Look up.

At Level B no benefit of repetition is provided:

Probe: I see a shooting star, so I tell my friend, what?
Target Response: Look up.

HELPSS uses the hierarchy of difficulty for aphasic production of syntactic forms established by Goodglass, Gleason, Bernholtz and Hyde (1972) and Gleason, Goodglass, Green, Ackerman and Hyde (1975). The patient progresses from the easiest level, the imperative intransitive, to the most difficult, the future.

Sentence Type	Exemplar
1. Imperative intransitive	"Watch out"
2. Imperative transitive	"Open the window"
3. WH interrogative	"Where are my shoes?"
4. Declarative transitive	"He smokes a pipe"
5. Declarative intransitive	"He smiles"
6. Comparative	"He's younger"
7. Passive	"The check was cashed"
8. Yes-No questions	"Did you brush your teeth?"
9. Direct and indirect object	"He gives his son a present."
10. Embedded sentence	"She wanted him to be neat"
11. Future	"He will diet"

The Manhattan VA Group Therapy Program. Schuell et al., (1964) argued that "individual therapy and group therapy are two entirely different classes of events, serve different purposes, and should not be confused" (p. 343). It was their thesis that treatment for aphasia had to be tailored for the individual patient. They believed that there were no mass methods, that each patient needed individual consideration as to the best way to facilitate response, that materials and methods had to be adapted to individual patient needs at successive stages of recovery. For these reasons they were opposed to group therapy as a basic method of treatment for aphasia. On the other hand, they felt that group therapy could be a good adjunct to individual treatment, helping the aphasic patient to feel less isolated, to observe other aphasic patients, and to become aware of other people and their problems.

Group therapy for the stroke patient has taken various directions within our medical center over time. On the one hand, it is used as an adjunct to individual therapy for aphasic patients. In this sense, the group process serves to facilitate speech and language abilities, and the emphasis within these groups is on maintaining and heightening functional communication skills. We still have at least one group that is specific for aphasic patients, and we refer patients to this group who are in particular need of a group structure to facilitate communication skills. Examples of patients referred to this group include a man who lives alone and has few opportunities for verbal interaction, a fluent aphasic who profits from the feedback the group can give him (since he is an especially loquacious and tangential talker, the group's feedback very often comes down to "talk less and listen more").

Activities for this group have always centered upon the practical. The members of the group are expected to discuss newspaper articles of interest to them from the preceding week (the group meets once weekly), they discuss the day's current news, and they spend time working on practical matters of their choice, for example, figuring out a strategy for ordering in a restaurant when you cannot read the menu and/or telling the waitress what you want, or a strategy for making change quickly and safely when your arithmetic processing is at best slow and laborious, and the like. Since the patients in this group tend to be chronic patients who have completed a course of individual treatment, we have not observed significant, measurable language changes, but what we think we *have* observed is consolidation and maintenance of the skills they have already recovered.

Esprit de corps in our group runs high. The members of the group are very supportive of one another and have been insightful in their appraisal of one another's weaknesses and strengths. For example, since we mix levels of severity and types of aphasia, we have patients who are almost speechless and patients who are very verbose within the same group. It was our loquacious patient described earlier who pointed out that our most impaired patient was perhaps the most efficient communicator in the group because he is to the point, supplements his verbal paucity with gestures and writing, and is blessedly brief. For him to gain the insight that he is able to communicate without oral speech raises his confidence that he can cope with a verbal and impatient world.

We try to be as nondirective as possible within the group so that the members decide topics for discussion, matters with which they wish assistance, and so forth. At one point they decided that they should start going to movies during the day, for the theatre nearest the hospital offered a daytime special of a dollar a movie for senior citizens. So confident of their abilities did they become that as a group they went off to see a pornographic movie in Times Square in spite of the objections of our feminist therapists.

One of the problems with such an ongoing group is that it tends to foster dependency on the hospital, on the therapist, and on one another. Such dependency has its advantages (we feel weekly attendance probably reduces hospitalization), but it has its disadvantages, too. One of the greatest of these is that even though we see the group as a maintenance program, the patients perceive it as an ongoing treatment program and expect it to go on forever. And one could make a sound argument for why it *should* go on "forever," for the group supplies important psychological support, it gives severely impaired patients a place where their limited communicative skills are valued, and it provides a focal point, a high point each week, to their very limited lives. Unfortunately, accountability is a very serious issue in any medical center these days, and we must provide justification for maintaining such patients in treatment. What we have evolved, with occupational therapy and social work services, is a three-stage program that includes a Discharge Planning Group, a Community Involvement Group, and a Stroke Club, and thus, we hope, circumventing hospital dependency.

The primary goals of the Discharge Planning Group and the Community Involvement Groups have been (1) to help the stroke patient accept altered physical and cognitive status; (2) to help the patient view progress and changed capacities more realistically; (3) to help find an alternative life-style within the family and community; (4) to use the group work to facilitate the individual work the patient might be receiving in his daily therapies; and finally, (5) to help the patient find community placement suited to modified abilities (West, O'Connor, and Bennett, 1981).

A patient is referred to Discharge Planning at the time he goes home for his first weekend from the rehabilitation ward. This is at about the period when he is approaching maximal hospital benefit. This group is very "issue" oriented, and its main theme is, "What will your life-style be like when you go home?" The emphasis is on very practical, prosaic topics such as, "When you were home for the weekend how did you get from the living room to the bathroom?" "What did you do when the phone rang?," "What happened when company arrived?," and so forth. We are very issue-oriented in this group because we find that the patients are not really able to accept discussion of their feelings about the changed life-style that is impending at discharge. While the patient is participating in Discharge Planning, the family is simultaneously in a group that is separate but has a similar focus.

Upon discharge, when the patient is actually in the situation experiencing the problems of living at home with his altered physical and cognitive being, he moves to our Community Involvement Group where the focus is on acceptance of the altered life-style and the development of alternative life-styles. What is meant by "development of alternative life-styles?" Two examples come to mind. One of our patients was a former policeman. He volunteered to work with his local youth group and was able to sit at the entrance of the youth group's club, checking people in and out. For another patient, it involved a change in his perception of roles within the family structure. His wife needed to begin to work outside the home and the husband was able to take on, accept, and even find enjoyable, household duties he had previously believed were sexually stereotyped.

Our Community Involvement Group does focus on discussions of feelings and attitudes based on incidents that have actually happened at home (e.g., the patient's wife is treating him like an infant, "babying" him excessively). To facilitate this psychological venting, we might introduce writing topics such as "write down a schedule of what you did yesterday," so that feelings and attitudes that have not come up in discussion may surface. Role-playing activities are stressed. For example, making a sandwich, riding a bus. Or the therapist might begin by saying, "I was in an elevator today and heard a doctor saying to a patient, 'you know it's time you went home; your arm's really not going to get much better.' Do you think the doctor should have said that to the patient? Why? What would you have said?," and so forth. The goal of this group is to "confront reality without destroying hope," a favorite saying of our Chief of Occupational Therapy.

Concurrently with the Community Involvement Group the therapists involved meet with the patient and the patient's family on an individual basis to determine what he can do and where he can go in his community. We often use the services of Community and Senior Citizen Centers. We help the patient to accept his discharge from the hospital and from outpatient treatment by finding alternative things to occupy him. The focus is on what he can do, not on what he cannot do. It is our belief that continuing to come to the hospital focuses on what the patient cannot do and becomes ultimately counterproductive to good rehabilitation.

The final stage in our group process is our Stroke Club, which is a monthly meeting with maintenance, supportive, and education goals. It evolved from the groups described above because the patients and their families still felt the need for a contact with the hospital. We see it not only as contributing to a support network for the patient and the family but also as an ongoing part of the rehabilitative process. Patients and their families may attend the Stroke Club from the beginning of this three-phase group process, but we find that it is most meaningful to them upon discharge from the other groups.

A patient is optimally in our active group treatment programs for four to six months, sometimes up to eight months, depending upon his ability to adjust. Thereafter, he attends only the Stroke Club. We believe that the sooner a patient is discharged from all therapies the quicker is his adjustment to what is his particular reality. We have found that as long as a patient is still receiving occupational or physical therapy, treatment from speech pathology, or the like, he tends not to come to grips with what his disability is and will continue to be.

Again, none of these latter three groups are centered on structured speech and language activities, per se. The emphasis is on using remaining abilities. "What will you do when you leave the hospital?" As such the groups tend to be extremely practical. A given patient, for example, may say that he cannot cook lunch for himself because he cannot open jars or cans with one hand. The group then will focus on finding alternative ways to open jars and cans.

Aphasic patients function very well in these groups. While there is no doubt that the severely impaired aphasic patient has a more difficult time within a group structure, and we have certainly found it difficult to place him in his community, overall we have had many positive examples of severe aphasics doing very well. We emphasize the use of visual aids, the group is maximally supportive, and we've usually managed to integrate the patient quite well within the group structure.

For the left brain-damaged patient, group therapy of this sort may well tap right hemisphere cognitive skills. A more holistic processing is required, a total communicative effort. Almost every group session gives an illustration of a patient with severe comprehension deficits responding to jokes and innuendos that would seem to be beyond his abilities as indicated on standard aphasia test batteries. We find that the left brain-damaged patient is more sympathetic and empathetic to the others in the group, more tuned in to the emotional nuances of what is happening in the group, and so forth, than is the right brain-damaged patient who ostensibly has no linguistic processing problems. Group therapy, we believe, heightens right hemisphere processing. We find that the left brain-damaged patients do seem to get the point of jokes more often than not, they are aware of the need to participate in a joke or a discussion, and they are aware of their responsibilities to the group as a social participant. Certainly, these are the patients that are sensitive to the physical situation of the group; they will arrange the chairs, assure that the group is set up properly, and the like; right brain-damaged patients are often oblivious to these "subtleties." A group structure allows the left brain-damaged patient to see that even though he's unable to talk, to say what he wants to say, he can still participate in a communicative effort. And in real life situations such as making a sandwich, or interacting with guests, these patients often do better than the right brain-damaged patient.

Overall, we feel that this particular structure of our group therapies "works" because it has evolved over time to suit our patients' particular problems and the problems that exist in our metropolitan community. We feel it contributes in a very positive manner to the total rehabilitation process and is a solution to the "chronic stroke patient" syndrome. Group programs such as these are cost effective, both in terms of dollars and in terms of improved quality of life, because they integrate the patient into existing family and community structures. This reduces hospital dependency and focuses on health rather than disability.

We have reviewed in this section a few of the therapeutic techniques used by aphasia therapists. Studies that evaluate the effectiveness of particular techniques are still needed. Research confirming the overall effectiveness of aphasia therapy has only recently been accepted as scientifically valid. Speech pathologists and aphasic patients have long been convinced of the value of aphasia therapy; the medical profession, until recently, has not.

EVALUATING THE OUTCOME OF TREATMENT
Review of Some Studies on Recovery

There is a deeply entrenched and widely taught adage among neurologists that therapy for aphasia is ineffective (Benson, 1979). Since almost every study published on the effects of speech and language therapy on recovery from aphasia (Frazier and

Ingham, 1920; Weisenburg and McBride, 1935; Butfield and Zangwill, 1946; Wepman, 1951; Marks, Taylor, and Rusk, 1957; Godfrey, 1959; Godfrey and Douglass, 1959; Schuell, et al., 1964; Vignolo, 1964; Smith, 1971; Hagan, 1973; Basso, Faglioni, and Vignolo, 1974; Basso, Capitani and Vignolo, 1979; Wertz et al., 1981) has shown positive results, this attitude is puzzling. One might conclude that neurologists have simply ignored the data if it weren't for the fact that the results of the one study (Sarno, Silverman, and Sands, 1970) that did show negative results *are* widely quoted. Admonishments as to the methodological limitations of the studies demonstrating positive effects of treatment abound ("Struggling with Aphasia," *Medical World News*, 1969; Benson, 1967b; Darley, 1972, 1975); the limitations of the Sarno, Silverman and Sands (1970) study, clearly indicated by the authors, are ignored.

The Sarno, Silverman and Sands study (1970) asked whether (1) severe aphasics can learn, and (2) whether programmed instruction is an effective method for teaching them. Both questions were answered negatively. However, the study used a group of patients who were so severely aphasic that they "had no speech function and little understanding of speech." Furthermore, the patients' aphasic symptoms were chronic; the number of months post-onset for the group as a whole approached three years, while the mean age was nearly sixty-five years. Thus, the patients studied were old, chronic, and severely impaired, all factors, as we have previously noted, which seriously mitigate against improvement. This study, then, tells us something about one particular type of aphasic patient and the outcome of a particular approach to treatment (although, as we've previously indicated, therapies such as VIC and VAT have proven more successful with the severely impaired aphasic.). What about studies of the outcome of treatment for other types of patients?

There is no question that the difficulties in evaluating the outcome of treatment are, as an editorial in the British journal, *Lancet*, put it, "daunting." Darley (1975) lists the following factors as being desirable to control or at least specify in a recovery study:

"1. Regarding the patients
  a. Specific nature of the language deficits and their severity
  b. Age at onset of aphasia
  c. Intelligence, educational level, and premorbid language proficiency
  d. Social status
  e. Premorbid personality characteristics
  f. Prior health and health during recovery
  g. Etiology
  h. Site of lesion
  i. Extent of lesion
  j. Number of patients studied
 2. Regarding the treatment
  a. Interval between onset of aphasia and beginning of treatment
  b. Treatment procedures used
  c. Intensity of treatment
  d. Quality of treatment (competence of clinicians; relevance of materials and content)
 3. Regarding measurement of results
  a. Reliability, validity, and objectivity of test instruments used
  b. Comprehensiveness of behavioral measures

c. Quantification of measures
4. Use of an untreated control group" (p. 126)

The more recent recovery studies control or specify at least some of the variables listed by Darley. Hagan (1973) studied the effects of treatment versus no treatment in a group of twenty aphasic patients. The ten treated patients were matched in severity and type of aphasia to ten untreated patients. All entered the study at three months post-onset; the first ten admitted to the hospital who met the study's criteria were designated as the treatment group and the second ten as the control group. Hagan justified the ethical considerations of withholding treatment by pointing out that because of the high patient-to-therapist ratio, a large number of patients would not have received treatment regardless of whether a study had been conducted.

The study was conducted in two phases. During the first phase, which lasted for three months, no subject received speech and language therapy; all were engaged instead in physical rehabilitation. Upon their discharge from the physical rehabilitation program, at six months post-onset, each study patient was assigned to a long-term care ward. The control subjects received all of the hospital medical and non-medical services except communication therapy, while the subjects in the experimental group received the same service plus intensive communication therapy. Each experimental subject received four hours of individual therapy, eight hours of group therapy, and six hours of independent therapy per week. The results indicate that while both groups showed spontaneous recovery during the first three months of the program (when neither group received speech and language therapy), only the treatment group continued to progress beyond the point of spontaneous recovery.

Basso, Capitani, and Vignolo (1979) studied 281 aphasic patients (162 treated and 119 controls) who were reevaluated on a standard language examination no less than six months after having had a first evaluation. The interactive effects of the following four independent variables on the one dependent variable, namely, improvement in language skills (speaking, understanding, writing, and reading) were studied: (a) time between onset and first examination (less than two months, two to six months, more than six months); (b) type of aphasia (e.g., fluent versus nonfluent); (c) overall severity of aphasia (severe or moderate); (d) rehabilitation between the first and second examination (presence or absence). Variables such as sex, age, education, nature of the lesion were reviewed; their distribution in the two groups was random, except for age, the nontreated subjects being slightly older than the treated subjects. The 119 control subjects were prevented from attending therapy by extraneous factors such as family or transportation problems, and this lack of strict randomization may have created inadvertent bias (Benson, 1979b). The results showed "that formal language rehabilitation in aphasics does have a positive effect on the improvement of the ability to communicate through speaking, listening, writing, and reading, provided that it is carried out at least six months and at a rate of no less than three individual sessions per week. The gains in these specific language modalities are significantly more frequent in treated than in nontreated patients" (Basso, et al., 1979, p. 195). Time since onset and overall severity of aphasia were negative factors that significantly influenced the subsequent course of nontreated as well as that of treated patients.

Although their earlier study (Basso, Faglioni, and Vignolo, 1974) had shown that type of aphasia played a role in prognosis (the nonfluent aphasics doing worse), that result was not substantiated in this larger study. Other things being equal, all types of

Measure	Purpose
Neurologic Examination	Determine neurologic status and severity
Sensory Screening	Determine auditory, visual, and tactile acuity
Porch Index of Communicative Ability	Determine overall, gestural, verbal, and graphic communication abilities
Token Test	Determine auditory comprehension ability
Word Fluency Measure	Determine word-finding ability
Motor Speech Evaluation	Determine presence and severity of apraxia of speech and dysarthria
Coloured Progressive Matrices	Determine "nonverbal intelligence"
Conversational Rating	Determine conversational ability
Informant's Rating	Determine functional language use

**Table 8–6. Periodic Evaluation Measures Administered at 4,
15, 26, 37, and 48 Weeks Post-Onset—VA Cooperative Study**

aphasics were equally good candidates for treatment; but patients with severe and longstanding deficits on the first examination were those with the poorest prognosis. The rank order of the four language modalities with respect to improvement was about the same in treated and nontreated patients, suggesting that "rehabilitation accelerates the natural course of restitution without altering its pattern" (p. 196).

The VA Cooperative Study

Because no single aphasia clinic sees a sufficient sample of patients to control for all the potential influences that may interact with a patient's response to treatment, the Veterans Administration Cooperative Study (Wertz et al., 1981) was undertaken in an attempt to pool patients and control for as many of the biographical and medical variables as possible, to ensure uniformity of diagnosis by employing standardized measures of aphasia, and to specify the type and amount of treatment administered. Five VA medical centers participated in the study. Ethical considerations prevented having a non-treatment group. Instead, individual and group therapy were compared. Patients who met the selection criteria were assigned randomly to one of two treatment groups, Group A, which received traditional, individual therapy, or Group B, which received traditional group therapy; at entry into the study, all patients were four weeks post-onset (plus or minus three days).

A comprehensive battery of measures (table 8–6) was administered to both groups at intake and every eleven weeks thereafter up to forty-eight weeks post-onset or until a patient dropped out of the study. To eliminate any testing bias, the treatment therapist administered only the initial test battery; thereafter the test battery was administered by another speech-language pathologist especially trained for the study. All evaluations were videotaped in the treatment center; the tapes were then forwarded to the study center and scored "blind" by two speech-language pathologists who did not know the patient's treatment group assignment.

The treatment therapist administered all therapy given to both treatment groups. All patients received eight hours of treatment for each week that they participated in

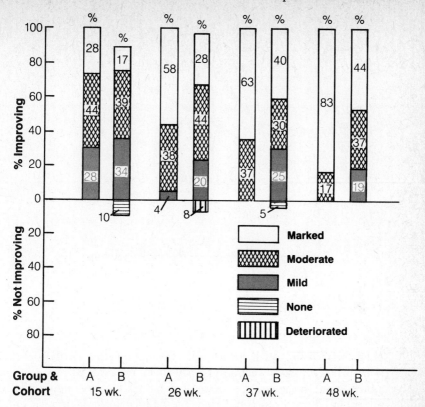

Figure 8–7. Percent of Patients in Each Cohort Improving, Not Improving, or Deteriorated on PICA Overall Percentile Score

the study. Each patient in Group A received four hours of direct therapist contact in traditional, individual stimulation therapy, plus four hours of supplemental machine-administered treatment specifically designed for him. Group B received four hours a week of group therapy; no direct manipulation of speech and language skills was permitted, the group's goals instead being to facilitate language in a social setting. This was supplemented by four hours each week of group recreational activities. The therapists as a group participated in writing a Treatment Protocol to serve as a guideline for treatment for the two groups and to ensure that essentially the same treatment was provided in the five medical centers. In addition, detailed treatment logs were maintained on each patient entered into the study.

Both groups showed significant improvement on all measures, and when the improvement of individual patients is reviewed, it is evident that most patients improved on most measures (figure 8–7). Much of the total improvement occurred during the first eleven weeks, but there was a significant time factor and those patients in therapy the longest continued improvement over time. Group A (individual therapy) resulted in more improvement than Group B (group therapy) on almost all measures at almost all points in time, but there were few statistically significant differences, although individual treatment resulted in significantly better overall performance (figure 8–8) on the Porch Index of Communicative Ability, perhaps the

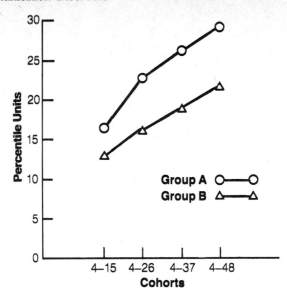

Figure 8–8. PICA Overall Percentile Group Mean Change Scores

most comprehensive measure used. Finally, the authors felt that "if the belief that significant spontaneous recovery was complete by six months was correct, continued significant improvement in the patients treated beyond six months implies that both individual and group treatment are efficacious means for managing aphasia".

Other Issues

It would seem, then, that the issue of proving the efficacy of aphasia therapy may finally be laid to rest. It would be better if we could finally focus our energies on developing new approaches to treatment, as well as elucidating which patients do best with which treatment. One could never control for all the variables that "should" be controlled in a study involving human beings, particularly human beings as complicated as those with aphasia. But it is perhaps comforting to note that a neurologist such as Benson who once said in a Medical World News interview, "Struggling with Aphasia" (1969):

> The classic aphasic patient comes in on a stretcher and isn't talking. When he leaves, he is walking but not talking.

more recently (1979a) said:

> aphasia therapy has already proved valuable in the total rehabilitation of appropriate brain-damaged patients and the future holds considerable promise of increasing help from aphasia therapists (p. 181).

On the other hand, now that it's documented that aphasia therapy does help, Benson says that this warrants serious interest in the process by neurologists. While he agrees (1979b) that "Most neurologists (and most other physicians) have little knowledge of aphasia therapy and are unable to either prescribe or monitor the procedure competently," nonetheless, "The course of treatment should be monitored by the physician in collaboration with the therapist and any decision to alter or discontinue therapy should be based on combined clinical judgment" (1979b, p. 188).

Aphasic patients *should* be managed by a team of specialists. Each specialist contributes his or her particular expertise to aphasia management. The aphasia therapist maintains perhaps the longest and closest relationship with the patient; the therapist typically sees the patient daily on an individual basis and can thus provide feedback to the other team members as to the patient's total well-being. One would hope, then, that the neurologist is as interested in taking advice about the proper levels of medication (to use a practical example) for a given patient from the aphasia therapist (who, after all, knows relatively little about medication, but can certainly observe its effect on behavior), as the neurologist is in giving advice about aphasia rehabilitation!

ON BECOMING AN APHASIA THERAPIST

Aphasia therapy is among the most challenging of human interactions. It can be demanding, exhausting, stimulating, and fun. Aphasic patients can be a trying population to deal with therapeutically, for their linguistic deficit often seems to be overwhelmingly difficult to remediate, and the personality traits associated with brain damage seem to mitigate against that remediation. The patients themselves can be very funny, they are almost always grateful for the effort spent in their behalf, and the therapeutic process itself is fascinating. If you can convey to a patient the sense that the two of you are engaged in mutual exploration of his cognitive and linguistic assets and limitations, if you can heighten the ability to laugh with you over linguistic boggles, and if you can foster the notion that the responsibility for remediation must be shared with you, significant therapeutic gain will have been made.

It is the relationship that the therapist establishes with the aphasic patient that probably matters most to rehabilitation. Strangers to the therapeutic process often comment that it must take a great deal of patience to treat an aphasic patient, but patience is not really the essential ingredient. Perhaps what it takes most is flexibility and a willingness to explore. As a therapist you must constantly be so tuned into a patient that you sense the cognitive processes underlying responses and be flexible enough to adapt the stimulus, or the response requirements, or both, to facilitate that responsiveness. You may begin with one goal in mind at the start of a therapy session and then find that you must concentrate on quite another process because the patient's needs for that particular day are quite different from what was planned. It is for this reason that many experienced clinicians prefer to work with what the patient brings to the session rather than with preconceived therapy plans. At issue is the patient's communication or emotional needs, and, with that in mind, an experienced clinician can build a therapeutic session around what is happening at the moment while still incorporating good learning principles into the session.

The notion that more therapy will make someone better and better, and that therapy should go on until one is completely better is on the surface a logical extension of the American drive for self-improvement. If a patient has not recovered from aphasia, how will it ever occur if therapy is terminated? How can a therapist cut off therapy when recovery isn't "complete"? There is almost always a discrepancy between what the aphasia therapist believes to be excellent recovery and what the patient and the family expected. At least initially, all concerned usually expect the patient to return to "normal." But the advantage of the long-term process that is aphasia therapy is that as treatment evolves, so do the patient and the family, and both usually begin to accept the limitations. The family who originally said to us, "When will the patient return to work?" moves through that phase to face the "possibility" of less demanding work, to finally the acceptance that the patient will never return to gainful employment again. Most families are resilient and the final stage in their acceptance is to say more or less that the patient is accepted and loved as a person who has once been someone different, is changed, but is still loved. How wise they have all become at this point, and how much they have lived through!

SUMMARY

Since Broca's description in 1861, lesions in the third left frontal convolution have been known to produce nonfluent, effortful, agrammatic verbal output with comprehension relatively better preserved. Broca's aphasia contrasts with the fluent aphasia first described by Wernicke in 1874; here the causative lesion lies in the left temporal lobe, the patient's speech is fluent and effortless yet full of paraphasic (substitution) errors, and comprehension is significantly compromised. Throughout the long and varied history of aphasia, many other types have been described, and many classification systems have evolved. For most aphasics all language modalities are impaired to some degree; as the patient moves through the period of spontaneous recovery, severity of the symptoms will abate to varying degrees. Many variables influence the amount of recovery: initial severity of the symptoms, etiology, site of lesion, age, education, intelligence, motivation. Speech therapy administered early in the recovery period at sufficient intensity will make a significant impact on the amount of recovery made. A wide variety of diagnostic test batteries are available to help assess the nature and the severity of the aphasic deficits and to document the changes that occur over time.

Aphasic comprehension and/or production of language is strongly influenced by variables such as frequency of occurrence or word familiarity, concreteness, imageability, complexity, redundancy, length, part of speech. How material is presented and how the patient is asked to respond will also make a difference in how readily a response is given and how accurate it is.

There have been two major approaches to aphasia rehabilitation. One is labeled "the stimulation approach" and advocates strong, controlled auditory stimulation to facilitate language recovery. The other, the programmed operant approach, systematically applies operant procedures to specify and measure carefully defined behaviors as they change over time. Some specific intervention techniques for aphasia rehabilitation have been described; group therapy and family counseling are important adjuncts. Although aphasia rehabilitation is a difficult and demanding profession, it is also among the most rewarding.

BIBLIOGRAPHY

Alajouanine, T. E., Verbal realization in aphasia. *Brain*, **79**, 1–28 (1956).
Albert, M. L., Goodglass, H., Helm, N. A., Rubens, A. B., and Alexander, M. P., *Clinical aspects of dysphasia*. New York: Springer-Verlag (1981).

Albert, M. L., Sparks, R., and Helm, N. A., Melodic intonation therapy for aphasia. *Archives of Neurology*, **29**, 130–131 (1973).

Altman, M., *Visual imagery as a facilitator of pair-associate learning with adult aphasics*. Unpublished Master's thesis, Hunter College, City University of New York (1977).

Baker, N. E., and Holland, A. L., Aphasic comprehension of related statements. In A. L. Holland (Ed.), *Psycholinguistics and behavioral variables underlying recovery from aphasia*. Project report submitted to Social and Rehabilitative Service, DHEW (1971).

Basso, A., Capitani, E., and Vignolo, L. A., Influence of rehabilitation of language skills in aphasic patients: A controlled study. *Archives of Neurology*, **36**, 190–196 (1979).

Basso, A., Faglioni, P., and Vignolo, L. A., Étude controlée de la rééducation due langage dans l'aphasic: comparaison entre aphasiques traités et non-traités. *Revue Neurologique* (Paris), **131**, 607–614 (1974).

Benson, D. F., Fluency in aphasia; correlation with radioactive scan localization, *Cortex*, **3**, 373–394 (1967).

Benson, D. F., *Aphasia, alexia, and agraphia*. New York: Churchill Livingstone (1979a).

Benson, D. F., Editorial: aphasia rehabilitation. *Archives of Neurology*, **36**, 187–189 (1979b).

Beyn, E., and Shokhor-Trotskaya, M., The preventive method of speech rehabilitation in aphasia. *Cortex*, **2**, 96–108 (1966).

Blumstein, S., and Cooper, W. E., Hemispheric processing of intonation contours. *Cortex*, **10**, 146–158 (1974).

Boller, F., Cole, M., Vrtunski, P. B., Patterson, M., and Kim, Y., Paralinguistic aspects of auditory comprehension in aphasia. *Brain and Language* **7**, 164–174 (1979).

Boller, F., and Green, E., Comprehension in severe aphasia. *Cortex*, **8**, 382–394 (1972).

Boller, F., and Vignolo, L. A., Latent sensory aphasia in hemisphere-damaged patients: an experimental study with the Token Test. *Brain*, **89**, 815–830 (1966).

Bousefield, W. A., The occurrence of clustering in the free recall of randomly arranged associates. *Journal of General Psychology*, **49**, 229–240 (1953).

Bricker, A. L., Schuell, H. M., and Jenkins, J. J., Effect of word frequency and word length on aphasic spelling errors. *Journal of Speech and Hearing Research*, **7**, 183–192 (1964).

Broca, P., Remarques sur le siége de la faculté du langage articulé, suives d'un observation d'aphémie. *Paris Bulletin de la Société d'Anatomie*, **6**, 330–357(a) (1861).

Broca, P., Nouvelle observation d'aphémie produite par une lésion de la moitié postérieure des deuxième et troisième circonvolutions frontales. *Paris Bulletin de la Société d'Anatomie*, **6**, 398–407(b) (1861).

Butfield, E., and Zangwill, O., Reeducation in aphasia: A review of 70 cases. *Journal of Neurology, Neurosurgery, and Psychiatry*, **9**, 75–79 (1946).

Carpentar, P. A., and Just, M. A., Sentence comprehension: A psycholinguistic processing model of verification. *Psychological Review*, **82**, 45–73 (1975).

Clark, H. H., and Chase, W. G., On the process of comparing sentences against pictures. *Cognitive Psychology*, **3**, 427–517 (1972).

Costello, J., Programmed instruction. *Journal of Speech and Hearing Disorders*, **42**, 3–28 (1977).

Culton, G. L., Spontaneous recovery from aphasia. *Journal of Speech and Hearing Research*, **12**, 825–832 (1969).

Culton, G. L., Reaction to age as a factor in chronic aphasia in stroke patients. *Journal of Speech and Hearing Disorders*, **36**, 563–564 (1971).

Dabul, B. L., *Apraxia battery for adults*. Tigard, Oregon: C.C. Publications (1979).

Darley, F. L., The efficacy of language rehabilitation in aphasia. *Journal of Speech and Hearing Disorders*, **37**, 3–21 (1972).

Darley, F. L., Treatment of acquired aphasia. In W. J. Friedlander (Ed.), *Advances in neurology* (Vol. 7). New York: Raven Press (1975).

Darley, F. L., *Aphasia*. Philadelphia: W.B. Saunders (1982).

Darley, F. L., Aronson, A. E., and Brown, J. R., Differential diagnostic patterns of dysarthria. *Journal of Speech and Hearing Research*, **12**, 246–269 (1969).

Darley, F. L., Aronson, A. E., and Brown, J. R., Clusters of deviant speech dimensions in the dysarthrias. *Journal of Speech and Hearing Research*, **12**, 462–496 (1969).

Darley, F. L., Aronson, A. E., and Brown, J. R., *Motor speech disorders*. Philadelphia: W. B. Saunders (1975).

Davis, A. *A Survey of Adult Aphasia*. Englewood Cliffs, N.J.: Prentice-Hall (1983).

Davis, G. A., and Wilcox, M. J., Incorporating parameters of natural conversation in aphasia treatment. In R. Chapey (Ed.), *Language Intervention Strategies in Adult Aphasia*. Baltimore: Williams & Wilkins (1981).

Deale, J. L., and Darley, F. L., The influence of linguistic and situational variables on phonemic accuracy in apraxia of speech. *Journal of Speech and Hearing Research*, **15**, 639–653 (1972).

DeRenzi, E., and Faglioni, P., The comparative efficiency of intelligence and vigilance tests in detecting hemispheric cerebral damage. *Cortex*, **1**, 410–433 (1965).

DeRenzi, E., and Faglioni, P., Normative data and screening power of a shortened version of the Token Test. *Cortex*, **14**, 41–49 (1978).

DeRenzi, E., and Vignolo, L. A., The Token Test: a sensitive test to detect receptive disturbances in aphasics. *Brain*, **85**, 665–678 (1962).

Dorland's Illustrated Medical Dictionary (24th ed.). New York: W. B. Saunders (1965).

Duffy, J. R., Schuell's stimulation approach to rehabilitation. In R. Chapey (Ed.), *Language Intervention Strategies in Adult Aphasia*. Baltimore: Williams & Wilkins (1981).

Ebbin, J. B., and Edwards, A. E., Speech sound discrimination of aphasics when intersound interval is varied. *Journal of Speech and Hearing Research*, **10**, 120–125 (1967).

Edelstein, D. A., *Visual imagery and recognition memory in aphasia*. Unpublished Master's thesis, Hunter College, City University of New York (1977).

Ellis, H. D., and Shepherd, J. W., Recognition of abstract and concrete words presented in left and right visual fields. *Journal of Experimental Psychology*, **103**, 1035–1036 (1974).

Estabrooks, N. H., *Helm Elicited Language Program for Syntax Stimulation*. Austin, Texas: Exceptional Resources (1981).

Frazier, C. H., and Ingham, S. D., A review of effects of gunshot wounds of the head: Based on the observation of two hundred cases at U.S. General Hospital No. 11, Cape May, N.J. *Archives of Neurology*, **3**, 17–40 (1920).

Gardner, H., Albert, M. L., and Weintraub, S., Comprehending a word: the influence of speed and redundancy on auditory comprehension in aphasia. *Cortex*, **11**, 155–162 (1975).

Gardner, H., Zurif, E., Berry, T., and Baker, E., Visual communication in aphasia. *Neuropsychologia*, **14**, 275–292 (1976).

Geschwind, N. Disconnexion syndromes in animals and man. *Brain*, **88**, 237–294; 585–644, (1965).

Geschwind, N. The apraxias: neural mechanisms of disorders of learned movement. *American Scientist*, **63**, 184–194, (1975).

Gleason, J. B., Goodglass, H., Green, F., Ackerman, N., and Hyde, M. K., The retrieval of syntax in Broca's aphasia. *Brain and Language* **24**, 451–471, (1975).

Gloning, I., Gloning, K., and Haub, G., Comparison of verbal behaviour in right-handed and non-right-handed patients with anatomically verified lesions of one hemisphere. *Cortex*, **5**, 43–52 (1969).

Godfrey, C. M., A dysphasia rehabilitation clinic. *Canadian Medical Association Journal*, **80**, 616–618 (1959).

Godfrey, C. M., and Douglass, E., The recovery process in aphasia. *Canadian Medical Association Journal*, **80**, 618–624 (1959).

Goldfarb, R., Operant conditioning and programmed instruction in aphasia rehabilitation. In R. Chapey (Ed.), *Language Intervention Strategies in Adult Aphasia*. Baltimore: Williams & Wilkins (1981).

Goldstein, K., *Language and Language Disturbances*. New York: Grune & Stratton (1948).

Goodglass, H., The syndromes of aphasia: similarities and differences in neurolinguistic features. *Topics in Language Disorders*, **1**, 1–14 (1981).

Goodglass, H., Symposium: classification in aphasia. Annual meeting of the Academy of Aphasia, Lake Mohonk, New York (1982).

Goodglass, H., and Berko, J., Agrammatism and inflectional morphology in English. *Journal of Speech and Hearing Research*, **3**, 257–267 (1960).

Goodglass, H., Blumstein, S. E., Gleason, J. B., Hyde, M. R., Green, E., and Statlender, S., The effect of syntactic encoding on sentence comprehension in aphasia. *Brain and Language*, **7**, 201–209 (1979).

Goodglass, H., Gleason, J. B., Bernholtz, N. D., and Hyde, M. K., Some linguistic structures in the speech of a Broca's aphasic. *Cortex*, **8**, 191–212 (1972).

Goodglass, H., Gleason, J. B., and Hyde, M. R., Some dimensions of auditory language comprehension in aphasia. *Journal of Speech and Hearing Research*, **13**, 596–606 (1970).

Goodglass, H. and Kaplan, E., *The assessment of aphasia and related disorders*. Philadelphia: Lea & Febiger (1972).

Goodglass, H., Klein, B., Carey, P., Jones, K., Specific semantic word categories in aphasia. *Cortex*, **2**, 74–89 (1966).

Goodglass, H., Klein, B., Weintraub, S., and Ackerman, N., The tip-of-the-tongue phenomenon in aphasia. *Cortex*, **12**, 145–153, (1976).

Goodglass, H., Quadfasel, F., and Timberlake, W., Phrase length and the type and severity of aphasia. *Cortex*, **1**, 133–153 (1964).

Grossman, M., *The effect of verb type on linguistic processing by aphasic and normal subjects*. Unpublished Master's thesis, Hunter College, City University of New York (1979).

Hagan, C., Communicative abilities in hemiplegia: Effect of speech therapy. *Archives of Physical Medicine and Rehabilitation*, **54**, 454–463 (1973).

Haire, A. D., and Davis, G. A., Can the clinical interaction analysis system describe PACE therapy? In R.H. Brookshire (Ed.), *Clinical Aphasiology Conference Proceedings*. Minneapolis: BRK Publishers (1979).

Head, H., *Aphasia and Kindred Disorders of Speech*. New York: Hafner (1963). (Originally published, 1926).

Helm, N. A., Criteria for selecting aphasia patients for melodic intonation therapy. Paper presented at *Language Rehabilitation in Aphasia*, American Academy for the Advancement of Science Annual Meeting, Washington, D.C. (1977).

Helm, N. A., A program for stimulating recovery from agrammatism. Paper presented at the American Speech and Hearing Association Convention, Chicago, Illinois (1977).

Helm, N. A., and Benson, D. F., Visual action therapy for global aphasia. Paper presented at the Academy of Aphasia Meeting, Chicago, Illinois (1978).

Hines, D., Recognition of verbs, abstract nouns and concrete nouns from the left and right visual half-fields. *Neuropsychologia*, **14**, 211–216 (1976).

Holland, A. L., *Communicative Abilities in daily living*. Baltimore: University Park Press (1980).

Holland, A. L., and Sonderman, J., Effects of a program based on the Token Test for teaching comprehension skills to aphasics. *Journal of Speech and Hearing Research*, **17**, 589–598 (1974).

Howes, D., and Geschwind, N., Quantitative studies of aphasic language. In D.M. Rioch & E.A. Weinstein (Eds.), *Disorders of communication*. Baltimore: Williams & Wilkins (1964).

Jackson, J. H., On the nature of the duality of the brain. In J. Taylor (Ed.), *Selected writings of John Hughlings Jackson* (Vol. 2). London: Staples Press, 1958. (Originally published, 1874).

Jackson, J. H., On affectations of speech from disease of the brain. In J. Taylor (Ed.), *Selected writings of John Hughlings Jackson (Vol. 2)*. London: Staples Press, 1958. (Originally published, 1879–80).

Jakobson, R., *Toward a linguistic typology of aphasic impairments*. In A. DeReuck and M. O'Connor (Eds.), *Disorders of Language*. London: J. & A. Churchill (1964).

Johns, D. F., and Darley, F. L., Phonemic variability in apraxia of speech. *Journal of Speech and Hearing Research*, **13**, 556–583 (1970).

Johns, D. F., and LaPointe, L. L., Neurogenic disorders of output processing: apraxia of speech. In H. Whitaker and H.A. Whitaker (Eds.), *Studies in neurolinguistics* (Vol. 1). New York: Academic Press (1976).

Katz, A. N., and Paivio, A., Imagery variables in concept identification. *Journal of Verbal Learning and Verbal Behavior*, **14**, 284–293 (1975).

Keenan, S. S., and Brassell, E., A study of factors related to prognosis for individual aphasic patients. *Journal of Speech and Hearing Disorders*, **39**, 257–269 (1974).

Kertesz, A., *Aphasia and associated disorders: taxonomy, localization, and recovery*. New York: Grune & Stratton (1979).

Kertesz, A., Evolution of aphasic syndromes. *Topics in Language Disorders*, **1**, 15–27 (1981).

Kertesz, A., and McCabe, P., Recovery patterns and prognosis in aphasia. *Brain*, **100**, 1–18 (1972).

Kubler-Ross, E., *On death and dying*. New York: Macmillan (1969).

LaPointe, L. L., Base-10 programming stimulation: task specification, scoring, and plotting performance in aphasia therapy. *Journal of Speech and Hearing Disorders*, **42**, 90–105 (1977).

LaPointe, L. L., Aphasia therapy: Some principles and strategies for treatment. In D. F. Johns (Ed.), *Clinical Management of Neurogenic Communication Disorders*. Boston: Little, Brown (1978).

LaPointe, L. L., and Horner, J., *Reading Comprehension Battery for Aphasia*. Tigard, Oregon: C.C. Publications (1979).

Lasky, E. Z., Weidner, W. E., and Johnson, J. P., Influence of linguistic complexity, rate of presentation, and interpause time on auditory-verbal comprehension of adult aphasic patients. *Brain and Language*, **3**, 386–395 (1976).

Lassen, N. A., Ingvar, D. H., and Skinhj, E., Brain function and blood flow. *Scientific American*, **239**, 62–71 (1978).

Lebrun, Y., Neurolinguistic models of language and speech. In H. Whitaker and H. A. Whitaker (Eds.), *Studies in Neurolinguistics* (Vol. 1). New York: Academic Press (1976).

Levin, J. R., What have we learned about maximizing what children learn? In J. R. Levin and V. L. Allen (Eds.), *Cognitive learning in children: Theories and strategies*. New York: Academic Press (1976).

Levin, J. R., and Rowher, W. D., Verbal Organization and the facilitation of serial learning. *Journal of Educational Psychology*, **58**, 186–190 (1968).

Levine, D. N. and Calvanio, R., The neurology of reading disorders. In M. A. Arbin, D. Caplan and J. C. Marshall (Eds.), *Neural Models of Language Processes*. New York: Academic Press (1982).

Levy, C., and Holland, A., Influence of grammatical complexity and sentence length on comprehension with adult aphasics. In A. L. Holland (Ed.), *Psycholinguistics and Behavioral Variables Underlying Recovery from Aphasia*. Project report submitted to Social and Rehabilitative Service, DHEW (1971).

Levy, C. B., and Taylor, O. L., Transformational complexity and comprehension in adult aphasics. Paper presented at American Speech and Hearing Association Convention, Denver, Colorado (1968).

Liepmann, H., *Das Krankheitbild der Apraxia (Motorischenasymbolie)*. Berlin: Karger (1900).

Liles, B. Z., and Brookshire, R. H., The effects of pause time on auditory comprehension of aphasic subjects. *Journal of Communication Disorders*, **8**, 221–235 (1975).

Luria, A. R., *Higher Cortical Functions in Man*. New York: Basic Books, (1966). (Originally published in Russian, 1962).

Luria, A. R., Factors and forms of aphasia. In A. DeReuck and M. O'Connor (Eds.), *Disorders of Language*. London: J. & A. Churchill (1964).

Luria, A. R., *Traumatic Aphasia*. Hague: Mouton (1970).

Marie, P., The third left frontal convolution plays no special role in the function of language. In M. F. Cole and M. Cole, *Pierre Marie's Papers on Speech Disorders*. New York: Hafner (1971). (Originally published in *Semaine Medicale*, **26**, 241–247) (1906).

McNeil, M. R., and Prescott, T. E., *Revised Token Test*. Baltimore: University Park Press (1978).

Marks, M., Taylor, M., and Rusk, H. A., Rehabilitation of the aphasic patient: A summary of three years experience in a rehabilitation setting. *Archives of Physical Medicine and Rehabilitation*, **38**, 219–226 (1957).

Monakow, C. von, *Die lokalisation im grossbirn under der abbau der funktionen durch corticale herde*. Bergmann: Wiesbaden (1914).

Osgood, C. E., and Miron, M. S. (Eds.), *Approaches to the Study of Aphasia*. Urbana: University of Illinois Press (1963).

Paivio, A., Abstractness, imagery, and meaningfulness in paired-associate learning. *Journal of Verbal Learning and Verbal Behavior*, **4**, 32–38 (1965).

Paivio, A., Latency of verbal associations and imagery to noun stimuli as a function of abstractness and generality. *Canadian Journal of Psychology*, **20**, 378–387 (1966).

Paivio, A., *Imagery and Verbal Processes*. New York: Holt, Rinehart and Winston (1971).

Paivio, A., Imagery and long term memory. In A. Kennedy and A. Wilkes (Eds.), *Studies in Long Term Memory*. New York: John Wiley & Sons (1975).

Paivio, A. and Csapo, K., Concrete image and verbal memory codes. *Journal of Experimental Psychology*, **80**, 279–285 (1969).

Paivio, A., Yuille J. C., and Madigan, S., Concreteness, imagery, and meaningfulness values for 925 nouns. *Journal of Experimental Psychology Monograph*, **76** (1, Pt. 2) (1968).

Parkhurst, B. G., The effect of time-altered speech stimuli on the performance of right hemiplegic adult aphasics. Paper presented at American Speech and Hearing Association Convention, New York, New York (1970).

Pick, A., *Die Agrammatischen Sprachstorungen*. Berlin: Springer (1913).

Porch, B. E., *The Porch Index of Communicative Ability*. Palo Alto: Consulting Psychologists Press (1981).

Premack, D., Language in Chimpanzee? *Science*, **172**, 808–822 (1971).

Ravens, J. C., *Coloured Progressive Matrices*. London: Lewis (1962).

Sands, E., Sarno, M. T., and Shankweiler, D., Long-term assessment of language function in aphasia due to stroke. *Archives of Physical Medicine and Rehabilitation*, **50**, 202–206; 222 (1969).

Sarno, M. T., *The Functional Communication Profile*. New York: New York University Medical Center, The Institute of Rehabilitation Medicine (1969).

Sarno, M. T., Recovery and rehabilitation in aphasia. In M. T. Sarno (Ed.), *Acquired Aphasia*. New York: Academic Press (1981).

Sarno, M. T., and Levita, E., Natural course of recovery in severe aphasia. *Archives of Physical Medicine and Rehabilitation*, **52**, 175–179 (1971).

Sarno, M. T., Silverman, M., and Sands, E., Speech therapy and language recovery in severe aphasia. *Journal of Speech and Hearing Research*, **13**, 607–623 (1970).

Schuell, H., Auditory impairment in aphasia: Significance and retraining techniques. *Journal of Speech and Hearing Disorders*, **18**, 14–21 (1953a).

Schuell, H., Aphasic difficulties understanding spoken language. *Neurology*, **3**, 176–184 (1953).

Schuell, H., *Administrative Manual for the Minnesota Test for Differential Diagnosis of Aphasia*. Minneapolis: University of Minnesota (1965).

Schuell, H., *The Minnesota Test for Differential Diagnosis of Aphasia*. Minneapolis: University of Minnesota Press (1965).

Schuell, H. M., Carroll, V. A., and Street, B. S., Clinical treatment of aphasia. *Journal of Speech and Hearing Disorders*, **20**, 43–53 (1955).

Schuell, H. M., and Jenkins, J. J., Reduction of vocabulary in aphasia. *Brain*, **84**, 243–261 (1961).

Schuell, H., Jenkins, J. J., and Jiménez-Pabón, E., *Aphasia in Adults*. New York: Harper & Row (1964).

Schwartz, M. F., Saffran, E. M., and Marin, O. S., The word order problem in agrammatism. I. Comprehension. *Brain and Language*, **10**, 249–262, (1980).

Seamon, J. G., and Gazzaniga, M. S., Coding strategies and cerebral laterality effects. *Cognitive Psychology*, **5**, 249–256 (1973).

Senter, R. J., and Hoffman, R. R., Bizarreness as a nonessential variable in mnemonic imagery: A confirmation. *Bulletin of Psychonomic Society*, **7**, 163–164 (1976).

Shewan, C. M. and Canter, G., Effects of vocabulary, syntax, and sentence length on auditory comprehension in aphasic patients. *Cortex*, **7**, 209–226 (1971).

Siegel, C. M., Dysphasic speech responses to visual word stimuli, *Journal of Speech and Hearing Research*, **2**, 152–160 (1959).

Skelly, M., *Amer-Ind Gestural Code Based on Universal American Indian Hand Talk*. New York: Elsevier (1979).

Skelly, M., Schinsky, L., Smith, R. W., and Fust, R.S., American Indian sign (Amer-Ind) as a facilitator of verbalization for the oral verbal apraxic. *Journal of Speech and Hearing Disorders*, **39**, 446–456 (1974).

Skinner, B. F., *Verbal Behavior.* New York: Appleton-Century-Crofts (1957).

Skinner, B. F., *Cumulative Record*. (Rev. ed.) New York: Appleton (1961).

Smith, A., Objective indices of severity of chronic aphasia in stroke patients. *Journal of Speech and Hearing Disorders*, **36**, 167–207 (1971).

Sparks, R. W., Melodic intonation therapy. In R. Chapey (Ed.), *Language Intervention Strategies in Adult Aphasia*. Baltimore: Williams & Wilkins (1981).

Sparks, R., Helm, N., and Albert, M., Aphasia rehabilitation resulting from melodic intonation therapy. *Cortex*, **10**, 303–316 (1974).

Sparks, R. W., and Holland, A. L., Method: Melodic intonation therapy for aphasia. *Journal of Speech and Hearing Disorders*, **41**, 287–297 (1976).

Sperry, R. W., and Gazzaniga, M. S., Language following surgical disconnection of the hemispheres. In C. H. Millikan and F. L. Darley (Eds.), *Brain Mechanisms Underlying Speech and Language*. New York: Grune & Stratton (1967).

Spreen, O., and Benton, A.L., *Neurosensory Center Comprehensive Examination for Aphasia* (1977 revision). Victoria, B.C.: Neuropsychology Laboratory, University of Victoria (1977).

Springer, S. P. and Deutsch, G., *Left Brain, Right Brain*. San Francisco: W.H. Freeman & Co. (1981). Struggling with aphasia. *Medical World News*, **10**, 37–40 (1969).

Subirana, A., Handedness and cerebral dominance. In P. J. Vinken, and G. W. Bruyn (Eds.), *Handbook of Clinical Neurology* (Vol. 4). New York: Elsevier (1969).

Swinney, D. A. and Taylor, O. L., Short-term memory recognition search in aphasics. *Journal of Speech and Hearing Research*, **14**, 578–588 (1971).

Taylor, M. L., A measurement of functional communication in aphasia. *Archives of Physical Medicine and Rehabilitation*, **46**, 101–107 (1965).

Teaching Resources Catalog. Hingham, Massachusetts: Teaching Resources (1982).

Thorndike, E. L., and Lorge, I., *The Teacher's Word Book of 30,000 Words*. New York: Columbia University (1972). (Originally published, 1944).

Thurston, J. R., An empirical investigation of loss of spelling ability in dysphasics. *Journal of Speech and Hearing Research*, **6**, 329–337 (1963).

Tillman, D., and Gerstman, L. J., Clustering by aphasics in free recall. *Brain and Language*, 1977, **4**, 355–364 (1977).

Toglia, M. P., and Battig, W. F., *Handbook of semantic word norms*. Hillsdale, New Jersey: John Wiley (1978).

Tulving, E., Theoretical issues in free recall. In T. B. Dixon and D. C. Horton (Eds.), *Verbal Learning and Verbal Behavior*. New Jersey: Prentice-Hall (1968).

Underwood, B. J., Ten years of massed practice on distributed practice. *Psychological Review*, **68**, 229–247 (1961).

Underwood, B. J., Some correlates of item repetition in free recall learning. *Journal of Verbal Learning and Verbal Behavior*, **8**, 83–94 (1969).

Underwood, B. J., A breakdown of the total time law in free-recall learning. *Journal of Verbal Learning and Verbal Behavior*, **9**, 573–580 (1970).

Vignolo, L. A., Evolution of aphasia and language rehabilitation: A retrospective exploratory study. *Cortex*, **1**, 344–367 (1964).

Weigel-Crump, C., and Koenigsknecht, R. A., Tapping the lexical store of the adult aphasic: An analysis of the improvement made in word retrieval skills. *Cortex*, **9**, 411–418 (1973).

Weigl, E., On the problem of cortical syndromes: experimental studies. In M. L. Simmel (Ed.), *The Reach of Mind: Essays in Memory of Kurt Goldstein*. New York: Springer (1968).

Weisenburg, T., and McBride, K. E., *Aphasia*. New York: Hafner (1973). (Originally published, 1935).

Wepman, J. M., *Recovery from Aphasia*. New York: Ronald Press (1951).

Wepman, J. M., Bock, R. D., Jones, L. V., and Van Pelt, D., Psycholinguistic study of aphasia: A revision of the concept of anomia. *Journal of Speech and Hearing Disorders*, **21**, 468–477 (1956).

Wepman, J. M., and Jones, L. V., *Studies in Aphasia: An Approach to Testing*. Chicago: Education-Industry Service (1961).

Wepman, J. M., and Jones, L. V., Five aphasias: A commentary on aphasia as a regressive linguistic phenomenon. In D. Rioch and E. Weinstein (Eds.), *Disorders of Communication*. Baltimore: Williams & Wilkins (1964).

Wernicke, C., *Der Aphasische Symptomenkomplex*. Breslau: Cohn & Weigert (1874).

Wernicke, C., The symptom-complex of aphasia. In A. Church (Ed.), *Diseases of the Nervous System*. New York: Appleton (1908).

Wertz, R. T., Collins, M. J., Weiss, D., Kurtzke, J. F., Friden, T., Brookshire, R. H., Pierce, J., Holtzapple, P., Hubbard, D. J., Porch, B. E., West, J. A., Davis, L., Matovitch, V., Morely, G. K., and Resurreccion, E., Veterans Administration cooperative study on aphasia: A comparison of individual and group treatment. *Journal of Speech and Hearing Research*, **24**, 580–594 (1981).

Wertz, R. T., and Rosenbek, J. C., Appraising apraxia of speech. *Journal of the Colorado Speech and Hearing Association*, **5**, 18–36 (1971).

West, J. A., The effect of structure on aphasic responses to grammatical and nongrammatical sequences of words. Unpublished doctoral dissertation, The University of Michigan (1968).

West, J. A., Therapeutic approaches to agrammatism in aphasia: Application of psycholinguistic theory. Paper presented at the American Speech and Hearing Association Convention, New York, New York (1970).

West, J. F., Free recall of learning in adult aphasics: The effect of massed versus distributed practice. Paper presented at the American Speech and Hearing Association Convention, Chicago, Illinois (1971).

West, J. A., Auditory comprehension in aphasic adults: Improvement through training. *Archives of Physical Medicine and Rehabilitation*, **54**, 78–86 (1973).

West, J. F., Improvement of receptive functioning in adult aphasic patients. In R. H. Brookshire (Ed.), *Clinical Aphasiology, Collected Proceedings*, 1972–1976. Minneapolis: BRK Publishers (1978). (Originally published, 1972).

West, J. F., Imaging and Aphasia. In R. H. Brookshire (Ed.), *Proceedings of the Clinical Aphasiology Conference*. Minneapolis: BRK Publishers (1977).

West, J. F., Heightening visual imagery. In E. Perecman (Ed.), *Cognitive Processing in the Right Hemisphere*. New York: Academic Press (in press).

West, J. A., Gelfer, C. E., and Rosen, J. S., Processing of true and false affirmative sentences by aphasic subjects. In R. H. Brookshire (Ed.), *Clinical Aphasiology: Collected Proceedings, 1972–1976*. Minneapolis: BRK Publishers (1978). (Originally published, 1976).

West, J. F., and Grossman, M., The effect of verb type on linguistic processing by aphasic and normal subjects. Paper presented at the International Neuropsychological Society Meeting, Chicanciano-Terme, Italy (1980).

West, J. F., and Kaufman, G., Some effects of redundancy on the auditory comprehension of adult aphasics. Paper presented at American Speech and Hearing Association Convention, San Francisco, California (1972).

West, J. F., O'Connor, S., and Bennett, L., Group treatment programs for stroke patients. In R. H. Brookshire (Ed.), *Clinical Aphasiology: Conference Proceedings* (1981).

Wiig, E. H., and Globus, D., Aphasic word identification as a function of logical relationship and association strength. *Journal of Speech and Hearing Research*, **14**, 195–204 (1971).

Wilcox, M. J., and Davis, G. A., Procedures for promoting communicative effectiveness in aphasic adults. Paper presented at the American Speech and Hearing Association Convention, San Francisco, California (1978).

Witelson, S. F., Anatomic asymmetry in the temporal lobes: Its documentation, phylogenesis, and relationship to functional asymmetry. In S. J. Dimond and D. A. Blizard (Eds.), *Evolution and Lateralization of the Brain*. New York: The New York Academy of Sciences (1977).

Wolff, P., and Levin, J. R., The role of covert activity in children's imagery production. *Child Development*, **43**, 537–547 (1972).

Wolff, P., Levin, J. R., and Longobardi, E. T., Motoric mediation in children's paired-associated learning: Effects of visual and tactual contact. *Journal of Experimental Child Psychology*, **14**, 176–183 (1972).

Wolff, P., Levin, J. R., and Longobardi, E. T., Activity and children's learning. *Child Development*, **45**, 221–223 (1974).

Wollen, K. A., Weber, A., Lowry, D. H., Bizarreness vs. interaction of mental images as determinants of learning. *Cognitive Psychology*, **3**, 518–523 (1972).

Word Making Productions, Ltd. P.O. Box 15038. Salt Lake City, Utah, 84115.

Yorkston, K. M., and Beukelman, D. R., *Assessment of Intelligibility of Dysarthric Speech*. Tigard, Oregon: C.C. Publications (1981).

Yorkston, K. M., Marshall, R. C. and Butler, M. R., Imposed delay of response: Effects on aphasics' auditory comprehension of visually and non-visually cued material. *Perceptual Motor Skills*, **44**, 647–655 (1977).

Zurif, E. B. and Blumstein, S. E., Language and the brain. In M. Halle, J. Bresan, and G. Miller (Eds.), *Linguistic Theory and Psychological Reality*. Cambridge, MA: MIT Press (1978).

Zurif, E. B., Caramazza, A., and Myerson, R., Grammatical judgements of agrammatic patients. *Neuropsychologia*, **10**, 405–417 (1972).

9 Remedial Practices with the Hearing Impaired

Edgar L. Lowell
Doreen B. Pollack

The remediation of communication problems associated with severe hearing impairment is no small task, and one not likely to be described comprehensively in even a series of books. It involves mastery of the most important learning task that people ever face—the acquisition of language. This chapter shall present two remedial approaches. One gives primary emphasis to the development of residual hearing in the hearing impaired, while the other places primary emphasis on visual training in a program of language remediation for the deaf known as "oralism." In the latter, auditory training is included but is given secondary emphasis.

Similar auditory training procedures are suggested in the two approaches, but the benefits expected from the auditory remediation experience is different in each one. Whether the auditory emphasis should be primary or secondary cannot be resolved in this chapter, but the reader can be given a perspective on the two approaches. Before taking them up in turn, however, it is well to consider the problems and levels of hearing impairments and relate them to the development of hearing function.

HEARING AND HEARING LOSS[1]

The world we live in is full of sounds, those made by the environment and those made by ourselves. Hearing keeps us in contact with our environment and with each other, even in the dark. It contributes to space perception and homeostasis. It gives us both warning signals and security. It is uniquely designed to permit us to learn the spoken language system, as the blind have demonstrated, and it plays a major role in the development of abstract concepts and temporal sequence. There is no substitute for hearing.

The child who is born deaf, or who acquires a hearing loss within the first year of life, misses this association of sound with experience. Myklebust (1960) has said that a child who has to explore the world without certain cues because of sensory depriva-

---

[1] Doreen Pollack is the author of this section, and the one immediately following, which discusses principles and practices of auditory remediation.

tion begins to behave differently. Without normal hearing, he may make an adjustment to the world, but it is not the *same* world.

The effects of hearing loss upon adults are also not widely understood but are known to be a feeling of isolation, stress, and misunderstanding, with subsequent social withdrawal. Sudden hearing loss can cause severe emotional trauma.

The Normal Development of Hearing Function

There has been relatively little research on the development of hearing in humans. The cochlea seems to be functional about the twentieth week of intrauterine life, and the basic mechanisms for coding, intensity, and frequency are probably operant by the twenty-eight to thirtieth week. The newborn child usually responds to a loud sound with a startle response (Moro's reflex), a sharp eyeblink (the acousticopalpebral reflex), or by other body movements (Northern and Downs, 1978).

Differential responses to frequency, constancy, and patterning begin soon after birth. For example, low frequency signals are effective inhibitors of infant distress, and generally evoke gross motor activity; high frequencies tend to occasion distress and a high proportion of freezing reactions (Eisenberg, 1976).

Within a few weeks, an infant exhibits a listening attitude by anticipatory cessation of crying, and begins to recognize mother's voice. The child may stop being interested in loud sounds, and ignore them unless they are new or meaningful. The child begins instead to listen and respond to quiet sounds. The child develops an auditory feedback mechanism, hearing himself or herself as well as others, and soon begins to laugh.

During the second three months of life, a baby begins to turn the eyes, and later the head, toward the source of sound. Thus, hearing contributes to spatial awareness. The child enjoys producing sound, so we give the child rattles and squeaky toys, but at five months, the child is often more interested in visual stimuli and may ignore familiar sounds.

By the time a baby is able to sit up, sounds can be localized accurately when they are close to the meatus and on a horizontal plane running through the two ears. Gradually the child finds sounds below and above this plane, and behind the head. Localization, however, does require two similar ears.

From the sixth to the ninth month, an infant becomes very attentive to the pitch, rhythm, rate and inflection of voice (Crystal, 1973). The child often plays vocally using singing tones and practices babbling phonemes, as by saying "dadadadada" over and over. This interest in inflectional contour is significant because a baby's vocalizations resemble the mother tongue by ten months; that is, a German baby sounds German, a French one sounds French.

Recent studies by Eilers et al. (1975, 1977) suggest that speech discrimination is also fairly well developed by this age, and may begin as early as three to four months of age.

By the first birthday, the infant has reached a symbolic level and comes to understand, as a result of gesture, experience, and repetition, that a sequence of sounds represents, or is associated with, a specific object, activity, or emotion. For example, mother extends her hand and says: "Give it to me."

About the same time, an infant usually reaches an echolalic stage and begins to imitate words. It still takes two or three years before a child with normal hearing acquires a large vocabulary and can generate complete sentences, and it takes several more years before discrimination, neuromuscular coordination, and imitative ability result in mature articulation (Pollack, 1964).

All of these experiences are complex, but a normal infant separates meaningful sound from the background noise. Having learned to discriminate and recognize sounds, the child next learns to ignore a great deal. An excellent description of all these stages may be found in *Three Babies* (Church, 1966).

The development of an auditory function normally takes place during the first year of life, and the following skills are acquired:

1. perception of loud and quiet sounds
2. discrimination of sounds
3. localization
4. distance hearing
5. recognition of and appropriate response to sounds
6. auditory feedback and feed forward
7. auditory memory: short term and long term
8. auditory sequencing and blending

Although the development of speech and language are interrelated, and seem to develop simultaneously, separate skills are involved.

Speech involves the motor skills:

1. breath control
2. vocalization (loudness, pitch, rate, inflection, etc.)
3. babbling
4. echolalia
5. recall of motor patterns

For language, the skills are verbal and conceptual:

1. realization that sound is used for communication
2. association of sound with meaning
3. development of symbolic sounds or processing
4. perception of syntactical patterns
5. development of abstractions
6. pragmatics

(See the review of receptive and expressive language development in chapter 2.)

Critical Periods for the Development of Hearing Perception

It is now widely accepted that there are critical periods for developing perception (Illingsworth, 1964), and the first three years of life seem to be the most sensitive for learning to listen (Whetnall and Fry, 1964). An infant who misses these early listening opportunities because of deafness becomes visually-oriented and unresponsive to sound, and the voice quality becomes devoid of pleasing intonation or inflection. It is

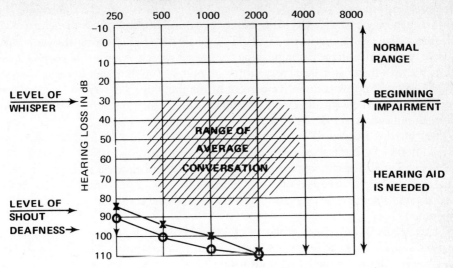

Figure 9–1. Comparison of Hearing Loss Curves for the Right Ear (o) and the Left Ear (x) with the Normal Range of Hearing for Speech. Audiometric measurement of the child's hearing showed that in the frequency range between 500 and 2000 Hz, the pure tone average for the right ear was 105 dB HTL, and for the left ear, 102 dB HTL. (See Figure 9–2 for the improvement in this child's hearing when he was fitted with two hearing aids).

always worthwhile to develop an auditory function, but it is difficult to integrate hearing into the deaf child's personality if detection of the hearing loss is greatly delayed. A hard-of-hearing child, on the other hand, develops an auditory function, albeit a defective and limited one, which may not be used because it is unreliable or inconsistent.

Loss of hearing at any age means a deterioration of auditory skills with subsequent loss of auditory information resulting in difficulties of communication in educational, social, and vocational situations.

Hearing Impairments

Measuring Levels of Hearing Loss. The population known as the "hearing impaired" is usually described in terms of audiometric measurement of the peripheral hearing mechanism (Darley, 1961).

The volume of the frequencies 125 to 8000 Hz. is increased from − 10 dB to 110 dB HTL (Hearing Threshold Level) (ANSI 1976 reference level) to determine the threshold of hearing, or the volume at which the sound becomes audible. Speech varies in intensity from a whisper at 30 dB SPL (Sound Pressure Level) to a loud shout at 80–90 dB SPL, with a comfortable conversational voice being at 60–70 dB SPL. The child with the audiogram shown in figure 9–1 is deaf to normal conversation.

The normal-hearing individual may be said to be one who can recognize all the distinguishing features of speech under good listening conditions without the aid of lipreading or other visual forms of communication. The threshold responses to the test frequencies occur at − 10 dB HTL to 20 dB HTL, while those of the hard-of-hearing individual fall between 25 dB HTL to 90 dB HTL, leaving the individual unable to recognize all the distinguishing features of speech. The deaf have thresholds greater than 90 dB and hear very little, or nothing of the human voice without amplification. Approximately five percent of the individuals described as "deaf" are totally deaf, with an equally small percentage being able to benefit only minimally from amplification.

Later in this chapter (Remedial Principles and Practices with Deaf Children) Lowell notes that the task of differentiating between hard-of-hearing and deaf children is obscured because some hard-of-hearing children behave as if they were deaf and some children behave as if they were hard-of-hearing. The critical variable which may account for this phenomenon may very well be the early auditory remediation program.

There seems to be a large group of children between the ages of one and seven years, who have sporadic losses of 15–40 dB which occur during those periods when they suffer from otitis media with effusion. These sporadic losses are nevertheless thought to result in significant delay in verbal language skills. Howie, Ploussard, and Sloyer (1975) found that 49 percent of the children they studied in Alabama had otitis before the first birthday, and 60 percent before the second birthday. Brooks (1981) reported that this high incidence decreased to 8 percent by age seven and 2 or 3 percent by age ten. Certain children are high-risk for conductive hearing losses of this kind, such as those with cleft palates, Down's syndrome and those born prematurely.

It is felt that the recurrent or persistent middle ear complications may cause educational retardation in some areas. Katz (1978) writes about auditory deprivation, and some animal studies suggest that lack of stimulation causes morphological deficiencies (Webster and Webster, 1977).

Audiometric descriptions by no means go to the heart of the problem since two individuals with similar audiograms will handle sounds in an entirely different way. An audiogram does not tell us exactly how much hearing exists, because the ear is capable of responding to loudness levels greater than those recorded by an audiometer. An audiogram also does not tell us how speech sounds when it reaches the brain, nor how the brain will process it.

In addition, other important factors enter into a description of hearing loss, such as age of onset, etiology, type and configuration of loss, present age of the individual, the presence of other handicaps, and so on.

Incidence of Hearing Impairment in Children. The incidence of limited hearing decreases as the severity of auditory impairment increases (Eagles et al., 1963). It is known that only 1 in every 2,000 babies born has a very severe hearing loss. In a study by Colorado State University (Willeford, 1971), a team tested 38,567 children in grades one through twelve and found that 170 children out of every 1,000 had a unilateral loss and 41 out of 1,000 had a bilateral loss. One out of five had a mild loss which was defined as 11 to 25 dB. Figures given by The National State Agencies Report show that 41,383 hard-of-hearing children were actually served, or one out of six, despite the recommendations in Public Law 94–142.

Percentages reported in the annual National Demographic Studies of children in

	1975–76 National Percent.	1977–78 National Percent.
"Normal" hearing (under 27 dB)	2.4	4.4
Mild (from 27 to 40 dB)	4.0	5.4
Moderate (from 41 to 55 dB)	8.2	8.8
Moderately Severe (from 56 to 70 dB)	13.3	13.0
Severe (from 71 to 90 dB)	26.3	24.7
Profound (from 91 dB and above)	45.8	43.7

Table 9–1. Percentage of Children with Varying Degrees of Hearing Loss in the United States

special education remain remarkably constant over a period of years (Office of Demographic Studies, Washington, D.C., 1974–78). (See table 9–1.)

Effects of Hearing Loss on Children and Adults. Although the effects of hearing impairment vary both in quantity and quality according to different individuals, it has been well documented that a hearing loss in childhood reduces the possibility of developing normal voice quality, intelligible speech (Ling, 1976a), good linguistic skills, and educational achievement levels commensurate with intellectual potential (Office of Demographic Studies, 1974–1978; Rodda, 1970).

A severe or profound congenital hearing loss also endangers the socio-emotional development of a young child because the quality of parenting changes when there is a lack of responsiveness to parental interaction. The mother's vocalization and verbalization decrease and the baby is surrounded by an atmosphere of grief and disappointment. Ninety percent of hearing impaired infants have normal-hearing parents. Later, impaired communication gives rise to a distorted or incorrect picture of the frames of reference and attitudes of normal hearing society. Cognitively, a hearing loss limits the source of information and causes a narrowing of social experiences, thus fostering greater dependency on normal hearing adults, who respond by overprotection (Northcott, 1973).

However, early intervention studies show significant improvement in speech skills (Ling, 1976b), spoken language (McConnell and Liff, 1975), reading and academic skills (Ernst, 1974; McClure, 1977), and personal-social development (Kennedy and Bruinkinks, 1974).

The effects of hearing loss upon adults will vary according to the age of onset. A clinician must be prepared to deal with educational, personal, social and other aspects of the patients' lives, and to help those adults who have never had normal hearing as well as those who have acquired a loss in later years (Johnson, 1978).

Studies of the adult deaf population generally show that they are underemployed or working for lower pay (Boatner et al., 1964). Five sixths of the deaf work in manual jobs as contrasted with only half of the hearing population. Their reading levels may be only third or fourth grade and the average graduate of a public residential school for the deaf at age twenty-one has an eighth grade education. This discrepancy between ability and achievement can be stress producing.

Severe hearing loss is a low incidence handicap resulting in a scattered population which may cause social isolation, especially in the one third of the deaf population that reports having only deaf friends. Social problems are reduced if a deaf person can use residual hearing and learn to speak.

In general, studies of the congenitally deaf seem to show a tendency toward egocentric, rigid personalities that are socially immature and naive (Levine, 1960; Rainer et al., 1969).

The adult who acquires a hearing loss loses not only communication skill but two major components to which we usually react without being aware of them:

1. warning signals (for example, being unable to locate sounds in the dark)
2. an auditory background

Hearing makes us feel part of a living world, and gives a background of feeling at a primitive level. Some adults complain that they feel in a vacuum and lose their sense of time when they lose their hearing. It is the unreality of pantomime. Adults may feel insecure and are tempted to talk too much. They may begin to distrust the normal hearing world and become discouraged, suspicious, and depressed. They miss "over-hearing" and are no longer at ease in a group situation, fearing rejection.

The hearing loss of the elderly may involve the discomfort of recruitment and tinnitus. Sixty percent of adults over sixty-five years of age (or twelve million people) are reported to have presbycusis with phonemic regression (Hull and Traynor, 1977). Thus they may hear someone speak but be unable to discriminate what is said. Unfortunately, low scores for discrimination do not always agree with the type and degree of the hearing loss, and one may have to deal with a deterioration of the intellect.

Problems Related to Hearing Loss. Hearing loss often accompanies severe diseases, such as those of the heart and kidneys, central nervous system dysfunctions, and so on. A high-risk register for hearing loss (Black et al., 1971) would take in a large percentage of the population whose main defects appear to be other than hearing loss. Conversely, those whose main defect appears to be hearing loss may be found to have other problems (Hardy, 1965). It is widely acknowledged that more defective children are surviving birth even after such handicapping disasters as rubella. The rubella epidemic, for example (1964–65), resulted in a large population of multiply handicapped children (McConnell, 1970; Murphy and Byrne, 1981).

A teacher or clinician faced with a limited-hearing child must be prepared to study the *whole* child. The teacher may find from thirty percent to almost fifty percent of the group classified as hearing-impaired have other problems in addition to the hearing loss. The National Demographic Study reports the following statistics for 1976 (Office of Demographic Studies, Washington, D.C., 1974–78):

Total number of students in special education classes	49,427
Number with additional handicaps	29,427
Additional handicapping conditions	21,424

The "handicaps" listed are brain damage, epilepsy, heart disorder, visual problems, retardation, emotional problems, and so on.

Additional problems besetting many of the children diagnosed as hearing impaired include:

1. Attention deficits, such as poor eye contact, hyperactivity and distractibility, and perseveration or inappropriate repetition and difficulty in shifting attention

2. Perceptual difficulties, such as avoidance of crossing the midline, inability to copy shapes appropriate to age, dislike of books because a relationship is not seen between picture and real life
3. Slow maturation of motor development, with abnormal reactions to touch (tactile defensiveness), feeding or sleeping problems, failure to develop a dominant hand, and difficulty with motor speech patterns, or dyspraxia
4. Symbolic learning problems, such as failure to understand gesture, failure to remember nouns, and problems in auditory sequencing and memory span

There is no panacea for their rehabilitation, and many solutions must be made available. Berg and Fletcher (1976) have suggested training a new specialist, the educational audiologist to isolate the parameters of hearing impairment, to identify the educational and psychological deficiencies as they relate to the unique problems of particular persons, and to develop educational programs which will foster effective functioning in a hearing world.

Because of these various consequences, participants in the Winnipeg conference on the early management of hearing loss (Mencher and Gerber, 1981) recommended that remediation of hearing impairment be accomplished by a team of professionals, including educators, developmentalists, geneticists, social workers, and so on.

The Decline of Auditory Function. There have been a number of studies to determine the decline of auditory function with age (Glorig, 1957). The twelve-year-old American boy is said to have the best hearing (although he appears to be the worst listener) whereas the fourteen-year-old already has a slight drop in acuity. Bergman (1971a) studied adults in each of the age decades from the twenties to the eighties and found a decline in hearing for the higher frequencies over each decade. More significantly, he found a sharp reduction in auditory performance under less favorable conditions as early as middle age. Apparently young people are able to tolerate more distortion.

Bergman (1971b) began with a baseline test for undistorted speech and then investigated such factors as:

1. time selection and synthesis (interrupted speech)
2. time scale distortion (speeded speech)
3. binaural fusion
4. binaural separation and identification
5. reverberation (poor acoustics)

Motivation appeared to keep older listeners more vigilant, but early language background influenced the scores.

Studies of the blind who develop hearing losses also showed that there are different kinds of auditory behavior (Bergman et al., 1965). The blind, because they do not have visual cues such as body language, eye contact, and so on, must rely on cues which the normal-sighted individual ignores or relegates to a lower level of consciousness. For example, they know by listening whether footsteps are going up or down the stairs.

Principles and techniques of remediation with the hearing-impaired will be presented in the following two sections, not with the suggestion that the reader will develop an expertise from reading about these techniques, but that the reader may have a basis for further exploration and experience, which are essential to the development of clinical competence.

PRINCIPLES AND PRACTICES OF AUDITORY REMEDIATION

The remedial approach discussed in this section emphasizes the development of residual hearing in hearing-impaired children. Some of the principles and procedures, however, are appropriate for use with adolescents and adults, and reference will be made to counseling procedures for persons in the older age groups.

The idea of utilizing residual hearing dates back to early time, but most of the remedial methods for the hearing-impaired are based upon the premise that the severity of a hearing handicap is irreversible, and that the main channels of communication must be visual and/or manual. Even when amplification is applied, lipreading, fingerspelling or signing are the methods used. O'Neill and Oyer (1961) pointed out that even the "Multisensory approach" emphasizes visual skills.

> In actual practice, major attention is directed toward the use of only one of the sensory modalities. . . . The existence of residual hearing is accepted but very little auditory training is provided. . . . Aural rehabilitation work should be directed toward the use of this residual hearing and not towards the determination of how well the individual can do without it (pp. 70–71).

In the 1940s, the advent of the new partnership of otology and audiology, together with tremendous progress in technology, opened the way to a new approach to hearing problems. Emphasis on the development of auditory abilities within the remedial effort gave new directions to clinical programs. Increased amplification, early identification of children with hearing losses, and improved professional services have all contributed to the effectiveness of programs for improving these children's communication skills.

General Principles of Remediation

With the recent gains in auditory habilitation for hearing-impaired children, some general principles of remediation have emerged as essential to the development of effective programs.

Early Detection. Screening programs for early detection of hearing loss now include neonatal (Mencher, 1974), preschool, public, and industrial testing (Darley, 1961) and are critical for the success of an auditory approach. It has even been stated that seventy percent of hearing problems can be treated medically if detected soon enough.

Program Planning. The clinician or teacher should try to develop a profile of each patient's auditory abilities and disabilities. One might do this by asking: What aspects of auditory behavior are defective? What are we going to train?

Alpiner (1978) gives excellent examples of evaluation forms to determine a profile of communicative function for adults.

The young child or adult with a total loss of hearing, or the school-age child who has never learned to communicate orally and auditorily, may be directed into a

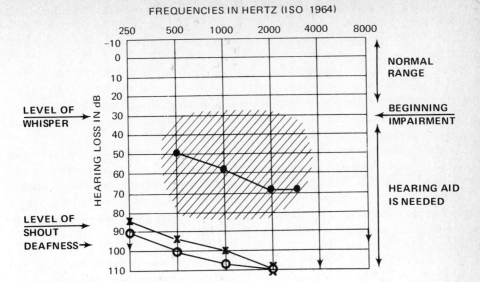

Figure 9–2. Comparison of Unaided Hearing with Aided Hearing. On being fitted with two separate hearing aids, the child whose audiogram was given in Figure 9–1 showed an improvement in pure tone average of 42 dB—going from 102 dB unaided PTA to 60 dB PTA for both ears with the aids. His aided threshold for voice awareness was 30 dB, and for speech reception, 65 dB in a sound field.

manual program (fingerspelling, signing, or cued speech). Individuals with mild or temporary problems and those with a precipitous loss (which sometimes precludes wearing a hearing aid) may be given a lipreading program and other support. Normally patients with moderate to profound losses should be fitted with hearing aids as soon as possible. A child today need spend very little time in a silent world, and many deaf adults are trying cochlear implants in lieu of a hearing aid (Balkany et al., 1981).

The auditory skills defined in the discussion of normal development of hearing function at the beginning of this chapter serve as parameters in designing a training program. Depending on the age of the patient, the training may involve the use of noisemakers, music, environmental sounds, speech, and language. All of this material can be given both live and recorded:

1. in a quiet room
   a. at close range,
   b. at increasing distances,
   c. from different parts of a room, and outside,
   d. without visual cues and with visual cues, if appropriate; and
2. against a background of noise.

Amplification. Within the last thirty years, hearing aids have changed from cumbersome and not very powerful boxes with separate batteries to very small but powerful monopacs which can give up to sixty-eight decibels of gain. The improvement obtained by one child is shown in figure 9–2.

The audiograms depict a sudden transition from deafness to the spoken word to partial ability to hear a quiet voice. This child can hear a whisper at close range implying a potential which does not seem to have been recognized by some schools for the deaf.

The modern aids—monaural, binaural, body aid, ear level, dichotic, in the ear, CROS and BICROS—offer such a variety of fittings that the hard-of-hearing no longer require long periods of orientation and lipreading. People who need the help of a communications specialist are the "hard core" who suffer from poor discrimination, tolerance problems, and/or deafness from an early age.

There is a new group of profoundly or totally deaf patients who are in need of innovative aural rehabilitation. These are adults who are wearing a microsurgically implanted prosthesis. The cochlear implant is designed to stimulate electrically the auditory nerve in response to sound. Although this does not achieve anything approaching normal hearing, it does provide auditory information about environmental sounds and vocalization (Balkany et al., 1981).

Instruction in the Use of Hearing Aids. All amplifiers need constant checking, and pamphlets should be dispensed which describe the maintenance and care of aids (Montgomery County Schools, 1975; Gauger, 1978). Arrangements should be made to test the hearing aids on an electroacoustical monitoring machine for distortion, preferably every three months, or whenever the aid is suspected or reported to be malfunctioning. In some states the State Department of Public Health provides this service; in others, it is obtainable from the state university or a local hearing aid dealer.

Unfortunately, training and maintenance efforts are inadequate (Northern et al., 1972). In a study of 130 school children, Gaeth and Lounsbury (1966) found that less than 20 percent were wearing aids which met their criteria for "satisfactory working condition of the aid," and they felt that the main deficiency in our auditory training programs was a lack of adequate follow-up and training in the use of the aids. In the classroom, one may decide to make use of the loop system, FM units, or other auditory media (Berg and Fletcher, 1976)—all of which require daily checking. If residual hearing is to be used to its maximum potential, it is essential to train residual hearing systematically and intensively. Hearing aids should be worn throughout the waking hours so that hearing is integrated into the personality: the aids should not be turned on and off. Two separate aids, one for each ear, are the fitting of choice if there is a reasonably similar loss in both ears, because binaural hearing greatly facilitates localization and speech discrimination, especially in noise, and gives a wider range as well as "stereophonic" sound (Ross, 1977; Libby, 1980).

Ongoing Evaluations. After early detection and medical treatment, the most important practice is to conduct a complete, ongoing evaluation. This may include audiologic, neurologic, psychologic, educational, perceptuomotor and other developmental assessments (Ruben and Rozycki, 1970). Although problems may not emerge until a particular learning task is encountered, it is now becoming possible to detect learning disabilities at an early age.

In chapter 2, the principles and procedures for assessing young children with language and learning difficulties are reviewed.

It should also be remembered that hearing may change which suggests the advisability of regular audiologic evaluations.

Although fluctuating hearing loss is seen more frequently in the presence of conductive impairments, there are a number of children who begin life with a mild to moderate sensorineural hearing loss which progresses rather suddenly and which may result eventually in profound or total deafness. Such a case was that of B.C., who entered a neighborhood preschool with the following audiogram:

	250	500	1000	2000	4000
Right Ear:	65	75	75	70	75
Left Ear:	65	70	75	70	80

One morning he awoke and reported that he could not hear. His hearing threshold had changed to the following:

	250	500	1000	2000	4000
Right Ear:	65	90	100	N.R.	N.R.
Left Ear:	70	85	95	N.R.	N.R.

After some delay, the diagnosis was Mondini Syndrome, and the insertion of endolymphatic shunts (Arenberg, 1980) stabilized the hearing and improved the acuity at 2000 Hz. It is to be hoped that regular evaluations and prompt referral by a clinician will result in early surgery, which will delay or prevent additional loss of hearing for this type of pathology in the future.

Remedial Techniques for the Young Child

Hearing Age Concept: Timetable for Expectations. In habilitation planning for children, the program should be based upon normal developmental milestones, remembering, however, to begin at the child's *hearing age* rather than at the chronologic age. That is to say, if a congenitally deaf infant is fit with hearing aids for the first time at age two, the *hearing age is zero,* and the child has to develop the basic auditory skills that normal hearing babies do—awareness, attention, localization, discrimination, and so on (Pollack, in Mencher and Gerber, 1981).

The time required for each child to acquire each skill will vary a great deal, but a general timetable of expectations can be found in Northcott (1977).

After fitting hearing aids upon a young child, there are three important steps to take:

1. focus the child's attention upon a sound stimulus
2. reward him by showing him the source or meaning of the sound
3. encourage feedback—that is, imitation of the activity or sound

Steps 2 and 3 develop motivation for the child to attend again.

Techniques for Developing Auditory Function. Some of the ways to develop an auditory function are illustrated in the following discussion.

Teaching Awareness of Loud Sounds. Loud noisemakers and music can be used in teaching the child with a new hearing aid to become aware of loud sounds. When using a noisemaker, the adult makes a loud sound several times out of the child's line of vision but close to the aid (for example, inside a box or under a table). The child holds his hands over his ears and says with a pleased, surprised expression, "I hear that. What's that?"

The teacher then shows the child the noisemaker, "That's what you heard."

Finally, the child is encouraged to make the sound again to elicit a reaction from the adult.

When using music, the adult can move the child rhythmically in time with it. (Suitable for the purpose is *Music for Exceptional Children*, available from Children's Music Center, Inc., 5373 West Pico Boulevard, Los Angeles, California 90019.)

Still another technique is to teach the distinction between on and off by saying, "I hear that" and patting the ears when a sound is heard, or "I don't hear that" and shaking the head when the sound ceases.

Teaching Awareness of Quiet Sounds. These procedures are the same as just described, but with quiet sounds, as the sounds are made, the adult points to his ear and says, "Listen" with an intent expression.

Teaching Awareness of Environmental Sounds. Going for listening walks gives the adult an opportunity to point out to the child the sounds being made and the sources of those sounds. The adult can show the child that the car horn sounding, the water running, the bird singing, and the dog barking can be heard. If sounds are not made meaningful for a young child, the child will ignore them.

In preparation for the real experience, the adult and child can play with toys or look at pictures together and make appropriate sounds for them. For example, the adult might say, "That's a doggie. The dog says 'bowowowowow.' I hear him."

Teaching Localization of Sounds. One technique is for the teacher to make a sound at the side of a baby's head, level with the ear. The parent then can turn the baby's head in the right direction to locate the source of the sound, and the teacher can change the location of the sound by moving to different parts of the room and outside the door.

The same method can be used in which the sound is that of the human voice, calling the baby's name.

Another method is to hide a music box or radio and look for it with the child.

Teaching Appropriate Response to Sound. The child should be taught to respond to the human voice and to environmental sounds.

A way of teaching a child to respond to the human voice is for the teacher (or another person) to look out the window, facing away from the child and his mother or father. The parent and child call the teacher's name, and the teacher turns around quickly, and says, "What?" Then the parent and child (together) change places with the teacher, facing away from the child. The teacher calls the child's name, and the parent turns the child around to the source of the sound. It is important always to call a child until the child turns around.

A way of teaching a child to respond to environmental sounds is to stand with the child close to the door on which someone knocks, and say, "I hear that. Open the door!" Then the child may stand at the other side of the door to knock or ring the bell and have it opened.

Developing Distance Hearing. The previous activities are again used but now the child is moved farther and farther from the source of the sound. Deaf children may have only a limited range, but they should be given every opportunity to develop that range. As pointed out elsewhere in these pages, it is important not to lower one's expectation of what they can do.

Teaching Discrimination of Sounds. Three noisemakers are placed upon the table and the child is allowed to play with them. One person sits with his back to the table. The parent and child make a sound with one of the noisemakers, place it back upon the table, and call the person's name, whereupon the person places his hands on his ears and turns around to identify the correct noisemaker. Then the child has a turn. There are many possible variations of this game.

Techniques for Developing Prelinguistic Skills. The voice of a young child retains a natural quality if hearing aids are fitted before sixteen months of age (approximately). Several strategies are useful in encouraging tendencies toward vocalization and verbalization.

Encouraging Vocal Play. The parents of a deaf infant should be instructed to echo back the sounds the baby makes and to play all of the vocal games families usually invent, such as, peekaboo, blowing raspberries, and so on. Parents should also encourage the baby to play with voice, imitating vowel sounds, shouting and whispering, singing high and low, and making all kinds of noises to accompany play. Humming on a kazoo is an excellent way to develop breath control for vocalization.

Encouraging Blowing. Paper balls, little candles, bubbles, and so on, are all good for this purpose.

Encouraging Babbling. As soon as a baby is vocalizing frequently with a natural, well-inflected, hearing-controlled voice, it is time to impose consonant production upon the vocalization. It has been assumed that certain types of hearing loss will impair an infant's ability to hear certain consonant sounds or phonemes, but it is not possible to predict what will be heard when wearing two hearing aids. If the child is unable to imitate after a sufficient period of stimulation, kinesthetic or other cues must be used, but all partially hearing infants should be given time to learn auditorily those phonemes which are babbled by an infant with normal hearing (Poole, 1934). Traditionally, a young child has been taught to imitate what is *seen* instead of what is *heard*, and this not only involves cross modality transfer, but reinforces a typical deaf voice quality.

The most helpful technique is to babble a phoneme frequently so that a clear auditory schema is formed, and to associate this sound with a motivating activity. One example would be to *hummmmmmm* while waving a toy airplane over one's head.

Special techniques are needed for the high frequency phonemes: p,/t,/f,/k,/and so on. After the child has learned to blow and whisper, these phonemes are also practiced as part of a motivating activity. That is, the child can practice producing *pppppp* when blowing a toy boat in the water; *kkkkkk* when cutting paper; *tttttt* when imitating a toy horse or clock, and so on. When introducing words containing these phonemes, such as *hot* or *stop it*, it is well to first whisper them, because amplified whispering retains excellent intelligibility, and the strong voiced components of a word do not mask out the high voiceless ones.

Encouraging Echolalia. If a child enjoys the activity, the child will imitate it. Thus, if the child and an adult are verbalizing, the child will echo the sounds that the adult is making. In this way the foundation for imitating words and sentences is laid, and the child is free to learn no matter where the child goes or what the child does. A way to encourage echolalia is to place one's hand in front of one's mouth during babbling and then to put the same hand in front of the child's mouth to indicate that the child should make the sound.

Developing Language Comprehension. Symbolic language begins in association with a highly motivating experience. For example: a parent lifts up the baby, saying, "Up, up you go." Later, the baby lifts up his or her arms to communicate that he or she wants up, and the parent says, "Pick me up." Then the baby hears the word used when they stack blocks together, go upstairs, throw the ball, look up at the airplane, and so on. A helpful parent verbalizes all these activities as they happen, and the baby begins to say "Up," and to transfer it to different situations.

An infant develops an understanding of many functional words, such as *bye-bye, all gone, more, no,* and *hot,* before acquiring a large vocabulary of nouns. A great deal of our language is very abstract and can only be learned auditorily at first. *Wait a minute!, You make me nervous,* and *Don't do that* are examples of abstract language understood by a young child.

The clinician must show the family and especially the mother, how to verbalize each activity—not once, but many times—speaking clearly, expressively, and in short sentences. (For other suggestions on teaching auditory skills to a young child, see Pollack, 1970 and Gordon, 1970. Pollack has also made a series of videotapes which can be rented from the Alexander Graham Bell Association in Washington, D.C.)

The tremendous change observed in 100 deaf infants who had received consistent early auditory stimulation and parent guidance has been described by Connor (1972) in reporting research done at the Lexington School. Evaluation of the children, five years after the start of training, showed that positive results went far beyond traditional expectations in hearing usage, speech and language progress, and overall child development. Over 50 percent of severely deafened children could be integrated into regular elementary schools. An average 40 to 50 dB difference was obtained between aided and unaided hearing for speech.

Similar reports have been published by Ernst (1974) and Northcott (1975).

Remedial Techniques for the Preschool Child

A preschool child whose hearing loss has been recently acquired, or detected after infancy, should receive training in the basic skills described in the infant program, but will require more intensive work to accelerate speech and language development.

A child with normal hearing learns an estimated 500 to 600 words a year, entering school with a vocabulary of about 2000 words, which subsequently increases at a rate of about 700 words per year. Moreover, by the fourth birthday, the normal hearing child has somehow acquired the knowledge of how words fit together into the syntax of language (McNeill, 1971). The child with a hearing loss, on the other hand, needs constant help in acquiring new vocabulary along with constant review. The child misses much of the input and reinforcement normally acquired from the radio, television, and casual conversation—all of which may not be heard at all.

With an infant, one stimulates, but does not demand, an immediate response. The preschool child, however, is required to respond to all auditory activities as described below.

Techniques for Developing Distance Hearing and Auditory Discrimination. The preschooler enjoys games which require a simple response. For example, the child holds a block to the ear. The teacher makes sounds with familiar noise-makers or with the voice from different parts of the room, beginning at close range. Every time the child hears something, the child puts the block upon the table, building a tower or a train. It becomes a challenge to hear the smallest sounds across the room.

The game of recognizing noisemakers on the table (described in the infant program) should be played with the child moving farther and farther away from the table.

A game of hide and seek also is greatly enjoyed. An adult hides, and constantly calls the child's name. The child finds the hiding place by listening.

Techniques for Developing a Vocabulary. It is best to plan vocabulary teaching in units, with a "core" of words in each unit which can be used immediately in many different situations. The vocabulary then is expanded in a circular manner around each core. For example, for parts of body, one might first teach eye, nose, hair, tummy and then add other words gradually. The core words of the clothing unit might be, *hat, shoe, coat,* and of the family, *mummy, daddy, baby.*

All of the words in each unit cannot be taught at the same time; the preschooler needs a few words with which to communicate in each activity. It is the teacher's responsibility to observe carefully and decide which words are needed first to develop understanding and speech.

The core should include functional words, verbs, and adjectives as well as nouns. Many verbs are necessary, and they usually require considerable emphasis.

At a certain age, color and number concepts become important, also pronouns, prepositions, and comparison of sizes (Pollack, 1970). Eventually, the child must be introduced to the fact that a word can have several meanings, such as *fly, trunk,* and so on. Ahead lie jokes, riddles, and puns.

Toys, picture charts, scrapbooks, flash cards, flannel-boards, inlay puzzles, children's word books, and card and table games can all be used to foster the growth of vocabulary in a dynamic, child-oriented program of highly motivating activities. The child must be encouraged to recognize all new vocabulary auditorily, that is, without visual cues. The teacher can hold a card in front of his or her face or sit behind the child. Rewards, in the form of signals from a buzz board (Pollack, 1970), or those provided by means of operant conditioning techniques, accelerate progress. Photographs of the child's activities promote a great deal of conversation and review.

No teacher can undertake this project alone. The family must take the major part of the responsibility to talk constantly and clearly, to review new vocabulary, to read aloud to the child daily and to stir up an interest in words. Parents should be reminded that when there is a hearing loss, the learning of language and the use of residual hearing can never be taken for granted.

Eventually, a child thus stimulated will reach the stage of demanding to know the meaning of the new words heard. Meanwhile, slow development of vocabulary, as illustrated by low scores on tests such as the Peabody Picture Vocabulary Test (Dunn, 1965) need not be discouraging as the following case history demonstrates:

S. was not fitted with a body aid until he was three years of age, several months after his parents suspected a hearing loss because he was not understanding speech. The etiology of his loss was not known. There was no familial history of deafness. Pregnancy and infancy had been normal, except for the child's having a high fever at fourteen months. He had several ear infections, two myringotomies, and allergies. Mumps had occurred at age five.

S. was a very frustrated child when first tested. He was enrolled in an acoupedic program (Pollack, 1964) until he entered regular kindergarten. He had to repeat third grade and from that point began to earn A's and B's. He needed tutoring in phonics, reading, word study skills, and speech until he entered a junior high school at age thirteen. In the sixth grade he was in a "team teaching" situation, and at the end of seventh grade, he had a B + average and was elected president of the student council. He has recently graduated from a four-year university program with a degree in business administration.

His Peabody scores remained low and increased slowly.

PPVT

C.A.	9–9	Derived scores:	5–6
C.A.	11–2	Derived scores:	6–10
C.A.	14–0	Derived scores:	9–10

These scores might be explained by the fact that S. was on every sports team and did not read for pleasure. He was able to learn the new vocabulary in school as he encountered it and maintain good grades. On the seventh grade report card was the comment: "He is one of our best listeners."

His audiogram was stable over the years, and he changed to two ear level aids.

Audiogram (I.S.O. 1964 level)

	250 Hz	500 Hz	1K	2K	4K	8K
Right Ear:	60	80	95	100	90	No response
Left Ear:	50	75	95	90	80	80

Pure Tone Average: 500–2000 Hz   Right Ear: 92 dB

Left Ear: 87 dB

Techniques for Developing Proper Syntax Usage. Although memory span depends largely on intelligence, all children can be helped to develop a longer auditory memory span, and this will foster their ability to remember sentence patterns.

Developing Auditory Memory Span and Sequencing. A preliminary drill for developing memory span includes review of vocabulary. Here, the teacher uses picture flash cards, asking the child to name the object depicted on each one as it is placed on the table in a column. Then the child is asked to give him one card at a time, two at a time, three, four, and so on, as the objects on the cards are named.

Preschool children enjoy all these activities more if they can change roles sometimes and make the teacher listen.

Within a meaningful context, the preschooler next must learn to memorize a two-word combination, such as *go bye-bye, yellow block, my shoe, mummy's shoe, new shoes, I'm tired, I'm hot, boy's jumping, he's jumping.*

Three-word combinations are sometimes easier to imitate because they are more rhythmic—*put it back, tie my shoe, where's my ball?*

Prepositional phrases can be learned as three-word spans—*where's my shoe?, under the bed, under the chair.*

Four-word spans can be introduced by going outside and saying *I hear a bird, I hear a car, I hear my shoes,* and so on.

The teacher needs to collect a large number of pictures to represent different sentence patterns and to promote questions and answers, for example, "What happened?" "The boy fell down." It is also important to use pictures portraying feelings—to say, for example, "He's feeling mad. Why?"

Teaching Sequence of Actions and Ideas. Here, it is well to begin with a motivating activity, such as planting a seed or having a birthday cake. Afterwards, a series of simple pictures can be drawn about the sequence of events with each one accompanied by a short sentence, and the child can be asked to place the pictures in the correct order. The teacher can stand at varying distances and describe each picture for the child to identify auditorily. Sequence picture cards can be obtained from Milton Bradley or Instructo.

Fostering Memorization. Finger plays, songs, nursery rhymes, and stories foster auditory memory. In particular, nursery stories include repetition of sentence patterns, such as:

> "Who will help me?" said the little red hen.
> "I won't," said the dog. "I'm tired."
> "I won't," said the pig. "I'm tired," and so on.

Auditory training is most successful when it is initiated in a one-to-one situation, based on an individual prescription. When group training is conducted, care should be taken that auditory rather than visual learning is reinforced. However, having learned to listen, a preschooler must integrate audition and vision. Most children with a hearing loss become natural lipreaders, but lipreading can be improved by training (Sanders, 1971). Inability to understand visual clues must be interpreted as a serious warning signal.

It will be realized that the auditory approach and the educational program have merged at this point, and a great deal of specialized work must be done to develop both receptive and expressive language. Northcott (1977) has written a curriculum guide, and lessons for parents have been prepared by Rushmer and Arpan (1977), and Stovall (1982).

The success of the training program can be measured by the Houston Test of Language Development for ages two to six (Crabtree, 1963) or the Preschool Language Scale (Zimmerman, 1969). Scores will show areas in which the child needs further training.

Remedial Techniques for the School-Age Child

With the advent of public law 94-142 which mandated placement of the handicapped child "in the least restrictive environment," school speech and language clinicians will see an increasing number of hearing-impaired children on their caseload.

Evaluation Program. Before a program of auditory training can be planned for the child who has reached school age, a comprehensive evaluation must take place. A battery of tests could include:

1. *Hearing Tests.* After the audiogram, the primary concern is aided response to speech testing. That is, how does the child function with the aid? The Test of Auditory Comprehension can be used (Los Angeles County, 1979).
2. *Speech Tests.* A developmental type of articulation test such as that described by Ling (1976) is used and articulation is checked in syllables, single words, and running speech. It is helpful to make tape recordings of the speech.
3. *Language Tests.* One might use the Peabody Picture Vocabulary Test (Dunn, 1965) for receptive vocabulary, the Northwestern Syntax Test (Lee, 1969), a Language Sample (Bloom and Lahey, 1978), a Spontaneous Language Analysis Procedure (Kretschmer and Kretschmer, 1978), and a Grammatical Analysis of Elicited Language (Moog and Geers, 1980).
4. *Social Performance Scales.* The Vineland Maturity Scale (Doll, 1947) can be used in making these measurements.
5. *Intelligence Tests.* The Goodenough Draw-a-Man Test (Goodenough, 1926), gives a base score against which to compare other scores in estimating intelligence. More precise measurements of intelligence may be obtained by the psychologist through the use of other IQ tests.
6. *Reading Tests.* Many public school systems use a reading inventory to score word recognition and comprehension. The material requires the child to formulate sentences and answer various types of questions which also gives a picture of language use.
7. *Written Language Tests.* A test should be used which requires a sample of the child's productivity, syntax, and language. The Picture Story Language Test (Myklebust, 1965) is one example, as is the test of Syntactic Ability (Quigley et al., 1976).
8. *Tests of Perception.* The Frostig (1966), ITPA (Kirk, McCarthy, and Kirk, 1968), and the Slingerland (1967) are tests which evaluate specific competencies.

Children who appear to have learning disabilities or developmental lags should be referred to the occupational therapist and the remedial specialists. In all areas, a remedial program must begin at the child's level of functioning.

Techniques for Teaching Auditory Discrimination and Related Skills.
Phonics. Children with hearing impairments require individual help with phonics—logically from the educational audiologist or the speech clinician. At the preschool

level instruction might begin with a speech notebook in which phonemes are associated with pictures such as *bbbbbbb* for the motorbike; *sssssss* for running water; and *sh!* for someone sleeping.

At the kindergarten level, a picture can be selected for each initial consonant—a picture of a ball for *b*, fish for *f*, and so on—and the child can find other objects whose names begin with these sounds and collect pictures for them, too. The child can be taught to write and recognize each symbol. The teacher should be careful at this stage to sound out each symbol. Later, children can be taught the name of the letter along with the way of writing the capital letters. A great deal of practice is required for the long and short vowels.

Houghton Mifflin manufactures a group of small toys and cardboard boxes which children enjoy using in many different ways. They can learn new vocabulary, sort the toys into the appropriate boxes for initial consonant sounds, try to recall which toys are in a box, and take turns in describing a toy or guessing which toy is being described.

- It is small.
- You wear it on your finger.
- It's for sewing, etc.
- It begins with "th."
- What is it? Answer: a thimble.

Pictures to foster recognition of phonemes in medial and final positions may then be used.

When the child can both discriminate and imitate each phoneme, the child is ready to move into a regular phonics program appropriate to his or her age.

Many children with a profound hearing loss are never given a strong phonics program, which is unfortunate. Admittedly, however, there are children with and without hearing loss, who find it extremely difficult to blend sounds into words (Rosewell and Chall, 1963) or to associate visual symbols with sounds (Katz, 1971).

Rhyming. Rhyming activities are excellent forms of auditory training. One activity centers upon a box of toys, from which the teacher picks out a toy (for example, a star) and holds it to the ear as the name is uttered. Then, picking out another toy, the teacher holds it to the other ear and says its name. The teacher shakes his or her head, and says, "No, that does not sound similar. That does not rhyme." And the teacher continues selecting toys until one is found whose name does rhyme (for example, car).

This activity can be followed by using rhyming picture cards, which are sometimes available at dime stores.

Vocabulary. The school child needs to recognize at first some basic vocabulary or "key" words which are then used in sentences, for example, numbers. The teacher can write the numbers 1–10 on the board and standing *behind* the student, call out one number at a time. When the student can recognize each number auditorily, the teacher gives information using those numbers:

- Turn to page 5.
- Draw 3 columns on your paper.
- That will cost 8 cents.
- My address is No. 10 Nevada Avenue.

The same activity can be used for colors, calendar dates, people's names, and so on. Other concepts which can be used are *before, after, next to, in the middle,* and so on.

Auditory Memory Span. The school-age child is required to constantly remember a stream of directions, questions, and facts, and therapy which extends the auditory memory span is of great benefit to the hearing-impaired youngster. It may also extend visual memory span. Children are motivated best by material which is relevant to their everyday lives, not by digit span activities. The adult can begin by giving one direction at a time, such as *sit on the floor,* and ask the child to repeat this aloud and then carry it out. Then the adult gives two directions at a time, and so on. It is also more fun for the child to take turns and give directions, too.

Other activities include such well-known games as "Twenty Questions" and "I packed my bag and in it I put . . ." which can be changed to fit any occasion: "Last night was Halloween and I saw . . ." (goblins, a ghost, a witch, etc.). Another activity is to read a short story and ask the child to pantomime what he remembers.

Auditory Tracking. School-age children benefit from practice in "tracking" because their classmates are frequently called upon to read aloud or the teacher may read aloud from the textbook.

The adult can read a few sentences and stop suddenly, and then the hearing-impaired child is expected to continue the sentence. Reading dialogue, riddles, or poems together is a similar activity.

Auditory Closure. This involves the ability to anticipate and supply missing words or word parts by using contextual clues. The teacher can use a variety of material for the child with a hearing loss to complete:

- s - t - ove
- The opposite of friend is _____.
- Grass is to green as sky is to _____.

Dictation. The hearing-impaired child needs practice in listening to and writing down what is heard—both in phonics and in spelling. The teacher may cover the mouth and speak very closely to the child and gradually move farther away. Word endings should be emphasized, as in plural *s,* past tense *ed,* and participle *ing.*

Listening to Recordings. It is a regrettable, but undeniable fact that the skills obtained by an early auditory approach are quickly lost if they are not continuously reinforced, or if too much emphasis is placed upon visual communication. School tends to be predominantly a visual learning experience, especially in the early grades, but recently there has been an attempt to introduce more auditory experiences in the schools by installing "listening corners" or laboratories. While some of this equipment can be used in an auditory training program, it may be advisable for the child to listen to the tapes or records through the child's own hearing aids, since many school headphone sets produce significant distortion.

The possibility that deaf children who have worn hearing aids since early infancy will be able to listen and understand recordings should not be dismissed. There is certainly nothing to lose and a great deal to gain through trying this form of auditory training. One by-product will be improved hearing for telephone conversations and television. An amplifier or speaker, obtainable from the telephone company, is essential for telephone reception, however.

Recordings of Environmental Noises. Most environmental sounds are taped for cassette recorders. Tape-recorded sounds are not as a realistic as sounds of actual happenings, but the tapes can help a hearing-impaired child associate sound with source, and prepare an adult for the noisy world which has become muffled.

Phonograph recordings are available in conjunction with a picture album (Utley, 1950). Also of value may be the tapes made by Bergman (et al., 1965) for training blind people to recognize the sequence of events in a number of situations. For example, someone is walking from the kitchen to the dining room, getting glasses, making an iced drink, setting the table, and so on. Bergman found that auditory discrimination of detail is a skill which can be "honed" even for normal hearing individuals. The latter are surprised, in fact, by the number of small and significant sounds they typically overlook, but become aware of following repeated presentations of the tape.

Speech Recordings. Listening to recorded speech is more difficult than listening to environmental noises.

It is more effective at first for the clinician to make his or her own tapes, because commercial recordings are often too fast or too detailed for the hearing-impaired person to follow.

A good way of proceeding with a child is to choose a book which has simple pictures on each page. Each picture should be described in a short sentence, which is written down, practiced aloud, and timed so as to leave a long enough interval for the child to turn the page. The child can play back the tape and turn the pages of the picture book or the pages of his or her own story. In this way, the speech, vocabulary, and speed are tailored to fit personal needs. Later, the child can write and record his or her own stories.

The school-age child needs to develop a one-to-one correspondence between words spoken or heard and words read. They must also recognize individual words embedded in phrases and sentences.

The itinerant teacher or school clinician will have to meet a continuing need for word study, beginning with the vocabulary most frequently encountered in the reading books at each level.

Flash cards should be made on index cards, one word to a card. The adult records these words (new words, from social studies, science, spelling, etc.) indicating syllables and stress. The child listens to the tape, selects each card as it is heard, and repeats it. Next, child and teacher formulate phrases or sentences using each word which they write on the back of the cards, and then record the sentences. Later, the child can learn to alphabetize the cards in a filebox for future reference.

Two programs which were developed for use in the public schools are the Auditory Skills Curriculum (Los Angeles County, 1979) which provides over 200 classroom activities for auditory discrimination, sequencing, feedback and figure-ground abilities, and the Barnell-Loft Reading Series (Boning, 1976).

Advanced Auditory Training for the Hard-of-Hearing

In addition to conducting an advanced program for older children similar to the type just described for preschoolers, an educational audiologist often is called to help persons who have acquired hearing losses after the normal development of speech and language. The goals of this kind of program are improving or preserving their auditory discrimination ability and teaching them to use a hearing aid in noise (Sanders, 1971; Alpiner, 1978).

Both auditory training and speech reading or lipreading are necessary to overcome phonemic-regression and discrimination problems. Studies have shown that improvement can be obtained with either visual or auditory training (Binnie et al., 1976; Walden et al., 1981).

A program could include the following activities:

1. listening to everyday information such as telephone numbers, birthdates, prices, people's names
2. listening to syllables: "Which word am I saying: morning or disappear?"
3. listening to directions and carrying them out
4. listening to descriptions of objects placed on the table and identifying them
5. listening to questions and answering them
6. listening to someone reading aloud and answering questions about the material, using *What People Say* by Ordman and Ralli (1976)
7. listening to the same material from different parts of the room and outside the room
8. listening from different distances
9. listening to recordings
10. repetition of all this material against a background of environmental noise

For teenagers and adults there is an excellent series of workbooks and tapes by Whitehurst (1958). These are designed to develop the following auditory skills:

1. listening to male and female voices
2. learning new vocabulary (the theme of each unit is a foreign country, but a few units emphasize experiences, such as going to a bank)
3. listening for similarities and differences in words, such as, loan, stone, phone, cone
4. listening for sequential clues (as in stories and informational paragraphs)
5. listening for a clue or sentence which will identify a vocabulary word
6. listening for clues from synonyms
7. listening to pairs of sentences in order to distinguish fine differences by associational clues

Whitehurst recommends that individuals with *severe* discrimination problems be encouraged to listen first with a script and then to withdraw it gradually. Progress may be slow and limited and hearing may only be a supplement to their lipreading and especially when an implant is worn. In any event, both lipreading and auditory skills are more quickly acquired when lessons are scheduled in rapid succession.

Another excellent device is the Language Master which utilizes cards which are placed in the unit to activate recordings of various types: environmental sounds, reading readiness exercises, specific vocabulary words, etc. The hearing-impaired person pushes one button to hear the recording, another to record an imitation of that recording, and a third button to listen to both. A simpler version of this machine is called the Voxcom. It can be attached to a standard cassette tape recorder.

Listening in Noise. A person with normal hearing, exposed from birth to a background of noise, learns gradually to discriminate between what he or she wishes to hear, and the background noise, which he or she comes to ignore. The ability to discriminate well in noise is known to be a function of binaural hearing. The slight differences in time and direction perceived by the two ears appear to enable the brain to accomplish the task of selective listening (Sullivan, 1965; Libby, 1980).

Exercises which should be part of the program for the new hearing aid use include listening to words, sentences, and directions against a competing background of noise, such as traffic, party conversations, and so on. People who have gradually lost their hearing acuity have the greatest difficulty because they have become used to a more silent world. Another common problem with which they and others have to cope is the distortion which accompanies a hearing loss, together with the distortion which a hearing aid adds to the experience. Consequently, hearing aid manufacturers are modifying their designs so as to reduce that ambient noise.

While listening in noise is somewhat difficult for people with a hearing loss, and especially for those who wear only one aid, a child who has worn two aids from infancy and has been taught by an auditory approach does not appear to experience abnormal difficulty with background noise. (The child may dislike wearing head-phones, because they isolate the child from background noises and change normal auditory perception.) The case is quite different for a child with learning disabilities, even one with normal hearing, because he or she experiences a dramatic increase in discrimination problems if there is background noise.

An advanced auditory training program should include listening to television, movies, radio, and the telephone. Moreover, there should be assignments to listen to group discussions, conversation in stores, people talking on the street, and so on.

The program should include speech correction and the preservation of voice quality—exercises for which can be found in speech pathology textbooks (Ling, 1976a and b).

The Counseling Program

Auditory remediation will not be successful unless the clinician views the hearing-impaired person as a member of a family and a community. This holistic concept reaches far beyond traditional "hearing aid orientation," with its emphasis upon information, and requires the clinician to function on a "feeling" level to facilitate the grief process of each family member until a coping mechanism has developed.

Disability has been described as a "spoiler of dreams and hopes," and it is now recognized that for both a hearing-impaired adult and the family of a deaf child, successful grieving involves feelings of denial, guilt, depression, anger, and anxiety. These feelings should be viewed as positive stages of growth toward acceptance of the permanence of the hearing loss, and the building of new expectations and lifestyle (Moses and Van Hecke-Wulatin, 1981; Clark, 1982).

For a child, the most important factors of a successful oral-auditory program are the child's parents' involvement in it and the goals they have. The parents' discovery that their child has a hearing loss is a traumatic experience, one often preceded by months of doubt, guilt, and fear. The average time lag between suspicion of a problem and the initiation of treatment seems to be at least two years. Parents all report the same stories—they are reassured, or they are told it is too early to test reliably. They even are told that nothing can be done about the hearing impairment until the child is six years old and can be sent away to a special school. Since everyone prefers normalcy, a search for a cure may be the next step.

When a diagnosis of permanent hearing loss is made, the implications of the handicap dawn slowly. At first the parents feel great sorrow, for the defect of a child is a defect of the family. Relatives and neighbors add to the problem with their often conflicting advice or opinions; or professional people might discuss different training philosophies, making the choice difficult. The general public exhibits ignorance of the nature of a hearing impairment and shows pity or rejection.

In the face of all this, parents need appropriate guidance and they need this support not just at the outset but on a continuing basis, because they reexperience some of the grieving states as their child matures and comes to a new major milestone. The difficulties encountered (as for example, problems with discipline, sibling rivalry, temper tantrums), are described fully in Gregory (1976). During the school years, the responsibility of participating in program planning, which has been mandated by P.L. 94-142, requires a broad educational program for parents (Mencher and Gerber, 1981).

Many children with hearing impairments are being integrated into schools for the normal hearing. A guidance program for staff, parents, and pupils is essential. Systems O.N.E. (Orientation to Normal Environment), a filmstrip presentation developed by, and available from, the University of Utah, is an excellent example of the materials available for this purpose. The classroom teacher needs to adjust his or her teaching methods somewhat and be willing to give the partially hearing child preferential seating, extra attention, and a measure of compassion (Northcott, 1973; Yater, 1977; Froehlinger, 1981).

There are now many different programs available to parents; some child-centered, others parent-centered. They may be found in a hospital, private agency, or school. In the early years, when the mother is the primary model for communication, mother and child should be taught together. Some clinicians visit homes or work in a demonstration home (McConnell, 1974).

Counseling the person with a hearing loss should be continuous, from childhood through adulthood. The hearing-impaired adult and the adolescent have a great need to sit down with an understanding person and discuss their feelings and experiences in coping with a normal hearing world. Our goal in counseling is to help them work with their handicap and not against it. They cannot be the same as a normal hearing person, but they do not have to be—they can build a life according to their own capabilities.

Individual and group counseling sessions should be part of every program for auditory remediation. Group sessions are effective because they are a vehicle for sharing feelings as well as for processing information. The group as helper is wiser than the individual. Luterman (1979) gives an excellent description of the group process, but warns that it may not be successful for all participants. For many families, individual counseling by a social worker, family therapist, or psychologist is of great benefit.

The Volta Bureau of the Alexander Graham Bell Association for the Deaf publishes books and pamphlets for parents and professionals, plus many helpful articles in the *Volta Review*. Books written by parents of the hearing impaired, or by adults who have experienced limited hearing are of inestimable value in the counseling effort

(Wright, 1969; Angus, 1974; Bitter, 1978; Star, 1980). So are meetings with adults and family members who have adjusted successfully to the problems associated with hearing loss. They can help a person who is trying to make that adjustment far more effectively than professional persons can. The latter, however, must be part of the picture by virtue of the breadth of professional information and experience. Clients look to the professionals for an understanding of the medical, audiologic, educational, and social implications of a hearing loss.

If the full consequences of deafness and its influence on mental growth, mental health, and social security are to be understood and remediated, it is necessary for the clinician to consider its effects in relation to every aspect of living.

REMEDIAL PRINCIPLES AND PRACTICES WITH DEAF CHILDREN[2]

In the learning of language, vision normally supplements hearing and vice versa, but in the person with a profound hearing impairment the learning must take place primarily through the eyes. It is a task for which the eyes are not well suited, because they have so many other functions to perform, and one in which they should derive all possible assistance from even a small residuum of hearing. Within this section dealing with remedial principles and practices with deaf children, therefore, we shall discuss auditory training, while stressing vision as the principal avenue of learning.

Focus of Discussion: The Prelingually Deaf

To even hope for a meaningful presentation, we must select a small segment of the hearing-impaired population and describe some of the remediation principles and practices appropriate for it. Therefore, we shall deal with the segment made up of prelingually deaf children. This is not to make less of the problems of older deaf children, hard-of-hearing teenagers, or seventy-five-year-old prebycusics, but simply to indicate that language acquisition, when it must be accomplished largely through a substitute modality, is an educational problem deserving of our primary attention.

Prelingual is used in referring to children who (1) were born deaf, or (2) became deaf before language and speech had developed through hearing. Today, the majority are of the first type because antibiotics and improved otologic and pediatric practices have reduced the number of the latter. For children who are "deafened" by infection or disease, it is difficult to set an exact cutoff period to define prelingual, but two years serves as a convenient landmark. If deafness occurs prior to age two, the child's education proceeds very much like that of a congenitally deaf child. If it occurs after age two, there is apparently enough language and auditory memory that the child may ultimately develop more normal language and speech than is generally possible for the congenitally deaf child.

We have described the focus population as *deaf* to distinguish it from the hard-of-hearing. It is difficult to provide exact definitions to distinguish the two categories because the pure tone air-conduction audiogram, although helpful, does not provide a reliable distinction. There is some consensus (O'Neill, 1964) that when the average

---

[2] This section was written by Edgar L. Lowell, who wishes to acknowledge the assistance in preparing the manuscript of associates at the John Tracy Clinic in Los Angeles.

threshold to 500, 1000, and 2000 Hz pure tones exceeds 90 dB (ISO 1964) the individual is *deaf*. Losses less severe than this characterize the hard-of-hearing. Yet in a language learning situation some hard-of-hearing children will behave as if they were deaf, and some children with average losses in excess of 90 dB will behave as if they had much more hearing.

Although a variety of as yet imperfectly understood factors cloud any attempt at a simple distinction between the deaf and the hard-of-hearing, for the purposes of this discussion a working definition of *deafness* will be "hearing impairment so severe that a person who manifests it must acquire language primarily through vision." *Hard-of-hearing* thus will apply to all of the remaining hearing-impaired population. They have enough residual hearing to be expected to acquire language through hearing if provided with amplification and special instruction. Note that our definition says "must *acquire* language primarily through vision," by way of emphasizing the prelingual period. In these terms, a child with a severe hearing loss acquired at age six would be considered "deafened" but not "deaf."

We might have used the term "profoundly hearing impaired" rather than "deaf." In fact, there appears to be growing sentiment for the use of hearing impaired as the generic term with the descriptors mild, moderate, severe, or profound used to indicate the degree of impairment. The emphasis on precision in terminology describing the hearing-impaired child is primarily to avoid faulty educational placement. "The improper application of the descriptive label 'deaf' can lead to an educational placement and therefore achievement and behavioral expectations consistent with the connotations of the label rather than the potential of the child" (Ross and Giolas, 1978).

Since the person with normal hearing develops most of his language and speech skills while still a child, we believe that the deaf child should have that same opportunity, and that any remediation program should begin at an early age. While we have little evidence related to critical periods for language development, we know that it is much easier for a young hearing child to acquire a second language and to speak it without a "foreign" accent than it is for an adult. We also know that hearing children, who begin the acquisition of language at an early age, have made great progress by the time they enter school. Remarkably, they accomplish this important learning task with little specific instruction. In the absence of any evidence to the contrary, then it would appear reasonable to start the deaf child's language experience as soon as possible.

There is general agreement about the primary importance of developing communication skill in the hearing impaired. A disagreement arises over the methods to be used. Essentially it has been an argument between oral (lipreading and speech) and manual (fingerspelling and signing) communication, although there are so many variations on these two general methods that describing it as a simple oral-manual controversy oversimplifies the issues. The controversy is not a new one. As early as 1880 the Congress of Milan debated the relative merits of the two methods and finally decided in favor of the oral method and agreed to ban sign language from the schools (Di Carlo, 1964). The controversy continues unabated to the present time. For background and a history of some of the interesting persons associated with the education of the deaf in general the reader is referred to Moores (1978), Di Carlo (1964), and Henderson (1975). Any attempt to describe the different varieties of communication methods used by the deaf will inevitably miss some, and will certainly fail to cover all of the merits claimed by the proponents of the different methods.

In the Oral group there is the multisensory approach which advocates the use of vision, residual hearing, and touch to develop language and speech. The Aural-Oral approach places greater emphasis on the use of residual hearing, in some cases covering the mouth to force the student to attend to the auditory signal. A good description of the status of the oral method is contained in the report of the First International Symposium on Oral Education held in the Netherlands in 1980. The Tadoma method (Vivian, 1966), designed primarily for deaf-blind students, places more emphasis on kinesthetic cues received by placing the hand on the speaker's face. While not widely used today, the Tadoma method has been used quite successfully in teaching deaf children.

The Manual group advocates the use of fingerspelling and signing. In finger-spelling each letter of the alphabet is represented by a hand position. Signs are defined by the place, handshape, movements of the hands, and facial expression. The most commonly used sign system is American Sign Language or Ameslan (Fant, 1972), which has about 4,000 signs. It meets all the requirements of a genuine language, but it differs from English in several important ways. Ameslan has a different syntax which results in a different word order than English. It also omits prepositions, articles, adverbial forms, prefixes, and suffixes. The most concrete or vivid element comes first in a sentence. Next come signs which explain or describe the situation (usually adjectives, adverbs, or verbs), followed by the result, the end product, or state of being. Plurals may be represented by repeating the sign. Tense indicators are used because Ameslan has no way to express tense in a verb sign. To sign the word "ate" you would use the sign for "eat" and add a tense indicator such as "finished" or "yesterday," yielding "finished eat" or "eat yesterday" (Solow, 1975).

Some Manualists feel that a manual communication system that followed the word order of English would be desirable because it would give the deaf student experience with the syntax used by the majority of communicators. SIGLISH (Signed English), Manual English, SEE I (Seeing Essential English), SEE II (Signing Exact English), and LOVE (Linguistics of Visual English) are some of the sign systems that represent attempts to cope with this problem. In general, each tries to use correct English syntatic and grammatical form using combinations of signs and fingerspelling, includ-ing spelled letter cues to modify a sign. (For example, working may be produced by the sign for "work" plus the fingerspelled "ing.") They have also created new signs and developed rules for compound words, such as "cowboy" which is produced by the two signs, "cow" and "boy." For more details the interested reader is referred to the papers by Anthony (1971), Fant (1972), Gustason (1972), Henderson (1975), Moores (1978), and Solow (1975).

Still another method is *Cued Speech* (Cornett, 1967), which combines hand configura-ration and placement used in conjunction with speech to give cues about the sounds that are either invisible (e.g., the /k/ sound, as in cat) or difficult to distinguish by lipreading (e.g., the /p/, /b/, /m/ sounds as in pat, bat, mat). Four of the cues indicate groups of vowel sounds, and are made by positioning the hand near the chin, cheek, throat, and mouth. The other eight identify groups of consonants, and are formed by different arrangement of the fingers of one hand (Miles, 1967).

The disagreement about communication philosophy is taken very seriously by many deaf people and professionals. The argument on one side runs that because lipreading and speech are so difficult to learn and use, that it is better for the deaf to use manual communication which is more visible and easier to learn. The opposite argument runs that the deaf person can only hope to achieve his or her full potential through lipreading and speech, that is, when the deaf person is not dependent on an interpreter, or limited to communicating with those people who understand manual communication.

The number of different communication methods reflects a general dissatisfaction with the results of our educational systems for the hearing impaired. When educators are dissatisfied with their results, it is only natural that they seek some new method or system. One of the newest and probably most widely used is called *Total Communication*. It is similar to an earlier Simultaneous Method which combined lipreading, speech, fingerspelling, and signing. Total Communication adds mime, gestures, body language, drawing, and anything else that will help transmit the message. Some do not classify Total Communication as a method, but rather a philosophy on communication.

While there has been considerable enthusiasm on the part of both educators and parents for Total Communication, it is not an easy system to implement. Teachers who have not been trained in the oral method are not able to suddenly modify their knowledge and skills to include lipreading and speech in their teaching, just because their school has adopted Total Communication. Similarly experienced Oral-Aural educators are not likely to be able to quickly incorporate fingerspelling and signing into their teaching. We have no programs to train teachers in the use and integration of mime and gestures and all of the other components that are called for by the concept of Total Communication. Any subsequent disappointment with the results of Total Communication programs may stem from the implementation rather than the concept.

With the great variety of methods available and in use in different schools, it would be difficult to describe remediation methods using all of them. The common objective of all methods is the development of communication skill. The examples of remedial principles and practices used here use the oral method, because of the author's experience. They can easily be modified for use with any of the other communication methods.

Remedial Techniques

Receptive Language Learning. The first step in remediation for the young deaf child is developing a receptive language foundation. By *receptive* language we are referring to the words that a person understands—as distinguished from *expressive* language, or the words used in ordinary conversation. Since we understand a great many more words than we use, our receptive vocabularies are larger than our expressive vocabularies.

For hearing children, receptive language development appears to be a prerequisite for expressive language and speech. During this receptive period a child is not particularly responsive to language. The child just listens. The child's later behavior shows that this was not a completely passive period and that there must have been some active cerebral organization going on which laid the foundation for his later rapid development of expressive language and speech.

A similar receptive period is necessary for the deaf child. The deaf child needs a receptive language period during which he or she is exposed over and over again to the visual stimuli of people's lips moving in relation to everything that is going on around him. No response should be expected. This is sometimes difficult for parents to understand, because one of their first questions when they learn that their child is deaf is "How soon will my child learn to talk?" They must be helped to realize that the first concern is not with speech but with language, or the understanding that precedes speech. You can teach a parrot to speak, but the parrot doesn't know what it is talking about. The deaf child has to learn to share our language system so that the child will have something to say before we become concerned with speech.

General Principles and Procedures for Teaching Lipreading. The development of receptive language begins with general lipreading. The importance of this beginning is perhaps best conveyed by the now-famous dictum of Mrs. Spencer Tracy, founder of the John Tracy Clinic: "Talk, talk, talk to the deaf child. . . . Give him a desire to talk, something to talk about, and someone to talk to" (Tracy, 1965). What this means is that parents need to acquire skill in recognizing and taking advantage of the child's interests in order to provide the child with receptive language experience; it means that they should show an interest in what the child is interested in, and talk to the child in short, simple sentences about that interest; and it means that they should follow some practices that make it easier for the child to see and ultimately understand what is being said. Such practices include:

1. using complete simple sentences or "carrier phrases," but not the same ones repeatedly;
2. emphasizing the key word, usually at the end of the phrase; and
3. using declarative sentences rather than questions, because the deaf child will probably not be aware of the rising inflection pattern characteristic of the question, nor at this stage be able to produce the verbal response that a question usually requires.

Some physical factors will make general lipreading easier, such as the following:

1. arranging the situation so that the light shines on the speaker's face rather than in the child's eyes;
2. getting down on the child's level so that the child doesn't have to be continually stretching his or her neck to see the speaker's face;
3. not talking with a cigarette in the mouth or with anything interfering with a clear view of the face; and
4. preventing other movement from competing for the child's attention. (Waving hands or bobbing the head while talking make it extremely difficult for the child to concentrate on the lips. If it is helpful to hold the object being talked about close to the mouth, the speaker should move it, stop, talk, and then move it away.)

There are other skills parents can develop in getting the child to look at them and to maintain eye contact. Some parents report that their children never seem to look at them, but experience shows that there are many times when a child will look. These are primarily when the child wants something, whether it be help, approval, permission, or praise. The skill is to be able to use those initially fleeting glances in such a way that the child learns that communication takes place when the child is watching the speaker's face—then the looks will be more purposive and for longer periods of time.

Some parents ask, "Why should I talk to him, when he can't hear me?" They should not expect the young deaf child to understand all, or even a fraction, of what they say at first. Gradually, with the hundreds and hundreds of pairings of the visual signal from the lips associated with the object or action that the child is interested in, he or she will begin to develop receptive language. The child also will learn that people do talk—that they communicate by moving their lips.

General lipreading should go on during the child's entire waking hours. Since the hearing child acquires language by "hearing" during all waking hours, the deaf child should be able to match that as closely as possible by a program that takes advantage of every opportunity for meaningful visual language input.

Specific Procedures for Teaching Lipreading. At the same time that a teacher or parent is talking to the deaf child about anything and everything of interest, one word should be selected for specific practice. We do not know how many times a child must be exposed to a word before learning it, but whatever the number, the child will reach it much sooner if there is a focus on a word for concentrated specific lipreading practice.

The word chosen should represent something in which the child has shown an interest. Generally, it should be a noun representing something that is readily available and encountered frequently. The word should be easy to lipread and not easily confused with another word that might sound different but look the same on the lips. When in doubt, a good way is to try the word before a mirror to see if it is easily visible and not likely to be confused with another word. *Cookie, flower*, and *water* are examples of words that are suitable—assuming that the child is interested in them.

After selecting a word for specific lipreading practice, parents should be advised to make plans for a variety of different play activities calling for repetitions of the word, yet still holding the child's interest. The following description of a planned activity for the word *water* was prepared for parents' use by the John Tracy Clinic.

PLANNED ACTIVITY: "WASHING UP"

Materials Needed:

You will need a shallow pan with a small amount of water in it, some facial tissues (cut in half) or toilet paper, and a snack that is guaranteed to leave your child's face and hands messy. This could be a jam sandwich, peanut butter and crackers, slices of orange, etc. You'll also want a chair or stool for your child to sit on and some newspaper to go under the pan.

Assemble the washing-up materials so that you are ready to wash up your child as soon as he has finished his snack. If this could be done close to a mirror, or if you could use a hand mirror at intervals, it would help maintain your child's interest.

What do do	*What to say*
After the snack, kneel down to your child and hold his messy hands, palms up, between you. Look at them. Hold still. When he looks to your face, say:	They're dirty.
Walk together to the area that you have selected. Hold a mirror so that he can see his dirty face. Remove the mirror. Hold still. When he looks to your face, say:	It's dirty.
Seat your child, get a bit of tissue, hold it near your mouth. Stop. When he looks to your face, say:	I'll get some water.
Dunk the tissue in the water. Spend a long enough time at it that your child sees the action of getting the tissue wet. While he is looking at the water in the pan, dip your hand into the water in the pan and dribble some of it off your fingers. Hold still. When your child looks to your face, say:	That's water.
Take the wet tissue and sponge off part of one of his cheeks. Show him the dirty tissue. When he looks to your face, say:	Your face is dirty.
Hold another tissue near your face and when your child looks to your face, say:	I'll get more water.
Dip it into the water so that it is quite wet. Hold it between you and your child—yet out of his reach. Let it drip water onto your other hand. Stop all motion and when he looks to your face, say:	That's water.
If he continues to look to your face, say again:	That's water.
Continue to sponge off the rest of the cheek area. Make it a pleasant activity. Have your child look into the mirror. Place your index finger on his clean cheek. When he looks to your face, say:	It's clean.

Go back to the washing. This time, take one of his hands and look at it as already described. Stop. When he looks to your face, say:	We'll put it in the water.
Place his hand in the pan and hold it there a moment. Stop. When he looks to your face, say:	It's in the water.
Rub his hand to get off the dirt. Lift it between you and let the water drip off to your own hand. Wait. When he looks to your face, say:	Look at the water.
Wipe his hand dry with tissue. Hold it up again and look at it. Wait. When he looks to your face, say:	The water's gone.
Drop his hand. Get another piece of tissue; hold it beside your face. Stop. When he looks, place his clean hand on your face for touch and say:	I'll get some water.
Drop his hand. Dip the tissue into the water; let it drip on your child's hand. Hold his hand still and the tissue away from his hand. When he looks to your face, say:	That's water.
Sponge off the rest of his face and have him look into the mirror to see his clean face. When he looks to your face, say:	It's clean.
Drop his hand. If your child remains interested, have him help you take the pan of water to the sink. Hold still just before you empty the pan and say:	Throw out the water.
Throw it out. Show the remaining water in the pan. Stop. When your child looks to your face, say:	I'll wipe out the water.
Wipe it out. Admire your clean child.	

Variations:

• Working from a water spigot instead of a pan of water.
• Using a wash cloth and towel instead of tissue.

An activity like the one for "Washing Up" provides many opportunities to present *water* in a meaningful fashion. Similar activities could be planned for watering the lawn, washing dishes or the car, or taking a bath. The teacher must develop skill in planning a variety of interesting activities for parent and child to do, as well as in taking advantage of the many unplanned opportunities that come up for meaningful repetitions of the specific lipreading word.

It should be remembered that general language practice proceeds concurrently with the specific practice. This is not an either-or situation—both must be carried on continuously.

Comprehension Checks. There is no agreement on how many repetitions it would take to learn a specific lipreading word, but after a great variety of planned and unplanned activities on the same word, there comes a time when it must be decided whether the child "knows" the word. "Knows" is misleading, because it implies that the deaf child shares the same full and elaborated meanings attached to a particular linguistic symbol that a normal-hearing person does. This is clearly not the case. At this stage, we can only check to see if the child has some simple comprehension of the linguistic concept.

Checking comprehension is more complicated than it may sound, because we cannot just ask the deaf child to define the word, and we cannot even accept his or her repeating it after us as evidence that it is comprehended. In the ideal situation, we try to remove all cues of time, place, and context and see if the child can give some behavioral evidence that the specific lipreading word is understood. If the first word was *airplane*, we would try to ask the child to get the airplane at a different time than usual. We might try it in a different room or out of doors, and we might try it with different toy airplanes to see if the child can generalize from one airplane to a broader class. It is not evidence of comprehension if at 11:55 the teacher says, "Wash for lunch," and the child goes to the sink to wash his or her hands. The child has probably done the same thing every day at that same time, and would continue to do so at 11:55 no matter what the teacher said.

The checks of comprehension should not resemble an examination. If the child does not understand, the incident should be treated as just another receptive repetition and the child should be shown what is being talked about. If he or she responds correctly, on the other hand, something should be done in response to the action. Several comprehension checks should be tried on the first word before going on to the second specific lipreading word.

Selection of the second specific lipreading word should follow the same rules suggested earlier, but the second word should be distinctively different from the first in as many visual dimensions as possible.

Expressive Language Learning. Another activity, which should be carried on concurrently with both general and specific lipreading activities, is the development of expressive language. As pointed out earlier, there is a difference between a person's receptive and expressive vocabularies, and this holds true for the young deaf child as well. The goals in expressive language training are to facilitate the child's communication with others and to help him develop an appreciation of language by seeing its influence on the environment. Note that we are not referring to speech *per se*, which was the parents' first concern. In speech training, the emphasis is on how intelligibly the language is produced, whereas in expressive language training, the primary concern is still on language.

Expressive language training follows many of the same procedures described for receptive language training. One major difference, however, is that the first expressive word should be an action verb rather than a noun. Verbs like *push, pull, stop, open,* and *up* are all good, for they cause something to happen in the environment, and thus help the young child begin to appreciate the power of language.

There are four stages in the development of an expressive language word—receptive, imitation, reminding, and spontaneous.

1. *The receptive stage.*   The first, or receptive, stage is so named because we must be certain that the child understands the word before we are concerned about expression. The practices would be very much the same as those for general and specific training of receptive language. The general practice has the advantage of frequently permitting generalization of the word in a variety of real-life experiences, while the specific practice accelerates the many repetitions required for mastery. As the word being worked on is an action word, it is frequently possible to have the child perform the action described, rather than be a passive observer. This practice should be continued until comprehension checks provide assurance that the child understands the word.

2. *The imitation stage.*   The second, or imitation stage, requires the participation of two adults. The goal is to give the child practice in meaningful imitation. The child first watches what one adult says to the other, and observes the second adult carry out the appropriate action. For example, in an activity on the word *push*, the first adult may place a toy car on a track and say to the other adult, "Give it a push," whereupon the second adult pushes the car. The child is then encouraged by the first adult to watch and to repeat the message to the second adult—who would again carry out the appropriate action. Although the child is merely imitating the first adult, the child can see that expressive language can produce the same result as that produced by adults.

3. *The reminding stage.*   In the reminding stage, the practices are much the same as in the imitation stage, except that the goal is to get the child to initiate the language. Although an activity from the imitation stage may be used, there will be no one to provide the child with an imitative model. For this stage to be successful, the adult must learn to pause with an "expectant look" and to give the child an opportunity to take the initiative. If the child does not respond after a few seconds, the incident should be treated as another receptive experience. Another technique is to occasionally use vibratory cues by placing the child's hand on his or her face as a reminder. The use of touch is described in more detail in relation to auditory training of deaf children (see sample activity *Waking Up*). Touch should be used only occasionally in the reminding stage or it will soon become ineffective.

4. *The spontaneous stage.*   The spontaneous stage, the final level of expressive word development, occurs when the child can consistently and spontaneously use the word in an appropriate situation. The main consideration thereafter is to react quickly so as to reinforce his experience with the power of language; and another is to hold him or her to that level of performance in future situations. After a number of words have been carried through to the spontaneous stage, it may be appropriate to begin with some of the words from the child's receptive vocabulary, as needs and interests dictate.

Soon the child may be at different stages with different words. The child may have one or more words in each of the transition stages that have been mentioned, plus a number in the spontaneous stage. The adult responsible for training must keep track of progress so that practice can be carried out with an appropriate level of expectancy, both in terms of effort and the response it is given. That is, it is wrong to respond to a child's language effort in a manner appropriate to the reminding stage if the child has already demonstrated mastery of that word at the spontaneous stage, just as it is wrong to expect a child to perform at the imitative stage before the word has been mastered at the receptive stage.

Pragmatics. This discussion has dealt with the semantic content of receptive language as though it was the first step in the development of communication. There has recently been considerable interest in the study of pragmatics, or communicative acts which precede (and overlap) semantic development. An example of a communicative act in a young child might be pointing at the milk bottle and making almost any kind of utterance, which the parent would understand as meaning that the child wanted more milk. Research with hearing impaired children has shown (Curtis, Prutting, and Lowell, 1979) that they develop pragmatic categories in much the same fashion as hearing children, although their semantic development is slower than for hearing children.

We believe that this is a fruitful area for further study. It has the potential of contributing new insights into the way language is acquired, and it has a positive psychological effect on the parents when they can see that they are able to (and regularly do) communicate with their young child despite deafness.

Advanced Language Learning. With continued practice, the deaf child will begin to put simple words together in two- and three-word combinations. These combinations may not follow the exact word order of English and they may reveal many omissions, particularly of function words, but they will be approximations of normal language. We know there is a great deal more to language than the vocabulary development we have described. There are countless rules or descriptions of the form-classes, constructions, and grammatical processes found in the language, knowledge of which the hearing child acquires with little formal instruction. That is, by merely being exposed to spoken language over and over, the child begins to internalize a set of implicit rules. The child demonstrates the mastery of these rules by applying them in novel situations. It is these rules that tell the child when a sentence is wrong. The child may not be able to tell what is wrong but the sentence sounds "funny." He or she also begins to "know" when a sentence is correct. The child also begins to incorporate this knowledge into his vocal productions. Linguists tell us that for hearing children, "Grammatical speech does not begin before one and one-half years of age; yet, as far as we can tell, acquisition is virtually complete by three and one-half or four years" (McNeill, 1966).

Much of our earlier teaching of language was based on learning a list of vocabulary words, which were built up into simple sentences by using formulas which covered the different English sentence structures. The Fitzgerald Key was one of these systems that was used widely in schools for the deaf.

The Fitzgerald Key. Because the deaf child is not exposed to language in the same way as the hearing child, the deaf child must acquire these complex rules of grammar in an artificial and less satisfactory way. A common way of teaching grammar has been with the Fitzgerald Key, which was introduced by the deaf teacher Fitzgerald (1954), who felt that correct sentences could aid the deaf child with "straight thinking" and "straight language." The Key, designed to provide guidelines for deaf children to use in developing sentences, is found in many classrooms written at the top of the blackboard:

WHAT	VERB	WHOM	WHERE	WHEN
WHO		WHAT		

By following the Fitzgerald Key, the deaf child has some help in combining words to produce a correct sentence. When skillfully employed, the Key is applicable to more complex sentences, and it undoubtedly has served as a useful tool. Criticism, however, has been leveled at the Key—partially because of its misuse (Di Carlo, 1964), but also because of its limitations. Linguistic studies have suggested (Tervoort and Verbeck, 1967) that teaching by the Key results in an oversimplified and formalized structure, which although useful in classroom situations, is not carried over to informal peer group communication.

The Natural Method. An alternative approach which gets away from the formal structure of the Fitzgerald Key is the *natural method* (Groht, 1958), which emphasizes language used in natural situations. The *conversational method* of van Uden (1968) uses natural language in a conversational format and de-emphasizes formal instruction on grammar. Others who advocate the use of the normal, natural flow of language for practice with deaf children are Simmons (1967) and Moog and Geers (1980). One problem with these methods is that it was not clear how much they help students internalize the rules of syntax.

Application of Transformational Generative Grammar. The more recent developments stem from Chomsky's (1965) transformational or generative grammar. "Rather than simply attempting to describe the structure of language as the structuralists had, Chomsky wanted to explain it, and for this reason proposed a 'generative' model of syntax which employed 'transformations' to link the underlying meaning of a sentence to the sentence as it was actually pronounced" (Russell, Quigley, and Power, 1976, pp. 14–15).

Transformational grammar is now being used in curriculum development and teaching methods for deaf children. The following are just a few: Hsu (1977) has developed a "Developmental Guide to English Syntax" at the St. Joseph's School for the Deaf; Blackwell et al. (1978) describe one developed at the Rhode Island School for the Deaf, Streng (1972) has a text on transformational grammar specifically for teachers of the hearing impaired.

At this time there is an increasing interest in the more linguistically oriented approaches to language instruction. While they are more complicated than some of the earlier methods, they are bringing much greater precision to our description and evaluation of language and, hopefully, will provide the foundation for a better understanding of the language acquisition process.

Auditory Training. In terms of our definition, the deaf child must rely on vision for his major avenue of communication, but this does not imply total deafness. Most deaf children have some residual hearing, generally in the low frequencies, which can be of great assistance in the development of language. To utilize this residual hearing requires both good quality amplification and appropriate auditory training.

The Goal of Auditory Training. The goal of auditory training is to develop good listening habits—a difficult process for the deaf child because the speech heard is not complete enough to be meaningful. Therefore, to foster the child's development of good listening habits, it is necessary to amplify sounds in a way that will make them meaningful. With loudness decreasing rapidly the farther the sound source is from the ear, the best amplification occurs when words are spoken in a normal voice close to the child's ear. But since this is not feasible for any length of time, amplification in the form of an auditory training unit or an individual hearing aid is indicated.

Use of Hearing Aids. The use of hearing aids sometimes causes misunderstanding among those who—unfamiliar with deafness—assume that a hearing aid can somehow "cure" the young deaf child. But a hearing aid and auditory training cannot improve the physiological capacity to hear; they only improve the child's awareness of and attention to sound.

It is probably fair to say that the hearing aid delivers both more and less than we expect. For even the deafest child, amplification can serve as a warning device and put the child in closer touch with the environment, giving some idea of which things make sounds and which do not. Amplification may also provide some sense of the rhythm patterns of speech, which contribute so much to intelligibility. These benefits, while not sufficient for the development of language and speech, are still of great importance to the hearing-impaired child. On the other hand, as we have said, the hearing aid does not reproduce sound for the deaf person with anything like the quality or clarity of normal hearing. For the deaf child with residual hearing in only the lower frequencies, no amount of amplification will deliver intelligible speech. The hearing loss acts as a filter through which pass only the low frequencies containing relatively little speech information.

Auditory Training Activities. As with all of the remediation practices described here, the introduction of amplified sound should be done in such a way as to interest the child and engage and hold his or her attention. The activities selected must be carefully tailored to the individual child's residual hearing, auditory discrimination ability, and experience with auditory training.

To assist in selecting appropriate activities, the staff of the John Tracy Clinic prepared an auditory training manual, *Play It by Ear* (Lowell and Stoner, 1960). This manual describes a series of simple auditory training activities suitable for the young deaf child. It is organized around common sounds to which the child is frequently exposed. There are exercises dealing with human, animal, and work sounds and noises; exercises dealing with music, including pitch, intensity, duration, and rhythm; and exercises dealing separately with vowels, consonants, pitch, intensity, duration, words, phrases, and stories. The final sections deal with distance and direction. Each exercise states an objective, the material needed for the activity, instructions on how to play the game, and variations to maintain the child's interest and to increase the difficulty of the auditory discrimination. An example of one of the activities, "Waking Up," follows.

SAMPLE ACTIVITY: "WAKING UP!"

The Purpose of This Activity:

To help the child discriminate between the "on" and "off" of sound, and furthermore, to make him more aware of the sounds around him.

Materials Needed:

An alarm clock with a fairly loud alarm.

A piece of cardboard cut in the shape of the clock, with the numbers written on it.

Some cereal.

How to Play:

You and the child sit facing each other. Tell him that you are both going to listen to the clock. Show him the clock and compare it to the cardboard one. Place pieces of the cereal on about six consecutive numbers on the cardboard clock.

Now place the child's fingertips on the alarm clock and tell him that you are both going to listen. Turn on the alarm and say to the child "It's on. I hear it." (Point to your ear.) Then take a piece of cereal and turn off the alarm. This is all done very quickly. Point to the next piece of cereal to be taken, telling the child that it is for him but that he must listen. Once more, place the child's fingertips on the alarm clock. Tell the child "It's off. I don't hear anything." (Point to your ear, shake your head to indicate "No.") Then turn on the alarm, go through the same procedure as described above, helping the child to make the response by taking the cereal when he hears the sound. He may then eat it.

Proceed in this manner until the child can respond accurately without assistance.

After the child can respond accurately with the help of touch, have him move his fingers away from the clock. If he cannot respond without feeling the clock, touch the table with the clock so that he cannot see you but can feel the vibration. You can also give the sound behind the child. If assistance is needed, you can gently touch his arm, the chair he is sitting on, or the floor, with the alarm clock.

If the child has enough hearing to do this activity without the help of touch, it is, of course, not necessary to have him touch the clock when playing this game.

Language expectancy will depend upon the expressive language level of the child.

Variations:

A. To Maintain Interest

1. Use marshmallows, raisins, etc., on the clock face numbers, or use any of the standard responses.
2. Place marbles on the clock face numbers and let the child put a marble into a container as his response.

3. Turn the cardboard clock face down and let the child turn it over as his response.
4. Let the child move one of the clock's hands an hour forward as his response.
5. Play the "fishing game," letting the child pick up small pictures of clocks.
6. Let the child put pictures on a flannel board.
7. Make a book. Let the child tape a picture of a clock into the book as his response.
8. Let the child drop pictures in a slot cut in a box resembling a clock. (Any square box will do. Stand it on end and draw a clock's face on the bottom.)
9. You might use a book made either by you or by the child, and let the child turn the pages of the book and find pictures of different clocks as his response.
10. If the child has a doll, he can pretend that the doll is asleep and let it make the same response. A hand puppet may be used in the same way.
11. Depending upon the child's language, you might work further on the association of an alarm clock with waking up by having the child tell you (or tell a doll) to "Wake up! It's time to get up!" etc. You might use a doll's bed and have the child tell the doll to get up and take the doll out of bed.
12. You and the child can take turns in ringing the alarm. When it is the child's turn to do so, you must then make the response.

B. To Increase the Difficulty of Auditory Discrimination

Move the alarm clock further away from the child.

There is some disagreement about how much benefit can be expected from auditory training. Although it is natural for a child to ignore residual hearing if it does not convey enough information to be valuable, and although auditory training can help him or her use residual hearing in conjunction with vision and touch, and enable the child to respond to efforts to associate meaning with sounds, opinions vary concerning the benefit to be expected from primary emphasis on amplification. This issue is obscured by the low predictive ability of our present hearing tests, the possibility that the deaf child's use of auditory information may be influenced by other neurological involvements, and the impossibility of determining retroactively what might have happened to a particular child if a different educational program had been employed. Much work is needed to clarify and resolve these questions.

A Multisensory Approach. The auditory training exercise "Waking Up" incorporates the use of touch and vision in a multisensory approach that takes advantage of all of the cues available to the child. Just as normal-hearing children use all of their senses in learning, the deaf child should have the same opportunities.

As the name implies, the multisensory approach calls for developing the child's use of touch, vision, and audition (TVA) as avenues of communication. Generally, all three will be used together, but occasionally each will be singled out for specific practice to prevent the child from starting to ignore one sense modality. The term *interweaving* is applied to the use of the three modalities in varying sequences and combinations; it will be described following a discussion of methods used to develop the child's use of touch.

Use of Touch. For touch we use certain set hand positions to provide additional sensory information.

In receptive language training, when face to face with the adult, the child places a hand directly across onto the adult's cheek without crossing the adult's face. Cupping half of the adult's chin in the hand, the child puts his or her little finger on the jaw line and the rest of the hand on the cheek. If child and adult are side by side facing into a mirror (which enables the child to see his or her own lips as well as the adult's), the child places his or her near hand on the far side of the adult's face in the same position.

In expressive language training, when face to face or side by side with the adult, the child has a hand placed in the same position as above but the hand is then moved back to his or her own face in the same manner to encourage expressive efforts and to enable the child to monitor his or her speech along with the adult's. Some children are reluctant to use touch, and they should not be pressured. For any child it should be used sparingly. Initially the adult may have to help the child get the hand in the right position, but physical intervention should be minimized as soon as possible.

Interweaving. The interweaving technique can be incorporated into general or specific lipreading activities. It may start with the use of only one sense, such as touch (by covering the mouth with a piece of cardboard and turning off the hearing aid or auditory training unit); vision alone (by turning off the amplification and not using touch); or audition alone (by covering the mouth and not using touch). This approach can be used in a purely receptive mode by providing for the use of all three senses the first time, reducing these to one, and then repeating with all three. It also may be used in a discrimination situation where only one modality is used for the initial presentation, a response is required, and then all three senses are used for confirmation of the correct response. Depending on the child, it may be necessary to add two modalities if the child cannot initially function with one. Varying the combination of modalities will give the instructor some appreciation of the contribution of each of the senses as well as an indication of where additional practice is needed. One word of caution: interweaving may be difficult for the child and so should be used sparingly.

Speech Remediation. Speech is by far the most difficult to learn of all the skills associated with remediation of the hearing impaired. It is a complex motor skill based on an understanding of language, and the language must be reproduced with sufficient similarity to a "normal" speech model—which the deaf child can never hear—so that it will be intelligible.

The Synthetic Approach. The approach used at the John Tracy Clinic is both synthetic and analytic, but it emphasizes the synthetic. The child is first encouraged to imitate whole words and phrases, and then is given practice in the elements of speech so that they can be used in improving or correcting the whole (Haycock, 1964). It has been demonstrated (Hudgins and Numbers, 1942) that intelligibility is not merely a function of precision of articulation, but is also influenced by breath control, rhythm, and stress. Training in these essentials of good speech can begin at an early age with exercises in pitch (high or low), loudness (loud or soft), and duration (long or short). Young children can also learn to distinguish between voiced, unvoiced, and nasal sounds, and to associate them with the colors red, blue, and brown as a help in later practice. With motor skills developing in these areas, it is possible by selective reinforcement to shape the child's expressive language vocabulary in the direction of more intelligible speech.

Because speech is such a complex motor skill, it requires a continuing effort in development, remediation, and maintenance. It is not something that once learned is always retained. Without auditory feedback the deaf person needs continuing help to monitor his or her speech production. The clinician must first know phonological production, then be able to recognize deviant speech production of the hearing impaired student, know what error is being made and how to remediate that error.

Ling (1976b) has presented a detailed system for teaching speech to the hearing impaired children that has attracted a wide following. Ling believes the most basic skills are those involving respiration and phonation—the ability to control breath and produce voice at will. Built on these basic skills, the ability to produce vowels, consonants and consonant blends, are developed sequentially with each stage providing a foundation for the next. Each stage requires the achievement of a number of specific speech production target behaviors. Underlying these target behaviors there is a range of subskills which the child may master through the use of whatever sense modality is most appropriate (Ling and Ling, 1978). (See also Calvert, 1980, and Calvert and Silverman, 1975.)

General Language, General Speech Pattern (GLGSP).

As the deaf child begins to acquire both language and speech, communication skill should be expected to increase rapidly. It does, but the child still faces a problem that can interfere with the development of positive attitudes about oral communication.

Consider this situation. The deaf child's language is still imperfect and the child's speech is not always intelligible, but the child wants to ask a question. He tries, and the adult frowns in return. What can the child interpret from that frown? Does it mean that the adult cannot answer the question, or that the speech was so unintelligible or the language so mixed up that the adult could not follow it? What kind of attitude toward communication would a person develop if almost every time the person spoke the other person signaled puzzlement, but did not let him or her know why? This is not a farfetched example; it happens more times than we like to recognize, and it undoubtedly has an adverse effect on the development of oral language skill.

In an attempt to overcome this kind of problem, the GLGSP was designed to put some structure into the communicative interaction with the deaf child. It provides a simple framework around which the teacher and the parent can organize their communication efforts.

Three Levels of Evaluation. The GLGSP calls for an evaluation of the deaf child's communication effort at one of three levels:

1. Understanding—could what the child was talking about be understood?
2. Language—was the child's language appropriate for the particular level of development?
3. Speech—was the child's speech as good as could have been expected?

The emphasis is on evaluation. We must determine what the child's level of mastery is and then always evaluate whether the performance is up to that level. This is not simple, for, as indicated earlier, a deaf child will be at different levels with different materials in both language and speech. To fail to hold the child to a reasonable level of performance is doing the child a disservice.

Evaluation begins at the lowest level—understanding. If the child cannot be understood, all other efforts must wait until he or she can be. The child should try again to show what he or she means, to draw a picture, or anything else that is necessary. When understanding occurs, the child should be shown it has, and should be given an appropriate response.

The next step is to evaluate language. If it is not up to expected levels, it may be desirable to give some assistance. It would then be appropriate to say, "I understand you, but let me help you with your language." This clears the air because it tells the child that the message was understood, and that what follows will be of some assistance in the language area. After helping the child—by providing a correct pattern or whatever else is required—and holding him or her to an improved attempt, it is important to give the child an appropriate response.

At the next level, the child's speech is evaluated. If there are speech errors the child can be helped with, it would be appropriate to say, "Your language is good, but let me help you with your speech." Again, he or she has had some positive reinforcement and knows what to expect. After the speech help, the child should again be given an appropriate response to the communication effort.

Advantages of GLGSP. That is all there is to the GLGSP, but it is well not to be misled by its simplicity. Consider the advantages it offers. The GLGSP:

1. gives the deaf child immediate and unambiguous feedback on the effectiveness of communication efforts;
2. provides an evaluation framework which makes it easy to hold to an appropriate level of performance;
3. gears the interaction to the child's interests, because any corrections or assistance will be related to something initiated, not something the adult thought the child would be interested in; and
4. provides for regularized reinforcement of the child's communication effort by indicating approval at one level and by responding. This benefit may be appreciated by recalling the all-too-common situation where the deaf child makes an error in speech and the teacher's first reaction is to help him with his speech. If repeated enough, this can only give the child the impression that the teacher is not interested in what he says but only in how he says it.

The GLGSP is also much more flexible than this brief description indicates. Utilizing the same ideas of approval and reinforcement at one level before going on to the next, it can be used to introduce variety into the language patterns. For example, "That was good language, but let's see if you can't say it another way." Experience has confirmed that once mastered, the GLGSP can become an effortless and routine part of adult-child communication.

Role of Parents in the Remedial Process

Many of the practices that we have described can and should be carried out by the parents because they are the only people around the child enough to have any significant impact on the acquisition of language. A deaf child must substitute eyes for ears to acquire language. This substitution is difficut because the eye is directional, whereas the ear is not. The hearing child can acquire language through listening whether he or she can see the speaker or not; the child can listen to people speaking behind him or her or in the next room. But for language to be acquired through the eyes, the visual field must be focused on the source of information; unless the deaf child looks at the speaker, there will be no communication. Much of the time his or her eyes are busy with other tasks, like watching where he or she is walking or guiding the spoon from a dish to the mouth. The eyes also tend to follow anything that moves, like a bird, a puppy, or a waving hand. To make any visual language experiences meaningful for the child requires having someone to take advantage of all possible opportunities for communication—a role for which the parents are obviously best suited. This point is better appreciated when we think how difficult learning English would be if instruction could take place only during school hours.

Some educators do not believe that parents should be involved in their child's education. They say that asking the parents to take on additional tasks may put them under too much pressure, and that if they are tense and nervous when they try to teach, the learning experience is likely to be unpleasant for the child and make the child less receptive to the parents' teaching efforts. This argument ignores the fact that parents *are* teachers, whether they realize it or not. All children learn a great deal from their parents. Our goal is to help parents develop skill in using every possible opportunity for language development. If we make them tense and nervous, then we are not doing our job properly. We must be certain that our instructions are understood and that our assignments are not unreasonable.

Involving parents requires special skills. It requires teaching adults as well as children; it requires an explanation and justification of the educational philosophy and program to be followed; it requires the preparation of lessons and assignments which are understandable and meaningful for the parents; and, most important, it requires convincing the parents of the important role they can play in their child's education. In return for this extra effort, the teacher has a highly motivated helper who can provide the many repetitions of visual and amplified language experience after school and on weekends, when the teacher is not available.

More recently the passage of Federal legislation entitled, *Education for All Handicapped Children Act*, or Public Law 94-142 has added a new dimension to the parents' involvement in their child's education. The law, among other things, calls for an *Individualized Educational Program* (IEP) for each handicapped child which the parents must agree to. If they do not agree, there are due process guarantees which insure that the parents' point of view will be reviewed at several levels beyond the local school jurisdiction if the parent and school are not in agreement on the most appropriate education for the individual child.

This Act brings into law new opportunities for parents' participation in the determination of their child's education. With those new privileges, however, there goes the concomitant responsibility for the parents to learn as much as possible about the educational program being offered their child, the alternative programs that might be available, and the desirability and availability of ancillary services. To become fully participating members in the IEP conference, the parents must become much better informed than in the past.

Although there is some question as to how long PL 94-142 will be maintained in its present form, either because of repeal of the legislation itself or failure to provide specific funding, the legislation has demonstrated the possibility of closer school-home cooperation. It has demonstrated the potential value of the Individualized Educational Program as a means of clarifying objectives and learning strategies so that both parents and teachers can evaluate the progress of an educational program.

Public Law 94-142 has also raised, and in many respects clarified the place of schools and programs exclusively for deaf children. The law requires that the handicapped child be educated in the *least restrictive environment*. For some, that meant "mainstreaming" for all deaf children and the end of the segregated school or program. Experience with the law has indicated that placing a deaf child in a regular classroom when the child cannot communicate with hearing peers is much more "restrictive" than the segregated school. There continues to be a need for the specialized program that can bring together large enough numbers of children so that graded classes are possible and where ancillary personnel, such as audiologists, speech therapists, etc., are practically and economically feasible.

Parent Counseling. In considering the role that parents can play in the remediation of communication disorders, we must also consider the impact of having a handicapped child on the parents. The professional responsible for implementing the remedial practices (or assisting the parents in administering them) can be much more effective if they are aware of and sensitive to the emotional trauma that the parents experience following the discovery that their child is deaf. Unfortunately, professional training programs rarely prepare the teacher or therapist for this dual role. In some settings there are trained counselors to work with the parents and their feelings, but inevitably the teacher or therapist will become involved, must develop an awareness and sensitivity, and be comfortable in dealing with parental reactions.

The initial response to the discovery or confirmation of the suspicion that a child is deaf is confusion. Deafness is such a low incidence disorder that relatively few parents have had experience with deafness or deaf people and so have little idea of what its consequences will be for them and their child. To complicate matters, imagine the further confusion of parents who hear their new situation described in terms of decibels, hertz, sensorineural, brain stem and the many other terms in common use in our professional jargon, but which are likely to be incomprehensible to the parent.

Parental reactions to having a hearing-impaired child have frequently been likened to the grief response described by Kubler-Ross (1969), Moses and Van Hecke-Wulatin (1981), and Luterman (1979).

Moses and Van Hecke-Wulatin (1981) describe grief as

> that process whereby an individual can separate from someone or something significant that has been lost. Grieving stimulates a reevaluation of one's social, emotional, and philosophic environment. Such shifts often lead to positive values and attitudes. Grieving facilitates growth. Without the ability to grieve, a person cannot separate from a lost person or "object," and thereby, in essence, "dies" with whatever or whomever is lost. These people lose a present and future orientation and focus only on the past; that is, only on the "good old days" before they sustained the loss. Grieving, therefore, is the catalyst of growth, for with all growth, there is loss, and continuous growth requires successful grieving. (p. 74)

The critical stages are denial, guilt, depression, anger, and anxiety. Each of these stages helps the parent to work through the grieving process and to develop the ability to cope with their situation. The stages do not occur in any set order and can occur simultaneously.

Professionals need to understand and accept the long term nature of the emotional process for parents and be prepared to offer assistance on a follow-up basis. In other words, this is not something that can be accomplished in a one- or two-visit contact. Professionals must develop the ability to listen to parents and to provide them with answers to the many questions which accompany this emotional state, and, most important, to develop the ability to accept and understand parental reactions. The anger, for example, that develops as a normal stage of the grief process may well be directed to the professional who is attempting to help. Moses and Van Hecke-Wulatin (1981) describe this:

> Parents who are frustrated by the birth of an impaired child, feel anger towards the deaf child who has intruded upon their lives and disrupted it in many realms. It is expensive, embarrassing, time consuming, energy consuming, exposing and shattering to have a hearing impaired child in your family. On a more psychologically primitive level, most parents feel that all this disruption and pain has emanated from the child . . . Since anger toward their child is considered heinous by most parents, they often displace these angry feelings upon others; most commonly, spouses, the deaf child's siblings, and, of course, professionals. (p. 74)

Parents of hearing impaired handicapped children often benefit from professional help dealing with their feelings. They also derive benefit from group activities with other parents of deaf children. It is hard to maintain the feeling that you are the only one that this tragedy has happened to if you are in a group of other parents in exactly the same situation. Parents also support each other both with information and emotional support. Parents of older deaf children have a credibility that is often reassuring to the new parent.

SUMMARY

In this chapter we have dealt with remedial principles and practices for the hearing impaired—a population which comprises the deaf and the hard-of-hearing. In the sections devoted to each of these major categories, limitations of space forced us to discuss techniques particularly appropriate for use with young children primarily, with less emphasis on teenagers and adults. This emphasis on remediation for preschool and school-age children seemed essential because the critical years of language and speech growth require an extensive remedial program if communication gains are to be accomplished.

Two remedial approaches have been presented—one giving primary emphasis to the development of residual hearing in the hearing impaired, and the other placing primary emphasis on visual training and secondary emphasis on auditory training in language remediation for the deaf.

In the section dealing with auditory remediation, the presence of usable or residual hearing suggested an emphasis on methods involving auditory skills to a degree consistent with the child's auditory potential. The goals of auditory remediation were shown to be early identification of the hearing loss, followed by intensive and consistent stimulation of the residual hearing. To accomplish these goals, a well-planned program is directed at teaching auditory skills, integrating hearing into the individual's total personality development, and educating the family and community on ways of helping develop communication proficiency. A variety of specific techniques were described for developing auditory function and linguistic skills in persons at age levels from prelinguistic through the school years.

The section dealing with remedial techniques for the deaf, with its focus on the training of prelingually deaf children in language acquisition primarily through the eyes, presented oralism as the method of choice. Oralism incorporates lipreading along with speech and auditory training, and unlike manual methods employing fingerspelling or signing, does not limit the deaf person's options for communicating within the range of those trained to communicate via the same manual method; the deaf person can communicate with a much wider segment of society. The section described techniques for developing the receptive, expressive, and advanced language abilities of the prelingually deaf, as well as techniques for their auditory and speech training and for evaluating their general language and speech patterns. Fostering a positive attitude toward communication when training the child, and helping the parents fulfill their role in the training are two extremely important aspects of the remedial program.

In spite of the space limitations on the development of subject matter within this chapter, it is hoped that the reader will have gained insight into the complex and challenging problems of developing communication skills in the deaf and the hard of hearing, and can appreciate the singular importance of providing the hearing impaired with training programs that will foster that development. Further reading and work in these areas will contribute to a professional expertise and the satisfaction of helping those with hearing impairments achieve more meaningful interaction with their worlds.

BIBLIOGRAPHY

Alpiner, J. G. (Ed.), *Handbook of Adult Rehabilitative Audiology.* Baltimore: Williams and Wilkins (1978).

Angus, J. R., *Watch My Words.* Cincinnati: Forward Movement Publications (1974).

Anthony, D. A., and Associates (Eds.), *Seeing Essential English.* Anaheim, CA.: Educational Services Division, Anaheim Union High School District (1971).

Arenberg, K. I., Unidirectional inner ear valve implant surgery. Otolaryngologic Clinics of North America, **13** (4), 745–765 (1980)

Balkany, T. J., Arenberg, K., Rucker, N., Pauley, J. D., and Northey, D. J., The cochlear prosthesis. *Colorado Medicine,* **1,** 11–14 (1981).

Berg, F. S., and Fletcher, S. G., *Educational Audiology.* New York: Grune and Stratton (1976).

Bergman, M., Changes in hearing with age. *The Gerontologist,* **2,** 148–151 (1971a).

Bergman, M., Hearing and aging. *Audiology,* **10,** 164–171 (1971b).

Bergman, M., Rusalem, H., Malles, I., Schiller, V., Cotton, H., and McKay, E., *Auditory Rehabilitation for Hearing-Impaired Blind Persons: ASHA Monographs* No. 12. Washington, D.C.: American Speech and Hearing Association (March, 1965).

Binnie, C., Jackson, P., and Montgomery, A., Visual intelligibility of consonants: a lipreading screening test with implications for aural rehabilitation. *JSHD,* **41,** 530–539 (1976).

Bitter, G. B., *Parents in Action.* Washington, D.C.: A. G. Bell (1978).

Black, F., Bergstrom, L., Downs, M., and Hemenway, W., *Congenital Deafness: A New Approach to Early Detection of Deafness Through a High Risk Register.* Denver, Colorado: Colo. Associated University Press (1971).

Blackwell, P. M., Engen, E., Fischgrund, J. E., and Zarcadoolas, C., *Sentences and Other Systems.* Washington, D.C.: The Alexander Graham Bell Association for the Deaf, Inc. (1978).

Bloom, L., and Lahey, M. *Language Development and Language Disorders.* New York: John Wiley and Sons (1978).

Boatner, E., Stuckless, E., and Moores, D., *Occupational Status of the Young Adult Deaf.* West Hartford, Conn.: Amer. Schl. for the Deaf (1964).

Boning, Richard A. *Specific Skill Series.* New York: Baldwin, Barnell and Loft (1976).

Brooks, D. N., *Otitis Media in Infancy in Early Management of Hearing Loss.* New York: Grune and Stratton (1981).

Calvert, D. R., *Descriptive Phonetics*. New York, New York: Brian C. Decker Division, Thieme-Stratton, Inc. (1980).

Calvert, D. R., and Silverman, S. R., *Speech and Deafness*. Washington, D.C.: Alexander Graham Bell Association for the Deaf (1975).

Chomsky, N., *Aspects of the Theory of Syntax*. Cambridge, Mass.: M.I.T. Press (1965).

Church, J., *Three Babies*. New York: Random House (1966).

Clark, J.: Counseling in a pediatric practice. *Asha*, **24**, 521–528 (1982).

Connor, L. E., *The President's Opinions: Early Intervention*. Washington, D.C.: The Volta Bureau (1972).

Cornett, R. O., The method explained. *Hearing and Speech News*, **35**, No. 5, 7–9 (1967).

Crabtree, M., *Houston Test for Language Development*, Parts 1 and 2. Obtainable from 10133 Bassoon, Houston, Texas (1963).

Crystal, D., Linguistic mythology and the first year of life. *Brit. J. Dis. Comm.*, **8**, 29–36 (1973).

Curtis, S., Prutting, C., Lowell, E., Pragmatic and semantic development in young children with impaired hearing, *Journal of Speech and Hearing Research*, **22**, No. 3, 534–552 (1979).

Darley, F. L. (Ed.), Identification audiometry. *J. Speech Hearing Dis. Mong.*, Supp. 9 (1961).

Di Carlo, L. M., *The Deaf*. Englewood Cliffs, N.J.: Prentice-Hall, Inc. (1964).

Doll, E. A., *Vineland Social Maturity Scale*. Minneapolis, Minn.: Minneapolis Educational Testing Bureau (1947).

Dunn, L., *The Peabody Picture Vocabulary Test*. Minneapolis, Minn.: American Guidance Service, Inc. (1965).

Eagles, E. L., Wishik, S. M., and Doerfler, L. G., *Hearing Sensitivity and Ear Disease and Children*. St. Louis, Mo.: The Laryngoscope (1963).

Eilers, R., and Minifie, F., Fricative discrimination in early infancy. *JSHR*, **18**, 158–167 (1975).

Eilers, R., Wilson, W., and Moore, J.: Developmental changes in speech discrimination in infants. *JSHR*, **20**, 766–781 (1977).

Eisenberg, R., *Auditory Competence in Early Life*. Baltimore: University Park Press (1976).

Ernst, M., Report of the Porter Hospital Study of Hearing-Impaired Children Born During 1964–65. Proceedings of the International Conference on Auditory Techniques. Springfield, Ill.: C. C. Thomas, 147–164 (1974).

Fant, L. J., Jr., *Ameslan: An Introduction to the American Sign Language*. Silver Spring, M.D.: National Association of the Deaf (1972).

Fellendorf, G. W. (Ed.), *Bibliography on Deafness*. Washington, D.C.: Alexander Graham Bell Association for the Deaf (1966).

Fitzgerald, E., *Straight Language for the Deaf: A System of Instruction for Deaf Children*. Washington, D.C.: The Volta Bureau (1954).

Froehlinger, V., *Into the Mainstream of Education*. Washington, D.C.: A. G. Bell Publications (1981).

Frostig, M., *Developmental Test of Visual Perception*. (Rev. ed.) Palo Alto, Calif.: Consulting Psychologists Press (1966).

Gaeth, J., and Lounsbury, E., Hearing aids and children in elementary schools. *J. Speech Hearing Dis.*, **31**, 283–289 (1966).

Gauger, J. S., *Orientation to Hearing Aids*. Rochester, New York: National Technical Institute for the Deaf (1978).

Glorig, A., Some medical implications of the 1954 Wisconsin State Fair hearing survey. *Trans. Amer. Acad. Opthal. Otolaryngol.*, **61**, 160–171 (1957).

Goodenough, F., *Measurement of Intelligence by Drawing*. Chicago: World Book Co. (1926).

Gordon, I. J., *Baby Learning Through Baby Play*. New York: St. Martin's Press (1970).

Gregory, S., *The Deaf Child and His Family*. New York: Wiley & Sons (1976).

Groht, M. A., *Natural Language for Deaf Children*. Washington, D.C.: The Volta Bureau (1958).

Gustason, G., Pfetzinger, D., and Zawolkow, E., *Signing Exact English*. Rossmoor, CA: Modern Signs Press (1972).

Hardy, J., Identification: Early postnatal tests. In H. Davis (Ed.), The young deaf child identification and management. *Acta Otolaryng*, Suppl. **206**, 34–75 (1965).

Haycock, G. S., *The Teaching of Speech*. Washington, D.C.: The Volta Bureau (1964).

Henderson, P. (Ed.), *Methods of Communication Currently Used in the Education of Deaf Children: Papers given at a Residential Seminar at Garnett College*, London, Royal National Institute for the Deaf (1975).

Howie, V. M., Ploussard, J. H., and Sloyer, J., The 'Otitis-prone' condition. *American Journal of the Disabled Child*, **129**, 676–678 (1975).

Hsu, J. R., *A Developmental Guide to English Syntax*. Bronx, N.Y., St. Joseph's School for the Deaf (1977).

Hudgins, C. V., and Numbers, F., An investigation of the intelligibility of the speech of the deaf. *Genet. Psych. Monog.*, **25**, 289–292 (1942).

Hull, R., and Traynor, R., Hearing impairment among aging persons in the health care facility: their diagnosis and rehabilitation. *Amer. Health Care Assoc.* **3,** 14–18 (1977).

Illingsworth, R., and Lister, J., The critical period. *J. Pediat.*, **65,** 839–848 (1964).

Johnson, D., The adult deaf client and rehabilitation. In J. Alpiner (Ed.), *Handbook of Adult Rehabilitative Audiology.* Baltimore: Williams and Wilkins (1978).

Katz, J., *Kindergarten Auditory Screening Test.* Chicago: Follett Educational Corporation (1971).

Katz, J., The effects of conductive hearing loss on auditory function. *Asha*, **20,** 879–886 (1978).

Kennedy, P., and Bruinkinks, R., Social status of hearing impaired children in the regular classrooms. *Except. Child.* **40,** 336–342 (1974).

Kirk, S., McCarthy, J., and Kirk, W., The Illinois Test of Psycholinguistic Abilities. (Rev. Ed.) Urbana, Ill.: Univ. Ill. Press (1968).

Kretschmer, R. R., Jr., and Kretschmer, L. W., *Language Development and Intervention with the Hearing Impaired.* Baltimore: University Park Press (1978).

Kubler-Ross, E., *On Death and Dying.* New York: Macmillan Publishing Co. (1969).

Lee, L., *The Northwestern Syntax Screening Test.* Evanston, Ill.: Northwestern Univ. Press (1969).

Levine, E., *The Psychology of Deafness.* New York: Columbia U. Pr. (1960).

Libby, E. R., *Binaural Hearing and Amplification.* Chicago, Ill.: Zenefron, Inc. (1980).

Ling, D., *Speech and the Hearing-Impaired Child.* Washington: A. G. Bell (1976a).

Ling, D., *Speech and the Hearing-Impaired Child: Theory and Practice.* Washington, D.C.: Alexander Graham Bell Association for the Deaf (1976b).

Ling, D., and Ling, A. H., *Aural Habilitation: The Foundations of Verbal Learning in Hearing-Impaired Children.* Washington, D.C.: Alexander Graham Bell Association for the Deaf (1978).

Los Angeles County, *The Test of Auditory Comprehension, and the Auditory Skills Curriculum.* Los Angeles, California: Foreworks (1979).

Lowell, E. L., and Stoner, M., *Play It by Ear.* Los Angeles: The John Tracy Clinic (1960).

Luterman, David, *Counseling Parents of Hearing Impaired Children.* Boston: Little, Brown & Co. (1979).

McClure, A., Academic achievement of mainstreamed hearing-impaired children with congenital rubella syndrome. *Volta Rev.,* **79,** 379–385 (1977).

McConnell, F., A new approach to the management of childhood deafness. *Ped. Clinics of N. Amer.,* **17,** 347–362 (1970).

McConnell, F., The parent teaching home: An early intervention program for hearing-impaired children. *Peabody J. of Educ.,* **51,** 162–171 (1974).

McConnell, F., and Liff, S., The rationale for early identification and intervention. *Otolaryng. Clinics of N. Amer.* **8,** 77–87 (1975).

McNeill, D., The capacity for language acquisition. *Volta Rev.,* **68,** 17–33 (1966).

McNeill, D., *The Acquisition of Language.* New York: Harper & Row (1971).

Mencher, G., A program for neonatal hearing screening. *Audiology,* **13,** 495–500 (1974).

Mencher, G. T., and Gerber, S. E., *Early Management of Hearing Loss.* New York: Grune and Stratton (1981).

Miles, A. C., Cued speech. *American Education,* **3,** 26 (1967).

Montgomery County Schools. *All About Hearing Aids.* Avail. from A. G. Bell Assn. in Washington, D.C. (1975).

Moog, J., and Geers, A., *Grammatical Analysis of Elicited Language.* St. Louis: Central Institute for the Deaf (1980).

Moores, D. F., *Educating the Deaf, Psychology, Principles, and Practices.* Boston: Houghton Mifflin Co. (1978).

Moses, K. L., and Van Hecke-Wulatin, M. The socio-emotional impact of infant deafness: A counseling model. In G. T. Mencher and S. E. Gerber (Eds.), *Early Management of Hearing Loss.* New York: Grune & Stratton (1981).

Murphy, K. P., and Byrne, D. J., The blind-deaf multiply disabled infant. In G. T. Mencher and S. E. Gerber (Eds.), *Early Management of Hearing Loss.* New York: Grune and Stratton (1981).

Myklebust, H., Picture story language test. In *Development and Disorders of Written Language.* New York: Grune and Stratton (1965).

Northcott, W., *The Hearing-Impaired Child in a Regular Classroom.* Washington, D.C.: The Volta Bureau (1973).

Northcott, W., Normalization of the preschool child with hearing-impairment. *Otolaryng. Clinics of N. Amer.*, **8,** (1) 159–186 (1975).

Northcott, W., *Curriculum Guide.* Washington, D.C.: A. G. Bell (1977).

Northern, J. L., and Downs, M. P., *Hearing in Children.* Baltimore: Williams and Wilkins (1978).

Northern, J. L., McChord, W., Fischer, E., and Evans, P., *Hearing Services in Residential Schools for the Deaf.* Maico Audiologic Library Services, Vol. II, Report 4 (1972).

Office of Demographic Studies. *Children in Special Education.* Washington: Gallaudet (1974–1978).

O'Connor, L., Early intervention. *Volta Review,* **73** (5), 270 (1971).

O'Neill, J. J., *The Hard of Hearing.* Englewood Cliffs, N.J.: Prentice-Hall, Inc. (1964).

O'Neill, J. J., and Oyer, H. J., *Visual Communication for the Hard-of-Hearing.* Englewood Cliffs: Prentice-Hall (1961).

Pollack, D., Acoupedics. *Volta Review,* **66** (7) 400–409 (1964).

Pollack, D., *Educational Audiology for the Limited Hearing Infant.* Springfield, Ill.: C. C. Thomas (1970).

Pollack, D., Acoupedics: An approach to early management. In G. T. Mencher and S. E. Gerber (Eds.), *Early Management of Hearing Loss.* New York: Grune and Stratton (1981).

Poole, I., The genetic development of the articulation of consonant sounds. *Elementary English Review,* **9,** 159–161 (1934).

Quigley, S., Wilbur, R., Montanelli, D., and Steinkamp, M., *Syntactic Structures in Language of Deaf Children.* Urbana, Ill.: Univ. Ill. Press (1976).

Rainer, J., Altshuler, K., and Kallman, F., *Family and Mental Health Problems in a Deaf Population.* Springfield, Ill.: C. C. Thomas (1969).

Rodda, M., *The Hearing Impaired School Leaver.* Springfield, Ill.: C. C. Thomas (1970).

Rosewell, F., and Chall, J., *Rosewell-Chall Auditory Blending Test.* New York: Essay Press (1963).

Ross, M., Hearing aids. In B. Jaffe (Ed.), *Hearing Loss in Children.* Baltimore: Univ. Park Press (1977).

Ross, M., and Giolas, T. G., *Auditory Management of Hearing Impaired Children: Principles and Prerequisites for Intervention.* Baltimore: University Park Press (1978).

Ruben, R. J., and Rozycki, D., Diagnostic screening for the deaf child. *Arch. Otolaryng.,* **91,** 429–432 (1970).

Russell, W. K., Quigley, S. P., and Power, D. J., *Linguistics and Deaf Children: Transformational Syntax and Its Applications.* Washington, D.C.: Alexander Graham Bell Association for the Deaf (1976).

Sanders, D., *Aural Rehabilitation.* Englewood Cliffs, New Jersey: Prentice-Hall (1971).

Simmons, A., Motivating language in the young child, *Proceedings of the International Conference on Oral Education of the Deaf.* Washington, D.C.: Alexander Graham Bell Association (1967).

Slingerland, B., *Slingerland Screening Tests for Identifying Children with Specific Language Disability.* Cambridge, Mass.: Educ. Pub. Service, Inc. (1967).

Solow, L. J., *American Sign Language and Related Sign Systems for the Deaf.* Northridge, CA: Center on Deafness, California State University, Northridge (1975).

Star, R., *We Can!* Vol. 1 and 2. Washington, D.C.: A. G. Bell (1980).

Stovall, D., *Teaching Speech to Hearing Impaired Infants and Children.* Springfield, Ill.: C. C. Thomas (1982).

Streng, A., *Syntax, Speech and Hearing: Applied Linguistics for Teachers of Children with Language and Hearing Disabilities.* New York: Grune and Stratton (1972).

Sullivan, R., Auditory localization. *Maico Audiological Library,* Vol. 3, Report 10 (1965).

Tervoort, B., and Verbeck, A. J. A., Analysis of communicative structure patterns in deaf children. Final report on project No. RD-467-64-65 of the Vocational Rehabilitation Administration, H.E.W. 385–387. Washington, D.C.: Groningen (1967).

Tracy, L. T., Talk, talk, talk to deaf children. *Am. Educ.,* **1,** 4–7 (1965).

Utley, J., *What's Its Name?* Urbana, Ill.: Univ. of Ill., (1950). Auditory Training Album obtainable from Maico Inc., Minneapolis, Minn.

van Uden, A., *A World of Language for Deaf Children.* St. Michelsgestel, Netherlands, Institute for the Deaf (1968).

Vivian, R. M., *The Tadoma Method: A Tactual Approach to Speech and Speechreading.* Washington, D.C.: The Alexander Graham Bell Association for the Deaf (1966).

Walden, B., Eerdman, S., Montgomery, A., Schwartz, D., and Porsek, R., Some effects of training on speech perception by hearing-impaired adults. *JSHR,* **24,** 207–217 (1981).

Webster, D. B., and Webster, M., Neonatal sound deprivation affects brainstem auditory nuclei. *Archives of Otolaryngology,* **103,** 392–396 (1977).

Whetnall, E., and Fry, D. B., *The Deaf Child*. Springfield, Ill.: C. C. Thomas (1964).

Whitehurst, M. W., *Integrated Lessons in Lipreading and Auditory Training*. Washington, D.C.: The Volta Bureau (1958).

Willeford, J., Hearing survey in schools. Unpublished study, Colorado State University, Fort Collins, Colorado (1971).

Wright, D., *Deafness*. New York: Stein and Day (1969).

Yater, V. V., *Mainstreaming of Children with a Hearing Loss*. Springfield, Ill.: C. C. Thomas (1977).

Zimmerman, I., Steiner, V., and Evatt, R., *The Preschool Language Scale*. Columbus, Ohio: Merrill (1969).

Appendix

REQUIREMENTS FOR THE CERTIFICATES OF CLINICAL COMPETENCE
(Revised January 1, 1981)

The American Speech-Language-Hearing Association issues Certificates of Clinical Competence to individuals who present satisfactory evidence of their ability to provide independent clinical services to persons who have disorders of communication (speech, language, and/or hearing). An individual who meets these requirements may be awarded a Certificate in Speech-Language Pathology or in Audiology, depending upon the emphasis of preparation; a person who meets the requirements in both professional areas may be awarded both Certificates.

I. Standards

The individual who is awarded either, or both of the Certificates of Clinical Competence must hold a master's degree or equivalent[1] with major emphasis in speech-language pathology, audiology, or speech-language and hearing science. The individual must also meet the following qualifications:

I,A. General Background Education

As stipulated below, applicants for a certificate should have completed specialized academic training and preparatory professional experience that provides an in-depth knowledge of normal communication processes, development and disorders

thereof, evaluation procedures to assess the bases of such disorders, and clinical techniques that have been shown to improve or eradicate them. It is expected that the applicant will have obtained a broad general education to serve as a background prior to such study and experience. The specific content of this general background education is left to the discretion of the applicant and to the training program attended. However, it is highly desirable that it include study in the areas of human psychology, sociology, psychological and physical development, the physical sciences (especially those that pertain to acoustic and biological phenomena) and human anatomy and physiology, including neuroanatomy and neurophysiology.

I,B. Required Education

A total of 60 semester hours[2] of academic credit must have been accumulated from accredited colleges or universities that demonstrate that the applicant has obtained a well-integrated program of course study dealing with the normal aspects of human communication, development thereof, disorders thereof, and clinical techniques for evaluation and management of such disorders.

Twelve (12) of these 60 semester hours must be obtained in courses that provide information that pertains to normal development and use of speech, language, and hearing.

Thirty (30) of these 60 semester hours must be in courses that provide (1) information relative to communication disorders, and

---

[1] Equivalent is defined as holding a bachelor's degree from an accredited college or university, and at least 42 post baccalaureate semester hours acceptable toward a master's degree, of which at least 30 semester hours must be in the areas of speech-language pathology, audiology, or speech-language and hearing science. At least 21 of these 42 semester hours must be obtained from a single college or university, none may have been completed more than 10 years prior to the date of application and no more than six semester hours may be credit offered for clinical practicum.

[2] In evaluation of credits, one quarter hour will be considered the equivalent of two-thirds of a semester hour. Transcripts that do not report credit in terms of semester or quarter hours should be submitted for special evaluation.

497

(2) information about and training in evaluation and management of speech, language and hearing disorders. At least 24 of these 30 semester hours must be in courses in the professional area (speech-language pathology or audiology) for which the certificate is requested, and no less than six (6) semester hours may be in audiology for the certificate in speech-language pathology or in speech-language pathology for the certificate in audiology. Moreover, no more than six (6) semester hours may be in courses that provide credit for clinical practice obtained during academic training.

Credit for study of information pertaining to related fields that augment the work of the clinical practitioner of speech-language pathology and/or audiology may also apply toward the total 60 semester hours.

Thirty (30) of the total 60 semester hours that are required for a certificate must be in courses that are acceptable toward a graduate degree by the college or university in which they are taken.[3] Moreover, 21 of those 30 semester hours must be within the 24 semester hours required in the professional area (speech-language pathology or audiology) for which the certificate is requested or within the six (6) semester hours required in the other area.

I,C. Academic Clinical Practicum

The applicant must have completed a minimum of 300 clock hours of supervised clinical experience with individuals who present a variety of communication disorders, and this experience must have been obtained within the training institution or in one of its cooperating programs.

I,D. The Clinical Fellowship Year

The applicant must have obtained the equivalent of nine (9) months of full-time professional experience (the Clinical Fellowship Year) in which bona fide clinical work has been accomplished in the major profes-

sional area (speech-language pathology or audiology) in which the certificate is being sought. The Clinical Fellowship Year must have begun after completion of the academic and clinical practicum experiences specified in Standards *I,A.*, *I,B.*, and *I,C.* above.

I,E. The National Examinations in Speech-Language-Pathology and Audiology

The applicant must have passed one of the National Examinations in Speech-Language-Pathology and Audiology, either the National Examination in Speech-Language-Pathology or the National Examination in Audiology.

II. Explanatory Notes

II,A. General Background Education

While the broadest possible general educational background for the future clinical practitioner of speech-language pathology and/or audiology is encouraged, the nature of the clinician's professional endeavors suggests the necessity for some emphasis in general education. For example, elementary courses in general psychology and sociology are desirable as are studies in mathematics, general physics, zoology, as well as human anatomy and physiology. Those areas of introductory study that do not deal specifically with communication processes are not to be credited to the minimum 60 semester hours of education specified in Standard *I,B.*

II,B. Required Education

II,B,1. Basic Communication Processes Area. The 12 semester hours in courses that provide information applicable to the normal development and use of speech, language, and hearing should be selected with emphasis on the normal aspects of human communication in order that the applicant has a wide exposure to the diverse kinds of information suggested by the content areas given under the three broad categories that follow: (1) anatomic and physiologic bases for the normal development and use of speech, language, and hearing, such as anatomy, neurology, and physiology of speech, language, and hearing mechanisms; (2) physical bases and processes of the production and perception of speech, language and hearing, such

---

[3] This requirement may be met by courses completed as an undergraduate providing the college or university in which they are taken specifies that these courses would be acceptable toward a graduate degree if they were taken at the graduate level.

as (a) acoustics or physics of sound, (b) phonology, (c) physiologic and acoustic phonetics, (d) perceptual processes, and (e) psychoacoustics; and (3) linguistic and psycholinguistic variables related to normal development and use of speech, language, and hearing, such as (a) linguistics (historical, descriptive, sociolinguistics, urban language), (b) psychology of language, (c) psycholinguistics, (d) language and speech acquisition, and (e) verbal learning or verbal behavior.

It is emphasized that the three broad categories of required education given above, and the examples of areas of study within these classifications, are not meant to be analogous with, or imply, specific course titles. Neither are the examples of areas of study within these categories meant to be exhaustive.

At least two (2) semester hours of credit must be earned in each of the three categories.

Obviously, some of these 12 semester hours may be obtained in courses that are taught in departments other than those offering speech-language pathology and audiology programs. Courses designed to improve the speaking and writing ability of the student will not be credited.

II,B,2. Major Professional Area, Certificate in Speech-Language-Pathology. The 24 semester hours of professional education required for the Certificate of Clinical Competence in Speech-Language-Pathology should include mastery of information pertaining to speech and language disorders as follows: (1) understanding of speech and language disorders, such as (a) various types of disorders of communication, (b) their manifestations, and (c) their classifications and causes; (2) evaluation skills, such as procedures, techniques, and instrumentation used to assess (a) the speech and language status of children and adults, and (b) the bases of disorders of speech and language, and (3) management procedures, such as principles in remedial methods used in habilitation and rehabilitation for children and adults with various disorders of communication.

Within these categories at least six (6) semester hours must deal with speech disorders and at least six (6) hours must deal with language disorders.

I,B,3. Minor Professional Area, Certificate in Speech-Language-Pathology. For the individual to obtain the Certificate in Speech-Language Pathology, no less than six (6) semester hours of academic credit in audiology is required. Where only this minimum requirement of six (6) semester hours is met, three (3) semester hours must be in habilitative/rehabilitative procedures with speech and language problems associated with hearing impairment, and three (3) semester hours must be in study of the pathologies of the auditory system and assessment of auditory disorders. However, when more than the minimum six (6) semester hours is met, study of habilitative/rehabilitative procedures may be counted in the Major Professional Area for the Certificate in Speech-Language-Pathology (see *Section II,B,8*).

II,B,4. Major Professional Area, Certificate in Audiology. The 24 semester hours of professional education required for the Certificate of Clinical Competence in Audiology should be in the broad, but not necessarily exclusive, categories of study as follows: (1) auditory disorders, such as (a) pathologies of the auditory system, and (b) assessment of auditory disorders and their effect on communication; (2) habilitative/rehabilitative procedures, such as (a) selection and use of appropriate amplification instrumentation for the hearing impaired, both wearable and group, (b) evaluation of speech and language problems of the hearing impaired, and (c) management procedures for speech and language habilitation and/or rehabilitation of the hearing impaired (that may include manual communication); (3) conservation of hearing, such as (a) environmental noise control, and (b) identification audiometry (school, military, industry); and (4) instrumentation, such as (a) electronics, (b) calibration techniques, and (c) characteristics of amplifying systems.

Not less than six (6) semester hours must be in the auditory pathology category, and not less than six (6) semester hours must be in the habilitation/rehabilitation category.

II,B,5. Minor Professional Area, Certificate in Audiology. For the individual to obtain the

Certificate in Audiology, not less than six (6) semester hours must be obtained in the areas of speech and language pathology, of these three (3) hours must be in the area of speech pathology and three (3) hours in the area of language pathology. It is suggested that where only this minimum requirement of six (6) semester hours is met, such study be in the areas of evaluation procedures and management of speech and language problems that are not associated with hearing impairment.

II,B,6. Related Areas. In addition to the 12 semester hours of course study in the Basic Communication Processes Area, the 24 semester hours in the Major Professional Area and the six (6) semester hours in the Minor Professional Area, the applicant may receive credit toward the minimum requirement of 60 semester hours of required education through advanced study in a variety of related areas. Such study should pertain to the understanding of human behavior, both normal and abnormal, as well as services available from related professions, and in general should augment the background for a professional career. Examples of such areas of study are as follows: (a) theories of learning and behavior, (b) services available from related professions that also deal with persons who have disorders of communication, and (c) information from these professions about the sensory, physical, emotional, social, and/or intellectual status of a child or an adult.

Academic credit that is obtained for practice teaching or practicum work in other professions will not be counted toward the minimum requirements.

In order that the future applicant for one of the certificates will be capable of critically reviewing scientific matters dealing with clinical issues relative to speech-language pathology and audiology, credit for study in the area of statistics, beyond an introductory course, will be allowed to a maximum of three (3) semester hours. Academic study of the administrative organization of speech-language pathology and audiology programs also may be applied to a maximum of three (3) semester hours.

II,B,7. Education Applicable to All Areas. Certain types of course work may be accept-able among more than one of the areas of study specified above, depending upon the emphasis. For example, courses that provide an overview of research, e.g., introduction to graduate study or introduction to research, that consist primarily of a critical review of research in communication sciences, disorders, or management thereof, and/or a more general presentation of research procedures and techniques that will permit the clinician to read and evaluate literature critically will be acceptable to a maximum of three (3) semester hours. Such courses may be credited to the Basic Communication Processes Area, or one of the Professional Areas or the Related Area, if substantive content of the course(s) covers material in those areas. Academic credit for a thesis or dissertation may be acceptable to a maximum of three (3) semester hours in the appropriate area. An abstract of the study must be submitted with the application if such credit is requested. In order to be acceptable, the thesis or dissertation must have been an experimental or descriptive investigation in the areas of speech, language and hearing science, speech-language pathology or audiology; that is, credit will not be allowed if the project was a survey of opinions, a study of professional issues, an annotated bibliography, biography, or a study of curricular design.

As implied by the above, the academic credit hours obtained for one course or one enrollment, may, and should, be in some instances divided among the Basic Communication Processes Area, one of the Professional Areas, and/or the Related Area. In such cases, a description of the content of that course should accompany the application. This description should be extensive enough to provide the Clinical Certification Board with information necessary to evaluate the validity of the request to apply the content to more than one of the areas.

II,B,8. Major Professional Education Applicable to Both Certificates. Study in the area of understanding, evaluation, and management of speech and language disorders associated with hearing impairment may apply to the 24 semester hours of Major Professional Area required for either certificate (speech-language pathology or audiology).

However, no more than six (6) semester hours of that study will be allowed in that manner for the certificate in speech-language pathology.

II,C. Academic Clinical Practicum

It is highly desirable that students who anticipate applying for one of the Certificates of Clinical Competence have the opportunity, relatively early in their training program, to observe the various procedures involved in a clinical program in speech-language pathology and audiology, but this passive participation is not to be construed as direct clinical practicum during academic training. The student should participate in supervised, direct clinical experience during that training only after the student has had sufficient course work to qualify for work as a student clinician and only after the student has sufficient background to undertake clinical practice under direct supervision. A minimum of 150 clock hours of the supervised clinical experience must be obtained during graduate study. Once this experience is undertaken, a substantial period of time may be spent in writing reports, in preparation for clinical sessions, in conferences with supervisors, and in class attendance to discuss clinical procedures and experiences; such time may not be credited toward the 300 minimum clock hours of supervised clinical experience required.

All student clinicians are expected to obtain direct clinical experience with both children and adults, and it is recommended that some of their direct clinical experience be conducted with groups. Although the student clinician should have experience with both speech-language and hearing disorders, at least 200 clock hours of this supervised experience must be obtained in the major professional area (speech-language pathology or audiology) in which certification is sought, and not less than 35 clock hours must be obtained in the minor area. A minimum of 50 supervised clock hours of the required 300 hours of clinical experience must be obtained in each of two distinctly different clinical settings. (The two separate clinical settings may be within the organizational structure of the same institution and may include the academic program's clinic and affiliated medical facilities, community clinics, public schools, etc.)

For certification in speech-language pathology, the student clinician is expected to have experience in both the evaluation and management of a variety of speech and language problems. The student must have no less than 50 clock hours of experience in evaluation of speech and language problems. The applicant must also have no less than 75 clock hours of experience in management of language disorders of children and adults, and no less than 25 clock hours each of experience in management of children and adults with whom disorders of (1) voice, (2) articulation, and (3) fluency are significant aspects of the communication handicap.[4]

Where only the minimum 35 clock hours of clinical practicum in audiology is met that is required for the persons seeking certification in speech-language pathology, that practicum must include 15 clock hours in assessment and/or management of speech and language problems associated with hearing impairment, and 15 clock hours must be in assessment of auditory disorders. However, where more than this minimum requirement is met, clinical practicum in assessment and/or management of speech and language problems associated with hearing impairment may be counted toward the minimum clock hours obtained with language and/or speech disorders.

For the student clinician who is preparing for certification in audiology, 50 clock hours of direct supervised experience must be obtained in identification and evaluation of hearing impairment, and 50 clock hours must be obtained in habilitation or rehabilitation of the communication handicaps of the hearing impaired. It is suggested that the 35 clock hours of clinical practicum in speech-language pathology required for certification in audiology be in evaluation and

---

[4] Work with multiple problems may be credited among these types of disorders. For example, a child with an articulation problem may also have a voice disorder. The clock hours of work with that child may be credited to experience with either articulation or voice disorders, whichever is most appropriate.

management of speech and language problems that are not related to a hearing impairment.

Supervisors of clinical practicum must be competent professional workers who hold a Certificate of Clinical Competence in the professional area (speech-language pathology or audiology) in which supervision is provided. This supervision must entail the personal and direct involvement of the supervisor in any and all ways that will permit the supervisor to attest to the adequacy of the student's performance in the clinical training experience. At least 25% of the therapy sessions conducted by a student clinician must be directly supervised, with such supervision being appropriately scheduled throughout the training period. (Direct supervision is defined as on-site observation or closed-circuit TV monitoring of the student clinician.) At least one-half of each diagnostic evaluation conducted by a student clinician must be directly supervised. (The amount of direct supervision beyond these minima should be adjusted upward depending on the student's level of competence.) The first 25 hours of a student's clinical practicum must be supervised by a qualified clinical supervisor who is a member of the program's professional staff (i.e., a primary employee of the training program). In addition to the required direct supervision, supervisors may use a variety of other ways to obtain knowledge of the student's clinical work such as conferences, audio- and videotape recordings, written reports, staffings, and discussions with other persons who have participated in the student's clinical training.[5]

II,D. The Clinical Fellowship Year

Upon completion of professional and clinical practicum education, the applicant must complete a Clinical Fellowship Year under the supervision of one who holds the Certificate of Clinical Competence in the professional area (speech-language pathology or audiology) in which that applicant is working (and seeking certification).

Professional experience is construed to mean direct clinical work with patients, consultations, record keeping, or any other duties relevant to a bona fide program of clinical work. It is expected, however, that a significant amount of clinical experience will be in direct clinical contact with persons who have communication handicaps. Time spent in supervision of students, academic teaching, and research, as well as administrative activity that does not deal directly with management programs of specific patients or clients will not be counted as professional experience in this context.

The Clinical Fellowship Year is defined as no less than nine months of full-time professional employment with full-time employment defined as a minimum of 30 clock hours of work a week. This requirement also may be fulfilled by part-time employment as follows: (1) work of 15–19 hours per week over 18 months; (2) work of 20–24 hours per week over 15 months; or, (3) work of 25–29 hours per week over 12 months. In the event that part-time employment is used to fulfill a part of the Clinical Fellowship Year, 100% of the minimum hours of the part-time work per week requirement must be spent in direct professional experience as defined above. The Clinical Fellowship Year must be completed within a maximum period of 36 consecutive months. Professional employment of less than 15 hours per week will not fulfill any part of this requirement. If the CFY is not initiated within two years of the date the academic and practicum education is completed, the applicant must meet the academic and practicum requirements current when the CFY is begun. Whether or not the Clinical Fellow (CF) is a member of ASHA, the CF must understand and abide by the ASHA Code of Ethics.

CFY supervision must entail the personal and direct involvement of the supervisor in any and all ways that will permit the CFY supervisor to monitor, improve, and evalu-

[5] An applicant whose application has been rejected may reapply if changes in the requirements make his application acceptable as a result of such changes. However, if the Clinical Fellowship Year is not initiated within two years of the time academic and practicum requirements are completed, the applicant must meet academic and practicum requirements that are current when the Clinical Fellowship Year is begun.

ate the CF's performance in professional clinical employment. The supervision must include on-site observations of the CF. Other monitoring activities such as conferences with the CF, evaluation of written reports, evaluations by professional colleagues, and so on may be executed by correspondence. The CFY supervisor must base the total evaluation on no less than 36 occasions of monitoring activities (a minimum of four hours each month). The monitoring activities must include at least 18 on-site observations (a minimum of two hours each month). Should any supervisor suspect that at any time during the Clinical Fellowship Year that the CF under supervision will not meet requirements, the CFY supervisor must counsel the CF both orally and in writing and maintain careful written records of all contacts and conferences in the ensuing months.[6]

II,E. The National Examinations in Speech-Language-Pathology and Audiology

The National Examinations in Speech-Language-Pathology and Audiology are designed to assess, in a comprehensive fashion, the applicant's mastery of professional concepts as outlined above to which the applicant has been exposed throughout professional education and clinical practicum. The applicant must pass the National Examination, in either Speech-Language Pathology or Audiology that is appropriate to the certificate being sought. An applicant will be declared eligible for the National Examination on notification of the acceptable completion of the educational and clinical practicum requirements. The Examination must be passed within three years after the first administration for which an applicant is notified of eligibility.

In the event the applicant fails the examination, it may be retaken. If the examination is not successfully completed within the above mentioned three years, the person's application for certification will lapse. If the examination is passed at a later date, the

person may reapply for clinical certification.[7]

III. Procedures for Obtaining the Certificates

III,A. The applicant must submit to the Clinical Certification Board, a description of professional education and academic clinical practicum on forms provided for that purpose.[8] The applicant should recognize that it is highly desirable to list upon this application form the entire professional education and academic clinical practicum training.

No credit may be allowed for courses listed on the application unless satisfactory completion is verified by an official transcript. *Satisfactory completion* is defined as the applicant's having received academic credit (i.e., semester hours, quarter hours, or other unit of credit) with a passing grade as defined by the training institution. If the majority of an applicant's professional training is received at a program accredited by the Education and Training Board (ETB) of the American Speech-Language-Hearing Association (ASHA), approval of educational and academic clinical practicum requirements will be automatic.

The applicant must request that the director of the training program where the majority of graduate training was obtained sign the application. In the case where that training program is not accredited by the ETB of ASHA, that director, by signature, (1) certifies that the application is correct, and (2) recommends that the applicant receive the certificate upon completion of all the requirements. In the case where the training program is accredited by the ETB of ASHA, that director (1) certifies that the applicant has met the educational and clini-

---

[6] Further requirements for the Clinical Fellowship Year are available, and, moreover, such requirements are provided with application material for certification.

[7] Upon such reapplication, the individual's application will be reviewed and current requirements will be applied. Appropriate fees will be charged for this review.

[8] Application material for certification, including a schedule of fees, may be obtained by writing to Information Services Section, American Speech-Language-Hearing Association, 10801 Rockville Pike, Rockville, Maryland 20852.

cal practicum requirements, and (2) recommends that the applicant receive the certificate upon completion of all the requirements.

In the event that the applicant cannot obtain the recommendation of the director of the training program, the applicant should send with the application a letter giving in detail the reasons for the inability to do so. In such an instance letters of recommendation from other faculty members may be submitted.

Application for approval of educational requirements and academic clinical practicum experiences should be made (1) as soon as possible after completion of these experiences, and (2) either before or shortly after the Clinical Fellowship Year is begun.

III,B. Upon completion of educational and academic clinical practicum training, the applicant should proceed to obtain professional employment and a supervisor for the Clinical Fellowship Year. Although the filing of a CFY Plan is not required, applicants may submit such a plan to the Clinical Certification Board (CCB) if they wish prior approval of the planned professional experience. Within one month following completion of the Clinical Fellowship Year, the CF and the CFY supervisor must submit a CFY Report to the Clinical Certification Board.

III,C. Upon notification by the Clinical Certification Board of approval of the academic course work and clinical practicum requirements the applicant will be sent registration material for the National Examinations in Speech-Language-Pathology and Audiology. Upon approval of the Clinical Fellowship Year, achieving a passing score on the National Examination, and payment of all fees the applicant will become certified.

III,D. As mentioned in Footnote 8, a schedule of fees for certification may be obtained, and payment of these fees is requisite for the various steps involved in obtaining a certificate. Checks should be made payable to the American Speech-Language-Hearing Association.

IV. Appeals

In the event that at any stage the Clinical Certification Board informs the applicant that the application has been rejected, the applicant has the right of formal appeal. In order to initiate such an appeal, the applicant must write to the Chairman of the Clinical Certification Board and specifically request a formal review of the application. If that review results, again, in rejection, the applicant has the right to request a review of the case by the Council on Professional Standards in Speech-Language Pathology and Audiology (COPS) by writing to the Chairman of the COPS at the National Office of the American Speech-Language-Hearing Association. The decision of the COPS will be final.

CODE OF ETHICS OF THE AMERICAN SPEECH-LANGUAGE-HEARING ASSOCIATION 1982
(Revised January 1, 1979)
Preamble

The preservation of the highest standards of integrity and ethical principles is vital to the successful discharge of the professional responsibilities of all speech-language pathologists and audiologists. This Code of Ethics has been promulgated by the Association in an effort to stress the fundamental rules considered essential to this basic purpose. Any action that is in violation of the spirit and purpose of this Code shall be considered unethical. Failure to specify any particular responsibility or practice in this Code of Ethics should not be construed as denial of the existence of other responsibilities or practices.

The fundamental rules of ethical conduct are described in three categories: Principles of Ethics, Ethical Proscriptions, Matters of Professional Propriety.

1. *Principles of Ethics.* Six Principles serve as a basis for the ethical evaluation of professional conduct and form the underlying moral basis for the Code of Ethics. Individ-

uals[1] subscribing to this Code shall observe these principles as affirmative obligations under all conditions of professional activity.

2. *Ethical Proscriptions*. Ethical Proscriptions are formal statements of prohibitions that are derived from the Principles of Ethics.

3. *Matters of Professional Propriety*. Matters of Professional Propriety represent guidelines of conduct designed to promote the public interest and thereby better inform the public and particularly the persons in need of speech-language pathology and audiology services as to the availability and the rules regarding the delivery of those services.

Principle of Ethics I

Individuals shall hold paramount the welfare of persons served professionally.

A. Individuals shall use every resource available, including referral to other specialists as needed, to provide the best service possible.

B. Individuals shall fully inform persons served of the nature and possible effects of the services.

C. Individuals shall fully inform subjects participating in research or teaching activities of the nature and possible effects of these activities.

D. Individuals' fees shall be commensurate with services rendered.

E. Individuals shall provide appropriate access to records of persons served professionally.

F. Individuals shall take all reasonable precautions to avoid injuring persons in the delivery of professional services.

G. Individuals shall evaluate services rendered to determine effectiveness.

Ethical Proscriptions
1. Individuals must not exploit persons in the delivery of professional services, includ-

[1] "Individuals" refers to all Members of the American Speech-Language-Hearing Association and non-members who hold Certificates of Clinical Competence from this Association.

ing accepting persons for treatment when benefit cannot reasonably be expected or continuing treatment unnecessarily.

2. Individuals must not guarantee the results of any therapeutic procedures, directly or by implication. A reasonable statement of prognosis may be made, but caution must be exercised not to mislead persons served professionally to expect results that cannot be predicted from sound evidence.

3. Individuals must not use persons for teaching or research in a manner that constitutes invasion of privacy or fails to afford informed free choice to participate.

4. Individuals must not evaluate or treat speech, language or hearing disorders except in a professional relationship. They must not evaluate or treat solely by correspondence. This does not preclude follow-up correspondence with persons previously seen, nor providing them with general information of an educational nature.

5. Individuals must not reveal to unauthorized persons any professional or personal information obtained from the person served professionally, unless required by law or unless necessary to protect the welfare of the person or the community.

6. Individuals must not discriminate in the delivery of professional services on any basis that is unjustifiable or irrelevant to the need for and potential benefit from such services, such as race, sex or religion.

7. Individuals must not charge for services not rendered.

Principle of Ethics II

Individuals shall maintain high standards of professional competence.

A. Individuals engaging in clinical practice shall possess appropriate qualifications which are provided by the Association's program for certification of clinical competence.

B. Individuals shall continue their professional development throughout their careers.

C. Individuals shall identify competent, dependable referral sources for persons served professionally.

D. Individuals shall maintain adequate records of professional services rendered.

Ethical Proscriptions
1. Individuals must neither provide services nor supervision of services for which they have not been properly prepared, nor permit services to be provided by any of their staff who are not properly prepared.

2. Individuals must not provide clinical services by prescription of anyone who does not hold the Certificate of Clinical Competence.

3. Individuals must not delegate any service requiring the professional competence of a certified clinician to anyone unqualified.

4. Individuals must not offer clinical services by supportive personnel for whom they do not provide appropriate supervision and assume full responsibility.

5. Individuals must not require anyone under their supervision to engage in any practice that is a violation of the Code of Ethics.

Principle of Ethics III

Individuals' statements to persons served professionally and to the public shall provide accurate information about the nature and management of communicative disorders, and about the profession and services rendered by its practitioners.

Ethical Proscriptions
1. Individuals must not misrepresent their training or competence.

2. Individuals' public statements providing information about professional services and products must not contain representations or claims that are false, deceptive or misleading.

3. Individuals must not use professional or commercial affiliations in any way that would mislead or limit services to persons served professionally.

Matters of Professional Propriety
1. Individuals should announce services in a manner consonant with highest professional standards in the community.

Principle of Ethics IV

Individuals shall maintain objectivity in all matters concerning the welfare of persons served professionally.

A. Individuals who dispense products to persons served professionally shall observe the following standards:

(1) Products associated with professional practice must be dispensed to the person served as a part of a program of comprehensive habilitative care.

(2) Fees established for professional services must be independent of whether a product is dispensed.

(3) Persons served must be provided freedom of choice for the source of services and products.

(4) Price information about professional services rendered and products dispensed must be disclosed by providing to or posting for persons served a complete schedule of fees and charges in advance of rendering services, which schedule differentiates between fees for professional services and charges for products dispensed.

(5) Products dispensed to the person served must be evaluated to determine effectiveness.

Ethical Proscriptions
1. Individuals must not participate in activities that constitute a conflict of professional interest.

Matters of Professional Propriety
1. Individuals should not accept compensation for supervision or sponsorship from the clinician being supervised or sponsored.

2. Individuals should present products they have developed to their colleagues in a manner consonant with highest professional standards.

Principle of Ethics V

Individuals shall honor their responsibilities to the public, their profession, and their relationships with colleagues and members of allied professions.

Matters of Professional Propriety

1. Individuals should seek to provide and expand services to persons with speech, language and hearing handicaps as well as to assist in establishing high professional standards for such programs.

2. Individuals should educate the public about speech, language and hearing processes, speech, language and hearing problems, and matters related to professional competence.

3. Individuals should strive to increase knowledge within the profession and share research with colleagues.

4. Individuals should establish harmonious relations with colleagues and members of other professions, and endeavor to inform members of related professions of services provided by speech-language pathologists and audiologists, as well as seek information from them.

5. Individuals should assign credit to those who have contributed to a publication in proportion to their contribution.

Principle of Ethics VI

Individuals shall uphold the dignity of the profession and freely accept the profession's self-imposed standards.

A. Individuals shall inform the Ethical Practice Board of violations of this Code of Ethics.

B. Individuals shall cooperate fully with the Ethical Practice Board inquiries into matters of professional conduct related to this Code of Ethics.

Acknowledgments

Figures 1–1, 1–2, 1–3, 1–4, 1–5, and 1–6 Courtesy of the Exceptional Children Educational Department at the State University College at Buffalo.

Figure 2–1 "A Receptive-Expression Language Model" from "Studies in Aphasia: Background and Theoretical Formulations" by J. Wepman, L. V. Jones, R. D. Bock, and D. Van Pelt in *Journal of Speech and Hearing Disorders*, Vol. 25, 1960. Copyright © 1960 by the American Speech-Language-Hearing Association.

Figure 2–2 "Speech and Language Processing Model" from *Diagnosis of Speech and Language Disorders* by James E. Nation and Dorothy M. Aram, 1977. Reprinted by permission of The C. V. Mosby Co., St. Louis, Missouri and the authors.

Table 2–1 "Looking at Language Learning" by Kathryn B. Horton, Janet E. Coscarelli and Patricia F. Casey. Copyright © 1977 by K. B. Horton and J. E. Coscarelli. Reprinted by permission.

Table 2–2 "Some Differences Between Nonstandard Black English (B.E.) and Standard English (S.E.)" from "A Linguistic Description of Social Dialects" prepared by R. Williams and W. Wolfram for the Committee of Communication Problems of the Urban and Ethnic Populations, American Speech and Hearing Association, 1974. Reprinted by permission of Walter Wolfram.

Table 2–3 After "Phonological Interference Points Between Spanish and English" by F. Williams, C. Cairns and H. Cairns and "Grammatical Interference Points Between Spanish and English" by A. Davis in *Introduction to Communication Disorders* by Thomas J. Hixon et al. Englewood Cliffs, New Jersey: Prentice-Hall, Inc., 1980.

Table 2–10 "The Developmental Sentence Scoring (DSS) Chart" from *Interactive Language Development Teaching* by Laura L. Lee, Roy Koenigsknecht and Susan Mulhern. Reprinted by permission of Northwestern University Press.

Figure 5–1 Adapted, by permission, from Von Leden, H., Moore, P., and Timcke, R., Laryngeal vibrations: Measurements of the glottic wave. III. The pathologic larynx. *Arch. Otolaryngol.*, 71, 29, January 1960. Copyright 1960 by the American Medical Association.

Figure 5–2 "Voice Profile" by Frank B. Wilson. Reprinted by permission of the author.

Figure 5–3 "The Buffalo Voice Profile" from *Voice Problems of Children*, 2nd ed., by D. Kenneth Wilson. Copyright © 1979. Reprinted by permission of William & Wilkins Co., Baltimore and the author.
The material on pages 258–259 is from "Counselling the Laryngectomee: A Study of the Surgeon's Approach" by Dr. Helene A. Kalfuss from a paper presented at the Ninth I.A.L. Voice Institute, University of Pittsburgh, July 17, 1969. Reprinted by permission of the author.

Figure 5–7 Picture of the Cooper-Rand Electronic Speech Aid reproduced with permission of the Luminaud Co., 8688 Tyler Blvd., Mentor, OH 44060; picture of the Aurex Neovox, courtesy of the Aurex Corp., 844 W. Adams St., Chicago, IL 60607; and picture of the Western Electric #5C Electrolarynx reproduced with permission of Western Electric, 222 Broadway, New York, NY 10038.

Figures 5–8, 5–9, 5–10, 5–11, and 5–12   From "Surgical Vocal Rehabilitation Following Total Laryngectomy: A State of the Art Report" by J. P. Dworkin and A. Spanker in *Clinical Otolaryngology*, Vol. 5, 1980. Copyright © 1983 by Blackwell Scientific Publications. Reprinted by permission.

Figure 5–13   "Blom and Singer's Tracheo-Esophageal Puncture Method" from *IAL News*, August 1980. Reprinted by permission of the International Association of Laryngectomees.

Figure 6–1   Courtesy of Dr. Betty Jane Philips, Boys Town Institute for Communication Disorders in Children, Omaha, Nebraska. With parental permission.

Figure 6–2   From S. Pruzansky, "Description, classification and analysis of unseparated clefts of the lip and palate." *American Journal of Orthodontics*, 39:590–611, August 1953. Reprinted with permission of S. Puzansky.

Figure 6–3   "The Eight Musculoskeletal Valves Produced by Oral and Pharyngeal Musculature During Articulation of Consonantal Sounds" from "Recent Cinefluorography Advances in Palatopharyngeal Roentgenography" by R. Sloan, S. Brummett, J. Westover, R. Ricketts, and F. Ashley in *American Journal of Roentgenology, Radium Therapy, and Nuclear Medicine*, November 1964. Reprinted by permission of Robert Ricketts.

Figure 6–5   "Weighted Values for Speech Symptoms Associated with Velopharyngeal Incompetence" from Velopharyngeal Incompetence by Betty J. McWilliams and Betty J. Philips, 1979. Reprinted by permission of W. B. Saunders Co. and the authors.

Figures 7–1, 7–2, and 7–3   Courtesy of the Program for the Orthopedically Handicapped, School #5, Rochester, New York.

Figures 7–4 and 7–5   "Sample of One-Minute Kymograms of Silent Breathing for Three Normal Children" and "Sample of One-Minute Kymograms of Silent Breathing for Four Cerebral-Palsied Children" from "Hearing and Speech Behavior Among Children with Cerebral Palsy" by Louis M. Di Carlo and Walter W. Amster in *Cerebral Palsy: Its Individual and Community Problems*, ed. by W. M. Cruickshank and G. M. Rause. Reprinted by permission of Syracuse University Press.

Figures 8–2 and 8–3   "Primary Language Areas of the Human Brain" and "Cerebral Arteries of the Human Brain" from "Language and the Human Brain" by Norman Geschwind in *Scientific American*, April 1972. Copyright © 1972 by Scientific American, Inc. All rights reserved. Reprinted by permission.

Figures 8–5 and 8–6   Poetry by Mr. Holopigian. Reprinted by permission of Joyce Fitch-West.

Table 8–2   "Aphasia Severity Rating Scale" and "Rating Scale Profile of Speech Characteristics" from *Boston Diagnostic Aphasia Examination* by H. Goodglass and E. Kaplan. Reprinted by permission of Lea & Fibiger and H. Goodglass.

Tables 8–3 and 8–4   "Porch Index of Communicative Ability" and "PICA Categories for Scoring Responses." Reproduced by special permission of the Publisher, Consulting Psychologists Press, Inc., Palo Alto, CA 94306, from PICA, *Administration, Scoring and Interpretation*, Vol. 2 by Bruce E. Porch, PhD. Copyright © 1981. Further reproduction is prohibited without the Publisher's consent.

Figures 8–7 and 8–8 and Table 8–6   "Periodic evaluation measures administered at 4, 15, 26, 37 and 48 weeks post-onset," "Percent of patients in each cohort improving, not improving, or deteriorated on PICA overall percentile score," and "PICA overall percentile group mean change scores" from "Veterans Administration Cooperative Study." Reprinted by permission of Robert T. Wertz.

Appendix   "Requirements for the Certificates of Clinical Competence" and "Code of Ethics of the American Speech-Language-Hearing Association." Reprinted by permission of American Speech-Language-Hearing Association.

Name Index

Subject Index